Comprehensive Study of Signal Transduction

Volume I

Comprehensive Study of Signal Transduction

Volume I

Edited by **Jim Salley**

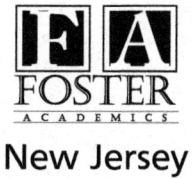

FOSTER
ACADEMICS

New Jersey

Published by Foster Academics,
61 Van Reypen Street,
Jersey City, NJ 07306, USA
www.fosteracademics.com

Comprehensive Study of Signal Transduction: Volume I
Edited by Jim Salley

International Standard Book Number: 978-1-63242-090-9 (Hardback)

Printed in the United States of America.

Contents

Preface

There are many thousands of processes that are going on inside the body of any given organism at any moment of the day. One of those processes is signal transduction. It refers to any process through which a cell converts any kind of stimulus or signal into another. These processes usually involve ordered sequences of biochemical responses and reactions inside the cellular body that are usually carried out by enzymes, and activated by messengers which results in what is usually known as 'signal transduction pathway'. This process of signal transduction is usually very fast and rapid, barely lasting milliseconds. The process is slightly different in the case of single cell organisms and multi-cellular organisms. Depending on the type of cell, the response in the signal transduction can alter the metabolism of a cell, or even its shape and gene expression. There are various steps and the signal can be amplified at any one of them and therefore there can be many responses to one single signalling molecule. This is quite a specialized field of study and thus the need for well qualified research scientists is more evident than ever. The future of signal transduction is quite exciting as new research is being done constantly and its application potential is great.

This book attempts to understand and collate under one aegis the various researches and data available on signal transduction. I am thankful to those who have put their effort and hard work into this compilation. I am also grateful to my family and friends who supported me in this endeavour.

Editor

Oxidative Stress Induced by MnSOD-p53 Interaction: Pro- or Anti-Tumorigenic?

Delira Robbins and Yunfeng Zhao

Department of Pharmacology, Toxicology & Neuroscience, Louisiana State University Health Sciences Center, Shreveport, LA 71130, USA

Correspondence should be addressed to Yunfeng Zhao, yzhao1@lsuhsc.edu

Academic Editor: Paolo Pinton

The formation of reactive oxygen species (ROS) is a result of incomplete reduction of molecular oxygen during cellular metabolism. Although ROS has been shown to act as signaling molecules, it is known that these reactive molecules can act as prooxidants causing damage to DNA, proteins, and lipids, which over time can lead to disease propagation and ultimately cell death. Thus, restoring the protective antioxidant capacity of the cell has become an important target in therapeutic intervention. In addition, a clearer understanding of the disease stage and molecular events that contribute to ROS generation during tumor promotion can lead to novel approaches to enhance target specificity in cancer progression. This paper will focus on not only the traditional routes of ROS generation, but also on new mechanisms via the tumor suppressor p53 and the interaction between p53 and MnSOD, the primary antioxidant enzyme in mitochondria. In addition, the potential consequences of the p53-MnSOD interaction have also been discussed. Lastly, we have highlighted clinical implications of targeting the p53-MnSOD interaction and discussed recent therapeutic mechanisms utilized to modulate both p53 and MnSOD as a method of tumor suppression.

1. Introduction

Oxidative stress has been defined as the cellular imbalance of prooxidants versus antioxidants that overwhelms the cell's capacity to scavenge the oxidative load and contributes to the pathogenesis of various diseases. Reactive oxygen species (ROS) are free radicals derived from molecular oxygen that play a key role in promoting oxidative stress. These radicals result from the incomplete reduction of oxygen mainly during mitochondrial respiration. There are several products of oxygen metabolism, both nonradicals and radicals that form ROS such as hydrogen peroxide (H_2O_2) and superoxide anions ($O_2{}^{\cdot-}$). Contributors of ROS can modify the intracellular redox status through unfavorable interactions with endogenous regulators of oxidative stress. Superoxide radicals can interact with mitochondrial nitric oxide to form peroxynitrite which can alter antioxidant enzymes such as aconitase and the mitochondrial complexes of the electron transport chain [1]. On the other hand, the presence of oxidative stress can alter normal cellular homeostasis by modifying proteins involved in DNA repair; activating signal transduction pathways involved in cell survival and inflammation; as well as, inducing cellular apoptotic pathways that are detrimental to the cell. For many years, scientists have tried to combat free radical generation and superoxide production through the utilization of the exogenous antioxidant supplementation, such as ascorbate, vitamin E, as well as linoleic acid. However, many of these trials have failed showing no significant decrease in cancer incidence, death, or major cardiovascular events [2]. Herein, we will focus on several novel signaling pathways affecting ROS generation, such as p53 signaling and the interaction between p53 and manganese superoxide dismutase (MnSOD) and how to potentially target these pathways for cancer therapy.

2. Oxidative Stress

Oxidative stress has been repeatedly shown to contribute to the progression of multiple diseases, such as cancer [3], diabetes [4], ulcerative colitis [5], cardiovascular disease [6], pulmonary disease [7] as well as neurodegenerative diseases [8]. Nevertheless, the biological significance of oxidative stress can be beneficial or detrimental depending on certain parameters such as concentration, duration of action, cell type exposed, the type of free radicals and reactive metabolites involved, and the activities of the associated signal transduction pathways.

The mitochondrial electron transport chain remains to be one of the main sources of intracellular oxidative stress [9]. During mitochondrial respiration, electrons flow through four integral membrane protein complexes to finally reduce molecular oxygen to water. However, approximately 1-2% of molecular oxygen undergoes incomplete reduction, resulting in the formation of superoxide anions and mitochondria-mediated ROS generation [10]. Though mainly produced from mitochondrial respiration, superoxide anions can be detoxified via endogenous antioxidant enzymes such as manganese superoxide dismutase (MnSOD) to hydrogen peroxide, which is further converted to water via the enzymatic actions of various antioxidant enzymes including glutathione reductases, peroxiredoxins, glutathione transferases, as well as catalase which all function in the removal of hydrogen peroxide.

Nevertheless, it is common for cells in response to stress to enhance ROS generation. Oxidoreductases are enzymes that are often activated during the cellular stress response and catalyze the transfer of electrons from the electron donor (reductant) to the electron acceptor (oxidant) [11] with associated formation of superoxide anions and ROS as byproducts. There are several enzymes that act as oxidoreductases and contribute to intracellular ROS generation, such as cyclooxygenase [12], lipoxygenase [12, 13], cytochrome P450 enzymes [14], nitric-oxide synthase [15], xanthine oxidase [16], and mitochondrial NADH: ubiquinone oxidoreductase (complex I) [17]. NAPDH oxidases of the Nox family are also oxidoreductases that produce superoxide anions as a primary product and one of the key sources of intracellular ROS formation. NADPH oxidases (Nox) are endogenous enzymatic heterogenic complexes that reduce molecular oxygen to superoxide, in conjunction with NADPH oxidation, which can be converted to various ROS. Nox can be activated by a myriad of cellular stress stimuli such as heavy metals [18, 19], organic solvents [20], UV and ionizing irradiation [21, 22]. Once the cellular stress response is initiated two cytosolic regulatory units of Nox, p47^{phox}, p67^{phox}, and the small G protein Rac translocate to the membrane and associate with cytochrome $b558$ (consisting of two subunits gp91phox (Nox2) and p22phox), which acts as a central docking site for complex formation [23]. Emerging evidence has linked Nox enzymes to oxidative stress that may contribute to disease progression [11, 17, 24, 25]. The radicals generated from Nox activation are capable of modulating various redox-sensitive signaling pathways involved in the activation of mitogen-activated protein kinases (MAPKs) and transcription factors (NF-κB) [26–28] causing regulation of Nox activation to be complex.

Oxidative stress can be generated endogenously, as well as promoted exogenously by multiple environmental factors. Ultraviolet irradiation (UV) is an environmental promoter of oxidative stress. UV is known to damage DNA and other intracellular proteins through direct and indirect mechanisms. UV exists in three forms UVA (400–320 nm), UVB (320–290 nm), and UVC (290–100 nm). UVA and UVB are the most biologically significant, with UVC being most absorbed by ozone [29]. UV is known to directly induce the cross-linking of neighboring pyrimidines to form pyrimidine dimers in DNA that result in mutagenic DNA lesions [30–35]. However, UV is known to promote ROS generation that can damage a large number of intracellular proteins and can indirectly damage DNA.

Associated with oxidative damage is lipid peroxidation. High levels of ROS are detrimental and can cause damage to various biomolecules, which include the fatty acid side chains of membrane lipids that form reactive organic products such as malondialdehyde and 4-hydroxynonenal, both of which can generate DNA adducts and point mutations [36]. Lipid peroxidation not only affects DNA stability, but can also alter lipid membrane proteins that are involved in signal transduction pathways to promote constitutive activation and downstream cellular proliferation. Furthermore, previous studies have shown that products of lipid peroxidation served as intermediates in the activation of signaling pathways that involved phospholipase A2 and the MAPK pathway, both associated with UV-induced carcinogenesis [37–39].

Although there are various sources of endogenous oxidative stress, mitochondria are the major cellular organelles that contribute to intracellular ROS generation. Mitochondria consume approximately 80–90% of the cell's oxygen for ATP synthesis via oxidative phosphorylation. In the early 1920s Otto Warburg and colleagues theorized that defective oxidative phosphorylation during cancer progression caused tumor cells to undergo a metabolic shift requiring high rates of glycolysis that promoted lactate production in the presence of oxygen. This phenomenon became known as aerobic glycolysis and later coined "The Warburg Effect." Some of the metabolic enzymes that are altered during cancer progression are involved in the mitochondrial electron transport chain [40, 41]. The electron transport chain consists of a constant flow of electrons through mitochondrial intermembrane complexes with molecular oxygen being the ultimate electron acceptor. The process of the electron transport chain is used to pump protons into the mitochondrial inner membrane creating an electrochemical gradient. The gradient that is created is coupled to ATP synthesis. However, leaking electrons contribute to the incomplete reduction of molecular oxygen, resulting in superoxide anion formation. Mitochondria are readily susceptible to oxidative damage for various reasons: (1) lack of effective base excision repair mechanisms; (2) the close proximity of mitochondrial DNA to ROS generation; (3) lack of mitochondrial DNA protective histones [42]. Therefore, alterations in mitochondrial ROS generation and protection via antioxidant expression are key in the detrimental effects of disease progression.

3. Manganese Superoxide Dismutase (MnSOD)

Maintaining a balance between free radicals and antioxidants is required for cellular homeostasis. However, when this balance is altered in favor of free radical generation, normal physiology is altered and the pathogenesis of disease is promoted. Antioxidants are endogenous defense mechanisms utilized by the cell to fight against fluctuations in free radical generation, which include both enzymatic and nonenzymatic contributors. Ascorbic acid (Vitamin C) and α-tocopherol (Vitamin E) are nonenzymatic antioxidants that have been previously shown to effectively scavenge free radicals. On the other hand, antioxidants such as glutathione peroxidase and superoxide dismutase are enzymatic antioxidants that catalyze the neutralization of free radicals into products that are nontoxic to the cell. Superoxide dismutase catalyzes the dismutation of superoxide anions leading to the formation of hydrogen peroxide and molecular oxygen. Hydrogen peroxide is further detoxified to water via catalase and other endogenous antioxidant enzymes. The superoxide dismutase family consists of metalloenzymes. Currently, there are three major superoxide dismutase enzymes within the human cell: manganese superoxide dismutase (MnSOD), copper-zinc superoxide dismutase (Cu, ZnSOD), and extracellular superoxide dismutase (ECSOD). MnSOD is localized in the mitochondrial matrix [43], Cu, ZnSOD is found primarily in the cytosol [44] and can be detected in the mitochondrial intermembrane space [45], and ECSOD is a homotetrameric glycosylated form of Cu, ZnSOD found in the extracellular space [46].

MnSOD is ubiquitously found in both prokaryotes and eukaryotes, and its increased activity is often associated with cytoprotection against oxidants. MnSOD can be induced by various mediators of oxidative stress such as tumor necrosis factor, lipopolysaccharide, and interleukin-1 [47]. This antioxidant enzyme is nuclear encoded by a gene localized to chromosome 6q25 [48], a region often lost in cancers such as melanoma [49]. MnSOD is synthesized in the cytosol as a larger precursor with a transit peptide on the N-terminus and imported to the mitochondrial matrix via proteolytic processing to the mature form [50]. Most cancer cells and in vitro transformed cell lines have diminished MnSOD activity compared to normal counterparts [51]. In addition, deficiencies in MnSOD may contribute to oxidative stress generation that promotes neoplastic transformation and/or maintenance of the malignant phenotype. In looking at the correlation between MnSOD expression and cancer progression, mutations within the MnSOD gene and its regulatory sequence have been observed in several types of human cancers [52, 53]. However, antioxidants can suppress carcinogenesis, particularly during the promotion phase. In addition, our laboratory as well as others has shown that overexpression of MnSOD reduces tumor multiplicity, incidence, and metastatic ability in various in vitro and in vivo models [54–57].

4. The Tumor Suppressor p53

p53 is a well-characterized transcription factor known to induce its tumor suppressor activity by activating genes known to play a role in cell cycle arrest, such as p21^{CIP1} and GADD45. These genes, once activated, arrest the cell cycle to allow for adequate DNA repair to restore normal cell proliferation. However, if the cell becomes overwhelmed by the stressor or the DNA damage cannot be repaired, p53 can ultimately induce apoptosis. The tumor suppressive activities of p53 can also be defined by the induction senescence. Senescence is characterized by irreversible loss of proliferative potential, acquisition of characteristic morphology, and expression of specific biomarkers such as senescence-associated β-galactosidase [58]. Nevertheless, how p53 regulates senescence is often contradictory and dependent on ROS generation. p53 can mediate cellular senescence via the transactivation of p21^{CIP1}. Nonetheless, emerging evidence suggests ROS as a common mediator of senescence with the involvement of superoxide dismutase and p53. Blander et al. reported that RNAi-mediated knockdown of SOD1 in primary human fibroblasts induced cellular senescence mediated by p53. However, senescence was not induced in p53-deficient human fibroblasts [59]. Furthermore overexpression of MnSOD induced growth arrest in the human colorectal cancer cell line HCT116 and increased senescence which required the induction of p53 [60]. On the contrary, p53 can suppress senescence through the inhibition of the mTOR pathway via multiple mechanisms [61–63]. Nevertheless, this diverse biological spectrum of p53 regulation of cellular function remains complex and is dependent on the source of activation and cell type.

There are various sources of p53 activators, which include nucleotide depletion, hypoxia, ultraviolet radiation, ionizing radiation, as well as many chemotherapeutic drugs can act as activators of p53 (i.e., Doxorubicin). In normal cells, p53 remains at a low level and is under strict control by its negative regulator Mdm2. p53 induces autoregulation via Mdm2. As a transcription factor, p53 can bind to the promoter region of the mdm2 gene to promote transcription of Mdm2 mRNA [64, 65]. Following proper translation into a functional protein, Mdm2 acts as an E3 ligase during p53 activation. Mdm2 can polyubiquitinate p53 leading to proteasomal degradation [66]. However, Mdm2 can also monoubiquinate p53 leading to intracellular trafficking [67]. The decisive role of p53 to induce cell cycle arrest, senescence, or apoptosis involves intricate posttranslational, as well as, transcription-dependent and transcription-independent mechanisms. The tumor suppressor p53 is a well-characterized transcription factor known to induce the transactivation of proapoptotic genes such as Bax, Puma, Noxa, Bid and represses the transcription of anti-apoptotic genes such as Bcl-2, Bcl-xL, and survivin [68, 69]. Nevertheless, p53 can induce apoptosis independent of its transcriptional activity. Many of the transcription-independent mechanisms of p53 were discovered through the use of inhibitors of transcription/translation, as well as p53 truncated mutants with altered subcellular localization, DNA binding, and cofactor recruitment. The p53 monomer consists of various multifunctional domains including the N-terminal transactivation domain (residues 1–73), a proline-rich region (residues 63–97), the highly conserved DNA-binding core domain (residues 94–312), a tetramerization domain located within the C-terminus (residues 324–355), and an unstructured basic domain (residues 360–393) [70] (Figure 1). There are multiple polymorphisms that occur within the TP3

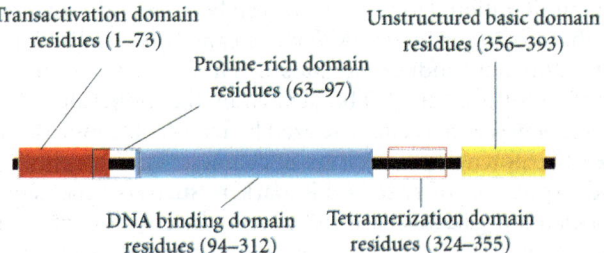

FIGURE 1: p53 Multifunctional domains. The p53 monomer consists of various multifunctional domains including the N-terminal transactivation domain (residues 1–73), a proline-rich region (residues 63–97), the highly conserved DNA-binding core domain (residues 94–312), a tetramerization domain located within the C-terminus (residues 324–355), and an unstructured basic domain (residues 360–393).

gene that may enhance or alter p53 functionality. Dumont et al. discovered functional differences in polymorphic variants that enhanced p53-mediated apoptosis independent of its transactivation abilities [71]. A common sequence polymorphism that occurs within the proline-rich domain encoding arginine at position 72 exhibited a fivefold increase in inducing apoptosis compared to the common proline (Pro72) variant. These results suggested two mechanisms of Arg 72 apoptotic enhancement: (1) increased mitochondrial localization; (2) enhanced binding of the Arg 72 variant to the negative p53 regulator E3 ligase, Mdm2. Although increased binding to Mdm2 did not augment p53 degradation, it was suggested that the altered confirmation of the p53 Arg 72 variant enhanced the binding ability and facilitated greater nuclear export [71]. This suggests the importance of understanding the regulation of structure-activity relationships in polymorphic forms of p53 in transcription-independent apoptosis.

During p53-mediated apoptosis, a distinct cytoplasmic pool of p53 translocates to the mitochondria. To promote mitochondrial translocation, the E3 ligase, Mdm2 monoubiquitinates p53 [72]. Since the p53 protein lacks a mitochondrial localization sequence, p53 interacts with Bcl-2 family proteins via Bcl-2 homology (BH) domains. The presence of the BH domain allows proteins to regulate and interact with other Bcl-2 members that consist of multiple BH domains [73]. Once p53 arrives at the mitochondrial outer membrane, p53 binds to Bak inducing a conformational change and Bak homo-oligomerization that results in mitochondrial outer membrane permeabilization (MOMP). MOMP allows for the release of pro-apoptotic signaling molecules from the outer and inner mitochondrial membranes into the cytosol triggering the intrinsic apoptotic signaling cascade. ROS generation has been suggested as an alternative p53 apoptotic target independent of cytochrome c release. Li et al. found that ROS generation regulated the mitochondrial membrane potential ($\Delta\psi$), which was found to be a key constituent in the induction of p53-mediated apoptosis [74]. Interestingly, during ROS generation, apoptosis occurred in the absence of Bax mitochondrial translocation, Bid activation, as well as cytochrome c release. Several studies

have suggested that the downstream effects of p53-mediated apoptosis are regulated by Bax expression. It has been shown that the introduction of recombinant Bax protein into isolated mitochondria induced cytochrome c release. The ability of Bax to initiate pore formation in synthetic membranes has been shown to regulate cytochrome c release resulting in the induction of apoptosis [75, 76]. However, discrepancies exist with *in vivo* studies showing Bax being localized in the cytosol, rather than within the mitochondrial membrane at physiological conditions [77].

Herein, we show how p53 has been shown to play a dual role in early-versus late-stage cancer progression. During the process of carcinogenesis, mutations can occur both upstream and downstream of p53 activation. For example, loss of upstream activators of p53, for example, ATM and Chk2, can prevent p53 activation, contributing to unregulated cell cycling and promoting tumorigenesis [78]. In addition, mutations within the p53 protein can alter necessary structure conformational changes and DNA binding properties needed for efficient p53 activation. Lastly, many of these mutations lead to loss of downstream genes such as Bax or NOXA which are pro-apoptotic and necessary for regulation of cellular proliferation and death signaling.

The process of tumor formation is a multistage process that involves both the activation of protooncogenes, and the inactivation of tumor suppressor genes, such as PTEN and p53. The multistage carcinogenesis paradigm consists of three well-characterized stages: initiation, promotion, and progression. During the initiation stage, there is the induction of mutations within critical target genes of stem cells, for example, H-ras; however in the skin carcinogenesis model, the epidermal layer remains phenotypically normal. During the tumor promotion stage, a noncarcinogenic agent such as a phorbol ester can be used to induce the clonal expansion of the initiated stem cells through epigenetic mechanisms. This stage is often used by investigators to identify potential therapeutic targets due to its reversibility. During the tumor progression stage, malignancy takes place, being characterized by enhanced invasiveness via the activation of proteases, and metastasizes via tumor cells entering into the lymphatics and loss of tumor suppressor activity (e.g., p53).

The two-stage skin carcinogenesis mouse model has been well characterized and used in numerous studies to screen anti cancer agents. An initiator, such as dimethylbenz[a]anthracene (DMBA), is applied to the skin to initiate DNA damage within skin cells. Following DMBA treatment, a tumor promoter such as 12-O-tetradecanoylphorbol-13-acetate (TPA) is applied topically to the same area repeatedly for the duration of the study to promote the clonal expansion of mutated cells during the promotion stage. Interestingly, during the early stages of DMBA/TPA-mediated tumor promotion both oncogenes and tumor suppressor genes are activated, resulting in increased cell proliferation being accompanied by increased cell death [79] (Figure 2). Both processes exist throughout skin tumor formation. Not surprising, these two opposing events are closely related.

Many of the tumor-promoting mechanisms utilized by phorbol esters are directly linked to the involvement of cell surface membranes [80, 81]. TPA can mediate its pleiotropic

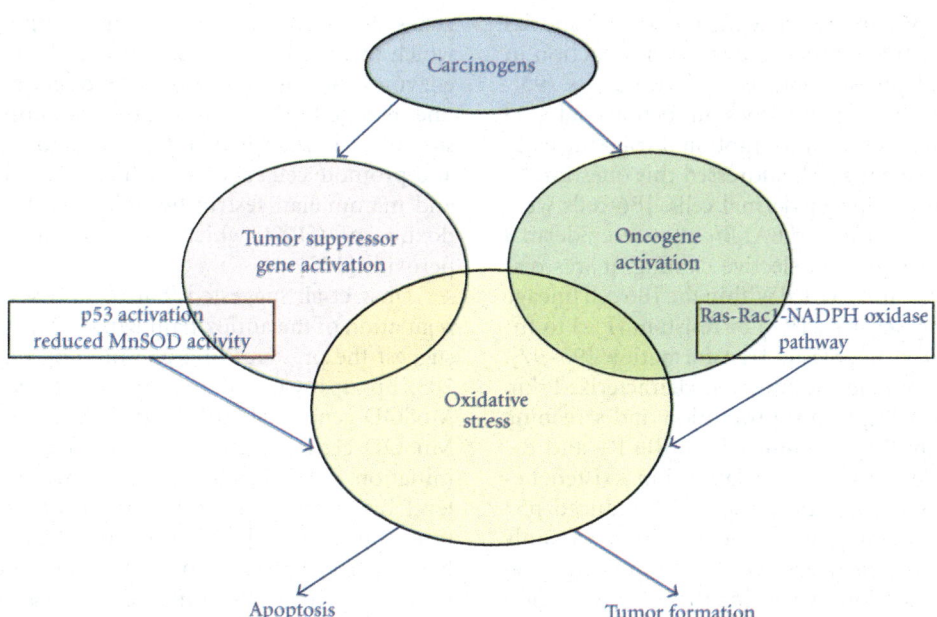

FIGURE 2: Mechanisms of carcinogens in early stage carcinogenesis. During the early stages of tumor promotion both oncogenes and tumor suppressor genes are activated, resulting in increased cell proliferation being accompanied by increased cell death.

actions through intercalating into the cellular membrane and inducing the activation of the Ca^{2+}-activated phospholipid-dependent protein kinase, protein kinase C (PKC) both *in vitro* and *in vivo*. TPA can directly activate PKC via molecular mimicry by substituting for diacylglycerol, the endogenous substrate, increasing the affinity of PKC for Ca^{2+} which leads to the activation of numerous downstream signaling pathways involved in a variety of cellular functions including proliferation and neoplastic transformation [82]. In addition, it is known that a direct correlation exists between phorbol ester-mediated tumor promotion and enzymatic activation of PKC [82, 83]. The PKC family consists of various highly conserved serine/threonine kinases. PKCs are involved in numerous cellular processes including cell differentiation, tumorigenesis, cell death, aging, and neurodegeneration [84]; however the induction of the signaling pathway is determined by the intracellular redox status and the isoform that is activated. The PKC family consists of a myriad of isoforms that have been divided into three classes: (a) classical or conventional PKCs (cPKC: α, βI, and βII, and γ); (b) novel PKCs (nPKC: δ, ε, η, and θ); (c) the atypical PKCs (aPKC: λ, ι, and ζ) which are classified based on sensitivity to Ca^{2+} and diacylglycerol (DAG) [84]. In various types of cancers PKCε has been shown to be upregulated while PKCα and PKCδ are downregulated. Interestingly, TPA activates the PKCε isoform in mouse skin tissues [85]. Furthermore, overexpression of PKCε has been shown to enhance the formation of skin carcinomas [86]. Moreover, TPA treatment leads to the concomitant activation of the redox-sensitive transcription factor activator protein-1 (AP-1) [85]. The AP-1 complex consists of both Jun and Fos oncoproteins. There are 3 jun isoforms (c-jun, jun-B, and jun-D) and 4 fos family members (c-fos, fra-1, fra-2, and fos-B) [87] whose activation is modulated by oxidants such as superoxide and

hydrogen peroxide, while DNA binding activities are modulated by the intracellular redox status [88–90]. Kiningham and Clair reported a reduction in tumorigenicity and AP-1 DNA binding activity following overexpression of MnSOD in transfected fibrosarcoma cells [91]. Furthermore, the protein expression of Bcl-xl, an antiapoptotic AP-1 target gene, was decreased, as well. In addition, PKCε activation was reduced in MnSOD transgenic mice treated with DMBA/TPA compared to their nontransgenic counterparts [85]. These results suggest a mechanistic linkage between MnSOD expression, mitogenic activation, and AP-1 binding activity.

5. MnSOD-p53 Mitochondrial Interaction

Another activated signaling pathway that has been defined following DMBA/TPA treatment is the Ras-Rac1-NADPH oxidase pathway, which leads to p53 mitochondrial translocation and apoptosis [92]. NADPH oxidase forms a stable heterodimer with the membrane protein p22^{phox}, which serves as a docking site for the SH3 domain-containing regulatory proteins p47^{phox}, p67^{phox}, and p40^{phox}. Upon TPA treatment, Rac, a small GTPase, binds to p67^{phox} which induces NADPH oxidase activation [11] and superoxide production. Mitochondrial p53 has been shown to interact with MnSOD, resulting in decreased enzymatic activity and promoting oxidative stress propagation [93].

The primary role of MnSOD is to protect mitochondria from oxidative damage. In 2005, Zhao et al. found that TPA treatment, both *in vitro* and *in vivo*, can induce p53 mitochondrial translocation [93]. In addition, p53 not only came in contact with the outer mitochondrial membrane but was able to localize to the mitochondrial matrix. Interestingly, following p53 mitochondrial translocation and matrix localization, p53 interacted with the mitochondrial antioxidant enzyme MnSOD that resulted in a reduction in MnSOD activity and propagation of oxidative stress [93]. However, the question remains: does mitochondrial p53 contribute to or suppress tumor promotion during the early stages of skin carcinogenesis? We addressed this question by utilizing the JB6 mouse skin epidermal cells. JB6 cells were originally derived from primary BALB/c mouse epidermal cell culture [94]. Through nonselective cloning, it was discovered that clonal variants existed within the JB6 cell lineage that were either stably sensitive (P+) or resistant (P−) to tumor promoter-induced neoplastic transformation [95–97]. In addition, JB6 cells remain the only well-characterized skin keratinocytes for studying tumor promotion and screening anti-cancer agents. In 2010, we utilized the JB6 P+ and P− clonal variants to determine if a relationship existed between tumor promotion and early-stage TPA-induced p53 activation [98]. Surprisingly, we found that p53 was only induced in promotion-sensitive P+ cells and not promotion resistant (P−) cells, therefore suggesting that p53 expression is highly associated with early stage tumor promotion. We then assessed Bax protein expression levels, as a marker for p53 transcriptional activity, and found that Bax expression is only induced in JB6 P+ cells and not P− cells, suggesting that p53 expression, as well as transcriptional activity, is highly associated with early-stage tumor promotion following TPA treatment. MnSOD expression was also measured in both JB6 P+ and P− cells and was found to be highly expressed in promotion-resistant P− cells compared to promotable P+ cells. TPA-mediated ROS generation was measured in P+ and P− cells (unpublished data), and promotion resistant cells contained significantly lower levels of ROS following TPA treatment when compared to their promotable counterparts. It is known that reduced MnSOD expression contributes to increased DNA damage, cancer incidence, and radical-caused diseases [99, 100]. Consistent with that, an increase of several markers of oxidative damage such as 4-HNE, 8-oxoDG, and lipid peroxidation has been seen in both *in vitro* and *in vivo* studies following TPA treatment [57, 85, 101, 102], suggesting the involvement of oxidative stress in the promotion of tumorigenesis. These results imply the importance of redox regulation in modulating cellular functions during the early stage of tumor promotion. We questioned whether the ROS generated from the MnSOD-p53 mitochondrial interaction was sufficient to promote tumorigenicity. Therefore, we utilized promotion-resistant JB6 P− cells that exhibited no p53 protein expression or transactivation following TPA treatment to address this question. Interestingly, we found that when JB6 promotion-resistant cells were transfected with wild-type p53, these cells were able to transform and form colonies in soft agar, in comparison to their control counterparts [98]. These results suggest a dual role of p53-mediated ROS generation during the early stages of skin carcinogenesis and how the presence of p53 is necessary for tumor promotion in skin (Figure 3).

The contradictory role of p53 in promoting cell survival or death is the result of the ability to regulate the expression of both pro- and antioxidant genes. For example, p53 can promote the generation of ROS through the induction of genes involved in mitochondrial injury and cell death which include Bax, Puma, and p66[SHC] and ROS-generating enzymes such as quinine oxidoreductase (NQO1) and proline oxidase [103]. However, p53 can upregulate the expression of various antioxidant enzymes to modulate ROS levels and promote cell survival such as aldehyde dehydrogenase 4 and mammalian sestrin homologues that encode peroxiredoxins and GPX1, which are major enzymatic removers of peroxide [103].

Dhar et al. suggested that p53 possessed "bidirectional" regulation of the antioxidant MnSOD gene. Previous reports suggest the presence of a p53 binding region at 328 bp and 2032 bp upstream of the transcriptional start site of the MnSOD gene [104, 105]. Others suggest that p53 represses MnSOD gene expression by interfering with transcription initiation [106], inhibiting gene activators at the promoter level by forming an inhibitory complex suppressing gene transcription [107] and protein-protein interactions [108]. Nevertheless, p53 can induce the gene expression of MnSOD [104]. p53-mediated MnSOD expression is regulated in conjunction with other cell proliferative transcription factors such as NF-κB. Kiningham and Clair demonstrated the presence of an NF-κB binding site within the intronic enhancer element of the MnSOD gene [91]. It was later shown that mutation of the NF-κB site within the enhancer element abrogated p53 induced MnSOD gene transcription. In addition, knockdown of p65 via siRNA reduced MnSOD gene transcription via p53 as well. Overall the effects of p53 on MnSOD gene expression have been suggested to be concentration dependent, with low concentrations of p53 increasing MnSOD expression via corroborative NF-κB binding promoting cell survival and high concentrations of p53 suppressing MnSOD expression by interfering with important transcriptional binding elements such as SP1.

6. Clinical Implications of the MnSOD-p53 Interaction

p53 is mutated in 50% of human cancers. However, the remaining human tumors contain wild-type p53 with defects in the downstream mediated p53-signaling pathways. This, in turn, provides novel areas of discovery in stabilization and restoration of wild-type p53 activity. Currently, many drug companies are focused on utilizing p53 interactions as targets for pharmacological intervention [78]. There are various protein-protein interactions that occur within the cell that positively or negatively regulate p53 expression and function. For example, Mdm2 is an E3 ligase of p53 that polyubiquitinates p53, priming the tumor suppressor for proteasomal degradation. Many have found that, by blocking this interaction through peptides or transcriptional inhibitors, longer durations of p53 activation have resulted. Some of the therapeutic strategies that are currently being utilized are peptides that increase p53 activation through inhibition of Mdm2 function [109]. Three-dimensional structural models [110] of the hdm2-p53 interaction along with biochemical data [111, 112] have identified three residues that are important to this interaction, Phe19, Trp23, and Leu26

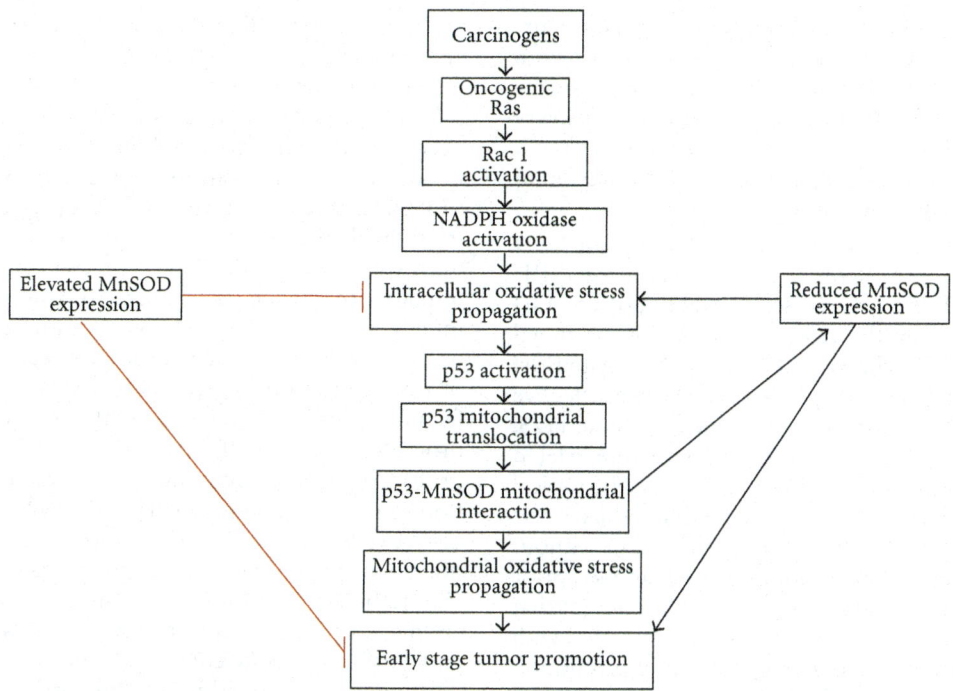

FIGURE 3: Mechanism involving the p53-MnSOD interaction during the early stage of tumor promotion. Following exposure to a carcinogen the Ras-Rac1-NADPH oxidase pathway is activated, which leads to p53 mitochondrial translocation. Mitochondrial p53 has been shown to interact with MnSOD, resulting in decreased enzymatic activity and promoting oxidative stress propagation contributing to the early stage of skin tumorigenicity. Elevated levels of MnSOD reduced oxidative stress propagation, suppressed p53 mitochondrial translocation, and decreased downstream skin tumor formation. Reduced levels of MnSOD have been shown to contribute to oxidative stress propagation and promote early-stage skin tumorigenicity.

[111, 112]. From this data, an 8-mer peptide was generated [113] and showed promising results in inducing apoptosis in tumor cells that overexpressed hdm2 [112]. However, these conditions were difficult to optimize with a smaller molecule therefore causing this peptide to be therapeutically inefficient. Also nutlins have been utilized to disrupt the mdm2-p53 interaction resulting in reactivation of the p53 response [114, 115]. Others have used antisense and transcription inhibitors to prevent the expression of Mdm2 [116].

Gene replacement therapy is another therapeutic modality that has been explored in treating tumors lacking or containing mutant p53. This technique utilizes adenoviruses, as well as retroviruses to achieve high expression of p53 in tumor cells. Promising results have been seen with retroviral vectors in patients with nonsmall cell lung cancers [117]. On the contrary, although we have seen the enhancement of tumorigenicity in our *in vitro* p53 transfection studies [98], we have not tested stably transfected cells in *in vivo* xenograft mouse models, nor have we tried other tissue types. Therefore, the reintroduction of the p53 gene into tumors may have contradictory outcomes depending on the cell type and tissue microenvironment. This concern has echoed through various studies, persuading investigators to opt to combine gene therapy with chemotherapy and radiotherapy [118–121].

For decades, it has been shown that p53 functions only as a tumor suppressor. In addition, p53-mediated ROS

generation has been limited to the induction of apoptosis. Currently, the ability of wild-type p53 to contribute to tumor promotion has received considerable attention. We have shown that the p53-MnSOD interaction contributes to the early stage of tumor promotion. In addition, it has been consistently shown that MnSOD activity is altered in human tumors. Therefore, designing diagnostic tools to assess MnSOD activity, as well as p53 activation, can be used to effectively design individualized treatments for cancer patients. For example, following chemotherapeutic treatment, patients that have higher levels of p53 expression and exhibit lower levels of MnSOD can receive an SOD mimetic that can upregulate MnSOD or synthetic compounds that can downregulate p53 activity to decrease ROS-mediated apoptosis and potential relapse within these patients.

Gene therapy has also been utilized to modulate MnSOD activity during cancer progression. Overexpression of MnSOD through gene therapy introducing genetically engineered DNA/liposomes containing the human MnSOD transgene into preclinical and clinical models has been shown to be protective in normal tissues against ionizing irradiation. The final product (VLTS-582) is a DNA/liposome formulation that consists of a double-stranded DNA bacterial plasmid containing human MnSOD cDNA in conjunction with two lipids {cholesterol and DOTIM (1-[2-[9-(2)-octadecenoyloxy]]-2-[8-(2)-heptadecenyl]-3-[hydroxyethyl] imidazolinium chloride)} [122]. Recent studies suggest that this formulation has been successful in murine models and has been administered orally to patients concurrently with a weekly chemotherapy regime exhibiting no dose-limiting toxicities. Although proven therapeutically efficacious, more studies are needed to improve (1) delivery of the transgene to the targeted tissue; (2) reducing rapid elimination of the transgene; (3) control of the expression of the transgene within targeted tissues.

On the other hand, a topical application of an SOD mimetic has also been described [123]. The Mn (III) porphyrin Mn^{III} TE-2-Pyp^{5+} possesses highly potent SOD activity as facilitated by the redox properties of the metal center and the positive charge to the ortho-N-ethylpyridyl nitrogens [124]. Mn^{III} TE-2-Pyp^{5+} has been proven effective *in vitro* and in various human diseases such as stroke [125, 126], diabetes [127, 128], and cancer and radiation-related treatment [129–132]. In preclinical animal models, topical application of Mn^{III} TE-2-Pyp^{5+} was shown to reduce levels of oxidative damage and reduced cell proliferation without interfering with p53-mediated apoptosis when applied prior to TPA treatment [129]. These data support the concept that overexpression of MnSOD when applied in conjunction with standard chemotherapeutics or during the tumor promotion stage is protective in both preclinical and clinical models.

Nevertheless, both p53 and MnSOD have been shown to posses reduced activity and/or mutated in most human diseases including cancer. Therefore, more therapeutic quests are needed to detect and restore both MnSOD and wild-type p53 activity. However, future therapeutic optimization strategies should have minimal nonspecific drug-related toxicities and be based on the stage of cancer progression which may reveal a therapeutic window for treatment intervention.

7. Concluding Remarks

In summary, reactive oxygen species have been implicated in the pathogenesis of various hyperproliferative and inflammatory diseases [133]. In addition, the tumor suppressor p53 has been shown to be activated during the early stage of skin carcinogenesis and contributed to the propagation of oxidative stress. Recent studies demonstrate a novel role of mitochondrial p53 activation. Once in the mitochondria, p53 physically interacts with MnSOD. As a result, this interaction reduces the free radical scavenging abilities of MnSOD, promoting enhanced ROS generation which has been shown to act as a tumorigenic stimulus during cancer progression. This suggests that wild-type p53 may play a direct role in promoting oxidative stress and contributing to the ROS-mediated tumor-proliferative stimuli. In addition, others have shown that mutant p53 can, in fact, translocate to the mitochondria and interact with MnSOD [134]. However, Lontz et al. observed following doxorubicin treatment of lymphoma cell lines with varying wt or mutant p53 levels, mitochondrial function, as evidenced by Complex I/II activities, was only compromised in lymphoma cells expressing wild-type and not mutant p53 [134]. Therefore, the continuation of deciphering mechanistic differences in tumors containing wild-type or mutant p53 can lead to the development of therapeutic p53-mediated interventions and

a clearer understanding of chemoresistance in both wild-type and mutant p53 human tumors.

Several studies have suggested that MnSOD may play a primary protective role against tissue injury. MnSOD has been found to be depleted in a variety of tumor cells, as well as *in vitro* transformed cell lines, suggesting that MnSOD may act as a novel tumor suppressor, protecting cells from oxidant-induced carcinogenesis [135]. Nevertheless, overexpression of MnSOD decreases the pathogenesis of human diseases such as cancer. Consistent with that, accumulating evidence suggests that a number of antioxidants or drugs with antioxidant properties can reduce mediators of tumor promotion [136]. Clair et al. showed that transfecting mouse 10T 1/2 cells with human MnSOD cDNA promoted differentiation with 5-azacytidine treatment and protected against neoplastic transformation [137]. In addition, transfecting human MnSOD cDNA into MCF-7 breast cancer cells and UACC-903melanoma cells suppressed their malignant phenotype and suppressed growth in nude mice [54, 138]. We have shown that the cumulative induction of endogenous antioxidant enzymes (i.e., catalase, total SOD and MnSOD) is efficient in reducing tumor incidence and multiplicity [57]. In addition, the induction of endogenous antioxidant enzymes via dietary administration can suppress p53 mitochondrial translocation [98]. TPA can induce p53 mitochondrial translocation; however, this phorbol ester also decreases the mitochondrial membrane potential, as well as mitochondrial complex activities and respiration. Other studies have shown that MnSOD overexpression in mice protects complex I from adriamycin-induced deactivation in cardiac tissue [139]. These results suggest that antioxidant expression protects against fluctuations in mitochondrial functions which suppress p53 mitochondrial translocation, p53-mediated ROS, and both downstream apoptotic and cell proliferation signaling pathways. On the contrary, Connor et al. suggest that overexpression of MnSOD in HT-1080 fibrosarcoma cells and 253J bladder tumor cells enhanced the migatory ability and invasiveness of tumor cells, through the upregulation of matrix metalloproteinases [140]. Although some tumors express higher levels of MnSOD, the downstream effects of enhanced antioxidant expression are dependent on the tumor type and susceptibility to oxidative damage, underlying oncogenic mutations and the stage of disease progression [140]. Nevertheless, these investigators stressed the need of refined regulation of H_2O_2 production. Therefore the question remains, are the effects of the p53-MnSOD interaction protumorigenic or anti-tumorigenic? To definitively answer this question further investigation of this interaction is needed. However, there are several factors that must be considered in determining the fate of the p53-MnSOD interaction, which include the stage of disease progression as well as tumor microenvironment. It has been shown that p53 activation is required in tumor promotion and can mediate ROS generation. However, the duration of enhanced ROS generation, severity of oxidative damage, and the status of the cellular antioxidant capacity can all contribute to the proliferative/apoptotic switch that occurs during the response to cellular stress. Overall, further studies are needed to clearly assess the status of MnSOD during the various stages of carcinogenesis to enhance the efficacy of standard treatment regimens currently being used.

Consistent with that, defining the downstream effects of the p53-MnSOD complex formation can expand our knowledge of the molecular mechanisms that contribute to the early stage of tumorigenesis and how they may be altered during cancer progression. With further knowledge, modulators of MnSOD, p53 and their associated regulators can be therapeutically useful in the treatment of cancer and various stages of tumor progression.

References

[1] R. Radi, A. Cassina, R. Hodara, C. Quijano, and L. Castro, "Peroxynitrite reactions and formation in mitochondria," *Free Radical Biology and Medicine*, vol. 33, no. 11, pp. 1451–1464, 2002.

[2] E. Lonn, J. Bosch, S. Yusuf et al., "Effects of long-term vitamin E supplementation on cardiovascular events and cancer: a randomized controlled trial," *Journal of the American Medical Association*, vol. 293, no. 11, pp. 1338–1347, 2005.

[3] M. M. Berger, "Can oxidative damage be treated nutritionally?" *Clinical Nutrition*, vol. 24, no. 2, pp. 172–183, 2005.

[4] D. Bonnefont-Rousselot, "The role of antioxidant micronutrients in the prevention of diabetic complications," *Treatments in Endocrinology*, vol. 3, no. 1, pp. 41–52, 2004.

[5] D. N. Seril, J. Liao, G. Y. Yang, and C. S. Yang, "Oxidative stress and ulcerative colitis-associated carcinogenesis: studies in humans and animal models," *Carcinogenesis*, vol. 24, no. 3, pp. 353–362, 2003.

[6] R. Stocker and J. F. Keaney Jr., "Role of oxidative modifications in atherosclerosis," *Physiological Reviews*, vol. 84, no. 4, pp. 1381–1478, 2004.

[7] A. M. Cantin, "Potential for antioxidant therapy of cystic fibrosis," *Current Opinion in Pulmonary Medicine*, vol. 10, no. 6, pp. 531–536, 2004.

[8] J. Viña, A. Lloret, R. Ortí, and D. Alonso, "Molecular bases of the treatment of Alzheimer's disease with antioxidants: prevention of oxidative stress," *Molecular Aspects of Medicine*, vol. 25, no. 1-2, pp. 117–123, 2004.

[9] G. Loschen, A. Azzi, and L. Flohe, "Mitochondrial H2O2 formation: relationship with energy conservation," *FEBS Letters*, vol. 33, no. 1, pp. 84–88, 1973.

[10] E. Cadenas, A. Boveris, C. I. Ragan, and A. O. M. Stoppani, "Production of superoxide radicals and hydrogen peroxide by NADH ubiquinone reductase and ubiquinol cytochrome c reductase from beef heart mitochondria," *Archives of Biochemistry and Biophysics*, vol. 180, no. 2, pp. 248–257, 1977.

[11] F. Jiang, Y. Zhang, and G. J. Dusting, "NADPH oxidase-mediated redoxsignaling: roles in cellular stress response, stress tolerance, and tissue repair," *Pharmacological Reviews*, vol. 63, no. 1, pp. 218–242, 2011.

[12] R. C. Kukreja, H. A. Kontos, M. L. Hess, and E. F. Ellis, "PGH synthase and lipoxygenase generate superoxide in the presence of NADH or NADPH," *Circulation Research*, vol. 59, no. 6, pp. 612–619, 1986.

[13] P. Roy, S. K. Roy, A. Mitra, and A. P. Kulkarni, "Superoxide generation by lipoxygenase in the presence of NADH and NADPH," *Biochimica et Biophysica Acta*, vol. 1214, no. 2, pp. 171–179, 1994.

[14] S. Puntarulo and A. I. Cederbaum, "Production of reactive oxygen species by microsomes enriched in specific human cytochrome P450 enzymes," *Free Radical Biology and Medicine*, vol. 24, no. 7-8, pp. 1324–1330, 1998.

[15] S. Pou, W. S. Pou, D. S. Bredt, S. H. Snyder, and G. M. Rosen, "Generation of superoxide by purified brain nitric oxide synthase," *Journal of Biological Chemistry*, vol. 267, no. 34, pp. 24173–24176, 1992.

[16] C. E. Berry and J. M. Hare, "Xanthine oxidoreductase and cardiovascular disease: molecular mechanisms and pathophysiological implications," *Journal of Physiology*, vol. 555, no. 3, pp. 589–606, 2004.

[17] K. K. Griendling, D. Sorescu, and M. Ushio-Fukai, "NAD(P)H oxidase: role in cardiovascular biology and disease," *Circulation Research*, vol. 86, no. 5, pp. 494–501, 2000.

[18] P. Rockwell, J. Martinez, L. Papa, and E. Gomes, "Redox regulates COX-2 upregulation and cell death in the neuronal response to cadmium," *Cellular Signalling*, vol. 16, no. 3, pp. 343–353, 2004.

[19] C. M. Yeh, P. S. Chien, and H. J. Huang, "Distinct signalling pathways for induction of MAP kinase activities by cadmium and copper in rice roots," *Journal of Experimental Botany*, vol. 58, no. 3, pp. 659–671, 2007.

[20] T. Hasegawa, M. Kikuyama, K. Sakurai et al., "Mechanism of superoxide anion production by hepatic sinusoidal endothelial cells and Kupffer cells during short-term ethanol perfusion in the rat," *Liver*, vol. 22, no. 4, pp. 321–329, 2002.

[21] P. K. Narayanan, E. H. Goodwin, and B. E. Lehnert, "α particles initiate biological production of superoxide anions and hydrogen peroxide in human cells," *Cancer Research*, vol. 57, no. 18, pp. 3963–3971, 1997.

[22] H. Wang and I. E. Kochevar, "Involvement of UVB-induced reactive oxygen species in TGF-β biosynthesis and activation in keratinocytes," *Free Radical Biology and Medicine*, vol. 38, no. 7, pp. 890–897, 2005.

[23] B. M. Babior, "NADPH oxidase: an update," *Blood*, vol. 93, no. 5, pp. 1464–1476, 1999.

[24] B. Lassègue and R. E. Clempus, "Vascular NAD(P)H oxidases: specific features, expression, and regulation," *American Journal of Physiology*, vol. 285, no. 2, pp. R277–R297, 2003.

[25] J. D. Lambeth, "Nox enzymes, ROS, and chronic disease: an example of antagonistic pleiotropy," *Free Radical Biology and Medicine*, vol. 43, no. 3, pp. 332–347, 2007.

[26] E. I. Azzam, S. M. De Toledo, D. R. Spitz, and J. B. Little, "Oxidative metabolism modulates signal transduction and micronucleus formation in bystander cells from α-particle-irradiated normal human fibroblast cultures," *Cancer Research*, vol. 62, no. 19, pp. 5436–5442, 2002.

[27] J. R. Collins-Underwood, W. Zhao, J. G. Sharpe, and M. E. Robbins, "NADPH oxidase mediates radiation-induced oxidative stress in rat brain microvascular endothelial cells," *Free Radical Biology and Medicine*, vol. 45, no. 6, pp. 929–938, 2008.

[28] Y. Tateishi, E. Sasabe, E. Ueta, and T. Yamamoto, "Ionizing irradiation induces apoptotic damage of salivary gland acinar cells via NADPH oxidase 1-dependent superoxide generation," *Biochemical and Biophysical Research Communications*, vol. 366, no. 2, pp. 301–307, 2008.

[29] R. M. Tyrrell, "UV activation of mammalian stress proteins," *EXS*, vol. 77, pp. 255–271, 1996.

[30] A. J. Varghese and S. Y. Wang, "Thymine-thymine adduct as a photoproduct of thymine," *Science*, vol. 160, no. 3824, pp. 186–187, 1968.

[31] A. J. Varghese and M. H. Patrick, "Cytosine derived heteroadduct formation in ultraviolet-irradiated DNA," *Nature*, vol. 223, no. 5203, pp. 299–300, 1969.

[32] A. J. Varghese, "Photochemistry of nucleic acids and their constituents," *Photophysiology*, no. 7, pp. 207–274, 1972.

[33] R. B. Setlow, "Cyclobutane-type pyrimidine dimers in polynucleotides," *Science*, vol. 153, no. 3734, pp. 379–386, 1966.

[34] R. B. Setlow and W. L. Carrier, "Pyrimidine dimers in ultraviolet-irradiated DNA's," *Journal of Molecular Biology*, vol. 17, no. 1, pp. 237–254, 1966.

[35] R. B. Setlow, "The photochemistry, photobiology, and repair of polynucleotides," *Progress in Nucleic Acid Research and Molecular Biology*, vol. 8, no. C, pp. 257–295, 1968.

[36] A. W. Girotti, "Lipid hydroperoxide generation, turnover, and effector action in biological systems," *Journal of Lipid Research*, vol. 39, no. 8, pp. 1529–1542, 1998.

[37] B. Halliwell and J. M. C. Gutteridge, "Role of free radicals and catalytic metal ions in human disease: an overview," *Methods in Enzymology*, vol. 186, pp. 1–85, 1990.

[38] Y. J. Suzuki, H. J. Forman, and A. Sevanian, "Oxidants as stimulators of signal transduction," *Free Radical Biology and Medicine*, vol. 22, no. 1-2, pp. 269–285, 1997.

[39] J. Rashba-Step, A. Tatoyan, R. Duncan, D. Ann, T. R. Pushpa-Rehka, and A. Sevanian, "Phospholipid peroxidation induces cytosolic phospholipase A2 activity: membrane effects versus enzyme phosphorylation," *Archives of Biochemistry and Biophysics*, vol. 343, no. 1, pp. 44–54, 1997.

[40] E. Cadenas and K. J. A. Davies, "Mitochondrial free radical generation, oxidative stress, and aging," *Free Radical Biology and Medicine*, vol. 29, no. 3-4, pp. 222–230, 2000.

[41] A. Navarro, "Mitochondrial enzyme activities as biochemical markers of aging," *Molecular Aspects of Medicine*, vol. 25, no. 1-2, pp. 37–48, 2004.

[42] S. Z. Imam, B. Karahalil, B. A. Hogue, N. C. Souza-Pinto, and V. A. Bohr, "Mitochondrial and nuclear DNA-repair capacity of various brain regions in mouse is altered in an age-dependent manner," *Neurobiology of Aging*, vol. 27, no. 8, pp. 1129–1136, 2006.

[43] R. A. Weisiger and I. Fridovich -, "Mitochondrial superoxide dismutase. Site of synthesis and intramitochondrial localization," *Journal of Biological Chemistry*, vol. 248, no. 13, pp. 4793–4796, 1973.

[44] J. M. McCord and I. Fridovich, "Superoxide dismutase. An enzymic function for erythrocuprein (hemocuprein)," *Journal of Biological Chemistry*, vol. 244, no. 22, pp. 6049–6055, 1969.

[45] A. Okado-Matsumoto and I. Fridovich, "Subcellular distribution of superoxide dismutases (SOD) in rat liver," *Journal of Biological Chemistry*, vol. 276, no. 42, pp. 38388–38393, 2001.

[46] S. L. Marklund, "Human copper-containing superoxide dismutase of high molecular weight," *Proceedings of the National Academy of Sciences of the United States of America*, vol. 79, no. 24 I, pp. 7634–7638, 1982.

[47] G. H. W. Wong and D. V. Goeddel, "Induction of manganous superoxide dismutase by tumor necrosis factor: possible protective mechanism," *Science*, vol. 242, no. 4880, pp. 941–944, 1988.

[48] S. L. Church, J. W. Grant, E. U. Meese, and J. M. Trent, "Sublocalization of the gene encoding manganese superoxide dismutase (MnSOD/SOD29 to 6q25 by fluorescence in situ hybridization and somatic cell hybrid mapping," *Genomics*, vol. 14, no. 3, pp. 823–825, 1992.

[49] D. Millikin, E. Meese, B. Vogelstein, C. Witkowski, and J. Trent, "Loss of heterozygosity for loci on the long arm of chromosome 6 in human malignant melanoma," *Cancer Research*, vol. 51, no. 20, pp. 5449–5453, 1991.

[50] J. R. Wispe, J. C. Clark, M. S. Burhans, K. E. Kropp, T. R. Korfhagen, and J. A. Whitsett, "Synthesis and processing of the precursor for human mangano-superoxide dismutase," *Biochimica et Biophysica Acta*, vol. 994, no. 1, pp. 30–36, 1989.

[51] L. W. Oberley and G. R. Buettner, "Role of superoxide dismutase in cancer: a review," *Cancer Research*, vol. 39, no. 4, pp. 1141–1149, 1979.

[52] Y. Xu, A. Krishnan, X. S. Wan et al., "Mutations in the promoter reveal a cause for the reduced expression of the human manganese superoxide dismutase gene in cancer cells," *Oncogene*, vol. 18, no. 1, pp. 93–102, 1999.

[53] H. J. Zhang, T. Yan, T. D. Oberley, and L. W. Oberley, "Comparison of effects of two polymorphic variants of manganese superoxide dismutase on human breast MCF-7 cancer cell phenotype," *Cancer Research*, vol. 59, no. 24, pp. 6276–6283, 1999.

[54] S. L. Church, J. W. Grant, L. A. Ridnour et al., "Increased manganese superoxide dismutase expression suppresses the malignant phenotype of human melanoma cells," *Proceedings of the National Academy of Sciences of the United States of America*, vol. 90, no. 7, pp. 3113–3117, 1993.

[55] M. Urano, M. Kuroda, R. Reynolds, T. D. Oberley, and D. K. St. Clair D.K., "Expression of manganese superoxide dismutase reduces tumor control radiation dose: gene-radiotherapy," *Cancer Research*, vol. 55, no. 12, pp. 2490–2493, 1995.

[56] W. Zhong, L. W. Oberley, T. D. Oberley, and D. K. St Clair, "Suppression of the malignant phenotype of human glioma cells by overexpression of manganese superoxide dismutase," *Oncogene*, vol. 14, no. 4, pp. 481–490, 1997.

[57] J. Liu, X. Gu, D. Robbins et al., "Protandim, a fundamentally new antioxidant approach in chemoprevention using mouse two-stage skin carcinogenesis as a model," *PloS One*, vol. 4, no. 4, article e5284, 2009.

[58] K. Itahana, J. Campisi, and G. P. Dimri, "Methods to detect biomarkers of cellular senescence: the senescence-associated β-galactosidase assay," *Methods in Molecular Biology*, vol. 371, pp. 21–31, 2007.

[59] G. Blander, R. M. De Oliveira, C. M. Conboy, M. Haigis, and L. Guarente, "Superoxide dismutase 1 knock-down induces senescence in human fibroblasts," *Journal of Biological Chemistry*, vol. 278, no. 40, pp. 38966–38969, 2003.

[60] L. Behrend, A. Mohr, T. Dick, and R. M. Zwacka, "Manganese superoxide dismutase induces p53-dependent senescence in colorectal cancer cells," *Molecular and Cellular Biology*, vol. 25, no. 17, pp. 7758–7769, 2005.

[61] Z. Feng, H. Zhang, A. J. Levine, and S. Jin, "The coordinate regulation of the p53 and mTOR pathways in cells," *Proceedings of the National Academy of Sciences of the United States of America*, vol. 102, no. 23, pp. 8204–8209, 2005.

[62] E. Drakos, V. Atsaves, J. Li et al., "Stabilization and activation of p53 downregulates mTOR signaling through AMPK in mantle cell lymphoma," *Leukemia*, vol. 23, no. 4, pp. 784–790, 2009.

[63] A. V. Budanov and M. Karin, "p53 target genes sestrin1 and sestrin2 connect genotoxic stress and mTOR signaling," *Cell*, vol. 134, no. 3, pp. 451–460, 2008.

[64] Y. Barak, E. Gottlieb, T. Juven-Gershon, and M. Oren, "Regulation of *mdm2* expression by p53: alternative promoters produce transcripts with nonidentical translation potential," *Genes and Development*, vol. 8, no. 15, pp. 1739–1749, 1994.

[65] Y. Barak, T. Juven, R. Haffner, and M. Oren, "*mdm2* Expression is induced by wild type p53 activity," *EMBO Journal*, vol. 12, no. 2, pp. 461–468, 1993.

[66] R. Honda, H. Tanaka, and H. Yasuda, "Oncoprotein MDM2 is a ubiquitin ligase E3 for tumor suppressor p53," *FEBS Letters*, vol. 420, no. 1, pp. 25–27, 1997.

[67] R. K. Geyer, Z. K. Yu, and C. G. Maki, "The MDM2 RING-finger domain is required to promote p53 nuclear export," *Nature Cell Biology*, vol. 2, no. 9, pp. 569–573, 2000.

[68] A. Vazquez, E. E. Bond, A. J. Levine, and G. L. Bond, "The genetics of the p53 pathway, apoptosis and cancer therapy," *Nature Reviews Drug Discovery*, vol. 7, no. 12, pp. 979–987, 2008.

[69] K. H. Vousden and C. Prives, "Blinded by the light: the growing complexity of p53," *Cell*, vol. 137, no. 3, pp. 413–431, 2009.

[70] O. Laptenko and C. Prives, "Transcriptional regulation by p53: one protein, many possibilities," *Cell Death and Differentiation*, vol. 13, no. 6, pp. 951–961, 2006.

[71] P. Dumont, J. I. J. Leu, A. C. Della Pietra, D. L. George, and M. Murphy, "The codon 72 polymorphic variants of p53 have markedly different apoptotic potential," *Nature Genetics*, vol. 33, no. 3, pp. 357–365, 2003.

[72] A. V. Vaseva and U. M. Moll, "The mitochondrial p53 pathway," *Biochimica et Biophysica Acta*, vol. 1787, no. 5, pp. 414–420, 2009.

[73] D. Speidel, "Transcription-independent p53 apoptosis: an alternative route to death," *Trends in Cell Biology*, vol. 20, no. 1, pp. 14–24, 2010.

[74] P. F. Li, R. Dietz, and R. Von Harsdorf, "p53 regulates mitochondrial membrane potential through reactive oxygen species and induces cytochrome c-independent apoptosis blocked by Bcl-2," *EMBO Journal*, vol. 18, no. 21, pp. 6027–6036, 1999.

[75] Y. T. Hsu, K. G. Wolter, and R. J. Youle, "Cytosol-to-membrane redistribution of Bax and Bcl-XL during apoptosis," *Proceedings of the National Academy of Sciences of the United States of America*, vol. 94, no. 8, pp. 3668–3672, 1997.

[76] B. Antonsson, F. Conti, A. Ciavatta et al., "Inhibition of Bax channel-forming activity by Bcl-2," *Science*, vol. 277, no. 5324, pp. 370–372, 1997.

[77] T. Rossé, R. Olivier, L. Monney et al., "Bcl-2 prolongs cell survival after Bax-induced release of cytochrome c," *Nature*, vol. 391, no. 6666, pp. 496–499, 1998.

[78] D. P. Lane and S. Lain, "Therapeutic exploitation of the p53 pathway," *Trends in Molecular Medicine*, vol. 8, no. 4, pp. S38–S42, 2002.

[79] Y. Zhao, T. D. Oberley, L. Chaiswing et al., "Manganese superoxide dismutase deficiency enhances cell turnover via tumor promoter-induced alterations in AP-1 and p53-mediated pathways in a skin cancer model," *Oncogene*, vol. 21, no. 24, pp. 3836–3846, 2002.

[80] I. B. Weinstein, L. S. Lee, and P. B. Fisher, "Action of phorbol esters in cell culture: mimicry of transformation, altered differentiation, and effects on cell membranes," *Journal of Supramolecular and Cellular Biochemistry*, vol. 12, no. 2, pp. 195–208, 1979.

[81] P. M. Blumberg, "In vitro studies on the mode of action of the phorbol esters, potent tumor promoters: part 1," *Critical Reviews in Toxicology*, vol. 8, no. 2, pp. 153–197, 1980.

[82] M. Castagna, Y. Takai, and K. Kaibuchi, "Direct activation of calcium-activated, phospholipid-dependent protein kinase by tumor-promoting phorbol esters," *Journal of Biological Chemistry*, vol. 257, no. 13, pp. 7847–7851, 1982.

[83] J. Yamanishi, Y. Takai, K. Kaibuchi et al., "Synergistic functions of phorbol ester and calcium in serotonin release from human platelets," *Biochemical and Biophysical Research Communications*, vol. 112, no. 2, pp. 778–786, 1983.

[84] C. Giorgi, C. Agnoletto, C. Baldini et al., "Redox control of protein kinase C: cell-and disease-specific aspects," *Antioxidants and Redox Signaling*, vol. 13, no. 7, pp. 1051–1085, 2010.

[85] Y. Zhao, Y. Xue, T. D. Oberley et al., "Overexpression of manganese superoxide dismutase suppresses tumor formation by modulation of activator protein-1 signaling in a multistage skin carcinogenesis model," *Cancer Research*, vol. 61, no. 16, pp. 6082–6088, 2001.

[86] P. J. Reddig, N. E. Dreckschmidt, J. Zou, S. E. Bourguignon, T. D. Oberley, and A. K. Verma, "Transgenic mice overexpressing protein kinase Cε in their epidermis exhibit reduced papilloma burden but enhanced carcinoma formation after tumor promotion," *Cancer Research*, vol. 60, no. 3, pp. 595–602, 2000.

[87] P. Angel and M. Karin, "The role of Jun, Fos and the AP-1 complex in cell-proliferation and transformation," *Biochimica et Biophysica Acta*, vol. 1072, no. 2-3, pp. 129–157, 1991.

[88] P. A. Amstad, G. Krupitza, and P. A. Cerutti, "Mechanism of c-fos induction by active oxygen," *Cancer Research*, vol. 52, no. 14, pp. 3952–3960, 1992.

[89] C. R. Timblin, Y. W. M. Janssen, and B. T. Mossman, "Transcriptional activation of the proto-oncogene c-jun by asbestos and H2O2 is directly related to increased proliferation and transformation of tracheal epithelial cells," *Cancer Research*, vol. 55, no. 13, pp. 2723–2726, 1995.

[90] C. Abate, L. Patel, F. J. Rauscher 3rd, and T. Curran, "Redox regulation of Fos and Jun DNA-binding activity in vitro," *Science*, vol. 249, no. 4973, pp. 1157–1161, 1990.

[91] K. K. Kiningham and D. K. S. Clair, "Overexpression of manganese superoxide dismutase selectively modulates the activity of jun-associated transcription factors in fibrosarcoma cells," *Cancer Research*, vol. 57, no. 23, pp. 5265–5271, 1997.

[92] Y. Zhao, L. Chaiswing, V. Bakthavatchalu, T. D. Oberley, and D. K. S. Clair, "Ras mutation promotes p53 activation and apoptosis of skin keratinocytes," *Carcinogenesis*, vol. 27, no. 8, pp. 1692–1698, 2006.

[93] Y. Zhao, L. Chaiswing, J. M. Velez et al., "p53 translocation to mitochondria precedes its nuclear translocation and targets mitochondrial oxidative defense protein-manganese superoxide dismutase," *Cancer Research*, vol. 65, no. 9, pp. 3745–3750, 2005.

[94] N. H. Colburn, B. F. Former, K. A. Nelson, and S. H. Yuspa, "Tumour promoter induces anchorage independence irreversibly," *Nature*, vol. 281, no. 5732, pp. 589–591, 1979.

[95] N. H. Colburn, B. A. Koehler, and K. J. Nelson, "A cell culture assay for tumor-promoter-dependent progression toward neoplastic phenotype: detection of tumor promoters and promotion inhibitors," *Teratogenesis Carcinogenesis and Mutagenesis*, vol. 1, no. 1, pp. 87–96, 1980.

[96] N.H. Colburn, L. D. Dion, and E. J. Wendel, "The role of mitogenic stimulation and specific glycoprotein changes in the mechanism of late-stage tumor promotion in JB6 epidermal cell lines," in *Carcinogenesis: A Comprehensive Survey*, E. Hecker, N. E. Fusening, W. Kunz, F. Marks, and H. W. Thielmann, Eds., pp. 231–235, Raven Press, New York, NY, USA, 1982.

[97] N. H. Colburn, L. Srinivas, and E. Wendel, "Responses of preneoplastic epidermal cells to tumor promoters and growth factors: use of promoter-resistant variants for mechanism studies," *Journal of Cellular Biochemistry*, vol. 18, no. 3, pp. 251–270, 1982.

[98] D. Robbins, X. Gu, R. Shi et al., "The chemopreventive effects of Protandim: modulation of p53 mitochondrial transloca- tion and apoptosis during skin carcinogenesis," *PLoS One*, vol. 5, no. 7, Article ID e11902, 2010.

[99] H. Van Remmen, Y. Ikeno, M. Hamilton et al., "Life-long reduction in MnSOD activity results in increased DNA dam- age and higher incidence of cancer but does not accelerate aging," *Physiological Genomics*, vol. 16, pp. 29–37, 2003.

[100] P. Storz, "Reactive oxygen species-mediated mitochondria- to-nucleus signaling: a key to aging and radical-caused diseases," *Science's STKE*, vol. 2006, no. 332, 2006.

[101] I. Manoli, S. Alesci, M. R. Blackman, Y. A. Su, O. M. Rennert, and G. P. Chrousos, "Mitochondria as key components of the stress response," *Trends in Endocrinology and Metabolism*, vol. 18, no. 5, pp. 190–198, 2007.

[102] X. M. Leverve, "Mitochondrial function and substrate avail- ability," *Critical Care Medicine*, vol. 35, no. 9, pp. S454–S460, 2007.

[103] B. Liu, Y. Chen, and D. K. S. Clair, "ROS and p53: a versatile partnership," *Free Radical Biology and Medicine*, vol. 44, no. 8, pp. 1529–1535, 2008.

[104] S. K. Dhar, Y. Xu, and D. K. S. Clair, "Nuclear factor κB- and specificity protein 1-dependent p53-mediated bi-directional regulation of the human manganese superoxide dismutase gene," *Journal of Biological Chemistry*, vol. 285, no. 13, pp. 9835–9846, 2010.

[105] P. Drane, A. Bravard, V. Bouvard, and E. May, "Recipro- cal down-regulation of p53 and SOD2 gene expression- implication in p53 mediated apoptosis," *Oncogene*, vol. 20, no. 4, pp. 430–439, 2001.

[106] S. P. Hussain, P. Amstad, P. He et al., "p53-induced up- regulation of MnSOD and GPx but not catalase increases oxidative stress and apoptosis," *Cancer Research*, vol. 64, no. 7, pp. 2350–2356, 2004.

[107] G. Farmer, P. Friedlander, J. Colgan, J. L. Manley, and C. Prives, "Transcriptional repression by p53 involves molecular interactions distinct from those with the TATA box binding protein," *Nucleic Acids Research*, vol. 24, no. 21, pp. 4281– 4288, 1996.

[108] J. Ho and S. Benchimol, "Transcriptional repression medi- ated by the p53 tumour suppressor," *Cell Death and Differen- tiation*, vol. 10, no. 4, pp. 404–408, 2003.

[109] M. Murphy, J. Ahn, K. K. Walker et al., "Transcriptional re- pression by wild-type p53 utilizes histone deacetylases, medi- ated by interaction with mSin3a," *Genes and Development*, vol. 13, no. 19, pp. 2490–2501, 1999.

[110] A. Böttger, V. Böttger, A. Sparks, W. L. Liu, S. F. Howard, and D. P. Lane, "Design of a synthetic Mdm2-binding mini pro- tein that activates the p53 response in vivo," *Current Biology*, vol. 7, no. 11, pp. 860–869, 1997.

[111] P. H. Kussie, S. Gorina, V. Marechal et al., "Structure of the MDM2 oncoprotein bound to the p53 tumor suppressor transactivation domain," *Science*, vol. 274, no. 5289, pp. 948– 953, 1996.

[112] V. Böttger, A. Böttger, S. F. Howard et al., "Identification of novel mdm2 binding peptides by phage display," *Oncogene*, vol. 13, no. 10, pp. 2141–2147, 1996.

[113] M. J. J. Blommers, G. Fendrich, C. Garcia-Echeverria, and P. Chene, "On the interaction between p53 and MDM2: trans- fer NOE study of a p53-derived peptide ligated to MDM2," *Journal of the American Chemical Society*, vol. 119, no. 14, pp. 3425–3426, 1997.

[114] C. Garcia-Echeverria, P. Chene, M. J. J. Blommers, and P. Furet, "Discovery of potent antagonists of the interaction between human double minute 2 and tumor suppressor p53," *Journal of Medicinal Chemistry*, vol. 43, no. 17, pp. 3205– 3208, 2000.

[115] L. T. Vassilev, "Small-molecule antagonists of p53-MDM2 binding: research tools and potential therapeutics," *Cell Cycle*, vol. 3, no. 4, pp. 419–421, 2004.

[116] L. T. Vassilev, B. T. Vu, B. Graves et al., "*In vivo* activation of the p53 pathway by small-molecule antagonists of MDM2," *Science*, vol. 303, no. 5659, pp. 844–848, 2004.

[117] H. Wang, L. Nan, D. Yu, S. Agrawal, and R. Zhang, "Antisense anti-MDM2 oligonucleotides as a novel therapeutic ap- proach to human breast cancer: in vitro and in vivo activities and mechanisms," *Clinical Cancer Research*, vol. 7, no. 11, pp. 3613–3624, 2001.

[118] J. A. Roth, D. Nguyen, D. D. Lawrence et al., "Retrovirus- mediated wild-type p53 gene transfer to tumors of patients with lung cancer," *Nature Medicine*, vol. 2, no. 9, pp. 985–991, 1996.

[119] K. F. Pirollo, Z. Hao, A. Rait et al., "P53 mediated sensi- tization of squamous cell carcinoma of the head and neck to radiotherapy," *Oncogene*, vol. 14, no. 14, pp. 1735–1746, 1997.

[120] F. R. Spitz, D. Nguyen, J. M. Skibber, R. E. Meyn, R. J. Cristiano, and J. A. Roth, "Adenoviral-mediated wild-type p53 gene expression sensitizes colorectal cancer cells to ionizing radiation," *Clinical Cancer Research*, vol. 2, no. 10, pp. 1665–1671, 1996.

[121] W. C. Broaddus, Y. Liu, L. L. Steele et al., "Enhanced radiosensitivity of malignant glioma cells after adenoviral p53 transduction," *Journal of Neurosurgery*, vol. 91, no. 6, pp. 997–1004, 1999.

[122] D. Cowen, N. Salem, F. Ashoori et al., "Prostate cancer ra- diosensitization in vivo with adenovirus-mediated p53 gene therapy," *Clinical Cancer Research*, vol. 6, no. 11, pp. 4402– 4408, 2000.

[123] A. A. Tarhini, C. P. Belani, J. D. Luketich et al., "A phase i study of concurrent chemotherapy (paclitaxel and carbo- platin) and thoracic radiotherapy with swallowed manga- nese superoxide dismutase plasmid liposome protection in patients with locally advanced stage III non-small-cell lung cancer," *Human Gene Therapy*, vol. 22, no. 3, pp. 336–342, 2011.

[124] Y. Zhao, L. Chaiswing, T. D. Oberley et al., "A mechanism- based antioxidant approach for the reduction of skin carcino- genesis," *Cancer Research*, vol. 65, no. 4, pp. 1401–1405, 2005.

[125] I. Spasojević, I. Batinić-Haberle, J. S. Rebouças, Y. M. Idemori, and I. Fridovich, "Electrostatic contribution in the catalysis of O_2^- dismutation by superoxide dismutase mimics Mn^{III}TE-2-Pyp^{5+} versus Mn^{III}Br$_8$T-2-Pyp$^+$," *Journal of Biological Chemistry*, vol. 278, no. 9, pp. 6831–6837, 2003.

[126] G. Burkhard Mackensen, M. Patel, H. Sheng et al., "Neu- roprotection from delayed postischemic administration of a metalloporphyrin catalytic antioxidant," *Journal of Neuro- science*, vol. 21, no. 13, pp. 4582–4592, 2001.

[127] H. Sheng, J. J. Enghild, R. Bowler et al., "Effects of met- alloporphyrin catalytic antioxidants in experimental brain ischemia," *Free Radical Biology and Medicine*, vol. 33, no. 7, pp. 947–961, 2002.

[128] J. D. Piganelli, S. C. Flores, C. Cruz et al., "A metallopor- phyrin-based superoxide dismutase mimic inhibits adoptive transfer of autoimmune diabetes by a diabetogenic T-cell clone," *Diabetes*, vol. 51, no. 2, pp. 347–355, 2002.

[129] R. Bottino, A. N. Balamurugan, S. Bertera, M. Pietropaolo, M. Trucco, and J. D. Piganelli, "Preservation of human islet

Oxidative Stress Induced by MnSOD-p53 Interaction: Pro- or Anti-Tumorigenic?

13

cell functional mass by anti-oxidative action of a novel SOD mimic compound," *Diabetes*, vol. 51, no. 8, pp. 2561–2567, 2002.

[130] I. Batinic-Haberle, I. Spasojevic, I. Fridovich, M. S. Anscher, and Z. Vujaskovic, "A novel synthetic superoxide dismutase mimetic manganese (III) tetrakis (N-ethylpyridinium-2-yl) porphyrin (MnIITE-2-PyP5+) protects lungs from radiation-induced injury," *International Journal of Radiation Oncology, Biology, Physics*, vol. 51, supplement 1, pp. 235–236.

[131] Z. Vujaskovic, I. Batinic-Haberle, I. Spasojevic et al., "A small molecular weight catalytic metalloporphyrin antioxidant with superoxide dismutase (SOD) mimetic properties protects lungs from radiation-induced injury," *Free Radical Biology and Medicine*, vol. 33, no. 6, pp. 857–863, 2002.

[132] Z. Vujaskovic, I. Batinic-Haberle, I. Spasojevic, I. Fridovich, M. S. Anscher, and M. W. Dewhirst, "Superoxide dismutase (SOD) mimetics in radiation therapy," *Free Radical Biology & Medicine*, vol. 31, p. S128, 2001.

[133] Z. Vujaskovic, I. Batinic-Haberle, Z. N. Rabbani et al., "A small molecular weight catalytic metalloporphyrin antioxidant with superoxide dismutase (SOD) mimetic properties protects lungs from radiation-induced injury," *Free Radical Biology and Medicine*, vol. 33, no. 6, pp. 857–863, 2002.

[134] W. Lontz, A. Sirsjo, W. Liu, M. Lindberg, O. Rollman, and H. Torma, "Increased mRNA expression of manganese superoxide dismutase in psoriasis skin lesions and in cultured human keratinocytes exposed to IL-1β and TNF-α," *Free Radical Biology and Medicine*, vol. 18, no. 2, pp. 349–355, 1995.

[135] F. Wang, J. Liu, D. Robbins et al., "Mutant p53 exhibits trivial effects on mitochondrial functions which can be reactivated by ellipticine in lymphoma cells," *Apoptosis*, vol. 16, pp. 301–310, 2010.

[136] H. Sumimoto, "Structure, regulation and evolution of Nox-family NADPH oxidases that produce reactive oxygen species," *FEBS Journal*, vol. 275, no. 13, pp. 3249–3277, 2008.

[137] D. K. St. Clair, T. D. Oberley, K. E. Muse, and W. H. St. Clair, "Expression of manganese superoxide dismutase promotes cellular differentiation," *Free Radical Biology and Medicine*, vol. 16, no. 2, pp. 275–282, 1994.

[138] J. J. Li, L. W. Oberley, D. K. St Clair, L. A. Ridnour, and T. D. Oberley, "Phenotypic changes induced in human breast cancer cells by overexpression of manganese-containing superoxide dismutase," *Oncogene*, vol. 10, no. 10, pp. 1989–2000, 1995.

[139] H. -C. Yen, T. D. Oberley, C. G. Gairola, L. I. Szweda, and D. K. St. Clair, "Manganese superoxide dismutase protects mitochondrial complex I against adriamycin-induced cardiomyopathy in transgenic mice," *Archives of Biochemistry and Biophysics*, vol. 362, no. 1, pp. 59–66, 1999.

[140] K. M. Connor, N. Hempel, K. K. Nelson et al., "Manganese superoxide dismutase enhances the invasive and migratory activity of tumor cells," *Cancer Research*, vol. 67, no. 21, pp. 10260–10267, 2007.

NPM-ALK: The Prototypic Member of a Family of Oncogenic Fusion Tyrosine Kinases

Joel D. Pearson,[1] Jason K. H. Lee,[1] Julinor T. C. Bacani,[1] Raymond Lai,[2] and Robert J. Ingham[1]

[1] *Department of Medical Microbiology and Immunology, University of Alberta, Edmonton, AB, Canada T6G 2E1*
[2] *Department of Laboratory Medicine and Pathology, University of Alberta, Edmonton, AB, Canada T6G 2B7*

Correspondence should be addressed to Robert J. Ingham, ringham@ualberta.ca

Academic Editor: Rudi Beyaert

Anaplastic lymphoma kinase (ALK) was first identified in 1994 with the discovery that the gene encoding for this kinase was involved in the t(2;5)(p23;q35) chromosomal translocation observed in a subset of anaplastic large cell lymphoma (ALCL). The NPM-ALK fusion protein generated by this translocation is a constitutively active tyrosine kinase, and much research has focused on characterizing the signalling pathways and cellular activities this oncoprotein regulates in ALCL. We now know about the existence of nearly 20 distinct ALK translocation partners, and the fusion proteins resulting from these translocations play a critical role in the pathogenesis of a variety of cancers including subsets of large B-cell lymphomas, nonsmall cell lung carcinomas, and inflammatory myofibroblastic tumours. Moreover, the inhibition of ALK has been shown to be an effective treatment strategy in some of these malignancies. In this paper we will highlight malignancies where ALK translocations have been identified and discuss why ALK fusion proteins are constitutively active tyrosine kinases. Finally, using ALCL as an example, we will examine three key signalling pathways activated by NPM-ALK that contribute to proliferation and survival in ALCL.

1. The ALK Receptor Tyrosine Kinase

Anaplastic lymphoma kinase (ALK) is a receptor tyrosine kinase of the insulin receptor superfamily, and in mice and humans, the normal expression of ALK is largely restricted to the brain and nervous system [1–4]. Mice deficient in ALK appear to have no overt developmental abnormalities [5–8]; however, behavioural abnormalities have been noted in these mice. ALK-deficient mice perform better on tests of cognitive ability and display less anxiety than their wild-type littermate controls [6, 7]. Behavioural tests also demonstrated increased alcohol consumption and altered sensitivity to alcohol in ALK-deficient mice compared to wild-type littermates [8]. Intriguingly, single-nucleotide polymorphisms (SNPs) in *ALK* have been identified in humans that correlate with decreased response to alcohol [8]. A correlation between *ALK* SNPs and schizophrenia has also been noted in a Japanese study [9].

In *Drosophila melanogaster*, the jelly belly protein (Jeb) has been characterized as an ALK ligand [10–12]. In mammals, there does not appear to be a Jeb homologue but two ligands for ALK have been described, pleiotrophin [13] and midkine [14]. However, there is not complete agreement regarding whether these are indeed ALK stimulating ligands [15, 16]. More recently, Perez-Pinera and colleagues proposed an alternative mechanism by which pleiotrophin could be stimulating ALK signalling. In their model, the binding of pleiotrophin to its known receptor, receptor tyrosine phosphatase β/ζ (RPTP β/ζ), relieves the inhibitory dephosphorylation of ALK by RPTP β/ζ, thereby turning on ALK signalling [17]. ALK has also been suggested to be a dependence receptor [18]. Dependence receptors induce apoptosis in their nonliganded state, but suppress apoptotic signalling in response to ligand binding [19].

2. The Identification of NPM-ALK and Other ALK Fusion Proteins

ALK-positive anaplastic large cell lymphomas (ALK+ ALCL) are a distinct subset of non-Hodgkin lymphomas with a T or null cell immunophenotype recognized by the World

Health Organization Classification Scheme for hematological neoplasms [58, 59]. These lymphomas express the CD30 (Ki-1) surface antigen, but the morphologic identification of ALK+ ALCL can be challenging, as the cytologic features of the tumor cells can be highly variable from case to case. Nevertheless, the identification of the so-called "hallmark cells," which are characterized by a horseshoe- or kidney-shaped nucleus and a prominent perinuclear Golgi body, can facilitate the diagnosis [58, 59]. Regarding the pathobiology of ALK+ ALCL, several groups in the late eighties and early nineties noted that these lymphomas possessed a recurrent chromosomal translocation, the t(2;5)(p23;q35) translocation [60–64]. In 1994, it was demonstrated that this translocation generates a fusion gene between a previously uncharacterized tyrosine kinase on chromosome 2, and the *nucleophosmin* (*NPM*) gene on chromosome 5 [20, 21]. This kinase was termed ALK owing to its association with ALCL and the expression of this kinase led to the identification of what is now considered to be a clinically distinct entity, ALK+ ALCL. In addition to NPM, several other ALK translocation partners have since been identified in ALK+ ALCL [23, 24, 27, 29–31, 33, 39, 42, 43, 45]. ALK fusion proteins have also been reported in other cancers (Table 1). These cancers include a portion of inflammatory myofibroblastic tumours (IMT) [25, 32, 34, 43, 44, 46, 55, 65], nonsmall cell lung carcinomas (NSCLC) [28, 49, 54, 57], diffuse large B-cell lymphomas (DLBCL) [22, 35–37, 47, 48, 51], colon cancers [50, 56], breast cancers [50], renal cell carcinomas [26, 52, 53], and extramedullary plasmacytomas [38]. Two papers also reported detecting tropomyosin 4- (TPM4-)ALK fusion protein expression in some cases of esophageal squamous cell carcinoma [40, 41]. Moreover, it has very recently been established that inhibitors of ALK are effective at treating patients with ALK+ ALCL [66] and other malignancies expressing ALK fusion proteins [67, 68]. Although not a focus of this paper, ALK has been reported to be highly expressed in breast cancer [69], and ALK gene amplifications and activating mutations have been identified in familial and sporadic neuroblastoma [70–75] and thyroid cancer [76].

The t(2;5)(p23;q35) translocation generates a fusion gene termed *NPM-ALK* whose transcription is under the control of *NPM* regulatory sites. NPM is a ubiquitously expressed protein that is predominately found in the nucleolus [77], but can shuttle between the cytoplasm and nucleus [78]. NPM is multifunctional and regulates several cellular activities including transcription, ribosome biogenesis, and the shuttling of proteins between the nucleus and cytoplasm [79]. The *NPM-ALK* fusion gene consists of the first four exons of *NPM* which encodes for the first 117 amino acids of the NPM protein, and the *ALK* portion of the fusion includes the exons encoding for the intracellular tail and kinase domain of ALK [20]. Importantly, the NPM part of the fusion includes the NPM dimerization/oligomerization domain [80, 81]. As we will discuss in the next section, this domain is critically important for NPM-ALK activity, and the presence of a dimerization/oligomerization domain is a common feature of other ALK fusion partners.

TABLE 1: Identified ALK fusion proteins and their associated malignancies. Known ALK fusion proteins and the cancers they have been identified in are indicated. ALCL: anaplastic large cell lymphoma; DLBCL: diffuse large B-cell lymphoma; IMT: inflammatory myofibroblastic tumour; NSCLC: nonsmall cell lung carcinoma; RCC: renal cell carcinoma; SCC: squamous cell carcinoma.

Fusion protein	Tumour type	Reference
NPM-ALK	ALCL, DLBCL	[20–22]
TPM3-ALK	ALCL, IMT, RCC	[23–26]
TFG-ALK	ALCL, NSCLC	[27, 28]
ATIC-ALK	ALCL, IMT	[29–32]
CLTC-ALK	ALCL, DLBCL, IMT, extramedullary plasmacytoma	[33–38]
TPM4-ALK	IMT, ALCL, SCC	[25, 39–41]
MSN-ALK	ALCL	[42]
ALO17-ALK	ALCL	[43]
CARS-ALK	IMT	[43]
RANBP2-ALK	IMT	[44]
MYH9-ALK	ALCL	[45]
SEC31L1-ALK	IMT, DLBCL	[46–48]
EML4-ALK	NSCLC, breast, colorectal, RCC	[26, 28, 49, 50]
SQSTM1-ALK	DLBCL	[51]
VCL-ALK	RCC	[52, 53]
KIF5B-ALK	NSCLC	[54]
PPFIBP1-ALK	IMT	[55]
C2orf44-ALK	Colorectal	[56]
KLC1-ALK	NSCLC	[57]

3. The Importance of Dimerization/Oligomerization Domains in ALK Fusion Proteins

An essential role for the NPM portion of NPM-ALK was first demonstrated by experiments showing that deletion of the entire NPM region of NPM-ALK generated a protein incapable of transforming NIH 3T3 cells [80]. Similarly, Bischof et al. demonstrated that NPM truncation or deletion mutants were not tyrosine phosphorylated and were unable to transform Fischer Rat 3T3 cells [81]. Since NPM has been reported to form hexamers and other oligomers [82, 83], researchers examined whether NPM could be providing an oligomerization domain in NPM-ALK. Indeed, gel filtration [80] and sucrose gradient [81] experiments demonstrated that NPM-ALK forms oligomeric complexes in an NPM-dependent manner. Moreover, NPM-ALK can dimerize with endogenous NPM, and it is believed that this accounts for why some NPM-ALK is observed in the nucleus [81].

The basic domain of Echinoderm microtubule-associated protein-like 4 (EML4) also functions as a dimerization domain in EML4-ALK [49], and this is likely mediated by

TABLE 2: Known or suspected dimerization/oligomerization domains in ALK fusion partners. Dimerization/oligomerization domains present ALK fusion partners that are postulated to mediate dimerization/oligomerization are indicated. With the exception of the basic domain of EML4-ALK, these domains have not been experimentally proven to mediate dimerization/oligomerization of the respective fusion proteins. The basic domain of EML4 also possesses a coiled-coil motif which is postulated to mediate dimerization.

Dimerization/oligomerization domain	Fusion protein	Reference
	TPM3-ALK	[23, 25]
	TPM4-ALK	[25]
	TFG-ALK	[27]
Coiled-coil	KIF5B-ALK	[54]
	PPFIBP1-ALK	[55]
	MYH9-ALK*	[45]
Leucine zipper	RANBP2-ALK	[44]
Basic domain/coiled-coil	EML4-ALK	[49]
PB1 domain	SQSTM1-ALK	[51]
WD40 repeats	SEC31L1-ALK	[46]
Triskelion assembly motifs	CLTC-ALK	[33]

*The MYH9 coiled-coil domain is truncated in the fusion protein and may not be functional.

a coiled-coil motif within the basic domain [84]. Most other ALK fusion partners possess known dimerization/oligomerization domains that are postulated to mediate dimerization/oligomerization of the fusion proteins (Table 2). MSN-ALK (a fusion between moesin and ALK) appears not to have an oligomerization domain and is postulated to be activated through the colocalization of MSN-ALK fusion proteins to cellular membranes [42]. Thus, dimerization, oligomerization, or colocalization of ALK fusion proteins appears to be a common and necessary requirement for these oncoproteins to signal.

4. Signalling Pathways Activated by NPM-ALK in ALK+ ALCL

NPM-ALK activates downstream signalling events that promote proliferation, prevent apoptosis, and enhance migration in ALK+ ALCL (reviewed in [5, 85, 86]). We will focus on the STAT3, MEK/ERK, and PI3K/Akt pathways, as much is known about the role these pathways play in ALK+ ALCL pathogenesis. In particular, we will discuss the cellular processes these pathways regulate in this lymphoma, and how they are regulated by NPM-ALK signalling.

5. The STAT3 Pathway

Members of the signal transducer and activator of transcription (STAT) family of transcription factors are activated by interferon, cytokine, and growth factor receptor signalling [87]. The tyrosine phosphorylation of STATs by tyrosine

kinases, particularly the Janus kinases (JAKs), facilitates the dimerization of STATs. This allows the STATs to translocate to the nucleus and promote the transcription of genes involved in proliferation, cell survival, and the immune response [87, 88]. In ALK+ ALCL, the activation of STAT3 has been strongly implicated in the pathogenesis of this lymphoma (Figure 1).

STAT3 is activated in ALK+ ALCL cell lines and patient samples [89–91], as well as cells isolated from NPM-ALK transgenic mice [92, 93], as measured by its phosphorylation on tyrosine 705. The inhibition of STAT3 in ALK+ ALCL cell lines, either through the overexpression of a dominant-negative STAT3 construct [94] or decreasing STAT3 expression using antisense oligonucleotides [93], resulted in decreased proliferation and the induction of apoptosis. STAT3 was also required for NPM-ALK to transform mouse embryo fibroblasts, and for the continued survival of T-cell lymphomas induced in mice by the expression of an NPM-ALK transgene [93].

STAT3 exerts its biological effects in ALK+ ALCL through regulating the expression of multiple genes. Microarray studies performed by Piva and colleagues demonstrated that knockdown of STAT3 altered the expression of ~1500 genes in a variant of the SUP-M2 ALK+ ALCL cell line [95]. Importantly, STAT3 functions both as an activator and repressor of transcription, and approximately 60% of the STAT3-regulated genes identified by Piva et al. were repressed by STAT3 [95]. Several additional studies have identified STAT3 regulated genes in ALK+ ALCL. Those genes found to be upregulated by STAT3 include: genes that promote proliferation such as Cyclin D1, Cyclin D3, c-Myc, ICOS, C/EBPβ [93–97]; those that promote survival such as Bcl-xL, Survivin, Bcl-2, Mcl-1, Bcl2A1, C/EBPβ [90, 93, 97, 98]; others including CD30, PD-L1, TIMP-1, Socs3, Hif1α, Twist1, IL10, and IL2Rα chain [94, 95, 99–104]. STAT3 is also responsible for repressing the expression of T-cell genes that are commonly not expressed in ALK+ ALCL including CD3ε, ZAP-70, LAT, and SLP-76, and it appears to do so in part through the upregulation of DNA methyltransferases (DNMTs) [105]. DNMTs methylate CpG motifs in promoter regions of genes, and this blocks the binding of some transcription factors and facilitates the recruitment of Methyl-C binding proteins to these promoters. methyl-C binding proteins can then recruit histone deacetylases and methyltransferases that convert promoter regions into transcriptionally inactive heterochromatin [106]. Zhang and colleagues demonstrated that STAT3 also promotes the binding of DNMTs 1–3 to the IL2Rγ promoter in order to repress IL2Rγ gene expression [107]. Silencing IL2Rγ chain expression appears to be critical in ALK+ ALCL as re-introduction of the IL2Rγ into ALK+ ALCL cell lines resulted in decreased NPM-ALK expression and reduced viability [107]. This study also demonstrated that STAT3 enhances DNMT1 expression through the suppression of the DNMT1-targeting microRNA, miR-21. STAT3 is also responsible for the epigenetic silencing of STAT5A in ALK+ ALCL, which prevents STAT5A from repressing NPM-ALK expression and thereby interfering with NPM-ALK signalling [108]. Given the importance of STAT3 transcriptional activity in ALK+

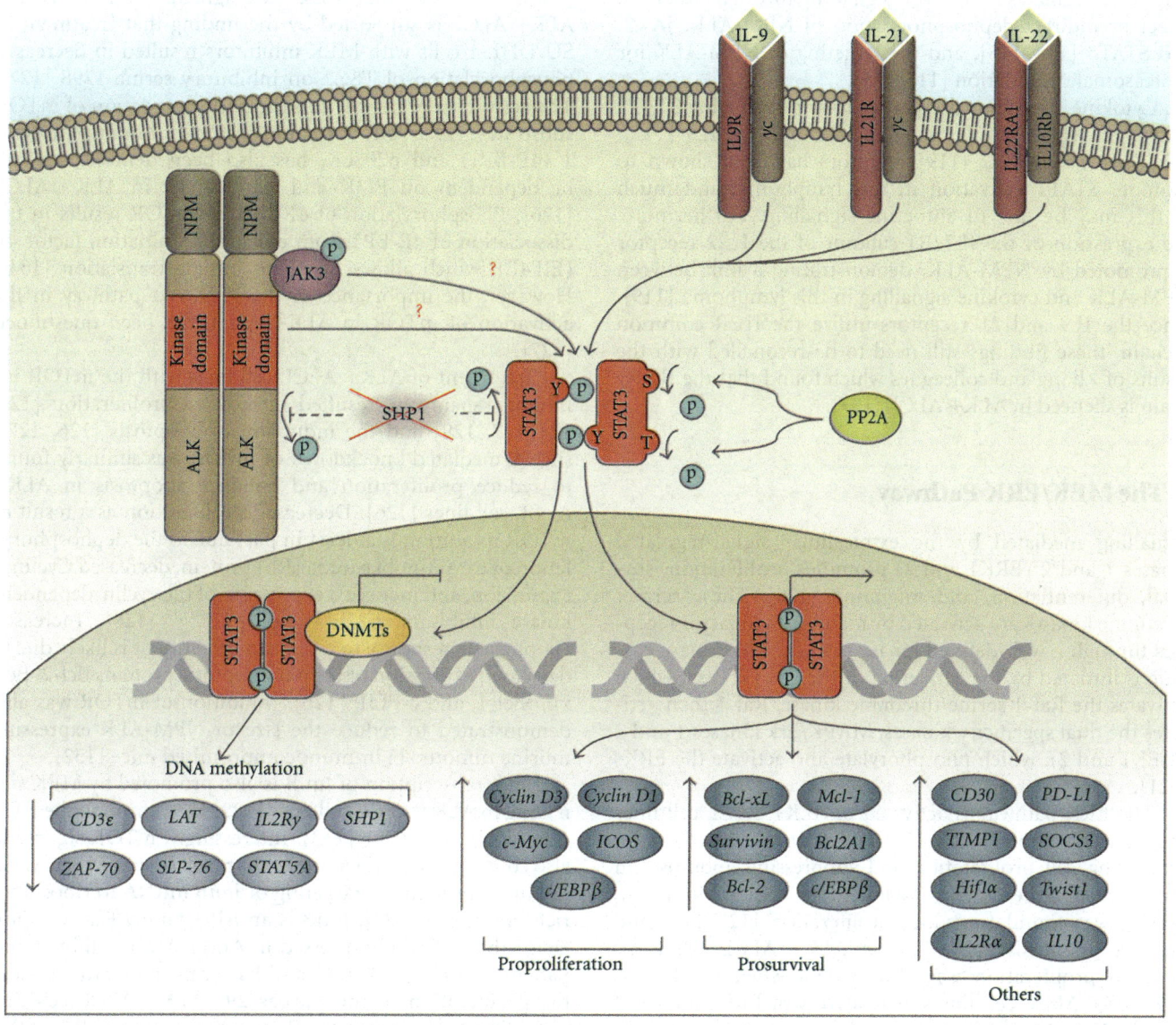

FIGURE 1: The STAT3 signalling pathway in ALK+ ALCL. STAT3 is activated by NPM-ALK signalling, but reports differ as to whether this is JAK3-dependent or independent. The phosphatase, PP2A, and signalling through the IL-9, IL-21, and IL-22 receptors also promote STAT3 activation in ALK+ ALCL. STAT3 promotes the expression of genes that suppress apoptosis and enhance proliferation in ALK+ ALCL. STAT3 can also repress a variety of genes in this malignancy through DNA methylation. Suppression of the SHP1 phosphatase by STAT3 is particularly important in ALK+ ALCL, as SHP1 inhibits NPM-ALK and STAT3 activity.

ALCL, it is not surprising that many mechanisms contribute to the activation of STAT3 in this lymphoma.

STAT3 [89, 109] and JAK3 [90] have both been shown to coimmunoprecipitate with NPM-ALK, and several studies have shown that NPM-ALK promotes the tyrosine phosphorylation of STAT3 [89, 90, 92, 93]. However, there is not complete agreement regarding whether STAT3 tyrosine phosphorylation is JAK3 dependent [94, 110], or whether STAT3 is tyrosine phosphorylated in a JAK3-independent manner, possibly through direct tyrosine phosphorylation by

NPM-ALK [111]. The serine/threonine phosphatase PP2A has also been implicated in positively regulating STAT3 activity in ALK+ ALCL, as inhibition of PP2A activity with Calyculin A was demonstrated to reduce STAT3 tyrosine phosphorylation [89]. STAT3 signalling is also likely enhanced in this lymphoma due to the fact that ALK+ ALCL cell lines do not express the STAT3 inhibitor, PIAS3 [89]. Moreover, the SHP-1 tyrosine phosphatase is often silenced by DNA methylation in ALK+ ALCL [112, 113], and this is likely due in part to the recruitment of DNMTs and histone deacetylases to the SHP-1 promoter by STAT3 [113]. Silencing SHP-1 in ALK+ ALCL is important as SHP-1 negative regulates NPM-ALK signalling through either the direct or indirect dephosphorylation of NPM-ALK, JAK2, and STAT3 [114–116], and the targeting of NPM-ALK for proteasomal degradation [115, 116].

Cytokine signalling also plays a role in regulating STAT3 activity in ALK+ ALCL. Signalling through the IL9 [117], IL21 [118], and IL22 [119] receptors has been shown to promote STAT3 activation in this lymphoma, and much of this may be due to autocrine signalling. Furthermore, the expression of the IL22R1 subunit of the IL22 receptor is promoted by NPM-ALK, demonstrating a link between NPM-ALK and cytokine signalling in this lymphoma [119]. Since the IL9 and 21 receptors utilize the IL2R common γ chain, these findings still need to be reconciled with the results of Zhang and colleagues which found that the IL2Rγ chain is silenced in ALK+ ALCL [107].

6. The MEK/ERK Pathway

Signalling mediated by the extracellular signal-regulated kinases 1 and 2 (ERK1 and 2) promotes proliferation, survival, differentiation, and migration [120]. These serine/threonine kinases are activated by many growth factor receptors through a well-defined kinase cascade. This kinase cascade is initiated by the activation of the Ras GTPase, which activates the Raf-1 serine/threonine kinase. Raf-1 then activates the dual specificity kinases, MAPK/Erk kinases 1 and 2 (MEK1 and 2), which phosphorylate and activate the ERKs [121].

The ERK pathway is activated in ALK+ ALCL cell lines and patient samples [122, 123] and plays a central role in promoting cell proliferation and suppressing apoptosis in this cancer (Figure 2). Treatment with the MEK1/2 inhibitor, U0126, was found to reduce proliferation [123–125] and enhance apoptosis [124, 125] in ALK+ ALCL cell lines. Reduced proliferation was also evident when the Karpas 299 ALK+ ALCL cell line was treated with ERK1 and/or 2 siRNA [124]. However, only the silencing of ERK1 in these cells was found to increase apoptosis [124]. Two important downstream mediators of MEK/ERK signalling in ALK+ ALCL are the serine/threonine kinase, mammalian target of rapamycin (mTOR), and the JunB transcription factor.

The mTOR pathway has been demonstrated to be activated in ALK+ ALCL patient samples, as measured by phosphorylation of mTOR [125, 126] and downstream targets of mTOR signalling [123, 125–127]. Marzec and colleagues found that treatment of the SU-DHL-1 ALK+ ALCL cell line with MEK inhibitors or ERK1/2 siRNA resulted in reduced phosphorylation of the ribosomal S6 protein (RPS6) [127]. RPS6 is a downstream target of mTOR signalling, and phosphorylation of RPS6 promotes cell growth [128]. The p70 S6 kinase (p70S6K), which is activated by mTOR and phosphorylates RPS6, is also inhibited in SU-DHL-1 cells treated with U0126 [129], but surprisingly not in the SR-786 ALK+ ALCL cell line [123]. MEK/ERK signalling was postulated to activate mTOR through inhibition of the tuberous sclerosis

complex (TSC) [127]. TSC is a GTPase-activating protein that inhibits mTOR through inactivating the Rheb GTPase [130]. The notion that MEK/ERK signalling inhibits TSC in ALK+ ALCL is supported by the finding that treatment of SU-DHL-1 cells with MEK inhibitors resulted in decreased phosphorylation of TSC2 on inhibitory serine 1798 [127]. The activation of mTOR and the phosphorylation of mTOR substrates, eukaryotic initiation factor 4E-binding protein-1 (4E-BP1) and p70S6K, has also been demonstrated to be dependent on PI3K and Akt activity in ALK+ ALCL [126]. Phosphorylation of 4E-BP1 by mTOR results in the dissociation of 4E-BP1 from eukaryotic initiation factor 4E (EIF4E), which allows EIF4E to initiate translation [131]. However, the importance of the PI3K/Akt pathway in the activation of mTOR in ALK+ ALCL has been questioned [127].

Treatment of ALK+ ALCL cell lines with the mTOR inhibitor, rapamycin, resulted in reduced proliferation [123, 125–127, 129] and the induction of apoptosis [126, 127]. siRNA-mediated knockdown of mTOR was similarly found to reduce proliferation and enhance apoptosis in ALK+ ALCL cell lines [126]. Decreased proliferation as a result of mTOR inhibition is at least in part due to the dephosphorylation of the retinoblastoma (Rb) protein, decreased Cyclin A expression, and increased expression of the cyclin-dependent kinase inhibitors, $p27^{kip1}$ and $p21^{waf1}$ [126]. Increased apoptosis in response to rapamycin treatment is likely due to decreased expression of the antiapoptotic proteins Bcl-2, Bcl-xL, Mcl-1, and c-FLIP [126]. Inhibition of mTOR was also demonstrated to reduce the size of NPM-ALK-expressing murine tumours in immunocompromised mice [132].

The transcription of JunB is also promoted by MEK signalling in ALK+ ALCL cell lines [122, 123], through the ETS-1 transcription factor [133]. Interestingly, mTOR signalling also contributes to enhanced JunB translation in ALK+ ALCL cell lines through the targeting of *JunB* mRNA to ribosome-rich polysomes [123]. JunB is an AP-1 family transcription factor that is highly expressed in ALK+ ALCL cell lines and patient samples [134–136] and has been shown to promote the proliferation of the Karpas 299 ALK+ ALCL cell line [123]. JunB also influences phenotypic characteristics of this lymphoma through promoting the transcription of CD30 [122, 137] and the Granzyme B serine protease [138]. CD30 signalling also activates MEK/ERK/JunB signalling in this lymphoma to further promote CD30 expression [122].

The activation of Raf-1, MEK, and ERK in ALK+ ALCL cell lines is dependent on NPM-ALK activity [124, 139], and the ectopic expression of NPM-ALK has also been demonstrated to induce the activation of these proteins [123, 124, 140, 141]. NPM-ALK can activate Ras when ectopically expressed in the Jurkat T leukemia cell line, and the expression of a dominant negative N17 Ras decreased NPM-ALK-dependent NF-AT/AP-1 luciferase activity in Jurkat cells. Furthermore, treatment of the SU-DHL-1 ALK+ ALCL cell line with the Ras inhibitor, FTI-277, resulted in increased apoptosis and decreased proliferation [125]. Several mechanisms for how NPM-ALK activates Ras have been postulated. The Ras activator, Son of Sevenless (SOS), has been argued to be recruited to NPM-ALK via the adapter

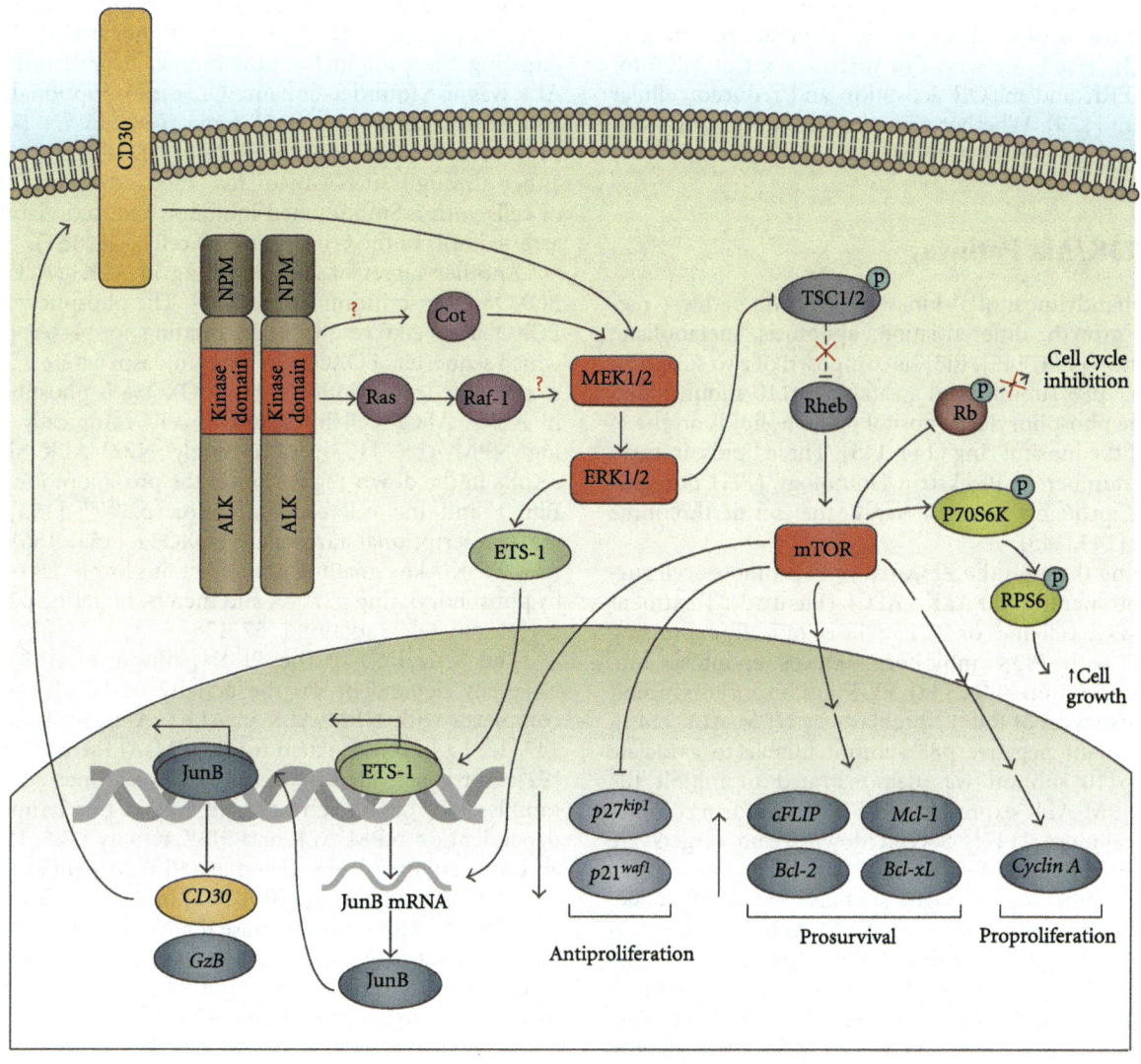

Figure 2: The MEK/ERK signalling pathway in ALK+ ALCL. NPM-ALK activates Ras, Raf-1, MEK1/2, and ERK1/2. The ability of NPM-ALK to activate MEK/ERK appears not to be dependent on Raf-1. Rather, another MAP3K, Cot, may be important for activation of MEK/ERK in ALK+ ALCL, but it is not known whether Cot is activated by NPM-ALK signalling. The activation of ERK1/2 promotes ALK+ ALCL proliferation and survival, largely through the JunB transcription factor and serine/threonine kinase, mTOR. ERK1/2 activates the ETS-1 transcription factor which promotes the transcription of *JunB*. JunB promotes the transcription of *CD30* and *Granzyme B* in this lymphoma, but likely has other important targets that have not yet been identified. ERK1/2 are thought to activate mTOR signalling in ALK+ ALCL by phosphorylating and inhibiting TSC1/2. mTOR phosphorylates and inhibits the cell cycle inhibitor, Rb. It also phosphorylates and activates p70S6K which phosphorylates RPS6 to promote cell growth. mTOR also influences the expression of genes that contribute to the survival and proliferation of ALK+ ALCL cells. MEK/ERK are also activated by signalling through CD30 in ALK+ ALCL, and this leads to enhanced CD30 expression.

protein Grb2 by molecules such as Shc, SHP2, and insulin receptor substrate-1 (IRS-1) [80, 141–143]. Ras activation has also been proposed to occur through a PLCγ-dependent activation of Ras guanyl nucleotide-releasing protein (Ras-GRP) [80]. While Raf-1 is activated by NPM-ALK, it does not appear to be required for ERK activation in ALK+ ALCL cell lines [124]. Another MAP3K, Cot/MAP3K8, may be the primary activator of MEK in this lymphoma. Treatment of the SU-DHL-1 cell line with Cot siRNA or a Cot inhibitor decreased ERK and mTOR activation and reduced cellular proliferation [129]. Whether Cot is regulated by NPM-ALK was not investigated in this study.

7. The PI3K/Akt Pathway

The phosphatidylinositol 3'-kinase (PI3K)/Akt pathway regulates cell growth, differentiation, apoptosis, metabolism, and migration [144, 145]. PI3K is composed of two subunits, a regulatory p85 subunit and a catalytic p110 subunit, and this enzyme phosphorylates inositol phospholipids on the 3' position of the inositol ring [144, 145]. These lipids, in turn, activate a number of Pleckstrin Homology (PH) domain-containing proteins; most notably the serine/threonine kinase Akt [144, 145].

Signalling through the PI3K pathway promotes cell survival and proliferation in ALK+ ALCL (Figure 3). Treatment of ALK+ ALCL cell lines or Ba/F3 cells ectopically expressing NPM-ALK with PI3K inhibitors induces apoptosis and reduces proliferation [146, 147]. PI3K inhibitors also inhibit the transformation of Rat-1 fibroblasts by NPM-ALK [146], and a dominant negative p85 subunit unable to associate with the p110 subunit was demonstrated to inhibit the ability of NPM-ALK-expressing Ba/F3 cells to form colonies in methylcellulose [147]. Several downstream targets are regulated by PI3K in ALK+ ALCL.

The Akt substrate, glycogen synthase kinase-3β (GSK-3β), is an important target of NPM-ALK signalling in ALK+ ALCL. Phosphorylation of GSK-3β on serine 9 by Akt inhibits GSK-3β activity [148], and in ALK+ ALCL this has been argued to be important for preventing GSK-3β from phosphorylating, and targeting for degradation, the antiapoptotic protein Mcl-1 and the positive cell cycle-regulator, phosphatase CDC25A [149]. Furthermore, this study showed that phosphorylation of GSK-3β on serine 9 correlated with elevated CDC25A levels in ALK+ ALCL patient tumour biopsies. A separate study also demonstrated that NPM-ALK promotes CDC25A expression through PI3K, through either transcriptional upregulation of CDC25A or enhanced CDC25A mRNA stability [150]. Further supporting the notion that inhibition of GSK-3β is an important target of NPM-ALK signalling, treatment of ALK+ ALCL cell lines with either GSK-3β shRNA or a GSK-3β inhibitor could partially rescue the decreased viability associated with ALK inhibitor treatment [149].

NPM-ALK/PI3K/Akt signalling also activates the sonic hedgehog (SHH) pathway in ALK+ ALCL [151]. SHH is a secreted molecule that, when bound to its receptor Patched, relieves inhibition of the Smoothened co-receptor by Patched. This allows Smoothened to activate glioma-associated homologue (GLI) transcription factors [152]. SHH and GLI1 were found to be highly expressed in primary ALK+ ALCL patient samples, and their expression in cell lines was dependent on NPM-ALK and PI3K activity [151]. It was argued in this study that PI3K-mediated activation of Akt is important for inhibiting GSK-3β in order to prevent GSK-3β from phosphorylating GLI1 and targeting the protein for proteasomal degradation. NPM-ALK was also found to enhance GLI1 transcriptional activity, and expression of the GLI1 target gene, cyclin D2 [151]. Moreover, the inhibition of GLI1 in ALK+ ALCL cell lines, either through siRNA-mediated knockdown or treatment of cells with a Smoothened inhibitor, reduced viability and arrested cells in the G1 stage of the cell cycle [151].

Another target of Akt signalling in ALK+ ALCL is the FOXO3a transcription factor [153]. The phosphorylation of FOXO3a by Akt results in its binding to 14-3-3 proteins, which sequesters FOXO3a in the cytoplasm where it is unable to promote transcription [154]. FOXO3a is phosphorylated in ALK+ ALCL cell lines and in cells ectopically expressing NPM-ALK [153]. Accordingly NPM-ALK signalling results in the down-regulation of the pro-apoptotic protein, Bim-1 and the cell cycle-inhibitor, p27^{kip1} [153], which are transcriptional targets of FOXO3a [155, 156]. NPM-ALK/PI3K/Akt signalling also maintains low levels of p27^{kip1} by phosphorylating p27^{kip1}, and thereby targeting p27^{kip1} for proteasomal degradation [157, 158].

The activation of the PI3K pathway in ALK+ ALCL is largely dependent on the activity of NPM-ALK. PI3K complexes with NPM-ALK in ALK+ ALCL cell lines [146, 147, 159] and cells isolated from NPM-ALK transgenic mice [92]. Akt is activated in ALK+ ALCL cell lines and patient samples [147]. The activation of Akt in this lymphoma is dependent on NPM-ALK and PI3K activity [126, 127, 160], and Akt activity is upregulated in a PI3K-dependent manner by ectopically expressed NPM-ALK in Ba/F3 cells [127, 146, 153]. PTEN, a lipid phosphatase that dephosphorylates PI3K lipid products [144, 145], is not expressed in some ALK+ ALCL patient samples, and this may be a contributing factor to Akt activation in these patients [161].

8. Conclusions and Future Perspectives

It has been over 15 years since the discovery of the NPM-ALK oncoprotein. In this time we have learned much about the signalling pathways activated by NPM-ALK in ALK+ ALCL, and how these pathways contribute to proliferation and survival of this lymphoma. This information has been critical in directing research towards understanding how ALK translocations signal and function in other malignancies. For example, STAT3 activation has been observed in clathrin heavy chain- (CTLC-)ALK-expressing DLBCL patient samples [162], and STAT3, ERK, and AKT are active in EML4-ALK-expressing NSCLC cell lines [163–165]; however, the importance of these pathways in NSCLC and their regulation by EML4-ALK appears to vary amongst NSCLC cell lines [163–165]. Yet, even if activation of

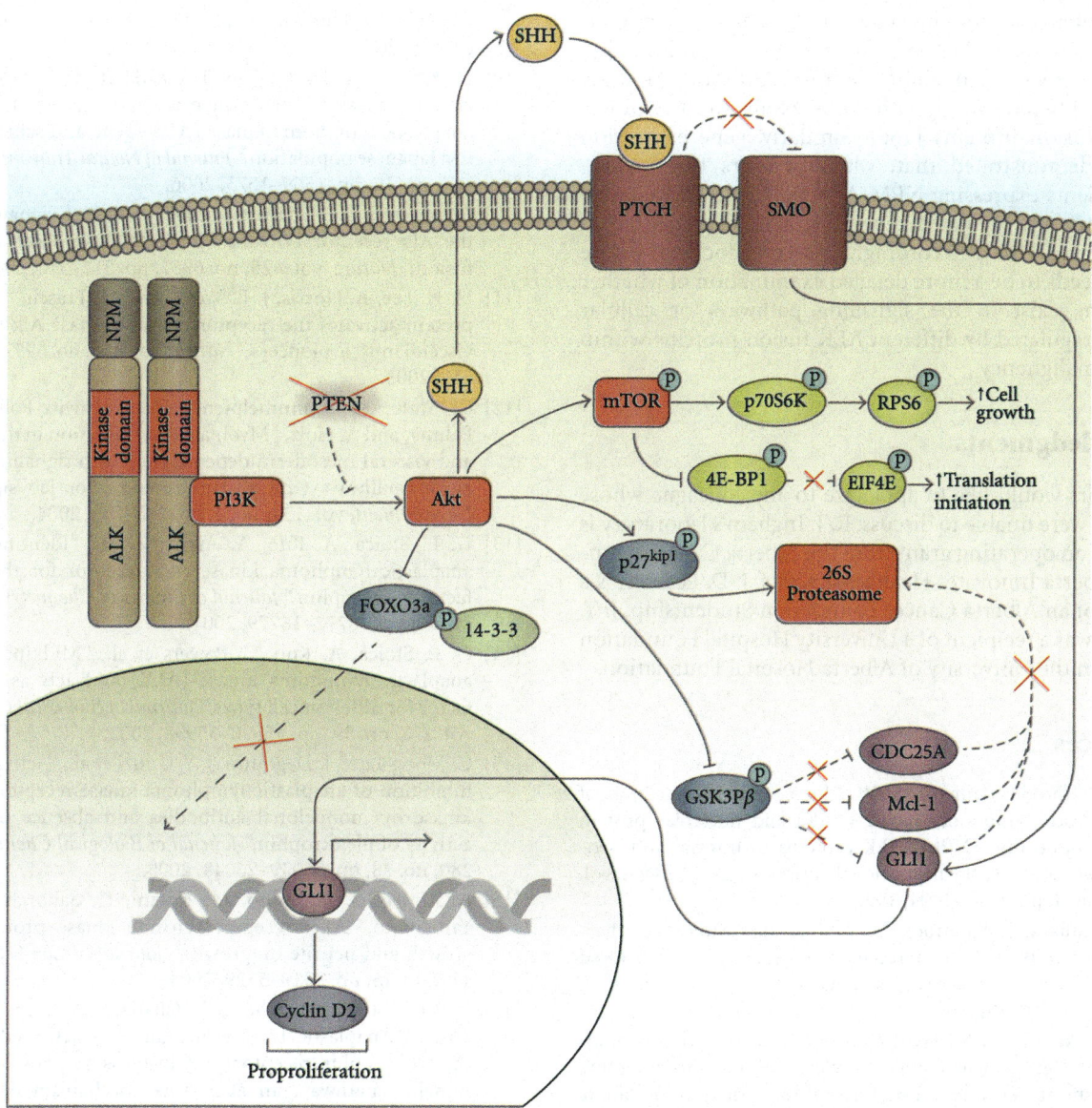

FIGURE 3: The PI3K/Akt signalling pathway in ALK+ ALCL. NPM-ALK associates with and activates PI3K, which, in turn, activates the serine/threonine kinase Akt. Expression of the PTEN lipid phosphatase, which inhibits PI3K signalling, is lost in some ALK+ ALCL tumour samples and likely contributes to Akt activation in cancers where PTEN is not expressed. Akt inhibits GSK3β activity in ALK+ ALCL, which protects GLI1, Mcl-1, and CDC25A from proteasomal degradation. Akt also phosphorylates the cell-cycle inhibitor, p27^{kip1}, in ALK+ ALCL and this results in the targeting of p27^{kip1} for proteasomal degradation. Phosphorylation of the FOXO3a transcription factor by Akt results in the binding of FOXO3a to 14-3-3 proteins. This sequesters FOXO3a in the cytoplasm, preventing it from translocating to the nucleus and transcribing pro-apoptotic and cell cycle inhibitory genes. In addition to being an important downstream target of MEK/ERK signalling in ALK+ ALCL, mTOR activity may also be promoted by PI3K/Akt signalling. NPM-ALK/Akt signalling also promotes the expression of SHH. When SHH binds its receptor, Patched (PTCH), this relieves the inhibition of the Smoothened (SMO) coreceptor by Patched. This allows Smoothened to activate the GLI1 transcription factor, which promotes the transcription of the proproliferation protein, *Cyclin D2*.

the STAT3, ERK, and PI3K/Akt pathways is common to malignancies expressing ALK fusion proteins, differences almost certainly exist in the genes regulated by these pathways in the individual cancers. Some of these differences may be important in the pathogenesis of their respective malignancies. Thus, a more thorough characterization of these signalling pathways in other ALK fusion protein-expressing malignancies needs to be a priority of future research.

While the information gained from elucidating how NPM-ALK signals in ALK+ ALCL has been, and will continue to be, beneficial for understanding how other ALK fusion proteins signal, it is clear that these fusion proteins are not identical in their signalling capability. In a study by Armstrong and colleagues, NIH 3T3 cells expressing the NPM-, Trk-fused gene (TFG)-, 5-aminoimidazole-4-carboxamide ribonucleotide formyltransferase/IMP cyclohydrolase (ATIC)-, tropomyosin 3 (TPM3)-, or CTLC-ALK fusion proteins at roughly equal levels, differed in their ability to activate STAT3 and Akt [166]. The proliferation rate, invasiveness, and ability to form tumours in nude mice also differed amongst the cells expressing the different ALK fusion proteins [166]. Similarly, gene expression profiling demonstrated that, while tumours from ALK+ ALCL patients expressing NPM-ALK or TPM3-ALK shared many commonly regulated genes, distinctly regulated genes were observed [167]. Accordingly, a second focus of future research needs to be a more detailed examination of whether distinctions exist in the signalling pathways or cellular processes regulated by different ALK fusion proteins within the same malignancy.

Acknowledgments

The authors would like to apologize to any colleague whose work they were unable to discuss. R. J. Ingham's laboratory is funded by an operating grant from the Alberta Cancer Foundation/Alberta Innovates Health Solutions. J. D. Pearson is a recipient of an Alberta Cancer Foundation Studentship. J. T. C. Bacani was a recipient of a University Hospital Foundation Grant from the University of Alberta Hospital Foundation.

References

[1] K. Pulford, L. Lamant, S. W. Morris et al., "Detection of anaplastic lymphoma kinase (ALK) and nucleolar protein nucleophosmin (NPM)-ALK proteins in normal and neoplastic cells with the monoclonal antibody ALK1," *Blood*, vol. 89, no. 4, pp. 1394–1404, 1997.

[2] T. Iwahara, J. Fujimoto, D. Wen et al., "Molecular characterization of ALK, a receptor tyrosine kinase expressed specifically in the nervous system," *Oncogene*, vol. 14, no. 4, pp. 439–449, 1997.

[3] S. W. Morris, C. Naeve, P. Mathew et al., "ALK the chromosome 2 gene locus altered by the t(2;5) in non-Hodgkin's lymphoma, encodes a novel neural receptor tyrosine kinase that is highly related to leukocyte tyrosine kinase (LTK)," *Oncogene*, vol. 14, no. 18, pp. 2175–2188, 1997.

[4] E. Vernersson, N. K. S. Khoo, M. L. Henriksson, G. Roos, R. H. Palmer, and B. Hallberg, "Characterization of the expression of the ALK receptor tyrosine kinase in mice," *Gene Expression Patterns*, vol. 6, no. 5, pp. 448–461, 2006.

[5] R. H. Palmer, E. Vernersson, C. Grabbe, and B. Hallberg, "Anaplastic lymphoma kinase: signalling in development and disease," *Biochemical Journal*, vol. 420, no. 3, pp. 345–361, 2009.

[6] J. B. Weiss, C. Xue, T. Benice, L. Xue, S. W. Morris, and J. Raber, "Anaplastic lymphoma kinase and leukocyte tyrosine kinase: functions and genetic interactions in learning, memory and adult neurogenesis," *Pharmacology, Biochemistry, and Behavior*, vol. 100, no. 3, pp. 566–574, 2012.

[7] J. G. Bilsland, A. Wheeldon, A. Mead et al., "Behavioral and neurochemical alterations in mice deficient in anaplastic lymphoma kinase suggest therapeutic potential for psychiatric indications," *Neuropsychopharmacology*, vol. 33, no. 3, pp. 685–700, 2008.

[8] A. W. Lasek, J. Lim, C. L. Kliethermes et al., "An evolutionary conserved role for anaplastic lymphoma kinase in behavioral responses to ethanol," *PLoS ONE*, vol. 6, no. 7, Article ID e22636, 2011.

[9] H. Kunugi, R. Hashimoto, T. Okada et al., "Possible association between nonsynonymous polymorphisms of the anaplastic lymphoma kinase (ALK) gene and schizophrenia in a Japanese population," *Journal of Neural Transmission*, vol. 113, no. 10, pp. 1569–1573, 2006.

[10] C. Englund, C. E. Lorén, C. Grabbe et al., "Jeb signals through the Alk receptor tyrosine kinase to drive visceral muscle fusion," *Nature*, vol. 425, no. 6957, pp. 512–516, 2003.

[11] H. H. Lee, A. Norris, J. B. Weiss, and M. Frasch, "Jelly belly protein activates the receptor tyrosine kinase Alk to specify visceral muscle pioneers," *Nature*, vol. 425, no. 6957, pp. 507–512, 2003.

[12] C. Stute, K. Schimmelpfeng, R. Renkawitz-Pohl, R. H. Palmer, and A. Holz, "Myoblast determination in the somatic and visceral mesoderm depends on Notch signalling as well as on milliways (miliAlk) as receptor for jeb signalling," *Development*, vol. 131, no. 4, pp. 743–754, 2004.

[13] G. E. Stoica, A. Kuo, A. Aigner et al., "Identification of anaplastic lymphoma kinase as a receptor for the growth factor pleiotrophin," *Journal of Biological Chemistry*, vol. 276, no. 20, pp. 16772–16779, 2001.

[14] G. E. Stoica, A. Kuo, C. Powers et al., "Midkine binds to anaplastic lymphoma kinase (ALK) and acts as a growth factor for different cell types," *Journal of Biological Chemistry*, vol. 277, no. 39, pp. 35990–35998, 2002.

[15] C. Moog-Lutz, J. Degoutin, J. Y. Gouzi et al., "Activation and inhibition of anaplastic lymphoma kinase receptor tyrosine kinase by monoclonal antibodies and absence of agonist activity of pleiotrophin," *Journal of Biological Chemistry*, vol. 280, no. 28, pp. 26039–26048, 2005.

[16] A. Motegi, J. Fujimoto, M. Kotani, H. Sakuraba, and T. Yamamoto, "ALK receptor tyrosine kinase promotes cell growth and neurite outgrowth," *Journal of Cell Science*, vol. 117, no. 15, pp. 3319–3329, 2004.

[17] P. Perez-Pinera, W. Zhang, Y. Chang, J. A. Vega, and T. F. Deuel, "Anaplastic lymphoma kinase is activated through the pleiotrophin/receptor protein-tyrosine phosphatase β/ζ signaling pathway: an alternative mechanism of receptor tyrosine kinase activation," *Journal of Biological Chemistry*, vol. 282, no. 39, pp. 28683–28690, 2007.

[18] J. Mourali, A. Bénard, F. C. Lourenço et al., "Anaplastic lymphoma kinase is a dependence receptor whose proapoptotic functions are activated by caspase cleavage," *Molecular and Cellular Biology*, vol. 26, no. 16, pp. 6209–6222, 2006.

[19] P. Mehlen and D. E. Bredesen, "The dependence receptor hypothesis," *Apoptosis*, vol. 9, no. 1, pp. 37–49, 2004.

[20] S. W. Morris, M. N. Kirstein, M. B. Valentine et al., "Fusion of a kinase gene, ALK, to a nucleolar protein gene, NPM, in non-Hodgkin's lymphoma," *Science*, vol. 263, no. 5151, pp. 1281–1284, 1994.

[21] M. Shiota, J. Fujimoto, T. Semba, H. Satoh, T. Yamamoto, and S. Mori, "Hyperphosphorylation of a novel 80 kDa protein-tyrosine kinase similar to Ltk in a human Ki-1 lymphoma cell line, AMS3," *Oncogene*, vol. 9, no. 6, pp. 1567–1574, 1994.

[22] D. A. Arber, L. H. Sun, and L. M. Weiss, "Detection of the t(2;5)(p23;q35) chromosomal translocation in large B-cell lymphomas other than anaplastic large cell lymphoma," *Human Pathology*, vol. 27, no. 6, pp. 590–594, 1996.

[23] L. Lamant, N. Dastugue, K. Pulford, G. Delsol, and B. Mariamé, "A new fusion gene TPM3-ALK in anaplastic large

cell lymphoma created by a (1;2)(q25;p23) translocation," *Blood*, vol. 93, no. 9, pp. 3088–3095, 1999.

[24] R. Siebert, S. Gesk, L. Harder et al., "Complex variant translocation t(1;2) with TPM3-ALK fusion due to cryptic ALK gene rearrangement in anaplastic large-cell lymphoma," *Blood*, vol. 94, no. 10, pp. 3614–3617, 1999.

[25] B. Lawrence, A. Perez-Atayde, M. K. Hibbard et al., "TPM3-ALK and TPM4-ALK oncogenes in inflammatory myofibroblastic tumors," *American Journal of Pathology*, vol. 157, no. 2, pp. 377–384, 2000.

[26] E. Sugawara, Y. Togashi, N. Kuroda et al., "Identification of anaplastic lymphoma kinase fusions in renal cancer: large-scale immunohistochemical screening by the intercalated antibody-enhanced polymer method," *Cancer*. In press.

[27] L. Hernández, M. Pinyol, S. Hernández et al., "TRK-fused gene (TFG) is a new partner of ALK in anaplastic large cell lymphoma producing two structurally different TFG-ALK translocations," *Blood*, vol. 94, no. 9, pp. 3265–3268, 1999.

[28] K. Rikova, A. Guo, Q. Zeng et al., "Global survey of phosphotyrosine signaling identifies oncogenic kinases in lung cancer," *Cell*, vol. 131, no. 6, pp. 1190–1203, 2007.

[29] M. Trinei, L. Lanfrancone, E. Campo et al., "A new variant anaplastic lymphoma kinase (ALK)-fusion protein (ATIC-ALK) in a case of ALK-positive anaplastic large cell lymphoma," *Cancer Research*, vol. 60, no. 4, pp. 793–798, 2000.

[30] Z. Ma, J. Cools, P. Marynen et al., "Inv(2)(p23q35) in anaplastic large-cell lymphoma induces constitutive anaplastic lymphoma kinase (ALK) tyrosine kinase activation by fusion to ATIC, an enzyme involved in purine nucleotide biosynthesis," *Blood*, vol. 95, no. 6, pp. 2144–2149, 2000.

[31] G. W. B. Colleoni, J. A. Bridge, B. Garicochea, J. Liu, D. A. Filippa, and M. Ladanyi, "ATIC-ALK: a novel variant ALK gene fusion in anaplastic large cell lymphoma resulting from the recurrent cryptic chromosomal inversion, inv(2)(p23q35)," *American Journal of Pathology*, vol. 156, no. 3, pp. 781–789, 2000.

[32] M. Debiec-Rychter, P. Marynen, A. Hagemeijer, and P. Pauwels, "ALK-ATIC fusion in urinary bladder inflammatory myofibroblastic tumor," *Genes Chromosomes and Cancer*, vol. 38, no. 2, pp. 187–190, 2003.

[33] C. Touriol, C. Greenland, L. Lamant et al., "Further demonstration of the diversity of chromosomal changes involving 2p23 in ALK-positive lymphoma: 2 cases expressing ALK kinase fused to CLTCL (clathrin chain polypeptide-like)," *Blood*, vol. 95, no. 10, pp. 3204–3207, 2000.

[34] J. A. Bridge, M. Kanamori, Z. Ma et al., "Fusion of the ALK gene to the clathrin heavy chain gene, CLTC, in inflammatory myofibroblastic tumor," *American Journal of Pathology*, vol. 159, no. 2, pp. 411–415, 2001.

[35] P. De Paepe, M. Baens, H. van Krieken et al., "ALK activation by the CLTC-ALK fusion is a recurrent event in large B-cell lymphoma," *Blood*, vol. 102, no. 7, pp. 2638–2641, 2003.

[36] R. D. Gascoyne, L. Lamant, J. I. Martin-Subero et al., "ALK-positive diffuse large B-cell lymphoma is associated with Clathrin-ALK rearrangements: report of 6 cases," *Blood*, vol. 102, no. 7, pp. 2568–2573, 2003.

[37] N. Chikatsu, H. Kojima, K. Suzukawa et al., "ALK+, CD30−, CD20− large B-cell lymphoma containing anaplastic lymphoma kinase (ALK) fused to clathrin heavy chain gene (CLTC)," *Modern Pathology*, vol. 16, no. 8, pp. 828–832, 2003.

[38] W. Y. Wang, L. Gu, W. P. Liu, G. D. Li, H. J. Liu, and Z. G. Ma, "ALK-positive extramedullary plasmacytoma with

expression of the CLTC-ALK fusion transcript," *Pathology, Research and Practice*, vol. 207, no. 9, pp. 587–591, 2011.

[39] S. J. Meech, L. McGavran, L. F. Odom et al., "Unusual childhood extramedullary hematologic malignancy with natural killer cell properties that contains tropomyosin 4—anaplastic lymphoma kinase gene fusion," *Blood*, vol. 98, no. 4, pp. 1209–1216, 2001.

[40] F. R. Jazii, Z. Najafi, R. Malekzadeh et al., "Identification of squamous cell carcinoma associated proteins by proteomics and loss of beta tropomyosin expression in esophageal cancer," *World Journal of Gastroenterology*, vol. 12, no. 44, pp. 7104–7112, 2006.

[41] X. L. Du, H. Hu, D. C. Lin et al., "Proteomic profiling of proteins dysregulted in Chinese esophageal squamous cell carcinoma," *Journal of Molecular Medicine*, vol. 85, no. 8, pp. 863–875, 2007.

[42] F. Tort, M. Pinyol, K. Pulford et al., "Molecular characterization of a new ALK translocation involving moesin (MSN-ALK) in anaplastic large cell lymphoma," *Laboratory Investigation*, vol. 81, no. 3, pp. 419–426, 2001.

[43] J. Cools, I. Wlodarska, R. Somers et al., "Identification of novel fusion partners of ALK, the anaplastic lymphoma kinase, in anaplastic large-cell lymphoma and inflammatory myofibroblastic tumor," *Genes Chromosomes and Cancer*, vol. 34, no. 4, pp. 354–362, 2002.

[44] Z. Ma, D. A. Hill, M. H. Collins et al., "Fusion of ALK to the Ran-binding protein 2 (RANBP2) gene in inflammatory myofibroblastic tumor," *Genes Chromosomes and Cancer*, vol. 37, no. 1, pp. 98–105, 2003.

[45] L. Lamant, R. D. Gascoyne, M. M. Duplantier et al., "Non-muscle myosin heavy chain (MYH9): a new partner fused to ALK in anaplastic large cell lymphoma," *Genes Chromosomes and Cancer*, vol. 37, no. 4, pp. 427–432, 2003.

[46] I. Panagopoulos, T. Nilsson, H. A. Domanski et al., "Fusion of the SEC31L1 and ALK genes in an inflammatory myofibroblastic tumor," *International Journal of Cancer*, vol. 118, no. 5, pp. 1181–1186, 2006.

[47] K. Van Roosbroeck, J. Cools, D. Dierickx et al., "ALK-positive large B-cell lymphomas with cryptic SEC31A-ALK and NPM1-ALK fusions," *Haematologica*, vol. 95, no. 3, pp. 509–513, 2010.

[48] C. Bedwell, D. Rowe, D. Moulton, G. Jones, N. Bown, and C. M. Bacon, "Cytogenetically complex SEC31A-ALK fusions are recurrent in ALK-positive large B-cell lymphomas," *Haematologica*, vol. 96, no. 2, pp. 343–346, 2011.

[49] M. Soda, Y. L. Choi, M. Enomoto et al., "Identification of the transforming EML4-ALK fusion gene in non-small-cell lung cancer," *Nature*, vol. 448, no. 7153, pp. 561–566, 2007.

[50] E. Lin, L. Li, Y. Guan et al., "Exon array profiling detects EML4-ALK fusion in breast, colorectal, and non-small cell lung cancers," *Molecular Cancer Research*, vol. 7, no. 9, pp. 1466–1476, 2009.

[51] K. Takeuchi, M. Soda, Y. Togashi et al., "Identification of a novel fusion, SQSTM1-ALK, in ALK-positive large B-cell lymphoma," *Haematologica*, vol. 96, no. 3, pp. 464–467, 2011.

[52] L. V. Debelenko, S. C. Raimondi, N. Daw et al., "Renal cell carcinoma with novel VCL-ALK fusion: new representative of ALK-associated tumor spectrum," *Modern Pathology*, vol. 24, no. 3, pp. 430–442, 2011.

[53] A. Mariño-Enríquez, W. B. Ou, C. B. Weldon, J. A. Fletcher, and A. R. Pérez-Atayde, "ALK rearrangement in sickle cell trait-associated renal medullary carcinoma," *Genes Chromosomes and Cancer*, vol. 50, no. 3, pp. 146–153, 2011.

[54] K. Takeuchi, L. C. Young, Y. Togashi et al., "KIF5B-ALK, a novel fusion oncokinase identified by an immunohistochemistry-based diagnostic system for ALK-positive lung cancer," *Clinical Cancer Research*, vol. 15, no. 9, pp. 3143–3149, 2009.

[55] K. Takeuchi, M. Soda, Y. Togashi et al., "Pulmonary inflammatory myofibroblastic tumor expressing a novel fusion, PPFIBP1-ALK: reappraisal of anti-ALK immunohistochemistry as a tool for novel ALK fusion identification," *Clinical Cancer Research*, vol. 17, no. 10, pp. 3341–3348, 2011.

[56] D. Lipson, M. Capelletti, R. Yelensky et al., "Identification of new ALK and RET gene fusions from colorectal and lung cancer biopsies," *Nature Medicine*, vol. 18, no. 3, pp. 382–384, 2012.

[57] Y. Togashi, M. Soda, S. Sakata et al., "KLC1-ALK: a novel fusion in lung cancer identified using a formalin-fixed paraffin-embedded tissue only," *PLoS ONE*, vol. 7, no. 2, Article ID e31323, 2012.

[58] G. Delsol, B. Falini, H. K. Muller-Hermelink et al., *Anaplastic Large Cell Lymphoma (ALCL), ALK-Positive*, International Agency for Research on Cancer (IARC), Lyon, France, 4th edition, 2008.

[59] A. Fornari, R. Piva, R. Chiarle, D. Novero, and G. Inghirami, "Anaplastic large cell lymphoma: one or more entities among T-cell lymphoma?" *Hematological Oncology*, vol. 27, no. 4, pp. 161–170, 2009.

[60] P. Fischer, E. Nacheva, D. Y. Mason et al., "A Ki-1 (CD30)-positive human cell line (Karpas 299) established from a high grade non-Hodgkin's lymphoma, showing a 2;5 translocation and rearrangement of the T-cell receptor β-chain gene," *Blood*, vol. 72, no. 1, pp. 234–240, 1988.

[61] R. Rimokh, J. P. Magaud, F. Berger et al., "A translocation involving a specific breakpoint (q35) on chromosome 5 is characteristic of anaplastic large cell lymphoma (Ki-1 lymphoma)," *British Journal of Haematology*, vol. 71, no. 1, pp. 31–36, 1989.

[62] Y. Kaneko, G. Frizzera, S. Edamura et al., "A novel translocation, t(2;5)(p23;q35), in childhood phagocytic large T-cell lymphoma mimicking malignant histiocytosis," *Blood*, vol. 73, no. 3, pp. 806–813, 1989.

[63] D. Y. Mason, C. Bastard, R. Rimokh et al., "CD30-positive large cell lymphomas (Ki-1 lymphoma) are associated with a chromosomal translocation involving 5q35," *British Journal of Haematology*, vol. 74, no. 2, pp. 161–168, 1990.

[64] M. M. Le Beau, M. A. Bitter, R. A. Larson et al., "The t(2;5)(p23;q35): a recurring chromosomal abnormality in Ki-1-positive anaplastic large cell lymphoma," *Leukemia*, vol. 3, no. 12, pp. 866–870, 1989.

[65] C. A. Griffin, A. L. Hawkins, C. Dvorak, C. Henkle, T. Ellingham, and E. J. Perlman, "Recurrent involvement of 2p23 in inflammatory myofibroblastic tumors," *Cancer Research*, vol. 59, no. 12, pp. 2776–2780, 1999.

[66] C. Gambacorti-Passerini, C. Messa, and E. M. Pogliani, "Crizotinib in anaplastic large-cell lymphoma," *The New England Journal of Medicine*, vol. 364, no. 8, pp. 775–776, 2011.

[67] E. L. Kwak, Y. J. Bang, D. R. Camidge et al., "Anaplastic lymphoma kinase inhibition in non-small-cell lung cancer," *The New England Journal of Medicine*, vol. 363, no. 18, pp. 1693–1703, 2010.

[68] J. E. Butrynski, D. R. D'Adamo, J. L. Hornick et al., "Crizotinib in ALK-rearranged inflammatory myofibroblastic tumor," *The New England Journal of Medicine*, vol. 363, no. 18, pp. 1727–1733, 2010.

[69] P. Perez-Pinera, Y. Chang, A. Astudillo, J. Mortimer, and T. F. Deuel, "Anaplastic lymphoma kinase is expressed in different subtypes of human breast cancer," *Biochemical and Biophysical Research Communications*, vol. 358, no. 2, pp. 399–403, 2007.

[70] L. Lamant, K. Pulford, D. Bischof et al., "Expression of the ALK tyrosine kinase gene in neuroblastoma," *American Journal of Pathology*, vol. 156, no. 5, pp. 1711–1721, 2000.

[71] I. Janoueix-Lerosey, D. Lequin, L. Brugières et al., "Somatic and germline activating mutations of the ALK kinase receptor in neuroblastoma," *Nature*, vol. 455, no. 7215, pp. 967–970, 2008.

[72] Y. Chen, J. Takita, Y. L. Choi et al., "Oncogenic mutations of ALK kinase in neuroblastoma," *Nature*, vol. 455, no. 7215, pp. 971–974, 2008.

[73] R. E. George, T. Sanda, M. Hanna et al., "Activating mutations in ALK provide a therapeutic target in neuroblastoma," *Nature*, vol. 455, no. 7215, pp. 975–978, 2008.

[74] H. Carén, F. Abel, P. Kogner, and T. Martinsson, "High incidence of DNA mutations and gene amplifications of the ALK gene in advanced sporadic neuroblastoma tumours," *Biochemical Journal*, vol. 416, no. 2, pp. 153–159, 2008.

[75] Y. P. Mossé, M. Laudenslager, L. Longo et al., "Identification of ALK as a major familial neuroblastoma predisposition gene," *Nature*, vol. 455, no. 7215, pp. 930–935, 2008.

[76] A. K. Murugan and M. M. Xing, "Anaplastic thyroid cancers harbor novel oncogenic mutations of the ALK gene," *Cancer Research*, vol. 71, no. 13, pp. 4403–4411, 2011.

[77] D. Wang, H. Umekawa, and M. O. J. Olson, "Expression and subcellular locations of two forms of nucleolar protein B23 in rat tissues and cells," *Cellular and Molecular Biology Research*, vol. 39, no. 1, pp. 33–42, 1993.

[78] R. A. Borer, C. F. Lehner, H. M. Eppenberger, and E. A. Nigg, "Major nucleolar proteins shuttle between nucleus and cytoplasm," *Cell*, vol. 56, no. 3, pp. 379–390, 1989.

[79] E. Colombo, M. Alcalay, and P. G. Pelicci, "Nucleophosmin and its complex network: a possible therapeutic target in hematological diseases," *Oncogene*, vol. 30, no. 23, pp. 2595–2609, 2011.

[80] J. Fujimoto, M. Shiota, T. Iwahara et al., "Characterization of the transforming activity of p80, a hyperphosphorylated protein in a Ki-1 lymphoma cell line with chromosomal translocation t(2;5)," *Proceedings of the National Academy of Sciences of the United States of America*, vol. 93, no. 9, pp. 4181–4186, 1996.

[81] D. Bischof, K. Pulford, D. Y. Mason, and S. W. Morris, "Role of the nucleophosmin (NPM) portion of the non-Hodgkin's lymphoma- associated NPM-anaplastic lymphoma kinase fusion protein in oncogenesis," *Molecular and Cellular Biology*, vol. 17, no. 4, pp. 2312–2325, 1997.

[82] P. K. Chan, "Cross-linkage of nucleophosmin in tumor cells by nitrogen mustard," *Cancer Research*, vol. 49, no. 12, pp. 3271–3275, 1989.

[83] B. Y. M. Yung and P. K. Chan, "Identification and characterization of a hexameric form of nucleolar phosphoprotein B23," *Biochimica et Biophysica Acta*, vol. 925, no. 1, pp. 74–82, 1987.

[84] H. Mano, "Non-solid oncogenes in solid tumors: EML4-ALK fusion genes in lung cancer," *Cancer Science*, vol. 99, no. 12, pp. 2349–2355, 2008.

[85] A. Barreca, E. Lasorsa, L. Riera et al., "Anaplastic lymphoma kinase in human cancer," *Journal of Molecular Endocrinology*, vol. 47, no. 1, pp. R11–R23, 2011.

[86] R. Chiarle, C. Voena, C. Ambrogio, R. Piva, and G. Inghirami, "The anaplastic lymphoma kinase in the pathogenesis of cancer," *Nature Reviews Cancer*, vol. 8, no. 1, pp. 11–23, 2008.

[87] D. E. Levy and J. E. Darnell, "STATs: transcriptional control and biological impact," *Nature Reviews Molecular Cell Biology*, vol. 3, no. 9, pp. 651–662, 2002.

[88] C. I. Santos and A. P. Costa-Pereira, "Signal transducers and activators of transcription-from cytokine signalling to cancer biology," *Biochimica et Biophysica Acta*, vol. 1816, no. 1, pp. 38–49, 2011.

[89] Q. Zhang, P. N. Raghunath, L. Xue et al., "Multilevel dysregulation of STAT3 activation in anaplastic lymphoma kinase-positive T/null-cell lymphoma," *Journal of Immunology*, vol. 168, no. 1, pp. 466–474, 2002.

[90] A. Zamo, R. Chiarle, R. Piva et al., "Anaplastic lymphoma kinase (ALK) activates Stat3 and protects hematopoietic cells from cell death," *Oncogene*, vol. 21, no. 7, pp. 1038–1047, 2002.

[91] J. D. Khoury, L. J. Medeiros, G. Z. Rassidakis et al., "Differential expression and clinical significance of tyrosine-phosphorylated STAT3 in ALK$^+$ and ALK$^-$ anaplastic large cell lymphoma," *Clinical Cancer Research*, vol. 9, no. 10, part 1, pp. 3692–3699, 2003.

[92] R. Chiarle, J. Z. Gong, I. Guasparri et al., "NPM-ALK transgenic mice spontaneously develop T-cell lymphomas and plasma cell tumors," *Blood*, vol. 101, no. 5, pp. 1919–1927, 2003.

[93] R. Chiarle, W. J. Simmons, H. Cai et al., "Stat3 is required for ALK-mediated lymphomagenesis and provides a possible therapeutic target," *Nature Medicine*, vol. 11, no. 6, pp. 623–629, 2005.

[94] H. M. Amin, T. J. McDonnell, Y. Ma et al., "Selective inhibition of STAT3 induces apoptosis and G1 cell cycle arrest in ALK-positive anaplastic large cell lymphoma," *Oncogene*, vol. 23, no. 32, pp. 5426–5434, 2004.

[95] R. Piva, L. Agnelli, E. Pellegrino et al., "Gene expression profiling uncovers molecular classifiers for the recognition of anaplastic large-cell lymphoma within peripheral T-cell neoplasms," *Journal of Clinical Oncology*, vol. 28, no. 9, pp. 1583–1590, 2010.

[96] Q. Zhang, H. Wang, K. Kantekure et al., "Oncogenic tyrosine kinase NPM-ALK induces expression of the growth-promoting receptor ICOS," *Blood*, vol. 118, no. 11, pp. 3062–3071, 2011.

[97] N. Anastasov, I. Bonzheim, M. Rudelius et al., "C/EBPβ expression in ALK-positiveanaplastic large cell lymphomas is required for cell proliferation and is induced by the STAT3 signaling pathway," *Haematologica*, vol. 95, no. 5, pp. 760–767, 2010.

[98] R. Piva, E. Pellegrino, M. Mattioli et al., "Functional validation of the anaplastic lymphoma kinase signature identifies CEBPB and BCl2A1 as critical target genes," *Journal of Clinical Investigation*, vol. 116, no. 12, pp. 3171–3182, 2006.

[99] M. Marzec, Q. Zhang, A. Goradia et al., "Oncogenic kinase NPM/ALK induces through STAT3 expression of immuno-suppressive protein CD274 (PD-L1, B7-H1)," *Proceedings of the National Academy of Sciences of the United States of America*, vol. 105, no. 52, pp. 20852–20857, 2008.

[100] R. Yamamoto, M. Nishikori, M. Tashima et al., "B7-H1 expression is regulated by MEK/ERK signaling pathway in anaplastic large cell lymphoma and Hodgkin lymphoma," *Cancer Science*, vol. 100, no. 11, pp. 2093–2100, 2009.

[101] R. Lai, G. Z. Rassidakis, L. J. Medeiros et al., "Signal transducer and activator of transcription-3 activation contributes

to high tissue inhibitor of metalloproteinase-1 expression in anaplastic lymphoma kinase-positive anaplastic large cell lymphoma," *American Journal of Pathology*, vol. 164, no. 6, pp. 2251–2258, 2004.

[102] M. Marzec, X. Liu, W. Wong et al., "Oncogenic kinase NPM/ALK induces expression of HIF1α mRNA," *Oncogene*, vol. 30, no. 11, pp. 1372–1378, 2011.

[103] J. Zhang, P. Wang, F. Wu et al., "Aberrant expression of the transcriptional factor Twist1 promotes invasiveness in ALK-positive anaplastic large cell lymphoma," *Cellular Signalling*, vol. 24, no. 4, pp. 852–858, 2012.

[104] M. Kasprzycka, M. Marzec, X. Liu, Q. Zhang, and M. A. Wasik, "Nucleophosmin/anaplastic lymphoma kinase (NPM/ALK) oncoprotein induces the T regulatory cell phenotype by activating STAT3," *Proceedings of the National Academy of Sciences of the United States of America*, vol. 103, no. 26, pp. 9964–9969, 2006.

[105] C. Ambrogio, C. Martinengo, C. Voena et al., "NPM-ALK oncogenic tyrosine kinase controls T-cell identity by transcriptional regulation and epigenetic silencing in lymphoma cells," *Cancer Research*, vol. 69, no. 22, pp. 8611–8619, 2009.

[106] N. Sasai and P. A. Defossez, "Many paths to one goal? The proteins that recognize methylated DNA in eukaryotes," *The International Journal of Developmental Biology*, vol. 53, no. 2-3, pp. 323–334, 2009.

[107] Q. Zhang, H. Y. Wang, X. Liu, G. Bhutani, K. Kantekure, and M. Wasik, "IL-2R common γ-chain is epigenetically silenced by nucleophosphin-anaplastic lymphoma kinase (NPM-ALK) and acts as a tumor suppressor by targeting NPM-ALK," *Proceedings of the National Academy of Sciences of the United States of America*, vol. 108, no. 29, pp. 11977–11982, 2011.

[108] Q. Zhang, H. Y. Wang, X. Liu, and M. A. Wasik, "STAT5A is epigenetically silenced by the tyrosine kinase NPM1-ALK and acts as a tumor suppressor by reciprocally inhibiting NPM1-ALK expression," *Nature Medicine*, vol. 13, no. 11, pp. 1341–1348, 2007.

[109] D. K. Crockett, Z. Lin, K. S. J. Elenitoba-Johnson, and M. S. Lim, "Identification of NPM-ALK interacting proteins by tandem mass spectrometry," *Oncogene*, vol. 23, no. 15, pp. 2617–2629, 2004.

[110] H. M. Amin, L. J. Medeiros, Y. Ma et al., "Inhibition of JAK3 induces apoptosis and decreases anaplastic lymphoma kinase activity in anaplastic large cell lymphoma," *Oncogene*, vol. 22, no. 35, pp. 5399–5407, 2003.

[111] M. Marzec, M. Kasprzycka, A. Ptasznik et al., "Inhibition of ALK enzymatic activity in T-cell lymphoma cells induces apoptosis and suppresses proliferation and STAT3 phosphorylation independently of Jak3," *Laboratory Investigation*, vol. 85, no. 12, pp. 1544–1554, 2005.

[112] J. D. Khoury, G. Z. Rassidakis, L. J. Medeiros, H. M. Amin, and R. Lai, "Methylation of SHP1 gene and loss of SHP1 protein expression are frequent in systemic anaplastic large cell lymphoma," *Blood*, vol. 104, no. 5, pp. 1580–1581, 2004.

[113] Q. Zhang, H. Y. Wang, M. Marzec, P. N. Raghunath, T. Nagasawa, and M. A. Wasik, "STAT3- and DNA methyltransferase 1-mediated epigenetic silencing of SHP-1 tyrosine phosphatase tumor suppressor gene in malignant T lymphocytes," *Proceedings of the National Academy of Sciences of the United States of America*, vol. 102, no. 19, pp. 6948–6953, 2005.

[114] J. F. Honorat, A. Ragab, L. Lamant, G. Delsol, and J. Ragab-Thomas, "SHP1 tyrosine phosphatase negatively regulates

NPM-ALK tyrosine kinase signaling," *Blood*, vol. 107, no. 10, pp. 4130–4138, 2006.

[115] Y. Han, H. M. Amin, B. Franko, C. Frantz, X. Shi, and R. Lai, "Loss of SHP1 enhances JAK3/STAT3 signaling and decreases proteosome degradation of JAK3 and NPM-ALK in ALK$^+$ anaplastic large-cell lymphoma," *Blood*, vol. 108, no. 8, pp. 2796–2803, 2006.

[116] Y. Han, H. M. Amin, C. Frantz et al., "Restoration of shp1 expression by 5-AZA-2′-deoxycytidine is associated with downregulation of JAK3/STAT3 signaling in ALK-positive anaplastic large cell lymphoma," *Leukemia*, vol. 20, no. 9, pp. 1602–1609, 2006.

[117] L. Qiu, R. Lai, Q. Lin et al., "Autocrine release of interleukin-9 promotes Jak3-dependent survival of ALK$^+$ anaplastic large-cell lymphoma cells," *Blood*, vol. 108, no. 7, pp. 2407–2415, 2006.

[118] J. D. Bard, P. Gelebart, M. Anand et al., "IL-21 contributes to JAK3/STAT3 activation and promotes cell growth in ALK-positive anaplastic large cell lymphoma," *American Journal of Pathology*, vol. 175, no. 2, pp. 825–834, 2009.

[119] J. D. Bard, P. Gelebart, M. Anand, H. M. Amin, and R. Lai, "Aberrant expression of IL-22 receptor 1 and autocrine IL-22 stimulation contribute to tumorigenicity in ALK$^+$ anaplastic large cell lymphoma," *Leukemia*, vol. 22, no. 8, pp. 1595–1603, 2008.

[120] C. R. Geest and P. J. Coffer, "MAPK signaling pathways in the regulation of hematopoiesis," *Journal of Leukocyte Biology*, vol. 86, no. 2, pp. 237–250, 2009.

[121] L. S. Steelman, R. A. Franklin, S. L. Abrams et al., "Roles of the Ras/Raf/MEK/ERK pathway in leukemia therapy," *Leukemia*, vol. 25, no. 7, pp. 1080–1094, 2011.

[122] M. Watanabe, M. Sasaki, K. Itoh et al., "JunB induced by constitutive CD30-extracellular signal-regulated kinase 1/2 mitogen-activated protein kinase signaling activates the CD30 promoter in anaplastic large cell lymphoma and Reed-Sternberg cells of Hodgkin lymphoma," *Cancer Research*, vol. 65, no. 17, pp. 7628–7634, 2005.

[123] P. B. Staber, P. Vesely, N. Haq et al., "The oncoprotein NPM-ALK of anaplastic large-cell lymphoma induces JUNB transcription via ERK1/2 and JunB translation via mTOR signaling," *Blood*, vol. 110, no. 9, pp. 3374–3383, 2007.

[124] M. Marzec, M. Kasprzycka, X. Liu, P. N. Raghunath, P. Wlodarski, and M. A. Wasik, "Oncogenic tyrosine kinase NPM/ALK induces activation of the MEK/ERK signaling pathway independently of c-Raf," *Oncogene*, vol. 26, no. 6, pp. 813–821, 2007.

[125] M. S. Lim, M. L. Carlson, D. K. Crockett et al., "The proteomic signature of NPM/ALK reveals deregulation of multiple cellular pathways," *Blood*, vol. 114, no. 8, pp. 1585–1595, 2009.

[126] F. Vega, L. J. Medeiros, V. Leventaki et al., "Activation of mammalian target of rapamycin signaling pathway contributes to tumor cell survival in anaplastic lymphoma kinase-positive anaplastic large cell lymphoma," *Cancer Research*, vol. 66, no. 13, pp. 6589–6597, 2006.

[127] M. Marzec, M. Kasprzycka, X. Liu et al., "Oncogenic tyrosine kinase NPM/ALK induces activation of the rapamycin-sensitive mTOR signaling pathway," *Oncogene*, vol. 26, no. 38, pp. 5606–5614, 2007.

[128] B. Magnuson, B. Ekim, D. C. Fingar et al., "Regulation and function of ribosomal protein S6 kinase (S6K) within mTOR signalling networks," *Biochemical Journal*, vol. 441, no. 1, pp. 1–21, 2012.

[129] M. Fernandez, R. Manso, F. Bernaldez, P. Lopez, A. Martin-Duce, and S. Alemany, "Involvement of Cot activity in the proliferation of ALCL lymphoma cells," *Biochemical and Biophysical Research Communications*, vol. 411, no. 4, pp. 655–660, 2011.

[130] B. D. Manning and L. C. Cantley, "Rheb fills a GAP between TSC and TOR," *Trends in Biochemical Sciences*, vol. 28, no. 11, pp. 573–576, 2003.

[131] X. M. Ma and J. Blenis, "Molecular mechanisms of mTOR-mediated translational control," *Nature Reviews Molecular Cell Biology*, vol. 10, no. 5, pp. 307–318, 2009.

[132] O. Merkel, F. Hamacher, D. Laimer et al., "Identification of differential and functionally active miRNAs in both anaplastic lymphoma kinase (ALK)$^+$ and ALK$^-$ anaplastic large-cell lymphoma," *Proceedings of the National Academy of Sciences of the United States of America*, vol. 107, no. 37, pp. 16228–16233, 2010.

[133] M. Watanabe, K. Itoh, T. Togano, M. E. Kadin, T. Watanabe, and R. Horie, "Ets-1 activates overexpression of JunB and CD30 in Hodgkin's lymphoma and anaplastic large-cell lymphoma," *The American Journal of Pathology*, vol. 180, no. 2, pp. 831–838, 2012.

[134] S. Mathas, M. Hinz, I. Anagnostopoulos et al., "Aberrantly expressed c-Jun and JunB are a hallmark of Hodgkin lymphoma cells, stimulate proliferation and synergize with NF-κB," *The EMBO Journal*, vol. 21, no. 15, pp. 4104–4113, 2002.

[135] A. P. Szremska, L. Kenner, E. Weisz et al., "JunB inhibits proliferation and transformation in B-lymphoid cells," *Blood*, vol. 102, no. 12, pp. 4159–4165, 2003.

[136] G. Z. Rassidakis, A. Thomaides, C. Atwell et al., "JunB expression is a common feature of CD30$^+$ lymphomas and lymphomatoid papulosis," *Modern Pathology*, vol. 18, no. 10, pp. 1365–1370, 2005.

[137] F. Y. Y. Hsu, P. B. Johnston, K. A. Burke, and Y. Zhao, "The expression of CD30 in anaplastic large cell lymphoma is regulated by nucleophosmin-anaplastic lymphoma kinase-mediated JunB level in a cell type-specific manner," *Cancer Research*, vol. 66, no. 18, pp. 9002–9008, 2006.

[138] J. D. Pearson, J. K. Lee, J. T. Bacani, R. Lai, and R. J. Ingham, "NPM-ALK and the JunB transcription factor regulate the expression of cytotoxic molecules in ALK-positive, anaplastic large cell lymphoma," *International Journal of Clinical and Experimental Pathology*, vol. 4, no. 2, pp. 124–133, 2011.

[139] J. G. Christensen, H. Y. Zou, M. E. Arango et al., "Cytoreductive antitumor activity of PF-2341066, a novel inhibitor of anaplastic lymphoma kinase and c-Met, in experimental models of anaplastic large-cell lymphoma," *Molecular Cancer Therapeutics*, vol. 6, no. 12, pp. 3314–3322, 2007.

[140] U. Ritter, C. Damm-Welk, U. Fuchs, R. M. Bohle, A. Borkhardt, and W. Woessmann, "Design and evaluation of chemically synthesized siRNA targeting the NPM-ALK fusion site in anaplastic large cell lymphoma (ALCL)," *Oligonucleotides*, vol. 13, no. 5, pp. 365–373, 2003.

[141] S. D. Turner, D. Yeung, K. Hadfield, S. J. Cook, and D. R. Alexander, "The NPM-ALK tyrosine kinase mimics TCR signalling pathways, inducing NFAT and AP-1 by RAS-dependent mechanisms," *Cellular Signalling*, vol. 19, no. 4, pp. 740–747, 2007.

[142] C. Voena, C. Conte, C. Ambrogio et al., "The tyrosine phosphatase Shp2 interacts with NPM-ALK and regulates anaplastic lymphoma cell growth and migration," *Cancer Research*, vol. 67, no. 9, pp. 4278–4286, 2007.

[143] L. Riera, E. Lasorsa, C. Ambrogio, N. Surrenti, C. Voena, and R. Chiarle, "Involvement of Grb2 adaptor protein in nucleophosmin-anaplastic lymphoma kinase (NPM-ALK)-mediated signaling and anaplastic large cell lymphoma growth," *Journal of Biological Chemistry*, vol. 285, no. 34, pp. 26441–26450, 2010.

[144] L. C. Cantley, "The phosphoinositide 3-kinase pathway," *Science*, vol. 296, no. 5573, pp. 1655–1657, 2002.

[145] P. Liu, H. Cheng, T. M. Roberts, and J. J. Zhao, "Targeting the phosphoinositide 3-kinase pathway in cancer," *Nature Reviews Drug Discovery*, vol. 8, no. 8, pp. 627–644, 2009.

[146] R. Y. Bai, T. Ouyang, C. Miething, S. W. Morris, C. Peschel, and J. Duyster, "Nucleophosmin-anaplastic lymphoma kinase associated with anaplastic large-cell lymphoma activates the phosphatidylinositol 3-kinase/Akt anti-apoptotic signaling pathway," *Blood*, vol. 96, no. 13, pp. 4319–4327, 2000.

[147] A. Slupianek, M. Nieborowska-Skorska, G. Hoser et al., "Role of phosphatidylinositol 3-kinase-Akt pathway in nucleophosmin/anaplastic lymphoma kinase-mediated lymphomagenesis," *Cancer Research*, vol. 61, no. 5, pp. 2194–2199, 2001.

[148] D. A. E. Cross, D. R. Alessi, P. Cohen, M. Andjelkovich, and B. A. Hemmings, "Inhibition of glycogen synthase kinase-3 by insulin mediated by protein kinase B," *Nature*, vol. 378, no. 6559, pp. 785–789, 1995.

[149] S. R. McDonnell, S. R. Hwang, V. Basrur et al., "NPM-ALK signals through glycogen synthase kinase 3beta to promote oncogenesis," *Oncogene*. In press.

[150] A. Fernandez-Vidal, A. Mazars, E. F. Gautier, G. Prévost, B. Payrastre, and S. Manenti, "Upregulation of the CDC25A phosphatase down-stream of the NPM/ALK oncogene participates to anaplastic large cell lymphoma enhanced proliferation," *Cell Cycle*, vol. 8, no. 9, pp. 1373–1379, 2009.

[151] R. R. Singh, J. H. Cho-Vega, Y. Davuluri et al., "Sonic hedgehog signaling pathway is activated in ALK-positive anaplastic large cell lymphoma," *Cancer Research*, vol. 69, no. 6, pp. 2550–2558, 2009.

[152] H. Zhu and H. W. Lo, "The human glioma-associated oncogene homolog 1 (GLI1) family of transcription factors in gene regulation and diseases," *Current Genomics*, vol. 11, no. 4, pp. 238–245, 2010.

[153] T. L. Gu, Z. Tothova, B. Scheijen, J. D. Griffin, D. G. Gilliland, and D. W. Sternberg, "NPM-ALK fusion kinase of anaplastic large-cell lymphoma regulates survival and proliferative signaling through modulation of FOXO3a," *Blood*, vol. 103, no. 12, pp. 4622–4629, 2004.

[154] H. Huang and D. J. Tindall, "Dynamic FoxO transcription factors," *Journal of Cell Science*, vol. 120, no. 15, pp. 2479–2487, 2007.

[155] P. F. Dijkers, R. H. Medema, J. W. J. Lammers, L. Koenderman, and P. J. Coffer, "Expression of the pro-apoptotic Bcl-2 family member Bim is regulated by the forkhead transcription factor FKHR-L1," *Current Biology*, vol. 10, no. 19, pp. 1201–1204, 2000.

[156] P. F. Dijkers, R. H. Medema, C. Pals et al., "Forkhead transcription factor FKHR-L1 modulates cytokine-dependent transcriptional regulation of p27^{KIP1}," *Molecular and Cellular Biology*, vol. 20, no. 24, pp. 9138–9148, 2000.

[157] A. Slupianek and T. Skorski, "NPM/ALK downregulates p27^{KIP1} in a PI-3K-dependent manner," *Experimental Hematology*, vol. 32, no. 12, pp. 1265–1271, 2004.

[158] G. Z. Rassidakis, M. Feretzaki, C. Atwell et al., "Inhibition of Akt increases p27^{KIP1} levels and induces cell cycle arrest in anaplastic large cell lymphoma," *Blood*, vol. 105, no. 2, pp. 827–829, 2005.

[159] D. Polgar, C. Leisser, S. Maier et al., "Truncated ALK derived from chromosomal translocation t(2;5)(p23;q35) binds to the SH3 domain of p85-PI3K," *Mutation Research*, vol. 570, no. 1, pp. 9–15, 2005.

[160] W. Wan, M. S. Albom, L. Lu et al., "Anaplastic lymphoma kinase activity is essential for the proliferation and survival of anaplastic large-cell lymphoma cells," *Blood*, vol. 107, no. 4, pp. 1617–1623, 2006.

[161] A. H. Uner, A. Saglam, U. Han, M. Hayran, A. Sungur, and S. Ruacan, "PTEN and p27 expression in mature T-cell and NK-cell neoplasms," *Leukemia and Lymphoma*, vol. 46, no. 10, pp. 1463–1470, 2005.

[162] S. Momose, J. I. Tamaru, H. Kishi et al., "Hyperactivated STAT3 in ALK-positive diffuse large B-cell lymphoma with clathrin-ALK fusion," *Human Pathology*, vol. 40, no. 1, pp. 75–82, 2009.

[163] Z. Chen, T. Sasaki, X. Tan et al., "Inhibition of ALK, PI3K/MEK, and HSP90 in murine lung adenocarcinoma induced by EML4-ALK fusion oncogene," *Cancer Research*, vol. 70, no. 23, pp. 9827–9836, 2010.

[164] Y. Li, X. Ye, J. Liu, J. Zha, and L. Pei, "Evaluation of eml4-alk fusion proteins in non-small cell lung cancer using small molecule inhibitors," *Neoplasia*, vol. 13, no. 1, pp. 1–11, 2011.

[165] K. Takezawa, I. Okamoto, K. Nishio, P. A. Jänne, and K. Nakagawa, "Role of ERK-BIM and STAT3-survivin signaling pathways in ALK inhibitor-induced apoptosis in EML4-ALK-positive lung cancer," *Clinical Cancer Research*, vol. 17, no. 8, pp. 2140–2148, 2011.

[166] F. Armstrong, M. M. Duplantier, P. Trempat et al., "Differential effects of X-ALK fusion proteins on proliferation, transformation, and invasion properties of NIH3T3 cells," *Oncogene*, vol. 23, no. 36, pp. 6071–6082, 2004.

[167] S. D. Bohling, S. D. Jenson, D. K. Crockett, J. A. Schumacher, K. S. J. Elenitoba-Johnson, and M. S. Lim, "Analysis of gene expression profile of TPM3-ALK positive anaplastic large cell lymphoma reveals overlapping and unique patterns with that of NPM-ALK positive anaplastic large cell lymphoma," *Leukemia Research*, vol. 32, no. 3, pp. 383–393, 2008.

3

Regulation of Adherens Junction Dynamics by Phosphorylation Switches

Cristina Bertocchi,[1] **Megha Vaman Rao,**[1] **and Ronen Zaidel-Bar**[1, 2]

[1] *Mechanobiology Institute Singapore, National University of Singapore, Singapore 117411*
[2] *Department of Bioengineering, Faculty of Engineering, National University of Singapore, Singapore 119077*

Correspondence should be addressed to Ronen Zaidel-Bar, biezbr@nus.edu.sg

Academic Editor: Donna Webb

Adherens junctions connect the actin cytoskeleton of neighboring cells through transmembrane cadherin receptors and a network of adaptor proteins. The interactions between these adaptors and cadherin as well as the activity of actin regulators localized to adherens junctions are tightly controlled to facilitate cell junction assembly or disassembly in response to changes in external or internal forces and/or signaling. Phosphorylation of tyrosine, serine, or threonine residues acts as a switch on the majority of adherens junction proteins, turning "on" or "off" their interactions with other proteins and/or their enzymatic activity. Here, we provide an overview of the kinases and phosphatases regulating phosphorylation of adherens junction proteins and bring examples of phosphorylation events leading to the assembly or disassembly of adherens junctions, highlighting the important role of phosphorylation switches in regulating their dynamics.

1. Introduction

Adherens junctions (AJs) are cell-cell adhesion sites where calcium-dependent cadherin receptors bind with their extracellular domains to cadherins on opposing cells and with their cytoplasmic tails connect—via adaptors—to filamentous actin [1, 2]. By essentially providing a physical link between the actin cytoskeleton of neighboring cells AJs facilitate the integration of individual cells into a tissue. Additionally, AJs are instrumental in setting up and maintaining the apicobasal polarity of epithelial cells [3, 4], they function as mechanosensors [5] and serve as a nexus for signaling affecting important cell decisions, such as survival and differentiation [6].

During the development and lifetime of an organism, cells frequently change shape and position relative to their neighbors. Hence, the ability of cells to regulate their adhesive interactions plays a key role during tissue morphogenesis, repair, and renewal [3, 7, 8]. Defects in the adhesive characteristics of epithelial cells are pathological signs and loss of cell-cell adhesion can generate dedifferentiation and invasiveness of human carcinoma cells [9]. Thus, there is

great interest in understanding the factors that affect assembly and disassembly of cell-cell adhesion at the molecular level.

When considering regulatory mechanisms controlling AJ proteins, we distinguish between three subsequent steps of regulation: synthesis, localization, and activation. First, a cell controls whether proteins are synthesized or not. Indeed, transcriptional regulation of E-cadherin, notably by the snail transcription factor, plays an important role in the breaking down of AJs accompanying epithelial to mesenchymal transition [10]. Once a protein is expressed the cell can determine its localization by controlling its transport. In fact, both exocytosis and endocytosis of E-cadherin are tightly controlled and the balance between the two processes has been shown to regulate AJ turnover both *in vitro* and *in vivo* [6]. Finally, a cell can control the activity and interactions of a protein at a given location by posttranslational modifications. These modifications include glycosylation, lipidation, ubiquitination, acetylation, proteolysis, and phosphorylation [11]. Phosphorylation of tyrosine (Y), serine (S), or threonine (T) residues, the topic of this review, is a rapid and reversible form of regulation affecting the majority of AJ proteins [12–16]. In some cases, posttranslational modifications have secondary effects on transcription and/or protein transport [17, 18]. However, here we will focus on the more direct mechanisms in which AJs are regulated by phosphorylation. First, we will introduce the enzymes responsible for phosphorylation and dephosphorylation at AJs and discuss how they are recruited into AJ and activated. Next, we will describe the targets of phosphorylation within AJ and by examining the consequences of specific phosphorylation events will show how phosphorylation is involved both in assembly and disassembly of AJ, essentially driving the dynamics of this highly responsive structure. In the end, we will point out open questions and suggest methods to address them.

2. Recruitment of Protein Kinases and Phosphatases into AJ

So far, twelve S/T kinases and one S/T phosphatase have been implicated in regulating phosphorylation of AJ proteins, and they are all cytoplasmic (Table 1). Prominent kinases in this group include PKC-α, cAMP-dependent protein kinase, Casein Kinase 1, Pak1, and ROCK1. Nine tyrosine kinases and twelve tyrosine phosphatases have been shown to be active in AJ, roughly half of them cytoplasmic and half part of a transmembrane receptor (Table 1). Prominent tyrosine kinases include the cytoplasmic Src, Fyn, Fer, and Abl, and the receptors of epidermal and hepatocyte growth factors. Major phosphatases involved are the cytoplasmic PTP-1B, PTP-PEST, SHP-1, SHP-2, and receptor-type tyrosine-protein phosphatases Mu, U, and Kappa.

Some of these kinases and phosphatases have been localized to AJ by immunofluorescence (e.g., [19–21]) and others have been shown to associate with AJ by coimmuno-precipitation (e.g., [21–23]), but the exact mechanism of recruitment into AJ of most of them is largely unknown. A few were shown to bind directly with cadherin, such as CSK with VE-cadherin and PTP-1B with E- and N-cadherin [19, 24, 25]; others bind one of the catenins (adaptor proteins linking cadherin with actin), such as MET and PTPRF with β-catenin [26, 27] and ROCK1 with p120-catenin [21]; some interact with other AJ adaptor proteins, such as PRKCA with vinculin and ROCK1 with Shroom3 [28, 29].

While it is most likely every kinase and phosphatase can recognize at least one docking site within the AJ, it is not currently known which of the kinases and phosphatases reside in AJ permanently and which are transient components, homing in to phosphorylate or dephosphorylate AJ proteins only under specific conditions. Even permanent residents may not always be active, as most kinases and phosphatases need themselves to be activated.

3. Activation of Kinases and Phosphatases in AJ

Receptor tyrosine kinases are commonly activated by an external ligand, such as a growth factor or cytokine, which induces dimerization, cis-phosphorylation or autophosphorylation and activation of the catalytic domain

[124, 125]. Receptor tyrosine phosphatases may be activated by homophilic association with their counterparts on neighboring cells [126], as well as by tyrosine phosphorylation [127]. Several S/T kinases are activated by binding of Rho GTPases, for example ROCK1 is activated by RhoA and PAK1 is activated by Rac1 and Cdc42 [128, 129]. S/T kinases are also regulated by tyrosine phosphorylation and tyrosine kinases and phosphatases are regulated by S/T phosphorylation, in a complex web of feedback and feedforward loops that is poorly understood (Figure 1). For example, Src phosphorylates PRKCD, which phosphorylates PTPN6, which in turn dephosphorylates SRC (feedback) [130–132]; PRKACA phosphorylates Src and Csk, and Csk also phosphorylates Src (feedforward) [133–135].

As will be discussed further below, some of the phosphorylation events serve to activate the kinases or phosphatases and others are inhibitory. One well-understood example of kinase activation is the mechanism of activation of Src. As reviewed in [136], the family of Src tyrosine kinases can be found in a nonactive "closed" conformation or in an "open" active conformation, depending on the phosphorylation status of a tyrosine residue at the C-terminus. When this residue is phosphorylated, it interacts with an SH2 domain in the middle of Src, blocking the catalytic site. Upon dephosphorylation of this specific tyrosine, the SH2 domain is released, and the protein unfolds, allowing autophosphorylation of another tyrosine residue situated within the enzyme's activation loop, rendering the kinase fully active [137]. It is important to point out that cadherin ligation and clustering may act as an activation signal for some kinases. Most notably, Src and Fer have been shown to be recruited to the membrane upon cadherin binding [138, 139], and EGFR signaling was shown to be stimulated by AJ formation independently of EGF ligand [140]. Furthermore, cadherin clustering has been found to indirectly induce activation of Rho GTPases [141], which in turn could activate S/T kinases.

4. Phosphorylation Targets within the AJ

The AJ can conceptually be divided into four layers (Table 2). The first, in the plane of the membrane, is where cadherins and other transmembrane proteins, such as nectin and AJAP1, reside. The next layer consists of membrane-bound adaptors, such as ERM proteins and MAGI1, and adaptors that directly bind transmembrane proteins, such as p120- and β-catenin (bind cadherin) and afadin (binds nectin). The following layer is composed of adaptor proteins, such as α-catenin and vinculin, which bind to the second layer adaptors and also bind F-actin. F-actin, along with actin-binding proteins, such as α-actinin, and actin regulators, such as cortactin, would be considered the last layer. Regulatory proteins, such as GAPs, GEFs, and GTPases, can be found throughout the AJ as reviewed in [14, 142].

There is evidence demonstrating both Y and S/T phosphorylation of proteins in all layers of the AJ (Table 2). As illustrated in Figure 1, often the same kinase will phosphorylate proteins from different layers. For example, Abl

TABLE 1: Kinases and phosphatases regulating phosphorylation of AJ proteins.

Gene symbol	Protein name	Phosphorylation type	Localization	Reference
Kinases				
SRC	Proto-oncogene tyrosine-protein kinase Src	Tyr	nonreceptor	[23, 30, 31]
CSK	c-src tyrosine kinase	Tyr	nonreceptor	[24, 32, 33]
FYN	Tyrosine-protein kinase Fyn	Tyr	nonreceptor	[34–36]
ABL1	Abl1	Tyr	nonreceptor	[37, 38]
SYK	Tyrosine protein kinase SYK	Tyr	nonreceptor	[39, 40]
PTK2B	Protein-tyrosine kinase 2-beta	Tyr	nonreceptor	[41–43]
FER	Tyrosine-protein kinase Fer	Tyr	nonreceptor	[44]
EGFR	Epidermal growth factor receptor	Tyr	Receptor	[45]
cMET/HGF	Hepatocyte growth factor receptor	Tyr	Receptor	[46]
PRKCA	Protein kinase C alpha type	Ser/Thr	nonreceptor	[47]
PRKACA	cAMP-dependent protein Kinase catalytic subunit alpha	Ser/Thr	nonreceptor	[48, 49]
ROCK1	Rho-associated, coiled-coil containing protein kinase 1	Ser/Thr	nonreceptor	[50]
PRKCD	Protein kinase C delta type	Ser/Thr	nonreceptor	[51, 52]
CSNK1E	Casein kinase I isoform epsilon	Ser/Thr	nonreceptor	[53]
CSNK2A1	Casein kinase 2	Ser/Thr	nonreceptor	[54]
PAK1	Serine/threonine-protein kinase PAK 1	Ser/Thr	nonreceptor	[55–57]
MAPK8	JNK	Ser/Thr	nonreceptor	[58]
PRKD1	Protein kinase D1	Ser/Thr	nonreceptor	[59]
PRKCI	Atypical protein kinase C-lambda/iota	Ser/Thr	nonreceptor	[60]
PRKCZ	Protein kinase C zeta type	Ser/Thr	nonreceptor	[60]
MARK2	MAP/microtubule affinity-Regulating kinase 2, Par-1	Ser/Thr	nonreceptor	[61]
Phosphatases				
PTPN1	Tyrosine-protein phosphatase non receptor type 1, PTP1B	Tyr	nonreceptor	[19, 62–64]
PTPN6	Tyrosine-protein phosphatase non receptor type 6, SHP1	Tyr	nonreceptor	[65]
PTPN11	Tyrosine-protein phosphatase non-receptor type 11, SHP2	Tyr	nonreceptor	[66]
PTPN12	Tyrosine-protein phosphatase non-receptor type 12, PTP-PEST	Tyr	nonreceptor	[67]
PTPN14	Tyrosine-protein phosphatase non-receptor type 14, PEZ	Tyr	nonreceptor	[68]
ACP1	Acid phosphatase of erythrocyte, LMW-PTP	Tyr	nonreceptor	[69, 70]
PTPRJ	Receptor-type tyrosine-protein phosphatase eta (R-PTP-eta), DEP1	Tyr	Receptor	[71]
PTPRM	Receptor-type tyrosine-protein phosphatase mu (RPTP mu)	Tyr	Receptor	[72–74]
PTPRT	Receptor-type tyrosine-protein phosphatase T (R-PTP-T)	Tyr	Receptor	[75]
PTPRU	Receptor-type tyrosine-protein phosphatase U (R-PTP-U)	Tyr	Receptor	[76, 77]
PTPRK	Receptor-type tyrosine-protein phosphatase kappa	Tyr	Receptor	[78, 79]
PTPRF	Receptor-type tyrosine-protein phosphatase F, LAR	Tyr	Receptor	[80–82]
PPP2CA	Serine/threonine-protein phosphatase 2A catalytic subunit alpha isoform	Ser/Thr	nonreceptor	[83–85]

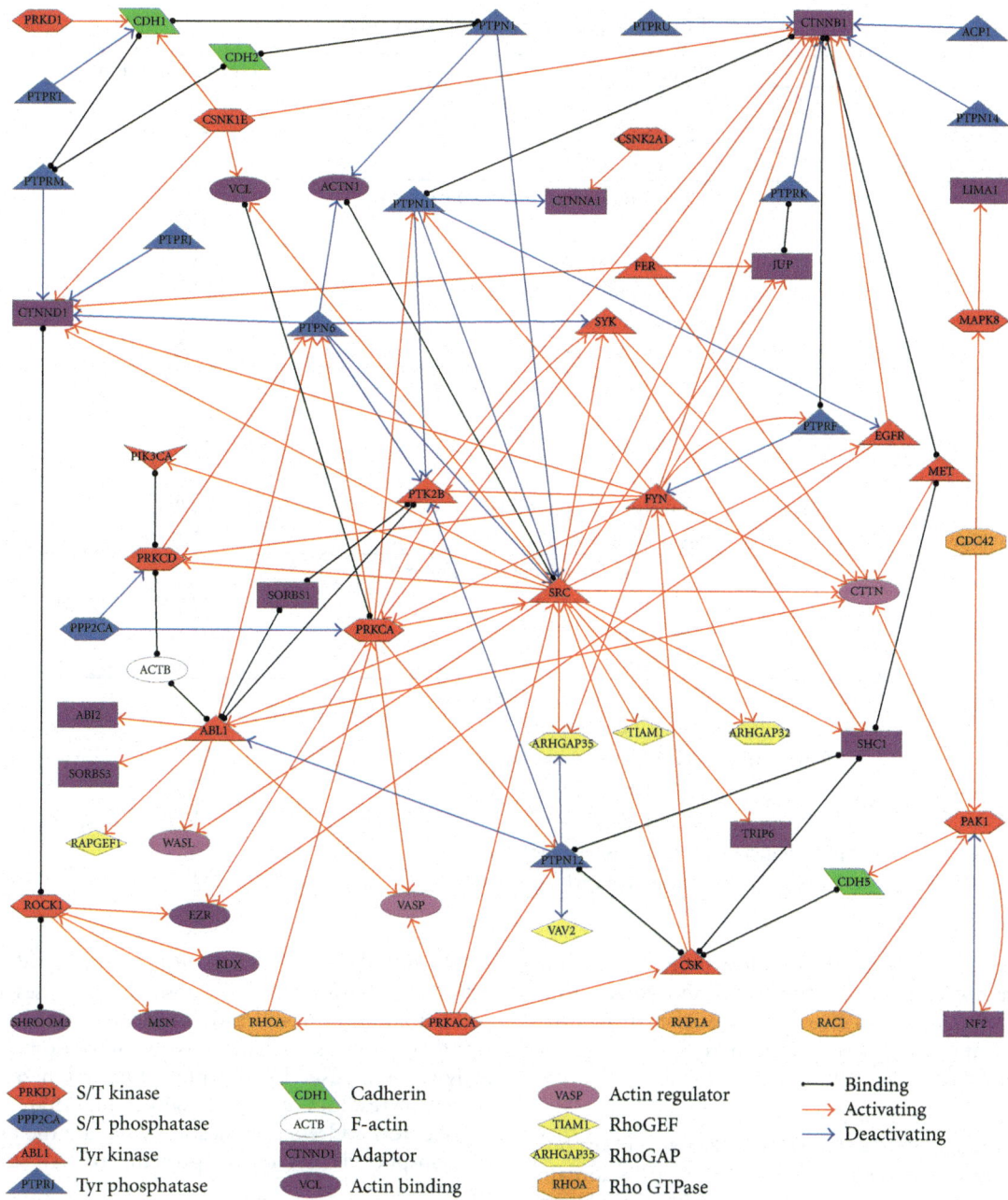

FIGURE 1: Network of phosphorylation enzymes and targets in the adherens junction.

phosphorylates actin regulators WASP and VASP [143, 144], as well as cadherin-bound adaptor δ-catenin [145] and second layer adaptors Abi2 and Vinexin (SORBS3) [146, 147].

Some AJ proteins have additional functions in the cell, and phosphorylation is also involved in regulating their non-AJ roles [148]. The most notable example is β-catenin, which plays an important role in the Wnt signaling pathway as a cotranscription factor of TCF/LEF [149]. Whether nonjunctional β-catenin will reach the nucleus or not depends on whether it is phosphorylated by GSK3 and Casein Kinse I in the "destruction complex" [150]. However,

such phosphorylation events taking place outside the context of AJ are beyond the scope of this paper.

For the phosphorylation events occurring within AJ an important question is how do they affect the target proteins?

5. Consequences of Phosphorylation on AJ Proteins

A phosphorylated tyrosine, serine, or threonine residue can affect a protein in three major ways: it can increase the affinity for another protein, it can inhibit a protein-protein

TABLE 2: Targets of phosphorylation in AJ.

Gene symbol	Protein name	Phosphorylated residue	Reference
Transmembrane			
CDH1	Ecadherin	S/Y	[54, 86, 87]
PVRL1	Nectin	Y	[88]
Cadherin- or membrane bound			
CTNNB1	β-catenin	S/T/Y	[16, 89, 90]
EZR, RDX, MSN	ERM proteins (ezrin/radixin/moesin)	S/T/Y	[91–93]
CTNND1	p_{120}-catenin	S/T/Y	[94, 95]
JUP	Gamma-catenin	Y	[96]
PARD3	Partitioning defective 3 homolog	S/T/Y	[97, 98]
Secondary adaptors			
CTNNA1	α-catenin	S/T/Y	[99, 100]
VCL	Vinculin	S/Y	[101, 102]
LIMA1	Eplin	S	[103]
VASP	Vasodilator-stimulated phosphoprotein	S/T/Y	[104–106]
SHC1	SHC-transforming protein 1	Y	[107, 108]
Actin and actin regulators			
ACTN1	α-actinin	S/Y	[109, 110]
CTTN	Cortactin	S/T/Y	[111, 112]
ACTB	F-actin	S/Y	[113–115]
GTPASE regulators			
PI3K	Phospho-inositide-3-kinase	Y	[116]
RAPGEF1	Rap guanine nucleotide exchange factor 1	Y	[117]
ARHGAP35	rho GAP p190A	Y	[118, 119]
ARHGAP32	p200RhoGAP	Y	[120, 121]
TIAM1	T-lymphoma invasion and metastasis-inducing protein 1	Y	[122]
VAV2	Vav 2 guanine nucleotide exchange factor	Y	[122, 123]

interaction, or it can activate enzymatic activity. In proteins with an intramolecular interaction, phosphorylation and dephosphorylation can elicit a conformational change in the protein. AJ components provide examples of each type of these outcomes, as detailed henceforth.

(1) Turn "on" Protein-Protein Interaction. Tyrosine phosphorylation can create a docking site for an SH2 or PTB domain of a partner protein. For example, tyrosine phosphorylation of cadherin creates docking sites for the SH2 domain of the adaptor SHC1 [151] and the PTB domain of the cell polarity protein Numb [152]. As mentioned earlier, SRC family kinases are inhibited by an intramolecular interaction between a central SH2 domain and a phosphorylated tyrosine at the C-terminus [137].

(2) Turn "off" Protein-Protein Interaction. Examples of interaction inhibition by phosphorylation are also found both between different proteins and intramolecularly: tyrosine phosphorylation of VE-cadherin at certain residues prevents the binding of p120-catenin and β-catenin [153]; phosphorylation of a threonine residue in the C-terminal actin binding domain of ERM proteins interferes with its interaction with the N-terminal FERM domain, helping to keep the protein in an active open conformation [154].

(3) Turn "on" Enzymatic Activity. Activation of the catalytic activity of tyrosine kinases and phosphatases by tyrosine phosphorylation has already been mentioned above [127]. Another important example is the activation of the motor activity of myosin by the phosphorylation of serine and threonine residues of myosin light chain [155].

We next address the question what are the ramifications of phosphorylation of AJ proteins on AJ structure and dynamics.

6. Global versus Specific Consequences of Phosphorylation on AJ Structure and Dynamics

Numerous experiments have been carried out over the years to address the role of Y and S/T phosphorylation in regulating AJ. Early experiments used broad-spectrum chemical inhibitors of kinases or phosphatases to conclude that phosphorylation negatively impacts cadherin function. For example, inhibition of S/T phosphatases by Okadaic acid or Calyculin-A was reported to lead to complete disassembly of AJ within an hour, and this disruption was attributed to an increase in S/T phosphorylation of β-catenin [89]. However, Calyculin-A has also been shown to increase actomyosin contractility in cells [156], suggesting that the disruption of

AJ in the above mentioned study may have been caused by mechanical tension at the junctions exceeding their adhesive strength. Inhibition of tyrosine phosphatases with sodium orthovanadate was reported to lead within minutes to a dramatic increase in phosphotyrosine signals at AJ, followed by the disassembly of AJ [157]. Consistent with the notion that excessive tyrosine phosphorylation in AJ causes their disassembly, cells expressing constitutively active Src kinase lost their AJ, and inhibition of tyrosine kinase activity by the drug tyrphostin was able to restore AJ in the Src-transformed cells [157]. These and similar experiments have led researchers in the late 90s of the previous century to the general conclusion that phosphorylation is a negative regulator of AJ.

However, in more recent years, there is accumulating evidence for a positive role of phosphorylation in AJ assembly, mainly coming out of loss-of-function experiments of specific kinases. For example, SRC and FYN were found to be essential for the formation of AJ in mouse keratinocytes [158]. Moreover, SRC activity was shown *in vitro* to be important for the recruitment of PI3K to AJ and the ability of cells to expand nascent cadherin-adhesive contacts [159]. Along the same lines, ABL1 tyrosine kinase activity was shown to be important for the maintenance of adherens junctions in epithelial cells [37], and S/T phosphorylation of E-cadherin by protein kinase D1 (PRKD1) was found to be associated with increased cellular adhesion and decreased cellular motility in prostate cancer [59].

Hence, the emerging view is that it is not possible to generalize the effect of phosphorylation on AJ. With some phosphorylation events leading to the switching "on" of a protein or interaction and other phosphorylation events, even on the same protein, serving as a switch "off", the effect of phosphorylation on AJ dynamics has to be examined on a residue-by-residue basis. After we delineate the effect of each individual phosphorylation event, we should be able to integrate this information into a single network of interconnected switches and perhaps then we can follow the global effects of a single phosphorylation switch, starting, for example, with hepatocyte growth factor stimulation [160].

7. Consequences of Specific Phosphorylation Events on AJ, Composition and Dynamics

We close this paper by giving a few examples of cases in which the consequences of specific phosphorylation events are known. The phosphorylation events presented occur on proteins from each layer of the AJ as well as one cell polarity protein.

(1) Cadherin. Serine phosphorylation of residues S840, S851 and S853 in the C-terminus of human E-cadherin (likely by CSNK1E or PRKD1) increases the binding affinity towards β-catenin, whereas phosphorylation of S846 is said to inhibit the same interaction [86]. Stronger binding of β-catenin to E-cadherin is conducive to a stronger AJ structure. Tyrosine phosphorylation of VE-cadherin at two critical tyrosines,

Y658 and Y731, is sufficient to prevent the binding of p120- and β-catenin, respectively [161]. Phosphorylation by Src of three tyrosines in position 753–755 on human E-cadherin creates a docking site for the E3-ligase Hakai [162]. Ubiquitination of E-cadherin by Hakai leads to internalization of E-cadherin facilitating disassembly of the AJ [162, 163].

(2) P120-Catenin. Eight tyrosine residues in the N-terminus of p120-catenin can be phosphorylated by Src [94]. Upon phosphorylation, these sites serve as docking sites for the recruitment of interacting proteins carrying SH2 domains, such as the tyrosine phosphatase SHP-1 [164]. Under certain conditions tyrosine phosphorylation of p120-catenin was shown to increase its affinity to cadherin, while in other instances such an increase was not observed (reviewed in [95]). The affinity of p120-catenin to cadherin is significant for AJ dynamics because p120-catenin protects cadherin from being internalized [165].

(3) Zyxin. Phosphorylation of S142 of zyxin is thought to result in the release of an intramolecular head-tail interaction [166]. Opening of the protein expose its ACTA repeats that recruit VASP, whose actin polymerization activity (see below) is important for AJ assembly and maintenance. Since zyxin-mediated recruitment of VASP has a positive effect on AJ [167, 168], it is not surprising that expression of a zyxin phosphomimetic mutant results in ultrastable AJ [166].

(4) VASP (Vasodilator Stimulated Phosphoprotein). As its name suggests, VASP is often found phosphorylated in cells. Three phosphorylation sites on residues S157, S239, and T274 are phosphorylated by PKA and PKG, as well as PKC [169, 170] and dephosphorylated by unknown phosphatase/s. The phosphorylation of VASP was shown to reduce its affinity towards actin [171] and essentially turn off its actin bundling and anticapping/elongation activity [171, 172]. VASP-mediated actin elongation is important for the formation of AJ and for the maintenance of actin structures associated with AJ [173, 174]. Thus, the consequence of VASP phosphorylation is to negatively regulate AJ assembly and maintenance.

(5) PARD3. In *Drosophila* epithelial cells the par-3 ortholog Bazooka is confined to AJ as a result of phosphorylation by either apical or basal polarity complexes [4]. At the apical side of cells Bazooka is phosphorylated by aPKC, resulting in its release from the cortex [175, 176]. In the basolateral membrane Par1 kinase phosphorylates Bazooka on unique sites that also lead to its cortical release [4]. Recently, it was shown that the ratio between Par-1 and aPKC determines the position of Bazooka and AJ along the lateral side and a reduction in Par-1 kinase activity leads to a basal shift of AJ followed by folding of the epithelial sheet [177].

8. Conclusions and Outlook

From the examples presented above, it is clear that phosphorylation switches play a pivotal role in regulating AJ assembly and disassembly dynamics. At the same time it is also clear that our knowledge is only scratching the surface of the phosphorylation network regulating AJ. For the majority of known phosphorylation events in AJ, we know either of a kinase or of a phosphatase involved, but rarely do we know both. Furthermore, while traditional biochemistry techniques have facilitated the characterization of a handful of phosphorylation events on AJ proteins, phosphoproteomic data indicates that the majority of AJ proteins are phosphorylated on multiple serine/threonine and tyrosine residues [178]. Phosphoproteomics, which utilizes a variety of techniques to label cells, enrich for phosphorylated peptides and identify them using mass-spectrometry (reviewed in [179–181]), not only highlights the hole in our knowledge but also offers the means to fill it.

Phospho-proteomics offers an unbiased and comprehensive snapshot of phosphorylation events, and several different approaches can be taken to elucidate phosphorylation switches in AJ: during normal assembly and maturation, following a signal for disassembly, or when a certain kinase or phosphatase is activated or missing (e.g., [39, 182–184]). The phospho-proteomic data obtained, especially if it is dynamic, can be used for a systems level analysis of phosphorylation switches in AJ [185, 186], but it seems likely to us that before the network can be modeled in a meaningful way more in depth characterization of specific phosphorylation events will be necessary, using cell biological techniques.

While for the discovery and mapping of phosphorylation events in AJ, one wants to be as comprehensive as possible, when it comes to characterizing a particular switch the more specific the tools, the better. One example of a specific tool is phosphorylation site-specific antibodies, such as those recognizing individual phosphorylation events on β-catenin and p-120-catenin [187, 188]. Another example are site-specific phospho-mimetic or nonphosphorylatable mutations, such as those successfully applied to the study of the effects of phosphorylation on cortactin, VASP, VE-cadherin, zyxin, and paxillin [153, 166, 189–191].

Facing an ever-changing landscape of forces and signaling cues, a cell must respond rapidly by adjusting the strength of its AJs according to need. For this it relies on continuous turnover and assembly of core AJ components. Phosphorylation is particularly suitable for regulating the balance between assembly and disassembly as it is rapid and affects the AJ proteins directly. Feedback loops must guarantee a combination of phosphorylated residues at AJ that matches the requirements for a given condition. Experiments have shown that when it comes to phosphorylation both "all on" and "all off" treatments are deleterious to AJ. The challenge now is to elucidate the mechanisms by which the cell maintains a "just right" level of phosphorylation in AJ. While phosphorylation is probably the most prominent regulatory switch controlling cell adhesion, other switches, such as GTPases, lipids and proteases, do exist [192]. A future challenge, therefore, will be to integrate the phosphorylation switch network with the other regulatory switches to facilitate a true understanding of how different signaling pathways and force regulate AJ dynamics.

Acknowledgment

This paper was made possible by an NRF fellowship awarded to R. Zaidel-Bar by the Singapore National Research Foundation.

References

[1] K. J. Green, S. Getsios, S. Troyanovsky, and L. M. Godsel, "Intercellular junction assembly, dynamics, and homeostasis," *Cold Spring Harbor Perspectives in Biology*, vol. 2, no. 2, p. a000125, 2010.

[2] M. Takeichi, "Cadherin cell adhesion receptors as a morphogenetic regulator," *Science*, vol. 251, no. 5000, pp. 1451–1455, 1991.

[3] B. Baum and M. Georgiou, "Dynamics of adherens junctions in epithelial establishment, maintenance, and remodeling," *Journal of Cell Biology*, vol. 192, no. 6, pp. 907–917, 2011.

[4] D. St Johnston and B. Sanson, "Epithelial polarity and morphogenesis," *Current Opinion in Cell Biology*, vol. 23, no. 5, pp. 540–546, 2011.

[5] S. Yonemura, Y. Wada, T. Watanabe, A. Nagafuchi, and M. Shibata, "α-Catenin as a tension transducer that induces adherens junction development," *Nature Cell Biology*, vol. 12, no. 6, pp. 533–542, 2010.

[6] T. Lecuit, "Adhesion remodeling underlying tissue morphogenesis," *Trends in Cell Biology*, vol. 15, no. 1, pp. 34–42, 2005.

[7] T. J. C. Harris, "Adherens junction assembly and function in the *Drosophila* embryo," *International Review of Cell and Molecular Biology*, vol. 293, pp. 45–83, 2012.

[8] A. M. Lynch and J. Hardin, "The assembly and maintenance of epithelial junctions in C. Elegans," *Frontiers in Bioscience*, vol. 14, no. 4, pp. 1414–1432, 2009.

[9] U. H. Frixen, J. Behrens, M. Sachs et al., "E-cadherin-mediated cell-cell adhesion prevents invasiveness of human carcinoma cells," *Journal of Cell Biology*, vol. 113, no. 1, pp. 173–185, 1991.

[10] J. Yoshino, T. Monkawa, M. Tsuji, M. Inukai, H. Itoh, and M. Hayashi, "Snail1 is involved in the renal epithelial-mesenchymal transition," *Biochemical and Biophysical Research Communications*, vol. 362, no. 1, pp. 63–68, 2007.

[11] R. S. B. Clark, H. Bayir, and L. W. Jenkins, "Posttranslational protein modifications," *Critical Care Medicine*, vol. 33, no. 12, pp. S407–S409, 2005.

[12] S. Roura, S. Miravet, J. Piedra, A. García De Herreros, and M. Duñachl, "Regulation of E-cadherin/catenin association by tyrosine phosphorylation," *Journal of Biological Chemistry*, vol. 274, no. 51, pp. 36734–36740, 1999.

[13] R. Michalides, T. Volberg, and B. Geiger, "Augmentation of adherens junction formation in mesenchymal cells by co-expression of N-CAM or short-term stimulation of tyrosine-phosphorylation," *Cell Adhesion and Communication*, vol. 2, no. 6, pp. 481–490, 1994.

[14] V. G. Brunton, I. R. J. MacPherson, and M. C. Frame, "Cell adhesion receptors, tyrosine kinases and actin modulators: a complex three-way circuitry," *Biochimica et Biophysica Acta*, vol. 1692, no. 2-3, pp. 121–144, 2004.

[15] J. M. Daniel and A. B. Reynolds, "Tyrosine phosphorylation and cadherin/catenin function," *BioEssays*, vol. 19, no. 10, pp. 883–891, 1997.

[16] J. Lilien and J. Balsamo, "The regulation of cadherin-mediated adhesion by tyrosine phosphorylation/dephosphorylation of β-catenin," *Current Opinion in Cell Biology*, vol. 17, no. 5, pp. 459–465, 2005.

[17] T. J. C. Harris and M. Peifer, "Decisions, decisions: β-catenin chooses between adhesion and transcription," *Trends in Cell Biology*, vol. 15, no. 5, pp. 234–237, 2005.

[18] M.-H. Park, D.-J. Kim, S.-T. You et al., "Phosphorylation of β-catenin at serine 663 regulates its transcriptional activity," *Biochemical and Biophysical Research Communications*, vol. 419, no. 3, pp. 543–549, 2012.

[19] J. Balsamo, T. Leung, H. Ernst, M. K. B. Zanin, S. Hoffman, and J. Lilien, "Regulated binding of a PTP1B-like phosphatase to N-cadherin: control of cadherin-mediated adhesion by dephosphorylation of β-catenin," *Journal of Cell Biology*, vol. 134, no. 3, pp. 801–813, 1996.

[20] S. Tsukita, K. Oishi, T. Akiyama, Y. Yamanashi, T. Yamamoto, and S. Tsukita, "Specific proto-oncogenic tyrosine kinases of src family are enriched in cell-to-cell adherens junctions where the level of tyrosine phosphorylation is elevated," *Journal of Cell Biology*, vol. 113, no. 4, pp. 867–879, 1991.

[21] A. L. Smith, M. R. Dohn, M. V. Brown, and A. B. Reynolds, "Association of Rho-associated protein kinase 1 with E-cadherin complexes is mediated by p120-catenin," *Molecular Biology of the Cell*, vol. 23, no. 1, pp. 99–110, 2012.

[22] J. Jiang, D. Dean, R. C. Burghardt, and A. R. Parrish, "Disruption of cadherin/catenin expression, localization, and interactions during HgCl2-induced nephrotoxicity," *Toxicological Sciences*, vol. 80, no. 1, pp. 170–182, 2004.

[23] N. P. Y. Lee and C. Y. Cheng, "Protein kinases and adherens junction dynamics in the seminiferous epithelium of the rat testis," *Journal of Cellular Physiology*, vol. 202, no. 2, pp. 344–360, 2005.

[24] U. Baumeister, R. Funke, K. Ebnet, H. Vorschmitt, S. Koch, and D. Vestweber, "Association of Csk to VE-cadherin and inhibition of cell proliferation," *EMBO Journal*, vol. 24, no. 9, pp. 1686–1695, 2005.

[25] P. Sheth, A. Seth, K. J. Atkinson et al., "Acetaldehyde dissociates the PTP1B-E-cadherin-β-catenin complex in Caco-2 cell monolayers by a phosphorylation-dependent mechanism," *Biochemical Journal*, vol. 402, no. 2, pp. 291–300, 2007.

[26] S. P. S. Monga, W. M. Mars, P. Pediaditakis et al., "Hepatocyte growth factor induces Wnt-independent nuclear translocation of β-catenin after Met-β-catenin dissociation in hepatocytes," *Cancer Research*, vol. 62, no. 7, pp. 2064–2071, 2002.

[27] B. Aicher, M. M. Lerch, T. Müller, J. Schilling, and A. Ullrich, "Cellular redistribution of protein tyrosine phosphatases LAR and PTPσ by inducible proteolytic processing," *Journal of Cell Biology*, vol. 138, no. 3, pp. 681–696, 1997.

[28] W. H. Ziegler, U. Tigges, A. Zieseniss, and B. M. Jockusch, "A lipid-regulated docking site on vinculin for protein kinase C," *Journal of Biological Chemistry*, vol. 277, no. 9, pp. 7396–7404, 2002.

[29] T. Nishimura and M. Takeichi, "Shroom3-mediated recruitment of Rho kinases to the apical cell junctions regulates epithelial and neuroepithelial planar remodeling," *Development*, vol. 135, no. 8, pp. 1493–1502, 2008.

[30] M. Shindo, H. Wada, M. Kaido et al., "Dual function of Src in the maintenance of adherens junctions during tracheal epithelial morphogenesis," *Development*, vol. 135, no. 7, pp. 1355–1364, 2008.

[31] D. W. Owens, G. W. McLean, A. W. Wyke et al., "The catalytic activity of the Src family kinases is required to disrupt cadherin-dependent cell-cell contacts," *Molecular Biology of the Cell*, vol. 11, no. 1, pp. 51–64, 2000.

[32] H. Jin, B. Garmy-Susini, C. J. Avraamides, K. Stoletov, R. L. Klemke, and J. A. Varner, "A PKA-Csk-pp60Src signaling pathway regulates the switch between endothelial cell invasion and cell-cell adhesion during vascular sprouting," *Blood*, vol. 116, no. 25, pp. 5773–5783, 2010.

[33] W. Rengifo-Cam, A. Konishi, N. Morishita et al., "Csk defines the ability of integrin-mediated cell adhesion and migration in human colon cancer cells: implication for a potential role in cancer metastasis," *Oncogene*, vol. 23, no. 1, pp. 289–297, 2004.

[34] J. Piedra, S. Miravet, J. Castaño et al., "p120 catenin-associated Fer and Fyn tyrosine kinases regulate β-catenin Tyr-142 phosphorylation and β-catenin-α-catenin interaction," *Molecular and Cellular Biology*, vol. 23, no. 7, pp. 2287–2297, 2003.

[35] R. Y. J. Huang, S. M. Wang, C. Y. Hsieh, and J. C. Wu, "Lysophosphatidic acid induces ovarian cancer cell dispersal by activating Fyn kinase associated with p120-catenin," *International Journal of Cancer*, vol. 123, no. 4, pp. 801–809, 2008.

[36] K. L. Hsu, H. J. Fan, Y. C. Chen et al., "Protein kinase C-Fyn kinase cascade mediates the oleic acid-induced disassembly of neonatal rat cardiomyocyte adherens junctions," *International Journal of Biochemistry and Cell Biology*, vol. 41, no. 7, pp. 1536–1546, 2009.

[37] N. L. Zandy, M. Playford, and A. M. Pendergast, "Abl tyrosine kinases regulate cell- cell adhesion through Rho GTPases," *Proceedings of the National Academy of Sciences of the United States of America*, vol. 104, no. 45, pp. 17686–17691, 2007.

[38] E. E. Grevengoed, J. J. Loureiro, T. L. Jesse, and M. Peifer, "Abelson kinase regulates epithelial morphogenesis in *Drosophila*," *Journal of Cell Biology*, vol. 155, no. 7, pp. 1185–1197, 2001.

[39] R. M. Larive, S. Urbach, J. Poncet et al., "Phosphoproteomic analysis of Syk kinase signaling in human cancer cells reveals its role in cell-cell adhesion," *Oncogene*, vol. 28, no. 24, pp. 2337–2347, 2009.

[40] X. Zhang, U. Shrikhande, B. M. Alicie, Q. Zhou, and R. L. Geahlen, "Role of the protein tyrosine kinase Syk in regulating cell-cell adhesion and motility in breast cancer cells," *Molecular Cancer Research*, vol. 7, no. 5, pp. 634–644, 2009.

[41] J. D. Van Buul, E. C. Anthony, M. Fernandez-Borja, K. Burridge, and P. L. Hordijk, "Proline-rich tyrosine kinase 2 (Pyk2) mediates vascular endothelial-cadherin-based cell-cell adhesion by regulating β-catenin tyrosine phosphorylation," *Journal of Biological Chemistry*, vol. 280, no. 22, pp. 21129–21136, 2005.

[42] F. De Amicis, M. Lanzino, A. Kisslinger et al., "Loss of proline-rich tyrosine kinase 2 function induces spreading and motility of epithelial prostate cells," *Journal of Cellular Physiology*, vol. 209, no. 1, pp. 74–80, 2006.

[43] R. J. Cain, B. Vanhaesebroeck, and A. J. Ridley, "The PI3K p110α isoform regulates endothelial adherens junctions via Pyk2 and Rac1," *Journal of Cell Biology*, vol. 188, no. 6, pp. 863–876, 2010.

[44] R. Rosato, J. M. Veltmaat, J. Groffen, and N. Heisterkamp, "Involvement of the tyrosine kinase Fer in cell adhesion," *Molecular and Cellular Biology*, vol. 18, no. 10, pp. 5762–5770, 1998.

[45] H. Hoschuetzky, H. Aberle, and R. Kemler, "β-Catenin mediates the interaction of the cadherin-catenin complex with epidermal growth factor receptor," *Journal of Cell Biology*, vol. 127, no. 5, pp. 1375–1380, 1994.

[46] G. Davies, W. G. Jiang, and M. D. Mason, "HGF/SF modifies the interaction between its receptor c-Met, and the E-cadherin/catenin complex in prostate cancer cells," *International Journal of Molecular Medicine*, vol. 7, no. 4, pp. 385–388, 2001.

[47] C. L. Williams and J. D. Noti, "Reduced expression of Wnt-1 and E-cadherin, and diminished beta-catenin stability in MCF-7 breast cancer cells that overexpress protein kinase C-alpha," *International Journal of Oncology*, vol. 19, no. 6, pp. 1227–1233, 2001.

[48] M. J. Boucher, P. Laprise, and N. Rivard, "Cyclic AMP-dependent protein kinase A negatively modulates adherens junction integrity and differentiation of intestinal epithelial cells," *Journal of Cellular Physiology*, vol. 202, no. 1, pp. 178–190, 2005.

[49] F. Leve, W. De Souza, and J. A. Morgado-Díaz, "A cross-link between protein kinase A and Rho-family GTPases signaling mediates cell-cell adhesion and actin cytoskeleton organization in epithelial cancer cells," *Journal of Pharmacology and Experimental Therapeutics*, vol. 327, no. 3, pp. 777–788, 2008.

[50] K. Taguchi, T. Ishiuchi, and M. Takeichi, "Mechanosensitive EPLIN-dependent remodeling of adherens junctions regulates epithelial reshaping," *Journal of Cell Biology*, vol. 194, no. 4, pp. 643–656, 2011.

[51] C. L. Chen and H. C. Chen, "Functional suppression of E-cadherin by protein kinase Cδ," *Journal of Cell Science*, vol. 122, no. 4, pp. 513–523, 2009.

[52] R. Singh, P. Lei, and S. T. Andreadis, "PKC-δ binds to E-cadherin and mediates EGF-induced cell scattering," *Experimental Cell Research*, vol. 315, no. 17, pp. 2899–2913, 2009.

[53] D. Casagolda, B. Del Valle-Pérez, G. Valls et al., "A p120-catenin-CK1ε complex regulates Wnt signaling," *Journal of Cell Science*, vol. 123, no. 15, pp. 2621–2631, 2010.

[54] H. Lickert, A. Bauer, R. Kemler, and J. Stappert, "Casein kinase II phosphorylation of E-cadherin increases E-cadherin/β- catenin interaction and strengthens cell-cell adhesion," *Journal of Biological Chemistry*, vol. 275, no. 7, pp. 5090–5095, 2000.

[55] C. Pirraglia, J. Walters, and M. M. Myat, "Pak1 control of E-cadherin endocytosis regulates salivary gland lumen size and shape," *Development*, vol. 137, no. 24, pp. 4177–4189, 2010.

[56] S. Elloul, O. Vaksman, H. T. Stavnes, C. G. Trope, B. Davidson, and R. Reich, "Mesenchymal-to-epithelial transition determinants as characteristics of ovarian carcinoma effusions," *Clinical and Experimental Metastasis*, vol. 27, no. 3, pp. 161–172, 2010.

[57] H. He, A. Shulkes, and G. S. Baldwin, "PAK1 interacts with β-catenin and is required for the regulation of the β-catenin signalling pathway by gastrins," *Biochimica et Biophysica Acta*, vol. 1783, no. 10, pp. 1943–1954, 2008.

[58] M. H. Lee, P. Koria, J. Qu, and S. T. Andreadis, "JNK phosphorylates β-catenin and regulates adherens junctions," *FASEB Journal*, vol. 23, no. 11, pp. 3874–3883, 2009.

[59] M. Jaggi, P. S. Rao, D. J. Smith et al., "E-cadherin phosphorylation by protein kinase D1/protein kinase Cμ is associated with altered cellular aggregation and motility in prostate cancer," *Cancer Research*, vol. 65, no. 2, pp. 483–492, 2005.

[60] A. Suzuki, T. Yamanaka, T. Hirose et al., "Atypical protein kinase C is involved in the evolutionarily conserved PAR protein complex and plays a critical role in establishing epithelia-specific junctional structures," *Journal of Cell Biology*, vol. 152, no. 6, pp. 1183–1196, 2001.

[61] M. Elbert, D. Cohen, and A. Müsch, "PAR1b promotes cell-cell adhesion and inhibits dishevelled-mediated transformation of Madin-Darby canine kidney cells," *Molecular Biology of the Cell*, vol. 17, no. 8, pp. 3345–3355, 2006.

[62] J. Balsamo, C. Arregui, T. Leung, and J. Lilien, "The nonreceptor protein tyrosine phosphatase PTP1B binds to the cytoplasmic domain of N-cadherin and regulates the cadherin-actin linkage," *Journal of Cell Biology*, vol. 143, no. 2, pp. 523–532, 1998.

[63] P. Pathre, C. Arregui, T. Wampler et al., "PTP1B regulates neurite extension mediated by cell-cell and cell-matrix adhesion molecules," *Journal of Neuroscience Research*, vol. 63, no. 2, pp. 143–150, 2001.

[64] M. V. Hernández, D. P. Wehrendt, and C. O. Arregui, "The protein tyrosine phosphatase PTP1B is required for efficient delivery of N-cadherin to the cell surface," *Molecular Biology of the Cell*, vol. 21, no. 8, pp. 1387–1397, 2010.

[65] J. Schnekenburger, J. Mayerle, B. Krüger et al., "Protein tyrosine phosphatase κ and SHP-1 are involved in the regulation of cell-cell contacts at adherens junctions in the exocrine pancreas," *Gut*, vol. 54, no. 10, pp. 1445–1455, 2005.

[66] J. A. Ukropec, M. K. Hollinger, S. M. Salva, and M. J. Woolkalis, "SHP2 association with VE-cadherin complexes in human endothelial cells is regulated by thrombin," *Journal of Biological Chemistry*, vol. 275, no. 8, pp. 5983–5986, 2000.

[67] R. Espejo, W. Rengifo-Cam, M. D. Schaller, B. M. Evers, and S. K. Sastry, "PTP-PEST controls motility, adherens junction assembly, and Rho GTPase activity in colon cancer cells," *American Journal of Physiology*, vol. 299, no. 2, pp. C454–C463, 2010.

[68] C. Wadham, J. R. Gamble, M. A. Vadas, and Y. Khew-Goodall, "The protein tyrosine phosphatase Pez is a major phosphatase of adherens junctions and dephosphorylates β-catenin," *Molecular Biology of the Cell*, vol. 14, no. 6, pp. 2520–2529, 2003.

[69] M. L. Taddei, P. Chiarugi, P. Cirri et al., "β-catenin interacts with low-molecular-weight protein tyrosine phosphatase leading to cadherin-mediated cell-cell adhesion increase," *Cancer Research*, vol. 62, no. 22, pp. 6489–6499, 2002.

[70] W. B. Fang, R. C. Ireton, G. Zhuang, T. Takahashi, A. Reynolds, and J. Chen, "Overexpression of EPHA2 receptor destabilizes adherens junctions via a RhoA-dependent mechanism," *Journal of Cell Science*, vol. 121, no. 3, pp. 358–368, 2008.

[71] L. J. Holsinger, K. Ward, B. Duffield, J. Zachwieja, and B. Jallal, "The transmembrane receptor protein tyrosine phosphatase DEP1 interacts with p120ctn," *Oncogene*, vol. 21, no. 46, pp. 7067–7076, 2002.

[72] G. C. M. Zondag, A. B. Reynolds, and W. H. Moolenaar, "Receptor protein-tyrosine phosphatase RPTPμ binds to and dephosphorylates the catenin p120(ctn)," *Journal of Biological Chemistry*, vol. 275, no. 15, pp. 11264–11269, 2000.

[73] S. M. Brady-Kalnay, T. Mourton, J. P. Nixon et al., "Dynamic interactions of PTPμ with multiple cadherins in vivo," *Journal of Cell Biology*, vol. 141, no. 1, pp. 287–296, 1998.

[74] S. Hiscox and W. G. Jiang, "Association of PTPμ with catenins in cancer cells: a possible role for E-cadherin," *International Journal of Oncology*, vol. 13, no. 5, pp. 1077–1080, 1998.

[75] J. A. Besco, R. Hooft van Huijsduijnen, A. Frostholm, and A. Rotter, "Intracellular substrates of brain-enriched receptor protein tyrosine phosphatase rho (RPTPρ/PTPRT)," *Brain Research*, vol. 1116, no. 1, pp. 50–57, 2006.

[76] H. X. Yan, Y. Q. He, H. Dong et al., "Physical and functional interaction between receptor-like protein tyrosine phosphatase PCP-2 and β-catenin," *Biochemistry*, vol. 41, no. 52, pp. 15854–15860, 2002.

[77] H. X. Yan, W. Yang, R. Zhang et al., "Protein-tyrosine phosphatase PCP-2 inhibits β-catenin signaling and increases E-cadherin-dependent cell adhesion," *Journal of Biological Chemistry*, vol. 281, no. 22, pp. 15423–15433, 2006.

[78] L. Novellino, A. De Filippo, P. Deho et al., "PTPRK negatively regulates transcriptional activity of wild type and mutated oncogenic β-catenin and affects membrane distribution of β-catenin/E-cadherin complexes in cancer cells," *Cellular Signalling*, vol. 20, no. 5, pp. 872–883, 2008.

[79] C. Wang, Z. Li, Z. Yang et al., "The effect of receptor protein tyrosine phosphatase kappa on the change of cell adhesion and proliferation induced by N-acetylglu-cosaminyltransferase V," *Journal of Cellular Biochemistry*, vol. 109, no. 1, pp. 113–123, 2010.

[80] R. M. Kypta, H. Su, and L. F. Reichardt, "Association between a transmembrane protein tyrosine phosphatase and the cadherin-catenin complex," *Journal of Cell Biology*, vol. 134, no. 6, pp. 1519–1529, 1996.

[81] J. R. Symons, C. M. Levea, and R. A. Mooney, "Expression of the leucocyte common antigen-related (LAR) tyrosine phosphatase is regulated by cell density through functional E-cadherin complexes," *Biochemical Journal*, vol. 365, no. 2, pp. 513–519, 2002.

[82] T. Müller, A. Choidas, E. Reichmann, and A. Ullrich, "Phosphorylation and free pool of β-catenin are regulated by tyrosine kinases and tyrosine phosphatases during epithelial cell migration," *Journal of Biological Chemistry*, vol. 274, no. 15, pp. 10173–10183, 1999.

[83] M. Nita-Lazar, I. Rebustini, J. Walker, and M. A. Kukuruzin-ska, "Hypoglycosylated E-cadherin promotes the assembly of tight junctions through the recruitment of PP2A to adherens junctions," *Experimental Cell Research*, vol. 316, no. 11, pp. 1871–1884, 2010.

[84] K. Suzuki and K. Takahashi, "Induction of E-cadherin endocytosis by loss of protein phosphatase 2A expression in human breast cancers," *Biochemical and Biophysical Research Communications*, vol. 349, no. 1, pp. 255–260, 2006.

[85] J. Götz, A. Probst, C. Mistl, R. M. Nitsch, and E. Ehler, "Distinct role of protein phosphatase 2A subunit Cα in the regulation of E-cadherin and β-catenin during development," *Mechanisms of Development*, vol. 93, no. 1-2, pp. 83–93, 2000.

[86] S. Dupre-Crochet, A. Figueroa, C. Hogan et al., "Casein kinase 1 is a novel negative regulator of E-cadherin-based cell-cell contacts," *Molecular and Cellular Biology*, vol. 27, no. 10, pp. 3804–3816, 2007.

[87] J. Qi, J. Wang, O. Romanyuk, and C. H. Siu, "Involvement of Src family kinases in N-cadherin phosphorylation and β-catenin dissociation during transendothelial migration of melanoma cells," *Molecular Biology of the Cell*, vol. 17, no. 3, pp. 1261–1272, 2006.

[88] M. Kikyo, T. Matozaki, A. Kodama, H. Kawabe, H. Nakanishi, and Y. Takai, "Cell-cell adhesion-mediated tyrosine phosphorylation of nectin-2δ, an immunoglobulin-like cell adhesion molecule at adherens junctions," *Oncogene*, vol. 19, no. 35, pp. 4022–4028, 2000.

[89] M. Serres, C. Grangeasse, M. Haftek, Y. Durocher, B. Duclos, and D. Schmitt, "Hyperphosphorylation of β-catenin on serine-threonine residues and loss of cell-cell contacts induced by calyculin A and okadaic acid in human epidermal cells," *Experimental Cell Research*, vol. 231, no. 1, pp. 163–172, 1997.

[90] H. S. Moon, E. A. Choi, H. Y. Park et al., "Expression and tyrosine phosphorylation of E-cadherin, β- and γ-catenin, and epidermal growth factor receptor in cervical cancer cells," *Gynecologic Oncology*, vol. 81, no. 3, pp. 355–359, 2001.

[91] L. Heiska and O. Carpén, "Src phosphorylates ezrin at tyrosine 477 and induces a phosphospecific association between ezrin and a kelch-repeat protein family member," *Journal of Biological Chemistry*, vol. 280, no. 11, pp. 10244–10252, 2005.

[92] R. Zhou, X. Cao, C. Watson et al., "Characterization of protein kinase A-mediated phosphorylation of ezrin in gastric parietal cell activation," *Journal of Biological Chemistry*, vol. 278, no. 37, pp. 35651–35659, 2003.

[93] J. Chen, J. A. Cohn, and L. J. Mandel, "Dephosphorylation of ezrin as an early event in renal microvillar breakdown and anoxic injury," *Proceedings of the National Academy of Sciences of the United States of America*, vol. 92, no. 16, pp. 7495–7499, 1995.

[94] D. J. Mariner, P. Anastasiadis, H. Keilhack, F. D. Böhmer, J. Wang, and A. B. Reynolds, "Identification of Src phosphorylation sites in the catenin p120 ctn," *Journal of Biological Chemistry*, vol. 276, no. 30, pp. 28006–28013, 2001.

[95] S. Alemà and A. M. Salvatore, "p120 catenin and phosphorylation: mechanisms and traits of an unresolved issue," *Biochimica et Biophysica Acta*, vol. 1773, no. 1, pp. 47–58, 2007.

[96] S. Miravet, J. Piedra, J. Castaño et al., "Tyrosine phosphorylation of plakoglobin causes contrary effects on its association with desmosomes and adherens junction components and modulates β-catenin-mediated transcription," *Molecular and Cellular Biology*, vol. 23, no. 20, pp. 7391–7402, 2003.

[97] Y. Wang, D. Du, L. Fang et al., "Tyrosine phosphorylated Par3 regulates epithelial tight junction assembly promoted by EGFR signaling," *EMBO Journal*, vol. 25, no. 21, pp. 5058–5070, 2006.

[98] A. Traweger, G. Wiggin, L. Taylor, S. A. Tate, P. Metalnikov, and T. Pawson, "Protein phosphatase 1 regulates the phosphorylation state of the polarity scaffold Par-3," *Proceedings of the National Academy of Sciences of the United States of America*, vol. 105, no. 30, pp. 10402–10407, 2008.

[99] J. Burks and Y. M. Agazie, "Modulation of α-catenin Tyr phosphorylation by SHP2 positively effects cell transformation induced by the constitutively active FGFR3," *Oncogene*, vol. 25, no. 54, pp. 7166–7179, 2006.

[100] H. Ji, J. Wang, H. Nika et al., "EGF-Induced ERK activation promotes CK2-mediated disassociation of α-catenin from β-catenin and transactivation of β-catenin," *Molecular Cell*, vol. 36, no. 4, pp. 547–559, 2009.

[101] S. Nakajo, K. Nakaya, and Y. Nakamura, "Phosphorylation of actin-binding proteins by casein kinases 1 and 2," *Biochemistry International*, vol. 15, no. 2, pp. 321–327, 1987.

[102] Z. Zhang, G. Izaguirre, S. Y. Lin, H. Y. Lee, E. Schaefer, and B. Haimovich, "The phosphorylation of vinculin on tyrosine residues 100 and 1065, mediated by Src kinases, affects cell spreading," *Molecular Biology of the Cell*, vol. 15, no. 9, pp. 4234–4247, 2004.

[103] M. Y. Han, H. Kosako, T. Watanabe, and S. Hattori, "Extracellular signal-regulated kinase/mitogen-activated protein kinase regulates actin organization and cell motility by phosphorylating the actin cross-linking protein EPLIN," *Molecular and Cellular Biology*, vol. 27, no. 23, pp. 8190–8204, 2007.

[104] M. Maruoka, M. Sato, Y. Yuan et al., "Abi-1-bridged tyrosine phosphorylation of VASP by Abelson kinase impairs association of VASP to focal adhesions and regulates leukaemic cell adhesion," *Biochemical Journal*, vol. 441, no. 3, pp. 889–899, 2012.

[105] D. M. Thomson, M. P. A. Ascione, J. Grange, C. Nelson, and M. D. H. Hansen, "Phosphorylation of VASP by AMPK alters actin binding and occurs at a novel site," *Biochemical and Biophysical Research Communications*, vol. 414, no. 1, pp. 215–219, 2011.

[106] A. Deguchi, J. W. Soh, H. Li, R. Pamukcu, W. J. Thompson, and I. B. Weinstein, "Vasodilator-stimulated phosphoprotein (VASP) phosphorylation provides a biomarker for the action of exisulind and related agents that activate protein kinase G.," *Molecular cancer therapeutics*, vol. 1, no. 10, pp. 803–809, 2002.

[107] S. F. Walk, M. E. March, and K. S. Ravichandran, "Roles of Lck, Syk and ZAP-70 tyrosine kinases in TCR-mediated phosphorylation of the adapter protein Shc," *European Journal of Immunology*, vol. 28, no. 8, pp. 2265–2275, 1998.

[108] P. Van Der Geer, S. Wiley, G. D. Gish, and T. Pawson, "The Shc adaptor protein is highly phosphorylated at conserved, twin tyrosine residues (Y239/240) that mediate protein-protein interactions," *Current Biology*, vol. 6, no. 11, pp. 1435–1444, 1996.

[109] M. Grønborg, T. Z. Kristiansen, A. Stensballe et al., "A mass spectrometry-based proteomic approach for identification of serine/threonine-phosphorylated proteins by enrichment with phospho-specific antibodies: identification of a novel protein, Frigg, as a protein kinase A substrate," *Molecular & Cellular Proteomics*, vol. 1, no. 7, pp. 517–527, 2002.

[110] H. Shao, C. Wu, and A. Wells, "Phosphorylation of α-actinin 4 upon epidermal growth factor exposure regulates its interaction with actin," *Journal of Biological Chemistry*, vol. 285, no. 4, pp. 2591–2600, 2010.

[111] W. Sangrar, Y. Gao, M. Scott, P. Truesdell, and P. A. Greer, "Fer-mediated cortactin phosphorylation is associated with efficient fibroblast migration and is dependent on reactive oxygen species generation during integrin-mediated cell adhesion," *Molecular and Cellular Biology*, vol. 27, no. 17, pp. 6140–6152, 2007.

[112] A. Grassart, V. Meas-Yedid, A. Dufour, J. C. Olivo-Marin, A. Dautry-Varsat, and N. Sauvonnet, "Pak1 phosphorylation enhances cortactin-N-WASP interaction in clathrin-caveolin-independent endocytosis," *Traffic*, vol. 11, no. 8, pp. 1079–1091, 2010.

[113] S. Van Delft, A. J. Verkleij, and J. Boonstra, "Epidermal growth factor induces serine phosphorylation of actin," *FEBS Letters*, vol. 357, no. 3, pp. 251–254, 1995.

[114] E. A. Papakonstanti and C. Stournaras, "Association of PI-3 kinase with PAK1 leads to actin phosphorylation and cytoskeletal reorganization," *Molecular Biology of the Cell*, vol. 13, no. 8, pp. 2946–2962, 2002.

[115] X. Liu, S. Shu, M. S. S. Hong, R. L. Levine, and E. D. Korn, "Phosphorylation of actin Tyr-53 inhibits filament nucleation and elongation and destabilizes filaments," *Proceedings of the National Academy of Sciences of the United States of America*, vol. 103, no. 37, pp. 13694–13699, 2006.

[116] A. Arcaro, M. Aubert, M. E. Espinosa del Hierro et al., "Critical role for lipid raft-associated Src kinases in activation of PI3K-Akt signalling," *Cellular Signalling*, vol. 19, no. 5, pp. 1081–1092, 2007.

[117] A. Mitra and V. Radha, "F-actin-binding domain of c-Abl regulates localized phosphorylation of C3G: role of C3G in c-Abl-mediated cell death," *Oncogene*, vol. 29, no. 32, pp. 4528–4542, 2010.

[118] R. M. Wolf, J. J. Wilkes, M. V. Chao, and M. D. Resh, "Tyrosine phosphorylation of p190 RhoGAP by Fyn regulates oligodendrocyte differentiation," *Journal of Neurobiology*, vol. 49, no. 1, pp. 62–78, 2001.

[119] R. W. Roof, M. D. Haskell, B. D. Dukes, N. Sherman, M. Kinter, and S. J. Parsons, "Phosphotyrosine (p-Tyr)-dependent and -independent mechanisms of p190 RhoGAP-p120 RasGAP interaction: Tyr 1105 of p190, a substrate for c-Src, is the sole p-Tyr mediator of complex formation," *Molecular and Cellular Biology*, vol. 18, no. 12, pp. 7052–7063, 1998.

[120] S. Taniguchi, H. Liu, T. Nakazawa, K. Yokoyama, T. Tezuka, and T. Yamamoto, "p250GAP, a neural RhoGAP protein, is associated with and phosphorylated by Fyn," *Biochemical and Biophysical Research Communications*, vol. 306, no. 1, pp. 151–155, 2003.

[121] S. Y. Moon, H. Zang, and Y. Zheng, "Characterization of a brain-specific Rho GTPase-activating protein, p200RhoGAP," *Journal of Biological Chemistry*, vol. 278, no. 6, pp. 4151–4159, 2003.

[122] J. M. Servitja, M. J. Marinissen, A. Sodhi, X. R. Bustelo, and J. S. Gutkind, "Rac1 function is required for Src-induced transformation: evidence of a role for Tiam1 and Vav2 in Rac activation by Src," *Journal of Biological Chemistry*, vol. 278, no. 36, pp. 34339–34346, 2003.

[123] S. K. Sastry, Z. Rajfur, B. P. Liu, J. F. Cote, M. L. Tremblay, and K. Burridge, "PTP-PEST couples membrane protrusion and tail retraction via VAV2 and p190RhoGAP," *Journal of Biological Chemistry*, vol. 281, no. 17, pp. 11627–11636, 2006.

[124] S. R. Hubbard and J. H. Till, "Protein tyrosine kinase structure and function," *Annual Review of Biochemistry*, vol. 69, pp. 373–398, 2000.

[125] A. W. Stoker, "Protein tyrosine phosphatases and signalling," *Journal of Endocrinology*, vol. 185, no. 1, pp. 19–33, 2005.

[126] G. C. M. Zondag and W. H. Moolenaar, "Receptor protein tyrosine phosphatases: involvement in cell-cell interaction and signaling," *Biochimie*, vol. 79, no. 8, pp. 477–483, 1997.

[127] S. Dadke, A. Kusari, and J. Kusari, "Phosphorylation and activation of protein tyrosine phosphatase (PTP) 1B by insulin receptor," *Molecular and Cellular Biochemistry*, vol. 221, no. 1-2, pp. 147–154, 2001.

[128] K. Fujisawa, A. Fujita, T. Ishizaki, Y. Saito, and S. Narumiya, "Identification of the Rho-binding domain of p160(ROCK), a Rho-associated coiled-coil containing protein kinase," *Journal of Biological Chemistry*, vol. 271, no. 38, pp. 23022–23028, 1996.

[129] W. Lu and B. J. Mayer, "Mechanism of activation of Pak1 kinase by membrane localization," *Oncogene*, vol. 18, no. 3, pp. 797–806, 1999.

[130] T. Rosenzweig, S. Aga-Mizrachi, A. Bak, and S. R. Sampson, "Src tyrosine kinase regulates insulin-induced activation

of protein kinase C (PKC) δ in skeletal muscle," *Cellular Signalling*, vol. 16, no. 11, pp. 1299–1308, 2004.

[131] K. Yoshida and D. Kufe, "Negative regulation of the SHPTP1 protein tyrosine phosphatase by protein kinase C δ in response to DNA damage," *Molecular Pharmacology*, vol. 60, no. 6, pp. 1431–1438, 2001.

[132] A. K. Somani, J. S. Bignon, G. B. Mills, K. A. Siminovitch, and D. R. Branch, "Src kinase activity is regulated by the SHP-1 protein-tyrosine phosphatase," *Journal of Biological Chemistry*, vol. 272, no. 34, pp. 21113–21119, 1997.

[133] Y. Obara, K. Labudda, T. J. Dillon, and P. J. S. Stork, "PKA phosphorylation of Src mediates Rap1 activation in NGF and cAMP signaling in PC12 cells," *Journal of Cell Science*, vol. 117, no. 25, pp. 6085–6094, 2004.

[134] T. Vang, K. M. Torgersen, V. Sundvold et al., "Activation of the COOH-terminal Src kinase (Csk) by cAMP-dependent protein kinase inhibits signaling through the T cell receptor," *Journal of Experimental Medicine*, vol. 193, no. 4, pp. 497–507, 2001.

[135] G. Superti-Furga, S. Fumagalli, M. Koegl, S. A. Courtneidge, and G. Draetta, "Csk inhibition of c-Src activity requires both the SH2 and SH3 domains of Src," *EMBO Journal*, vol. 12, no. 7, pp. 2625–2634, 1993.

[136] R. W. McLachlan and A. S. Yap, "Not so simple: the complexity of phosphotyrosine signaling at cadherin adhesive contacts," *Journal of Molecular Medicine*, vol. 85, no. 6, pp. 545–554, 2007.

[137] B. Nagar, O. Hantschel, M. A. Young et al., "Structural basis for the autoinhibition of c-Abl tyrosine kinase," *Cell*, vol. 112, no. 6, pp. 859–871, 2003.

[138] T. Y. El Sayegh, P. D. Arora, L. Fan et al., "Phosphorylation of N-cadherin-associated cortactin by Fer kinase regulates N-cadherin mobility and intercellular adhesion strength," *Molecular Biology of the Cell*, vol. 16, no. 12, pp. 5514–5527, 2005.

[139] N. L. Zandy and A. M. Pendergast, "Abl tyrosine kinases modulate cadherin-dependent adhesion upstream and downstream of Rho family GTPases," *Cell Cycle*, vol. 7, no. 4, pp. 444–448, 2008.

[140] C. K. Joo, H. S. Kim, J. Y. Park, Y. Seomun, M. J. Son, and J. T. Kim, "Ligand release-independent transactivation of epidermal growth factor receptor by transforming growth factor-β involves multiple signaling pathways," *Oncogene*, vol. 27, no. 5, pp. 614–628, 2008.

[141] T. Watanabe, K. Sato, and K. Kaibuchi, "Cadherin-mediated intercellular adhesion and signaling cascades involving small GTPases," *Cold Spring Harbor Perspectives in Biology*, vol. 1, no. 3, p. a003020, 2009.

[142] V. M. M. Braga and A. S. Yap, "The challenges of abundance: epithelial junctions and small GTPase signalling," *Current Opinion in Cell Biology*, vol. 17, no. 5, pp. 466–474, 2005.

[143] E. A. Burton, T. N. Oliver, and A. M. Pendergast, "Abl kinases regulate actin comet tail elongation via an N-WASP-dependent pathway," *Molecular and Cellular Biology*, vol. 25, no. 20, pp. 8834–8843, 2005.

[144] M. Martin, S. M. Ahern-Djamali, F. M. Hoffmann, and W. M. Saxton, "Abl tyrosine kinase and its substrate Ena/VASP have functional interactions with kinesin-1," *Molecular Biology of the Cell*, vol. 16, no. 9, pp. 4225–4230, 2005.

[145] Q. Lu, N. K. Mukhopadhyay, J. D. Griffin, M. Paredes, M. Medina, and K. S. Kosik, "Brain armadillo protein δ-catenin interacts with Abl tyrosine kinase and modulates cellular morphogenesis in response to growth factors," *Journal of Neuroscience Research*, vol. 67, no. 5, pp. 618–624, 2002.

[146] Z. Dai and A. M. Pendergast, "Abi-2, a novel SH3-containing protein interacts with the c-Abl tyrosine kinase and modulates c-Abl transforming activity," *Genes and Development*, vol. 9, no. 21, pp. 2569–2582, 1995.

[147] M. Mitsushima, H. Takahashi, T. Shishido, K. Ueda, and N. Kioka, "Abl kinase interacts with and phosphorylates vinexin," *FEBS Letters*, vol. 580, no. 17, pp. 4288–4295, 2006.

[148] P. D. McCrea, D. Gu, and M. S. Balda, "Junctional music that the nucleus hears: cell-cell contact signaling and the modulation of gene activity," *Cold Spring Harbor Perspectives in Biology*, vol. 1, no. 4, p. a002923, 2009.

[149] F. H. Brembeck, M. Rosário, and W. Birchmeier, "Balancing cell adhesion and Wnt signaling, the key role of β-catenin," *Current Opinion in Genetics and Development*, vol. 16, no. 1, pp. 51–59, 2006.

[150] W. J. Nelson and R. Nusse, "Convergence of Wnt, β-Catenin, and Cadherin pathways," *Science*, vol. 303, no. 5663, pp. 1483–1487, 2004.

[151] Y. Xu and G. Carpenter, "Identification of cadherin tyrosine residues that are phosphorylated and mediate Shc association," *Journal of Cellular Biochemistry*, vol. 75, no. 2, pp. 264–271, 1999.

[152] Z. Wang, S. Sandiford, C. Wu, and S. S. C. Li, "Numb regulates cell-cell adhesion and polarity in response to tyrosine kinase signalling," *EMBO Journal*, vol. 28, no. 16, pp. 2360–2373, 2009.

[153] M. D. Potter, S. Barbero, and D. A. Cheresh, "Tyrosine phosphorylation of VE-cadherin prevents binding of p120- and β-catenin and maintains the cellular mesenchymal state," *Journal of Biological Chemistry*, vol. 280, no. 36, pp. 31906–31912, 2005.

[154] S. Yonemura, T. Matsui, S. Tsukita, and S. Tsukita, "Rho-dependent and -independent activation mechanisms of ezrin/radixin/moesin proteins: an essential role for polyphosphoinositides in vivo," *Journal of Cell Science*, vol. 115, no. 12, pp. 2569–2580, 2002.

[155] M. Amano, M. Ito, K. Kimura et al., "Phosphorylation and activation of myosin by Rho-associated kinase (Rho-kinase)," *Journal of Biological Chemistry*, vol. 271, no. 34, pp. 20246–20249, 1996.

[156] J. H. Henson, S. E. Kolnik, C. A. Fried et al., "Actin-based centripetal flow: phosphatase inhibition by calyculin-A alters flow pattern, actin organization, and actomyosin distribution," *Cell Motility and the Cytoskeleton*, vol. 56, no. 4, pp. 252–266, 2003.

[157] T. Volberg, Y. Zick, R. Dror et al., "The effect of tyrosine-specific protein phosphorylation on the assembly of adherens-type junctions," *EMBO Journal*, vol. 11, no. 5, pp. 1733–1742, 1992.

[158] E. Calautti, S. Cabodi, P. L. Stein, M. Hatzfeld, N. Kedersha, and G. P. Dotto, "Tyrosine phosphorylation and Src family kinases control keratinocyte cell-cell adhesion," *Journal of Cell Biology*, vol. 141, no. 6, pp. 1449–1465, 1998.

[159] J. H. Pang, A. Kraemer, S. J. Stehbens, M. C. Frame, and A. S. Yap, "Recruitment of phosphoinositide 3-kinase defines a positive contribution of tyrosine kinase signaling to E-cadherin function," *Journal of Biological Chemistry*, vol. 280, no. 4, pp. 3043–3050, 2005.

[160] S. Shibamoto, M. Hayakawa, K. Takeuchi et al., "Tyrosine phosphorylation of β-catenin and plakoglobin enhanced by hepatocyte growth factor and epidermal growth factor in human carcinoma cells," *Cell Adhesion and Communication*, vol. 1, no. 4, pp. 295–305, 1994.

[161] K. Hatanaka, M. Simons, and M. Murakami, "Phosphorylation of VE-cadherin controls endothelial phenotypes via p120-catenin coupling and Rac1 activation," *American Journal of Physiology*, vol. 300, no. 1, pp. H162–H172, 2011.

[162] S. Pece and J. S. Gutkind, "E-cadherin and Hakai: signalling, remodeling or destruction?" *Nature Cell Biology*, vol. 4, no. 4, pp. E72–E74, 2002.

[163] Y. Fujita, G. Krause, M. Scheffner et al., "Hakai, a c-Cbl-like protein, ubiquitinates and induces endocytosis of the E-cadherin complex," *Nature Cell Biology*, vol. 4, no. 3, pp. 222–231, 2002.

[164] H. Keilhack, U. Hellman, J. Van Hengel, F. Van Roy, J. Godovac-Zimmermann, and F. D. Böhmer, "The protein-tyrosine phosphatase SHP-1 binds to and dephosphorylates p120 catenin," *Journal of Biological Chemistry*, vol. 275, no. 34, pp. 26376–26384, 2000.

[165] Y. Fukumoto, Y. Shintani, A. B. Reynolds, K. R. Johnson, and M. J. Wheelock, "The regulatory or phosphorylation domain of p120 catenin controls E-cadherin dynamics at the plasma membrane," *Experimental Cell Research*, vol. 314, no. 1, pp. 52–67, 2008.

[166] G. S. Call, J. Y. Chung, J. A. Davis et al., "Zyxin phosphorylation at serine 142 modulates the zyxin head-tail interaction to alter cell-cell adhesion," *Biochemical and Biophysical Research Communications*, vol. 404, no. 3, pp. 780–784, 2011.

[167] T. N. Nguyen, A. Uemura, W. Shih, and S. Yamada, "Zyxin-mediated actin assembly is required for efficient wound closure," *Journal of Biological Chemistry*, vol. 285, no. 46, pp. 35439–35445, 2010.

[168] M. D. H. Hansen and M. C. Beckerle, "Opposing roles of Zyxin/LPP ACTA repeats and the LIM domain region in cell-cell adhesion," *Journal of Biological Chemistry*, vol. 281, no. 23, pp. 16178–16188, 2006.

[169] E. Butt, K. Abel, M. Krieger et al., "cAMP- and cGMP-dependent protein kinase phosphorylation sites of the focal adhesion vasodilator-stimulated phosphoprotein (VASP) in vitro and in intact human platelets," *Journal of Biological Chemistry*, vol. 269, no. 20, pp. 14509–14517, 1994.

[170] K. Chitaley, L. Chen, A. Galler, U. Walter, G. Daum, and A. W. Clowes, "Vasodilator-stimulated phosphoprotein is a substrate for protein kinase C," *FEBS Letters*, vol. 556, no. 1-3, pp. 211–215, 2004.

[171] B. Harbeck, S. Hüttelmaier, K. Schlüter, B. M. Jockusch, and S. Illenberger, "Phosphorylation of the vasodilator-stimulated phosphoprotein regulates its interaction witn actin," *Journal of Biological Chemistry*, vol. 275, no. 40, pp. 30817–30825, 2000.

[172] M. Barzik, T. I. Kotova, H. N. Higgs et al., "Ena/VASP proteins enhance actin polymerization in the presence of barbed end capping proteins," *Journal of Biological Chemistry*, vol. 280, no. 31, pp. 28653–28662, 2005.

[173] V. Vasioukhin, C. Bauer, M. Yin, and E. Fuchs, "Directed actin polymerization is the driving force for epithelial cell-cell adhesion," *Cell*, vol. 100, no. 2, pp. 209–219, 2000.

[174] J. A. Scott, A. M. Shewan, N. R. Den Elzen, J. J. Loureiro, F. B. Gertler, and A. S. Yap, "Ena/VASP proteins can regulate distinct modes of actin organization at cadherin-adhesive contacts," *Molecular Biology of the Cell*, vol. 17, no. 3, pp. 1085–1095, 2006.

[175] E. Morais-de-Sá, V. Mirouse, and D. St Johnston, "aPKC phosphorylation of bazooka defines the apical/lateral border in *Drosophila* epithelial cells," *Cell*, vol. 141, no. 3, pp. 509–523, 2010.

[176] R. F. Walther and F. Pichaud, "Crumbs/DaPKC-dependent apical exclusion of bazooka promotes photoreceptor polarity remodeling," *Current Biology*, vol. 20, no. 12, pp. 1065–1074, 2010.

[177] Y.-C. Wang, Z. Khan, M. Kaschube, and E. F. Wieschaus, "Differential positioning of adherens junctions is associated with initiation of epithelial folding," *Nature*, vol. 484, no. 7394, pp. 390–393, 2012.

[178] P. V. Hornbeck, I. Chabra, J. M. Kornhauser, E. Skrzypek, and B. Zhang, "PhosphoSite: a bioinformatics resource dedicated to physiological protein phosphorylation," *Proteomics*, vol. 4, no. 6, pp. 1551–1561, 2004.

[179] A. M. E. Jones and T. S. Nühse, "Phosphoproteomics using iTRAQ," *Methods in Molecular Biology*, vol. 779, pp. 287–302, 2011.

[180] B. Eyrich, A. Sickmann, and R. P. Zahedi, "Catch me if you can: mass spectrometry-based phosphoproteomics and quantification strategies," *Proteomics*, vol. 11, no. 4, pp. 554–570, 2011.

[181] H. Imamura, N. Yachie, R. Saito, Y. Ishihama, and M. Tomita, "Towards the systematic discovery of signal transduction networks using phosphorylation dynamics data," *BMC Bioinformatics*, vol. 11, article 232, 2010.

[182] I. Martinez-Ferrando, R. Chaerkady, J. Zhong et al., "Identification of targets of c-Src tyrosine kinase by chemical complementation and phosphoproteomics," *Molecular and Cellular Proteomics*. In press.

[183] M. Hilger, T. Bonaldi, F. Gnad, and M. Mann, "Systems-wide analysis of a phosphatase knock-down by quantitative proteomics and phosphoproteomics," *Molecular and Cellular Proteomics*, vol. 8, no. 8, pp. 1908–1920, 2009.

[184] P. H. Huang, A. Mukasa, R. Bonavia et al., "Quantitative analysis of EGFRvIII cellular signaling networks reveals a combinatorial therapeutic strategy for glioblastoma," *Proceedings of the National Academy of Sciences of the United States of America*, vol. 104, no. 31, pp. 12867–12872, 2007.

[185] H. Kozuka-Hata, S. Tasaki, and M. Oyama, "Phosphoproteomics-based systems analysis of signal transduction networks," *Frontiers in Physiology*, vol. 2, no. 113, 2011.

[186] A. Derouiche, C. Cousin, and I. Mijakovic, "Protein phosphorylation from the perspective of systems biology," *Current Opinion in Biotechnology*. In press.

[187] E. Sadot, M. Conacci-Sorrell, J. Zhurinsky et al., "Regulation of S33/S37 phosphorylated β-catenin in normal and transformed cells," *Journal of Cell Science*, vol. 115, no. 13, pp. 2771–2780, 2002.

[188] M. V. Brown, P. E. Burnett, M. F. Denning, and A. B. Reynolds, "PDGF receptor activation induces p120-catenin phosphorylation at serine 879 via a PKCα-dependent pathway," *Experimental Cell Research*, vol. 315, no. 1, pp. 39–49, 2009.

[189] G. Ren, F. M. Helwani, S. Verma, R. W. McLachlan, S. A. Weed, and A. S. Yap, "Cortactin is a functional target of E-cadherin-activated Src family kinases in MCF7 epithelial monolayers," *Journal of Biological Chemistry*, vol. 284, no. 28, pp. 18913–18922, 2009.

[190] P. M. Benz, C. Blume, S. Seifert et al., "Differential VASP phosphorylation controls remodeling of the actin cytoskeleton," *Journal of Cell Science*, vol. 122, no. 21, pp. 3954–3965, 2009.

[191] R. Zaidel-Bar, R. Milo, Z. Kam, and B. Geiger, "A paxillin tyrosine phosphorylation switch regulates the assembly and form of cell-matrix adhesions," *Journal of Cell Science*, vol. 120, no. 1, pp. 137–148, 2007.

[192] R. Zaidel-Bar and B. Geiger, "The switchable integrin adhesome," *Journal of Cell Science*, vol. 123, no. 9, pp. 1385–1388, 2010.

4

MAP Kinases and Prostate Cancer

Gonzalo Rodríguez-Berriguete,[1] **Benito Fraile,**[1] **Pilar Martínez-Onsurbe,**[2]
Gabriel Olmedilla,[2] **Ricardo Paniagua,**[1] **and Mar Royuela**[1]

[1] *Department of Cell Biology and Genetics, University of Alcalá, Alcalá de Henares, 28871 Madrid, Spain*
[2] *Department of Pathology, Príncipe de Asturias Hospital, Alcalá de Henares, 28806 Madrid, Spain*

Correspondence should be addressed to Mar Royuela, mar.royuela@uah.es

Academic Editor: Fred Schaper

The three major mitogen-activated protein kinases (MAPKs) p38, JNK, and ERK are signal transducers involved in a broad range of cell functions including survival, apoptosis, and cell differentiation. Whereas JNK and p38 have been generally linked to cell death and tumor suppression, ERK plays a prominent role in cell survival and tumor promotion, in response to a broad range of stimuli such as cytokines, growth factors, ultraviolet radiation, hypoxia, or pharmacological compounds. However, there is a growing body of evidence supporting that JNK and p38 also contribute to the development of a number of malignances. In this paper we focus on the involvement of the MAPK pathways in prostate cancer, including the less-known ERK5 pathway, as pro- or antitumor mediators, through their effects on apoptosis, survival, metastatic potential, and androgen-independent growth.

1. Introduction

Mitogen-activated protein kinases (MAPKs) are serine/threonine kinases that mediate intracellular signaling associated with a variety of cellular activities including cell proliferation, differentiation, survival, death, and transformation [1, 2]. The three main members that integrate the MAPK family in mammalian cells are stress-activated protein kinase c-Jun NH2-terminal kinase (JNK), stress-activated protein kinase 2 (SAPK2, p38), and the extracellular signal-regulated protein kinases (ERK1/2, p44/p42) (Figure 1). In addition, other less-characterized MAPK pathways exist, such as the extracellular regulated kinase 5 (ERK5) pathway [3, 4] (Figure 1). Albeit with multiple exceptions, JNK and ERK5 are generally associated with apoptosis induction, while ERK1/2 are generally associated to mitogenesis, and inversely related to apoptosis [3, 4], and contradictory effects on cell death have been described to p38 [5–12].

In mammalian cells, ERK, p38, and JNK activities are, respectively, regulated by different MAPKs cascades, which provide a link between transmembrane signaling and changes in transcription and that are activated in response to different environmental or developmental signals [4] (Figure 1). Depending on the cell type, a particular MAPK

cascade may be involved in different cellular responses. The JNK and p38 signaling pathways are activated by proinflammatory (TNFα, IL-6 or IL-1) or anti-inflammatory (EGF, TGF-β) cytokines, but also in response to cellular stresses such as genotoxic, osmotic, hypoxic, or oxidative stress. The JNK pathway consists of JNK, an MAPKK such as SEK1 (also known as MEK4) or MEK7, and an MAPKKK such as ASK1, MEKK1, mixed-lineage kinase (MLK), or transforming growth factor-β-activated kinase 1 (TAK1) [13, 14]. In the p38 signaling pathway, distinct MAPKKs such as MEK3 and MEK6 activate p38, and these can be activated by the same MAPKKKs (such as ASK1 and TAK1) that function in the JNK pathway. In the ERK signaling pathway, ERK1 or ERK2 (ERK1/2) is activated by MEK1/2, which in turn is activated by a Raf isoform such as A-Raf, B-Raf, or Raf-1 (also known as C-Raf) and also by TRAF-2 and TRAF-6. The kinase Raf-1 is activated by the small Ras-like GTPase, whose activation is mediated by the receptor tyrosine kinase (RTK)-Grb2-SOS signaling axis [15]. Members of the Ras family of proteins, including K-Ras, H-Ras, and N-Ras, play a key role in transmission of extracellular signals into cells [16] (Figure 1).

The aim of this paper was to focus on the possible involvement of MAPKs in several transduction pathways

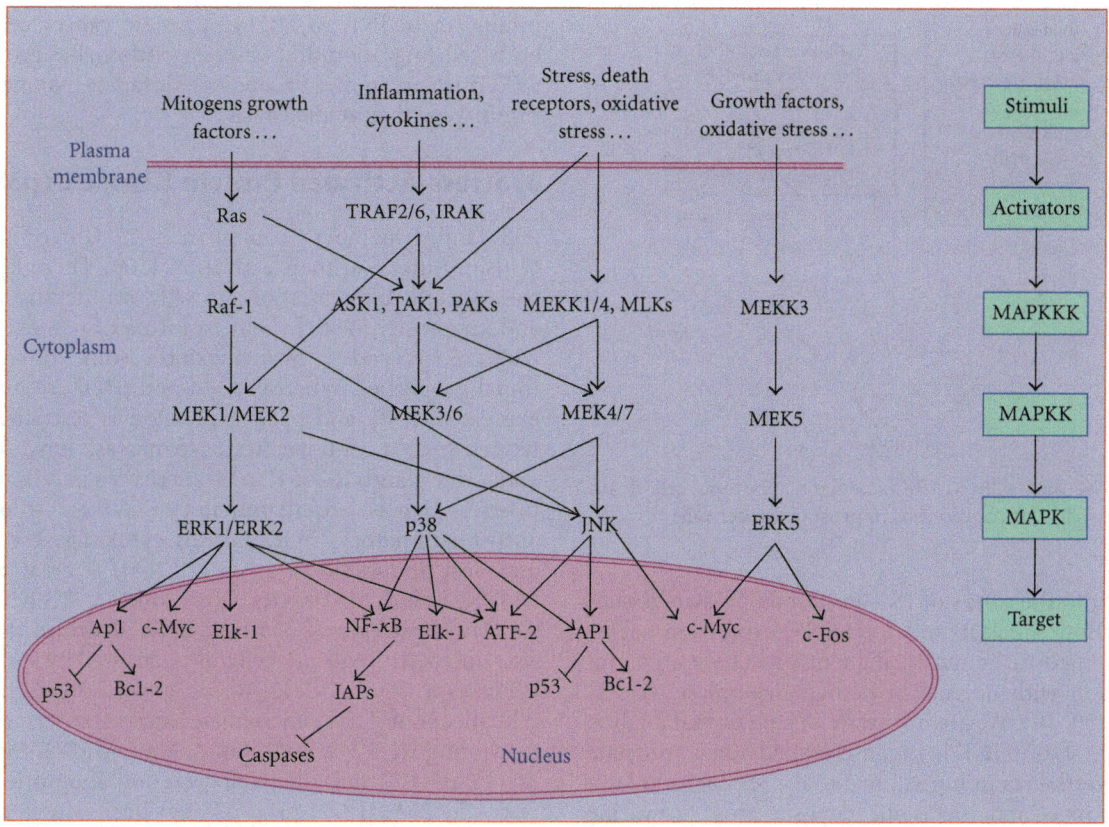

FIGURE 1: Mitogen-activated protein kinase (MAPK) signaling. MAP kinases are activated by upstream kinases such as MAP kinase kinase (MAPKK), that include MEKs 1, 2, 3, 4, 5, 6, and 7. In turn, MAPKKs are activated by several different MAP kinase kinase kinases (MAPKKKs). Numerous stimulatory factors such as cytokines, mitogens, or death receptors can activate MAPKKKs. Each MAPK, depending on the stimulus and cell type, can phosphorylate different transcription factors.

related with prostate cancer development as well as the possible functional role of MAPKs in cell death/survival/ proliferation decisions depending on the cell type, stage, and cell stimulus. We also discuss the possible value of members of these pathways as potential therapeutic targets.

2. Jun N-Terminal Kinase (JNK)

JNK proteins, also called stress-activated protein kinases (SAPKs), share a threonine-proline-tyrosine (TPY) motif within their activation loop [17]. They have been involved in development, morphogenesis, and cell differentiation [17]. The earliest discoveries included the identification of the three mammalian JNK genes, namely, JNK1, JNK2, and JNK3 (SAPK-γ, SAPK-α, and SAPK-β, resp.) which can generate 10 isoforms by alternative splicing [18, 19]. Alternative splicing further increases the diversity of JNK proteins; however apart from early biochemical studies on these splice forms [16] their functional significance *in vivo* remains largely unexplored [19]. The products of JNK1 and JNK2 are ubiquitously expressed in almost all cell types and tissues, whereas JNK3 is localized primarily in brain, heart, and testis. Due to their differential expression distribution it is thought that JNK3 presents different functions than

JNK1 and JNK2, whereas these latter may have redundant functions [20]. Investigations on JNKs have focused on their activation in response to diverse extracellular stimuli including ultraviolet (UV) and gamma radiation, inflammatory cytokines (IL-6, IL-1, and TNF), and cytotoxic drugs (Figure 2) [21, 22]. These stimuli are able to activate JNK through multiple and even overlapping cascades in which participate members of the small Ras-like GTPases or several MAPKKs (Figure 1). For its complete activation JNK requires dual phosphorylation of threonine and tyrosine residues. MEK4 and MEK7 preferentially phosphorylate at tyrosine and threonine, respectively [23–27], being both MAPKKs needed to fully activate JNK [4, 28]. Depending on the stimulus and cell type, JNKs phosphorylate different substrates, including transcription factors (AP-1, ATF-2, Elk-1, c-Myc, p53, MLK2) and several members of the Bcl-2 family, among others [17, 20, 29] (Figure 1).

Several authors suggest that JNK activity is chronically altered in various cancer types such as those of the prostate [30, 31], breast [32, 33], pancreas, or lung [34, 35]. Both JNK1 and 2 have been shown to exert pro- as well as antitumor actions in a number of *in vivo* and *in vitro* models of malignancies [6, 36]. A number of findings suggest that in apoptosis JNKs have opposite functions depending on the cellular stimulus and type or even the JNK isoform.

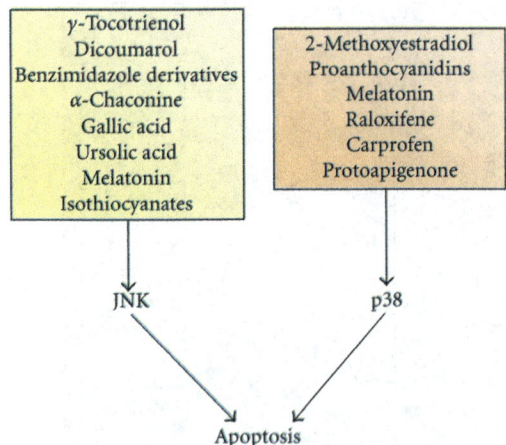

FIGURE 2: JNK and p38 MAPKs mediate apoptotic cell death induced by a variety of compounds in prostate cancer cells.

Studies into the status of JNK in human prostate tissues are scarce. Both nuclear and total JNK expression seems to be augmented in human malignant prostate epithelium in comparison with normal or benign hyperplasic (BPH) epithelium [30–40]. We are not aware of studies that analyze the activation state of JNK in organ-confined human prostate cancers. Nevertheless in human metastatic lesions, and late-stage carcinomas and metastatic deposits from a murine model of prostate cancer, JNK phosphorylated forms seem to be reduced [39, 41, 42].

In spite of its prominent role as a proapoptotic factor, as in other malignances, both pro- and antitumor actions have been attributed to JNK in prostate cancer. Hence, a great number of agents have been shown to trigger apoptosis through JNK. These include gamma-tocotrienol [43], dicoumarol [44], benzimidazole derivatives [45], alpha-chaconine, gallic acid [34], ursolic acid [35], melatonin [36], and isothiocyanates [46, 47] (Figure 2). It is of interest to note that androgen deprivation, the most common therapy used as treatment for advanced prostate cancer, may elicit apoptosis through JNK activation [48]. In the context of its proapoptotic role JNK has been linked to reactive oxygen species (ROS). Some works have highlighted the capability of JNK to trigger apoptosis through ROS production in prostate cancer cells [49, 50]. Conversely, ROS may induce apoptosis acting through JNK activation. For instance, both genipin- and guggulsterone-induced prostate cancer cell apoptoses are caused by ROS-dependent JNK activation [51, 52]. Regarding to its antiapoptotic function, JNKs have been involved in protection from serum starvation-, Fas-, and (at early phase) glucose deprivation-induced apoptosis [53–55].

Besides promoting prostate cancer development by protecting cells from apoptosis, JNK may be involved in prostate cancer metastasis, through its ability to regulate cell adhesion, invasion, and migration. Thus, JNK has been shown to promote the expression of some proteins responsible for extracellular matrix degradation during invasion in prostate cancer cells, such as matrix metalloproteinases (MMPs)-2 and -9, and urokinase-type plasminogen activator (u-PA) [56–58]. Moreover, Kwon et al. [56] reported that chemical inhibition of JNK in DU145 prostate cancer cells reduces both cell migration and vascular-endothelial growth factor (VEGF) expression, a proangiogenic factor that may facilitate tumor growth and metastasis.

3. Stress-Activated Protein Kinase 2 (p38)

p38 family members contain a TGY (threonine-glycine-tyrosine) motif in their activation loop. These kinases play roles in cell differentiation, growth, proliferation, survival, and apoptosis [59–61]. Four isoforms of p38 exist, namely, p38α, β, γ, and δ, which exhibit some different functional properties. Whereas p38α and p38β are ubiquitously expressed, p38γ and p38δ expression is restricted to some tissues such as muscle, testis, pancreas, lung, kidney, or endocrine glands [62–64]. p38 is activated in cells in response to stress signals, proinflammatory (TNFα, IL-6 or IL-1) or anti-inflammatory (EGF, TGF-β) cytokines, UV radiation, and heat and osmotic shock [59, 65]. A great number of MAPKKs and MAPKKKs (e.g., Mlk1-3, MEKK1-4, TAK, ASK1/2) upstream of p38 have been identified. Both MAP-KKs and MAPKKKs are generally activated by small Ras-like GTPases as Rac1, Cdc42, RhoA, and RhoB [64]. Activated p38 phosphorylates and regulates many transcription factors (including ATF-2, NF-κB, Elk-1, Max, MEF-2, Mac, p53, or Stat1) [65–67] and other cell cycle and apoptotic mediators (e.g., Cdc25A, Bcl-2) [61]. p38 has been shown to enhance cell survival in response to stress stimuli, for instance, in response to DNA damage [61–68]. Triggering of pro- or antiapoptotic p38-mediated response seems to depend on the stimulus, the cell system, and the p38 isoform involved [64].

Several studies suggest that p38 play an important role in leukemia [64], lymphomas [69], and a number of solid malignances such as breast [65], prostate [70], gastric [71], or lung [72] cancers.

Both p38 and its active form p-p38, as well as some upstream kinases (PAK1, MEK6, MEK4), are overexpressed in human cancerous prostatic epithelium [11, 30, 41]. This agrees with the enhanced levels of the phosphorylated form of the well-established p38 substrates Elk-1 and ATF-2 at the same compartment [11]. Uzgare et al. [41], using a transgenic mouse model for prostate cancer, described that p-p38 is overexpressed in prostatic intraepithelial neoplasia (PIN), well-differentiated and moderately differentiated cancers while was reduced or absent in late-stage adenocarcinomas and metastatic deposits. However, like in other tissues, studies focused on p38 function in the prostate malignancy reveal that this MAPK can elicit multiple and even opposite responses, which seem to vary depending on the cell system and context.

A proapoptotic role for p38 has been established in a number of prostate cancer in vitro models and conditions. p38 promotes apoptosis induced by 2-methoxyestradiol [5], melatonin [6], proanthocyanidins [7], raloxifene [8], carprofen [9], or protoapigenone [10] (Figure 2). By contrast, p38 exerts a protective effect in TNF-induced apoptosis in LNCaP cells, which represents a good model of well-differentiated tumor [11].

In spite of having a prominent proapoptotic role p38 may contribute to prostate cancer progression by promoting tumor growth, androgen independence acquisition, and metastasis. It has been proposed that IL-6 may support androgen-independent tumor growth by enhancing androgen receptor (AR) expression/activity. Lin et al. [73] demonstrated that, in turn, the IL-6-induced androgen response depends on p38 activity. p38 seems to play a critical role in hypoxia-reoxygenation-induced increase in AR activity, as well as increased survival, clonogenicity, and invasiveness in prostate cancer cells [74], thus providing additional support for a role for p38 in androgen dependence acquisition. Huang et al. [75] showed in PC3 cells that p38 MAPK is necessary for TGF-β-mediated activation of MMP-2 and cell invasion in prostate cancer. Moreover, p38 has been involved in the invasion and migration abilities of the prostate cancer DU145 cells, by enhancing the expression of MMPs-2 and -9, and urokinase-type plasminogen activator (u-PA) [76]. Xu et al. [77] also described MEK4 as a regulator and activator of MMP-2. In agreement, Tang and Lu [78] found that p38 activity contributes to adiponectin-induced integrin expression and migration capability of human prostate cancer cells. Therefore, and in spite of displaying proapoptotic functions, p38 may constitute a target for prostate cancer treatment given its demonstrated contribution to some prostate cancer hallmarks, as androgen dependence and metastatic phenotype acquisition.

4. Extracellular Signal-Regulated Protein Kinases (ERK1/2)

ERK has a threonine-glutamic acid-tyrosine (Thr-Glu-Tyr) motif [79, 80] that plays a central role in stimulation of cell proliferation [81, 82]. The biological consequences of phosphorylation of ERK substrates include increased proliferation, differentiation, survival [83], angiogenesis [84], motility [85], and invasiveness [86]. The two isoforms of ERK, referred to as ERK1 (or p44) and ERK2 (or p42), share 85% amino acid identity and represent a convergence point for mitogenic signaling from a diverse array of pathways [87–89]. Both are ubiquitously expressed, although their relative abundance in tissues is variable. For example, in many immune cells ERK2 is the predominant species, while in several cells of neuroendocrine origin they may be equally expressed [90].

The ERK pathway is triggered mainly by mitogens and cytokines (Figure 1), acting through receptor tyrosine kinases, G-protein-coupled receptors, and nonnuclear activated steroid hormone receptors [4, 65]. Most of the signals activating the ERK pathway are initiated through receptor-mediated activation of Ras [4] by stimulating the exchange of GDP bound to Ras for GTP [91]. Then, Ras phosphorylates Raf-1. Then, a MAPK cascade is initiated in which Raf-1 sequentially phosphorylates MEK1/2 and ERK1/2. Later, ERK1/2 translocate to the nucleus in a process that culminates in modulation of gene transcription through the activation of several transcription factors such as Ets-1 [4], ATF-2, c-Fos, c-Myc, Elk-1 [92], or NF-κB [29]

(Figure 1). At the same time, ERK1/2 can also phosphorylate cytoplasmic and nuclear kinases, such as MNK1, MNK2, MPKAP-2, RSK, or MSK1 [90].

TGF-β and EGF are growth factors that can induce tumor progression by means of the ERK pathway [93–96]. Several studies showed that these factors are overexpressed in prostate cancer in comparison with normal tissue [95–98]. In different tumor cells, expression of some EGF family members such as EGF or TGF-α is associated with poor patient prognosis or resistance to chemotherapeutics [94–99]. IGF-1 and EGF stimulate intracellular signaling pathways converging at the level of ERK2 [100], which is a key kinase mediator of growth-factor-induced mitogenesis in prostate cancer cells [101]. The two major substrates of the IGF-1 receptor, insulin receptor substrate-1 [102] and Shc, are known to contribute to IGF-1-induced activation of ERK [103].

The ERK signaling pathway plays a role in several steps of tumor development [14]. In fact, some components of the Raf-MEK-ERK pathway are activated in solid tumors (such as prostate or breast cancer) and hematological malignances [104–106]. In approximately 30% of human breast cancers, mutations are found in the ERK1/2 MAPK pathway [65]. ERK1/2 and downstream ERK1/2 targets are hyperphosphorylated in a large subset of mammary tumors [107]. Mutations of K-Ras appear frequently in many cancers including those of the lung and colon [108]. Mutations in the B-Raf gene are responsible for 66% of malignant melanomas [109]. Increased expressions of Raf pathway has been associated with advanced prostate cancer, hormonal independence, metastasis, and a poor prognosis [110]. Moreover, prostate cancer cell lines isolated from patients with advanced cancer (LNCaP, PC3, DU145) expressed low levels of active Raf kinase inhibitors [105]. TNF-α acts as an ERK activator in some cases related to inflammation and cell proliferation. In this way, Ricote et al. [11] showed that ERK phosphorylation was notably increased by TNF-α in a dose-dependent manner in LNCaP cells. In prostate cancer, presence of Raf-1 and MEK1 in conjunction with elevated ERK1 and ERK2, and their phosphorylated forms, suggests that stimulation of cell proliferation could be triggered by IL-6 via the ERK pathway [104]. In fact, IL-6 expression increased in prostate cancer in comparison with normal tissue [104, 111]. Moreover, LNCaP cells which produce IL-6 show increased proliferation, at least in part, due to ERK activation [112]. Recently, a phase I clinical trial has revealed the ability of an anti-IL-6 antibody (siltuximab) to inhibit ERK1/2 phosphorylation in prostate tumors [113].

Several investigators suggest associations between decline in ERK activity and advanced malignancy [114, 115]. Conversely Gioeli et al. [116] demonstrated that ERK activation is correlated with tumor malignancy. Junttila et al. [4] demonstrated in the TRAMP mouse model that ERK activation is linked to prostatic epithelial proliferation and initiation of prostate cancer development, while ERK inactivation is correlated with the emergence of a poorly differentiated metastatic and androgen-independent phenotype. Activated ERK mediates activation of the androgen receptor and/or PSA secretion through the growth factor receptor tyrosine kinase, Her2/Neu (also known as erbB2) in androgen-independent prostate cancer cells [117]. Other important issue of this pathway in tumor development is that the phosphorylation by ERK of proteins such as myosin, calpain, focal adhesion kinase, and paxillin promotes cancer cell migration. Also, ERK can promote the degradation of extracellular matrix proteins and consequent tumor invasion [14].

ERK may also induce the phosphorylation of apoptotic regulatory molecules including bcl-2 family members (e.g., Bad, Bim, and controversially Bcl-2) and caspase 9 [93]. There are pieces of evidence suggesting a protective effect in cells by NF-κB activation via ERK [118, 119]. Upon cell stimulation NF-κB is translocated into the nucleus [120], where it promotes the expression of several antiapoptotic genes such as inhibitors of apoptosis proteins (IAPs) [121] and bcl-2 family members [122].

5. ERK5

The fourth MAPK of interest in this paper is ERK5. ERK5 is a large molecular size kinase [123] identified independently by two groups. One used a two-hybrid screen with an upstream activator MEK5 as the bait; the other used a degenerate PCR strategy to clone novel MAPK [123, 124]. ERK5 is activated by growth factors [125], integrin engagement [126], and cell stress [111] and contributes to expression induction of Ap1 (cJun [127] and Fos [128]), MEF family group (e.g., MEF2C, a well-characterized target [129], and c-Myc [130] transcription factors).

In an *in vitro* study on androgen-independent PC3 cells, McCracken et al. [131] described ERK5 overexpresion related to proliferative, migrative, and invasive capabilities, establishing the potential importance of ERK5 in aggressive prostate cancer. In other study, Sawhney et al. [126] hypothesized that ERK5 activation could promote cancer metastasis through its ability to regulate cell adhesion and motility.

6. New Perspectives

The literature reviewed in this paper suggests that the MAPK transduction pathways are involved in prostate cancer development. The ability of JNK, p38, and ERK to act either as prostate cancer suppressors or promoters depends on the cell type, developmental stage, and specific stimuli. Nevertheless, the molecular roles of these proteins are not known at all. The aim of future studies might be directed towards revealing the factors and mechanisms that account for the differential function of JNK, p38, and ERK MAPKs as pro- or antitumor factors. It may lead to the development of therapeutic approaches to effectively target the protumor effects of the MAPK pathways.

Acknowledgments

This paper is supported by grants from the "Fundación Mutua Madrileña, 2010 (AP76182010)" (Spain) and the "University of Alcalá-Comunidad Autónoma de Madrid, Spain (CCG10-UAH/BIO-5985). G. Rodríguez-Berriguete had a predoctoral fellowship from the Alcalá University (Madrid, Spain) during the course of this work.

References

[1] J. A. McCubrey, M. M. LaHair, and R. A. Franklin, "Reactive oxygen species-induced activation of the MAP kinase signaling pathways," *Antioxidants and Redox Signaling*, vol. 8, no. 9-10, pp. 1775–1789, 2006.

[2] B. N. Kholodenko and M. R. Birtwistle, "Four-dimensional dynamics of MAPK information processing systems," *Wiley Interdisciplinary Reviews. Systems Biology and Medicine*, vol. 1, pp. 28–44, 2009.

[3] M. Hayashi and J. D. Lee, "Role of the BMK1/ERK5 signaling pathway: lessons from knockout mice," *Journal of Molecular Medicine*, vol. 82, no. 12, pp. 800–808, 2004.

[4] M. R. Junttila, S. P. Li, and J. Westermarck, "Phosphatase-mediated crosstalk between MAPK signaling pathways in the regulation of cell survival," *FASEB Journal*, vol. 22, no. 4, pp. 954–965, 2008.

[5] K. Shimada, M. Nakamura, E. Ishida, and N. Konishi, "Molecular roles of MAP kinases and FADD phosphorylation in prostate cancer," *Histology and Histopathology*, vol. 21, no. 4–6, pp. 415–422, 2006.

[6] S. S. Joo and Y. M. Yoo, "Melatonin induces apoptotic death in LNCaP cells via p38 and JNK pathways: therapeutic implications for prostate cancer," *Journal of Pineal Research*, vol. 47, no. 1, pp. 8–14, 2009.

[7] P. K. Vayalil, A. Mittal, and S. K. Katiyar, "Proanthocyanidins from grape seeds inhibit expression of matrix metalloproteinases in human prostate carcinoma cells, which is associated with the inhibition of activation of MAPK and NF kappa B," *Carcinogenesis*, vol. 25, no. 6, pp. 987–995, 2004.

[8] Y. X. Zhang and C. Z. Kong, "The role of mitogen-activated protein kinase cascades in inhibition of proliferation in human prostate carcinoma cells by raloxifene: an in vitro experiment," *Zhonghua Yi Xue Za Zhi*, vol. 88, no. 4, pp. 271–275, 2008.

[9] F. S. Khwaja, E. J. Quann, N. Pattabiraman, S. Wynne, and D. Djakiew, "Carprofen induction of p75NTR-dependent apoptosis via the p38 mitogen-activated protein kinase pathway in prostate cancer cells," *Molecular Cancer Therapeutics*, vol. 7, no. 11, pp. 3539–3545, 2008.

[10] H. L. Chang, Y. C. Wu, J. H. Su, Y. T. Yeh, and S. S. F. Yuan, "Protoapigenone, a novel flavonoid, induces apoptosis in human prostate cancer cells through activation of p38 mitogen-activated protein kinase and c-Jun NH2-terminal kinase 1/2," *Journal of Pharmacology and Experimental Therapeutics*, vol. 325, no. 3, pp. 841–849, 2008.

[11] M. Ricote, I. García-Tuñón, B. Fraile et al., "P38 MAPK protects against TNF-α-provoked apoptosis in LNCaP prostatic cancer cells," *Apoptosis*, vol. 11, no. 11, pp. 1969–1975, 2006.

[12] G. Rodríguez-Berriguete, B. Fraile, R. Paniagua, P. Aller, and M. Royuela, "Expression of NF-κB-related proteins and their modulation during TNF-α-provoked apoptosis in prostate cancer cells," submitted to *Prostate*.

[13] R. J. Davis, "Signal transduction by the JNK group of MAP kinases," *Cell*, vol. 103, no. 2, pp. 239–252, 2000.

[14] E. K. Kim and E. J. Choi, "Pathological roles of MAPK signaling pathways in human diseases," *Biochimica et Biophysica Acta*, vol. 1802, no. 4, pp. 396–405, 2010.

[15] A. S. Dhillon, S. Hagan, O. Rath, and W. Kolch, "MAP kinase signalling pathways in cancer," *Oncogene*, vol. 26, no. 22, pp. 3279–3290, 2007.

[16] B. B. Ancrile, K. M. O'Hayer, and C. M. Counter, "Oncogenic ras-induced expression of cytokines: a new target of anti-cancer therapeutics," *Molecular Interventions*, vol. 8, no. 1, pp. 22–27, 2008.

[17] L. E. Heasley and S. Y. Han, "JNK regulation of oncogenesis," *Molecules and Cells*, vol. 21, no. 2, pp. 167–173, 2006.

[18] B. Derijard, M. Hibi, I. H. Wu et al., "JNK1: a protein kinase stimulated by UV light and Ha-Ras that binds and phosphorylates the c-Jun activation domain," *Cell*, vol. 76, no. 6, pp. 1025–1037, 1994.

[19] M. A. Bogoyevitch, K. R. W. Ngoei, T. T. Zhao, Y. Y. C. Yeap, and D. C. H. Ng, "c-Jun N-terminal kinase (JNK) signaling: recent advances and challenges," *Biochimica et Biophysica Acta*, vol. 1804, no. 3, pp. 463–475, 2010.

[20] A. M. Bode and Z. Dong, "The functional contrariety of JNK," *Molecular Carcinogenesis*, vol. 46, no. 8, pp. 591–598, 2007.

[21] H. Khalaf, J. Jass, and P. E. Olsson, "Differential cytokine regulation by NF-kappaB and AP-1 in Jurkat T-cells," *BMC Immunology*, vol. 11, article 26, 2010.

[22] F. De Graeve, A. Bahr, K. T. Sabapathy et al., "Role of the ATFa/JNK2 complex in Jun activation," *Oncogene*, vol. 18, no. 23, pp. 3491–3500, 1999.

[23] I. Sanchez, R. T. Hughes, B. J. Mayer et al., "Role of SAPK/ERK kinase-1 in the stress-activated pathway regulating transcription factor c-jun," *Nature*, vol. 372, no. 6508, pp. 794–800, 1994.

[24] S. Lawler, Y. Fleming, M. Goedert, and P. Cohen, "Synergistic activation of SAPK1/JNK1 by two MAP kinase kinases in vitro," *Current Biology*, vol. 8, no. 25, pp. 1387–1390, 1998.

[25] Y. Fleming, C. G. Armstrong, N. Morrice, A. Paterson, M. Goedert, and P. Cohen, "Synergistic activation of stress-activated protein kinase 1/c-Jun N-terminal kinase (SAPK1/JNK) isoforms by mitogen-activated protein kinase kinase 4 (MKK4) and MKK7," *Biochemical Journal*, vol. 352, no. 1, pp. 145–154, 2000.

[26] T. Wada, K. Nakagawa, T. Watanabe et al., "Impaired synergistic activation of stress-activated protein kinase SAPK/JNK in mouse embryonic stem cells lacking SEK1/MKK4," *Journal of Biological Chemistry*, vol. 276, no. 33, pp. 30892–30897, 2001.

[27] X. Wang, B. Nadarajah, A. C. Robinson et al., "Targeted deletion of the mitogen-activated protein kinase kinase 4 gene in the nervous system causes severe brain developmental defects and premature death," *Molecular and Cellular Biology*, vol. 27, no. 22, pp. 7935–7946, 2007.

[28] C. Tournier, C. Dong, T. K. Turner, S. N. Jones, R. A. Flavell, and R. J. Davis, "MKK7 is an essential component of the JNK signal transduction pathway activated by proinflammatory cytokines," *Genes and Development*, vol. 15, no. 11, pp. 1419–1426, 2001.

[29] A. G. Turjanski, J. P. Vaqué, and J. S. Gutkind, "MAP kinases and the control of nuclear events," *Oncogene*, vol. 26, no. 22, pp. 3240–3253, 2007.

[30] M. Royuela, M. I. Arenas, F. R. Bethencourt, B. Fraile, and R. Paniagua, "Regulation of proliferation/apoptosis equilibrium by mitogen-activated protein kinases in normal, hyperplastic, and carcinomatous human prostate," *Human Pathology*, vol. 33, no. 3, pp. 299–306, 2002.

[31] J. Meshki, M. C. Caino, V. A. von Burstin, E. Griner, and M. G. Kazanietz, "Regulation of prostate cancer cell survival by protein kinase Cε involves bad phosphorylation and modulation of the TNFα/JNK pathway," *Journal of Biological Chemistry*, vol. 285, no. 34, pp. 26033–26040, 2010.

[32] H. Y. Wang, Z. Cheng, and C. C. Malbon, "Overexpression of mitogen-activated protein kinase phosphatases MKP1, MKP2 in human breast cancer," *Cancer Letters*, vol. 191, no. 2, pp. 229–237, 2003.

[33] J. Wang, I. Kuiatse, A. V. Lee, J. Pan, A. Giuliano, and X. Cui, "Sustained c-Jun-NH2-kinase activity promotes epithelial-mesenchymal transition, invasion, and survival of breast cancer cells by regulating extracellular signal-regulated kinase activation," *Molecular Cancer Research*, vol. 8, no. 2, pp. 266–277, 2010.

[34] G. H. Su, W. Hilgers, M. C. Shekher et al., "Alterations in pancreatic, biliary, and breast carcinomas support MKK4 as a genetically targeted tumor suppressor gene," *Cancer Research*, vol. 58, no. 11, pp. 2339–2342, 1998.

[35] J. J. Lee, J. H. Lee, Y. G. Ko, S. I. Hong, and J. S. Lee, "Prevention of premature senescence requires JNK regulation of Bcl-2 and reactive oxygen species," *Oncogene*, vol. 29, no. 4, pp. 561–575, 2010.

[36] O. Potapova, M. Gorospe, F. Bost et al., "c-Jun N-terminal kinase is essential for growth of human T98G glioblastoma cells," *Journal of Biological Chemistry*, vol. 275, no. 32, pp. 24767–24775, 2000.

[37] N. Chen, M. Nomura, Q. B. She et al., "Suppression of skin tumorigenesis in c-Jun NH(2)-terminal kinase-2-deficient mice," *Cancer Research*, vol. 61, no. 10, pp. 3908–3912, 2001.

[38] Q. B. She, N. Chen, A. M. Bode, R. A. Flavell, and Z. Dong, "Deficiency of c-Jun-NH(2)-terminal kinase-1 in mice enhances skin tumor development by 12-O-tetradecanoylphorbol-13-acetate," *Cancer Research*, vol. 62, no. 5, pp. 1343–1348, 2002.

[39] H. Takahashi, H. Ogata, R. Nishigaki, D. H. Broide, and M. Karin, "Tobacco smoke promotes lung tumorigenesis by triggering IKKbeta- and JNK1-dependent inflammation," *Cancer Cell*, vol. 17, no. 1, pp. 89–97, 2010.

[40] C. Magi-Galluzzi, R. Mishra, M. Fiorentino et al., "Mitogen-activated protein kinase phosphatase 1 is overexpressed in prostate cancers and is inversely related to apoptosis," *Laboratory Investigation*, vol. 76, no. 1, pp. 37–51, 1997.

[41] A. R. Uzgare, P. J. Kaplan, and N. M. Greenberg, "Differential expression and/or activation of p38MAPK, erk1/2, and jnk during the initiation and progression of prostate cancer," *Prostate*, vol. 55, no. 2, pp. 128–139, 2003.

[42] R. L. Grubb, J. Deng, P. A. Pinto et al., "Pathway biomarker profiling of localized and metastatic human prostate cancer reveal metastatic and prognostic signatures," *Journal of Proteome Research*, vol. 8, no. 6, pp. 3044–3054, 2009.

[43] W. N. Yap, P. N. Chang, H. Y. Han et al., "γ-tocotrienol suppresses prostate cancer cell proliferation and invasion through multiple-signalling pathways," *The British Journal of Cancer*, vol. 99, no. 11, pp. 1832–1841, 2008.

[44] J. Watanabe, H. Nishiyama, Y. Matsui et al., "Dicoumarol potentiates cisplatin-induced apoptosis mediated by c-Jun N-terminal kinase in p53 wild-type urogenital cancer cell lines," *Oncogene*, vol. 25, no. 17, pp. 2500–2508, 2006.

[45] W. L. Chang, C. S. Chang, P. C. Chiang et al., "2-Phenyl-5-(pyrrolidin-1-yl)-1-(3,4,5-trimethoxybenzyl)-1H-benzimidazole, a benzimidazole derivative, inhibits growth of human prostate cancer cells by affecting tubulin and c-Jun

N-terminal kinase," *The British Journal of Pharmacology*, vol. 160, no. 7, pp. 1677–1689, 2010.

[46] Y. R. Chen, J. Han, R. Kori, A. N. Tony Kong, and T. H. Tan, "Phenylethyl isothiocyanate induces apoptotic signaling via suppressing phosphatase activity against c-Jun N-terminal kinase," *Journal of Biological Chemistry*, vol. 277, no. 42, pp. 39334–39342, 2002.

[47] C. Xu, G. Shen, X. Yuan et al., "ERK and JNK signaling pathways are involved in the regulation of activator protein 1 and cell death elicited by three isothiocyanates in human prostate cancer PC-3 cells," *Carcinogenesis*, vol. 27, no. 3, pp. 437–445, 2006.

[48] P. I. Lorenzo and F. Saatcioglu, "Inhibition of apoptosis in prostate cancer cells by androgens is mediated through downregulation of c-Jun N-terminal kinase activation," *Neoplasia*, vol. 10, no. 5, pp. 418–428, 2008.

[49] J. Antosiewicz, W. Ziolkowski, J. J. Kaczor, and A. Herman-Antosiewicz, "Tumor necrosis factor-α-induced reactive oxygen species formation is mediated by JNK1-dependent ferritin ç degradation and elevation of labile iron pool," *Free Radical Biology and Medicine*, vol. 43, no. 2, pp. 265–270, 2007.

[50] A. M. Sánchez, S. Malagarie-Cazenave, N. Olea, D. Vara, A. Chiloeches, and I. Díaz-Laviada, "Apoptosis induced by capsaicin in prostate PC-3 cells involves ceramide accumulation, neutral sphingomyelinase, and JNK activation," *Apoptosis*, vol. 12, no. 11, pp. 2013–2024, 2007.

[51] S. V. Singh, S. Choi, Y. Zeng, E. R. Hahm, and D. Xiao, "Guggulsterone-induced apoptosis in human prostate cancer cells is caused by reactive oxygen intermediate dependent activation of c-Jun NH2-terminal kinase," *Cancer Research*, vol. 67, no. 15, pp. 7439–7449, 2007.

[52] H. Y. Hong and B. C. Kim, "Mixed lineage kinase 3 connects reactive oxygen species to c-Jun NH2-terminal kinase-induced mitochondrial apoptosis in genipin-treated PC3 human prostate cancer cells," *Biochemical and Biophysical Research Communications*, vol. 362, no. 2, pp. 307–312, 2007.

[53] S. Yang, M. Lim, L. K. Pham et al., "Bone morphogenetic protein 7 protects prostate cancer cells from stress-induced apoptosis via both Smad and c-Jun NH2-terminal kinase pathways," *Cancer Research*, vol. 66, no. 8, pp. 4285–4290, 2006.

[54] J. F. Curtin and T. G. Cotter, "JNK regulates HIPK3 expression and promotes resistance to Fas-mediated apoptosis in DU 145 prostate carcinoma cells," *Journal of Biological Chemistry*, vol. 279, no. 17, pp. 17090–17100, 2004.

[55] H. Yun, H. S. Kim, S. Lee et al., "AMP kinase signaling determines whether c-Jun N-terminal kinase promotes survival or apoptosis during glucose deprivation," *Carcinogenesis*, vol. 30, no. 3, pp. 529–537, 2009.

[56] G. T. Kwon, H. J. Cho, W. Y. Chung, K. K. Park, A. Moon, and J. H. Y. Park, "Isoliquiritigenin inhibits migration and invasion of prostate cancer cells: possible mediation by decreased JNK/AP-1 signaling," *Journal of Nutritional Biochemistry*, vol. 20, no. 9, pp. 663–676, 2009.

[57] S. H. Hung, K. H. Shen, C. H. Wu, C. L. Liu, and Y. W. Shih, "α-mangostin suppresses PC-3 human prostate carcinoma cell metastasis by inhibiting matrix metalloproteinase-2/9 and urokinase-plasminogen expression through the JNK signaling pathway," *Journal of Agricultural and Food Chemistry*, vol. 57, no. 4, pp. 1291–1298, 2009.

[58] C. S. Chien, K. H. Shen, J. S. Huang, S. C. Ko, and Y. W. Shih, "Antimetastatic potential of fisetin involves

inactivation of the PI3K/Akt and JNK signaling pathways with downregulation of MMP-2/9 expressions in prostate cancer PC-3 cells," *Molecular and Cellular Biochemistry*, vol. 333, no. 1-2, pp. 169–180, 2010.

[59] J. Raingeaud, S. Gupta, J. S. Rogers et al., "Pro-inflammatory cytokines and environmental stress cause p38 mitogen-activated protein kinase activation by dual phosphorylation on tyrosine and threonine," *Journal of Biological Chemistry*, vol. 270, no. 13, pp. 7420–7426, 1995.

[60] L. Hui, L. Bakiri, E. Stepniak, and E. F. Wagner, "p38α: a suppressor of cell proliferation and tumorigenesis," *Cell Cycle*, vol. 6, no. 20, pp. 2429–2433, 2007.

[61] T. M. Thornton and M. Rincon, "Non-classical p38 map kinase functions: cell cycle checkpoints and survival," *International Journal of Biological Sciences*, vol. 5, no. 1, pp. 44–51, 2009.

[62] Y. Jiang, Z. Li, E. M. Schwarz et al., "Structure-function studies of p38 mitogen-activated protein kinase. Loop 12 influences substrate specificity and autophosphorylation, but not upstream kinase selection," *Journal of Biological Chemistry*, vol. 272, no. 17, pp. 11096–11102, 1997.

[63] X. S. Wang, K. Diener, C. L. Manthey et al., "Molecular cloning and characterization of a novel p38 mitogen-activated protein kinase," *Journal of Biological Chemistry*, vol. 272, no. 38, pp. 23668–23674, 1997.

[64] Y. Feng, J. Wen, and C. C. Chang, "p38 mitogen-activated protein kinase and hematologic malignancies," *Archives of Pathology and Laboratory Medicine*, vol. 133, no. 11, pp. 1850–1856, 2009.

[65] J. Whyte, O. Bergin, A. Bianchi, S. McNally, and F. Martin, "Key signalling nodes in mammary gland development and cancer. Mitogen-activated protein kinase signalling in experimental models of breast cancer progression and in mammary gland development," *Breast Cancer Research*, vol. 11, no. 5, p. 209, 2009.

[66] M. Zhao, L. New, V. V. Kravchenko et al., "Regulation of the MEF2 family of transcription factors by p38," *Molecular and Cellular Biology*, vol. 19, no. 1, pp. 21–30, 1999.

[67] M. Royuela, G. Rodríguez-Berriguete, B. Fraile, and R. Paniagua, "TNF-α/IL-1/NF-κB transduction pathway in human cancer prostate," *Histology and Histopathology*, vol. 23, no. 10, pp. 1279–1290, 2008.

[68] C. D. Wood, T. M. Thornton, G. Sabio, R. A. Davis, and M. Rincon, "Nuclear localization of p38 MAPK in response to DNA damage," *International Journal of Biological Sciences*, vol. 5, no. 5, pp. 428–437, 2009.

[69] B. Zheng, P. Flumara, Y. V. Li et al., "MEK/ERK pathway is aberrantly active in Hodgkin disease: a signaling pathway shared by CD30, CD40, and RANK that regulates cell proliferation and survival," *Blood*, vol. 102, no. 3, pp. 1019–1027, 2003.

[70] M. Ricote, I. García-Tuñón, F. Bethencourt et al., "The p38 transduction pathway in prostatic neoplasia," *Journal of Pathology*, vol. 208, no. 3, pp. 401–407, 2006.

[71] X. Guo, N. Ma, J. Wang et al., "Increased p38-MAPK is responsible for chemotherapy resistance in human gastric cancer cells," *BMC cancer*, vol. 8, p. 375, 2008.

[72] C. Zhang, H. Zhu, X. Yang et al., "P53 and p38 MAPK pathways are involved in MONCPT-induced cell cycle G2/M arrest in human non-small cell lung cancer A549," *Journal of Cancer Research and Clinical Oncology*, vol. 136, no. 3, pp. 437–445, 2010.

[73] D. L. Lin, M. C. Whitney, Z. Yao, and E. T. Keller, "Interleukin-6 induces androgen responsiveness in prostate cancer cells through up-regulation of androgen receptor expression," *Clinical Cancer Research*, vol. 7, no. 6, pp. 1773–1781, 2001.

[74] L. Khandrika, R. Lieberman, S. Koul et al., "Hypoxia-associated p38 mitogen-activated protein kinase-mediated androgen receptor activation and increased HIF-1α levels contribute to emergence of an aggressive phenotype in prostate cancer," *Oncogene*, vol. 28, no. 9, pp. 1248–1260, 2009.

[75] X. Huang, S. Chen, L. Xu et al., "Genistein inhibits p38 map kinase activation, matrix metalloproteinase type 2, and cell invasion in human prostate epithelial cells," *Cancer Research*, vol. 65, no. 8, pp. 3470–3478, 2005.

[76] K. H. Shen, S. H. Hung, L. T. Yin et al., "Acacetin, a flavonoid, inhibits the invasion and migration of human prostate cancer DU145 cells via inactivation of the p38 MAPK signaling pathway," *Molecular and Cellular Biochemistry*, vol. 333, no. 1-2, pp. 279–291, 2010.

[77] L. Xu, Y. Ding, W. J. Catalona et al., "MEK4 function, genistein treatment, and invasion of human prostate cancer cells," *Journal of the National Cancer Institute*, vol. 101, no. 16, pp. 1141–1155, 2009.

[78] C. H. Tang and M. E. Lu, "Adiponectin increases motility of human prostate cancer cells via AdipoR, p38, AMPK, and NF-κB pathways," *Prostate*, vol. 69, no. 16, pp. 1781–1789, 2009.

[79] T. Hunter, "Signaling—2000 and beyond," *Cell*, vol. 100, no. 1, pp. 113–127, 2000.

[80] Y. Liu, L. Formisano, I. Savtchouk et al., "A single fear-inducing stimulus induces a transcription-dependent switch in synaptic AMPAR phenotype," *Nature Neuroscience*, vol. 13, no. 2, pp. 223–231, 2010.

[81] R. Marais and C. J. Marshall, "Control of the ERK MAP kinase cascade by ras and raf," *Cancer Surveys*, vol. 27, pp. 101–125, 1996.

[82] S. Peng, Y. Zhang, J. Zhang, H. Wang, and B. Ren, "ERK in learning and memory: a review of recent research," *International Journal of Molecular Sciences*, vol. 11, no. 1, pp. 222–232, 2010.

[83] G. Pearson, F. Robinson, T. B. Gibson et al., "Mitogen-activated protein (MAP) kinase pathways: regulation and physiological functions," *Endocrine Reviews*, vol. 22, no. 2, pp. 153–183, 2001.

[84] G. Pagès, J. Milanini, D. E. Richard et al., "Signaling angiogenesis via p42/p44 MAP kinase cascade," *Annals of the New York Academy of Sciences*, vol. 902, pp. 187–200, 2000.

[85] E. J. Joslin, L. K. Opresko, A. Wells, H. S. Wiley, and D. A. Lauffenburger, "EGF-receptor-mediated mammary epithelial cell migration is driven by sustained ERK signaling from autocrine stimulation," *Journal of Cell Science*, vol. 120, no. 20, pp. 3688–3699, 2007.

[86] D. J. Price, S. Avraham, J. Feuerstein, Y. Fu, and H. K. Avraham, "The invasive phenotype in HMT-3522 cells requires increased EGF receptor signaling through both PI 3-kinase and ERK 1,2 pathways," *Cell Communication and Adhesion*, vol. 9, no. 2, pp. 87–102, 2002.

[87] P. J. Cullen and P. J. Lockyer, "Integration of calcium and Ras signalling," *Nature Reviews Molecular Cell Biology*, vol. 3, no. 5, pp. 339–348, 2002.

[88] D. A. Eisinger and H. Ammer, "δ-opioid receptors activate ERK/MAP kinase via integrin-stimulated receptor tyrosine kinases," *Cellular Signalling*, vol. 20, pp. 2324–2331, 2008.

[89] L. Gao, L. Chao, and J. Chao, "A novel signaling pathway of tissue kallikrein in promoting keratinocyte migration: activation of proteinase-activated receptor 1 and epidermal growth factor receptor," *Experimental Cell Research*, vol. 316, no. 3, pp. 376–389, 2010.

[90] A. Zebisch, A. P. Czernilofsky, G. Keri, J. Smigelskaite, H. Sill, and J. Troppmair, "Signaling through RAS-RAF-MEK-ERK: from basics to bedside," *Current Medicinal Chemistry*, vol. 14, no. 5, pp. 601–623, 2007.

[91] J. S. Silver and C. A. Hunter, "gp130 at the nexus of inflammation, autoimmunity, and cancer," *Journal of Leukocyte Biology*, vol. 88, no. 6, pp. 1145–1156, 2010.

[92] G. Werlen, B. Hausmann, D. Naeher, and E. Palmer, "Signaling life and death in the thymus: timing is everything," *Science*, vol. 299, no. 5614, pp. 1859–1863, 2003.

[93] N. Thakur, A. Sorrentino, C. H. Heldin, and M. Landström, "TGF-β uses the E3-ligase TRAF6 to turn on the kinase TAK1 to kill prostate cancer cells," *Future Oncology*, vol. 5, no. 1, pp. 1–3, 2009.

[94] K. J. Wilson, J. L. Gilmore, J. Foley, M. A. Lemmon, and D. J. Riese, "Functional selectivity of EGF family peptide growth factors: implications for cancer," *Pharmacology and Therapeutics*, vol. 122, no. 1, pp. 1–8, 2009.

[95] M. P. De Miguel, M. Royuela, F. R. Bethencourt, L. Santa-maria, B. Fraile, and R. Paniagua, "Immuno-expression of tumor necrosis factor-a and its receptors 1 and 2 correlates with proliferation/apoptosis equilibrium in normal, hyperplasic and carcinomatous human prostate," *Cytokine*, vol. 5, pp. 535–538, 2000.

[96] M. Royuela, M. P. De Miguel, F. R. Bethencourt, M. Sanchez-Chapado, B. Fraile, and R. Paniagua, "Transforming growth factor β1 and its receptor types I and II. Comparison in human normal prostate, benign prostatic hyperplasia, and prostatic carcinoma," *Growth Factors*, vol. 16, no. 2, pp. 101–110, 1998.

[97] I. Leav, J. E. McNeal, J. Ziar, and J. Alroy, "The localization of transforming growth factor alpha and epidermal growth factor receptor in stromal and epithelial compartments of developing human prostate and hyperplastic, dysplastic, and carcinomatous lesions," *Human Pathology*, vol. 29, no. 7, pp. 668–675, 1998.

[98] M. R. Cardillo, E. Petrangeli, L. Perracchio, L. Salvatori, L. Ravenna, and F. Di Silverio, "Transforming growth factor-beta expression in prostate neoplasia," *Analytical & Quantitative Cytology & Histology*, vol. 22, pp. 1–10, 2000.

[99] N. Eckstein, K. Servan, L. Girard et al., "Epidermal growth factor receptor pathway analysis identifies amphiregulin as a key factor for cisplatin resistance of human breast cancer cells," *Journal of Biological Chemistry*, vol. 283, no. 2, pp. 739–750, 2008.

[100] T. Putz, Z. Culig, I. E. Eder et al., "Epidermal growth factor (EGF) receptor blockade inhibits the action of EGF, insulin-like growth factor I, and a protein kinase A activator on the mitogen-activated protein kinase pathway in prostate cancer cell lines," *Cancer Research*, vol. 59, no. 1, pp. 227–233, 1999.

[101] P. L. De Souza, M. Castillo, and C. E. Myers, "Enhancement of paclitaxel activity against hormone-refractory prostate cancer cells in vitro and in vivo by quinacrine," *The British Journal of Cancer*, vol. 75, no. 11, pp. 1593–1600, 1997.

[102] H. Y. Chang, H. Nishitoh, X. Yang, H. Ichijo, and D. Baltimore, "Activation of apoptosis signal-regulating kinase 1 (ASK1) by the adapter protein Daxx," *Science*, vol. 281, no. 5384, pp. 1860–1863, 1998.

[103] M. Dews, M. Prisco, F. Peruzzi, G. Romano, A. Morrione, and R. Baserga, "Domains of the insulin-like growth factor I receptor required for the activation of extracellular signal-regulated kinases," *Endocrinology*, vol. 141, no. 4, pp. 1289–1300, 2000.

[104] G. Rodriguez-Berriguete, A. Prieto, B. Fraile et al., "Relationship between IL-6/ERK and NF-κB: a study in normal and pathological human prostate gland (benign hyperplasia, intraepithelial neoplasia and cancer)," *European Cytokine Network*, vol. 21, no. 4, pp. 241–250, 2010.

[105] J. A. McCubrey, L. S. Steelman, W. H. Chappell et al., "Roles of the Raf/MEK/ERK pathway in cell growth, malignant transformation and drug resistance," *Biochim Biophys Acta*, vol. 1773, pp. 1263–1284, 2007.

[106] S. Grant, "Cotargeting survival signaling pathways in cancer," *Journal of Clinical Investigation*, vol. 118, no. 9, pp. 3003–3006, 2008.

[107] H. Mueller, N. Flury, S. Eppenberger-Castori, W. Kueng, F. David, and U. Eppenberger, "Potential prognostic value of mitogen-activated protein kinase activity for disease-free survival of primary breast cancer patients," *International Journal of Cancer*, vol. 89, no. 4, pp. 384–388, 2000.

[108] S. Schubbert, K. Shannon, and G. Bollag, "Hyperactive ras in developmental disorders and cancer," *Nature Reviews Cancer*, vol. 7, no. 4, pp. 295–308, 2007.

[109] E. Halilovic and D. B. Solit, "Therapeutic strategies for inhibiting oncogenic BRAF signaling," *Current Opinion in Pharmacology*, vol. 8, no. 4, pp. 419–426, 2008.

[110] E. T. Keller, Z. Fu, K. Yeung, and M. Brennan, "Raf kinase inhibitor protein: a prostate cancer metastasis suppressor gene," *Cancer Letters*, vol. 207, no. 2, pp. 131–137, 2004.

[111] B. Wegiel, A. Bjartell, Z. Culig, and J. L. Persson, "Interleukin-6 activates PI3K/Akt pathway and regulates cyclin A1 to promote prostate cancer cell survival," *International Journal of Cancer*, vol. 122, no. 7, pp. 1521–1529, 2008.

[112] J. Karkera, H. Steiner, W. Li et al., "The anti-interleukin-6 antibody siltuximab down-regulates genes implicated in tumorigenesis in prostate cancer patients from a phase I study," *Prostate*, vol. 71, pp. 1455–1465, 2011.

[113] H. Steiner, S. Godoy-Tundidor, H. Rogatsch et al., "Accelerated in vivo growth of prostate tumors that up-regulate interleukin-6 is associated with reduced retinoblastoma protein expression and activation of the mitogen-activated protein kinase pathway," *The American Journal of Pathology*, vol. 162, no. 2, pp. 655–663, 2003.

[114] C. P. Pjaweletz, L. Charboneau, V. E. Bichsel et al., "Reverse phase protein microarrays which capture disease progression show activation of pro-survival pathways at the cancer invasion front," *Oncogene*, vol. 20, no. 16, pp. 1981–1989, 2001.

[115] S. N. Malik, M. Brattain, P. M. Ghosh et al., "Immunohistochemical demonstration of phospho-Akt in high Gleason grade prostate cancer," *Clinical Cancer Research*, vol. 8, no. 4, pp. 1168–1171, 2002.

[116] D. Gioeli, J. W. Mandell, G. R. Petroni, H. F. Frierson, and M. J. Weber, "Activation of mitogen-activated protein kinase associated with prostate cancer progression," *Cancer Research*, vol. 59, no. 2, pp. 279–284, 1999.

[117] M. E. Grossmann, H. Huang, and D. J. Tindall, "Androgen receptor signaling in androgen-refractory prostate cancer," *Journal of the National Cancer Institute*, vol. 93, no. 22, pp. 1687–1697, 2001.

[118] Y. Zhu, C. Culmsee, S. Klumpp, and J. Krieglstein, "Neuroprotection by transforming growth factor-β1 involves activation of nuclear factor-κB through phosphatidylinositol-3-OH kinase/Akt and mitogen-activated protein kinase-extracellular-signal regulated kinase1,2 signaling pathways," *Neuroscience*, vol. 123, no. 4, pp. 897–906, 2004.

[119] L. F. Chu, W. T. Wang, V. K. Ghanta, C. H. Lin, Y. Y. Chiang, and C. M. Hsueh, "Ischemic brain cell-derived conditioned medium protects astrocytes against ischemia through GDNF/ERK/NF-κB signaling pathway," *Brain Research*, vol. 1239, pp. 24–35, 2008.

[120] M. Karin, "Nuclear factor-κB in cancer development and progression," *Nature*, vol. 441, no. 7092, pp. 431–436, 2006.

[121] G. Rodriguez-Berriguete, B. Fraile, F. R. de Bethencourt et al., "Role of IAPs in prostate cancer progression: immunohistochemical study in normal and pathological (benign hyperplastic, prostatic intraepithelial neoplasia and cancer) human prostate," *BMC Cancer*, vol. 10, p. 18, 2010.

[122] B. B. Aggarwal, "Tumour necrosis factors receptor associated signalling molecules and their role in activation of apoptosis, JNK and NF-κB," *Annals of the Rheumatic Diseases*, vol. 59, no. 1, pp. i6–i16, 2000.

[123] J. D. Lee, R. J. Ulevitch, and J. Han, "Primary structure of BMK1: a new mammalian map kinase," *Biochemical and Biophysical Research Communications*, vol. 213, pp. 715–724, 1995.

[124] G. Zhou, Zhao Qin Bao, and J. E. Dixon, "Components of a new human protein kinase signal transduction pathway," *Journal of Biological Chemistry*, vol. 270, no. 21, pp. 12665–12669, 1995.

[125] Y. Kato, R. I. Tapping, S. Huang, M. H. Watson, R. J. Ulevitch, and J. D. Lee, "Bmk1/Erk5 is required for cell proliferation induced by epidermal growth factor," *Nature*, vol. 395, no. 6703, pp. 713–716, 1998.

[126] R. S. Sawhney, W. Liu, and M. G. Brattain, "A novel role of ERK5 in integrin-mediated cell adhesion and motility in cancer cells via Fak signaling," *Journal of Cellular Physiology*, vol. 219, no. 1, pp. 152–161, 2009.

[127] M. Kayahara, X. Wang, and C. Tournier, "Selective regulation of c-jun gene expression by mitogen-activated protein kinases via the 12-o-tetradecanoylphorbol-13-acetate-responsive element and myocyte enhancer factor 2 binding sites," *Molecular and Cellular Biology*, vol. 25, no. 9, pp. 3784–3792, 2005.

[128] S. Kamakura, T. Moriguchi, and E. Nishida, "Activation of the protein kinase ERK5/BMK1 by receptor tyrosine kinases. Identification and characterization of a signalling pathway to the nucleus," *Journal of Biological Chemistry*, vol. 274, no. 37, pp. 26563–26571, 1999.

[129] Y. Kato, V. V. Kravchenko, R. I. Tapping, J. Han, R. J. Ulevitch, and J. D. Lee, "BMK1/ERK5 regulates serum-induced early gene expression through transcription factor MEF2C," *EMBO Journal*, vol. 16, no. 23, pp. 7054–7066, 1997.

[130] J. M. English, G. Pearson, R. Baer, and M. H. Cobb, "Identification of substrates and regulators of the mitogen-activated protein kinase ERK5 using chimeric protein kinases," *Journal of Biological Chemistry*, vol. 273, no. 7, pp. 3854–3860, 1998.

[131] S. R. C. McCracken, A. Ramsay, R. Heer et al., "Aberrant expression of extracellular signal-regulated kinase 5 in human prostate cancer," *Oncogene*, vol. 27, no. 21, pp. 2978–2988, 2008.

5

Protein-Tyrosine Kinase Signaling in the Biological Functions Associated with Sperm

Takashi W. Ijiri,[1] A. K. M. Mahbub Hasan,[1, 2] and Ken-ichi Sato[1]

[1] *Laboratory of Cell Signaling and Development, Department of Molecular Biosciences, Faculty of Life Sciences, Kyoto Sangyo University, Kyoto 603-8555, Japan*
[2] *Laboratory of Gene Biology, Department of Biochemistry and Molecular Biology, University of Dhaka, Dhaka 1000, Bangladesh*

Correspondence should be addressed to Ken-ichi Sato, kksato@cc.kyoto-su.ac.jp

Academic Editor: Alakananda Basu

In sexual reproduction, two gamete cells (i.e., egg and sperm) fuse (fertilization) to create a newborn with a genetic identity distinct from those of the parents. In the course of these developmental processes, a variety of signal transduction events occur simultaneously in each of the two gametes, as well as in the fertilized egg/zygote/early embryo. In particular, a growing body of knowledge suggests that the tyrosine kinase Src and/or other protein-tyrosine kinases are important elements that facilitate successful implementation of the aforementioned processes in many animal species. In this paper, we summarize recent findings on the roles of protein-tyrosine phosphorylation in many sperm-related processes (from spermatogenesis to epididymal maturation, capacitation, acrosomal exocytosis, and fertilization).

1. Introduction

Protein-tyrosine kinase (PTK) activity and tyrosine phosphorylation of cellular protein were initially discovered by Hunter and colleagues [1–3]; they analyzed the protein kinase activity associated with the protein complex of polyoma virus middle T antigen and viral Src gene product, a cellular counterpart of which is the cellular Src protein. At that time, phosphorylation events on amino acids other than tyrosine (i.e., serine and threonine residues) were already known as posttranslational modifications of physiological importance. However, the discovery of tyrosine phosphorylation for the first time opened a window to understand the relationship between protein phosphorylation (including serine/threonine phosphorylation) and malignant cell transformation (e.g., development of cancer) [4]. In addition, a growing body of evidence has demonstrated that tyrosine phosphorylation catalyzed by cellular Src and other PTKs expressed in normal cells and tissues regulates a variety of cellular functions such as developmental processes, disorder of normal cell functions, immunological responses, neuronal differentiation and transmission, pathological infection, and senescence. Thus, protein-tyrosine phosphorylation has

emerged as a signal transduction mechanism of fundamental importance in all eukaryotic cells and, in some cases, prokaryotic cell behavior [5–7].

In the sexual reproduction system, two different kinds of gamete cell: egg and sperm, interact and fuse with each other to accomplish fertilization that gives rise to a newborn [8]. In this fundamental biological event, both egg and sperm undergo a number of biochemical and cell biological reactions that culminate in successful embryogenesis and early development. Especially in the case of multicellular organisms including humans, egg and sperm are special cells in view of their appearance as a single cell. To become such a specialized type of cell, the ancestor of the gametes, that is, primordial germ cell (PGC), along with sex determination in the host, must undergo meiotic cell division [9]. Moreover, to become fully competent for fertilization, egg and sperm must undergo a series of "differentiation" or "maturation" events [10–12]. During the past several decades, a number of studies have dealt with the cellular and molecular mechanisms of gametogenesis, fertilization, and embryogenesis. Among these are characterizations of protein-tyrosine phosphorylation in these events that involved identification of the responsible PTKs (e.g., Src), their regulators and substrates, and

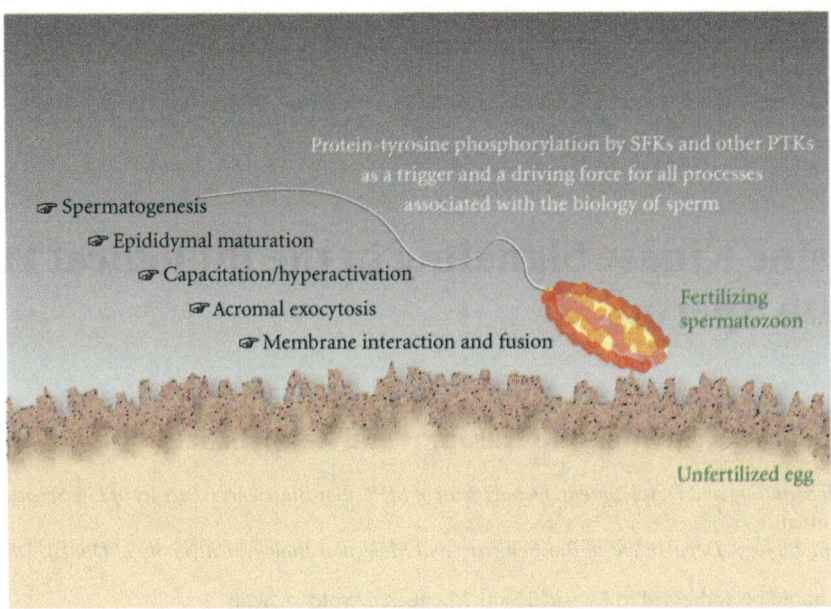

FIGURE 1: Protein-tyrosine phosphorylation and the biology of sperm. A sequence of events in the sperm must be done to facilitate a successful fertilization. The events include spermatogenesis and epididymal maturation that occur in the male reproductive organs, capacitation/hyperactivation and acrosomal exocytosis (or acrosome reaction, AE) in the female reproductive tract (in the case of species employing internal fertilization: e.g., mammals) or in the extracellular space (in the case of species employing external fertilization: e.g., frogs and fishes), and gamete interaction and fusion at the plasma membranes. In all of these processes, protein-tyrosine phosphorylation catalyzed by SFKs (e.g., Src) and/or other PTKs (e.g., EGFR, Abl) is suggested to play an important role. For details, see text.

evaluation of their roles for cellular functions [13–19]. In this paper, we will briefly discuss the biology of sperm (gametogenesis, differentiation, maturation, and fertilization), recent achievements in understanding the involvement of PTKs and protein-tyrosine phosphorylation in the biology of sperm, and future directions for this research field (Figure 1).

2. General View of Sperm Biology

Spermatogenesis is a highly specialized process of cellular differentiation in which diploid progenitor cells of the testis differentiate into haploid spermatozoa [20]. The entire process is divided into three sequential mitotic, meiotic, and postmeiotic stages. In the male meiotic stage, after PGCs migrate into the genital ridges, they become gonocytes and start differentiation into spermatogonia at the basement of seminiferous tubules. Some of them, spermatogonial stem cells (SSCs), also retain the ability for self-renewal [21]. Owing to the role of SSCs, sperm are produced continually (more than 50,000,000 a day in humans) almost throughout the lifetime. Meiosis is the event in which chromosome pairing and genetic recombination occur in the functional tetraploid pachytene spermatocytes [22]. In this process, the genes are shuffled between homologous chromosomes, which results in genetic diversity. This helps the species to survive through natural selection.

Most of the components found in mature spermatozoa are primarily produced at the postmeiotic phase in mammals, and developing spermatids display a variety of

morphological and biochemical changes [23]. Many of the organelles in spermatids are transformed into specific structures; the acrosome originates from Golgi body and the main part of the flagellum is composed of spindle-shaped body. The flagellum contains cytoskeletal components and signal transduction mediators. The fibrous sheath, a unique mammalian cytoskeletal structure surrounding the axoneme, serves as a scaffold for constituents of signaling cascades in the regulation of sperm motility [24]. The nucleus is also changed into the tightly compacted shape and size of sperm head by the sequential replacement of the histones with transition proteins and protamines [25].

All stages in spermatogenesis are regulated by the stage-specific expression of a wide variety of genes. Other factors that influence spermatogenesis are the interactions between Sertoli cells and testosterone produced from Leydig cells [26]. In female animals, however, the limited numbers of oogonia differentiate, progress through the first meiotic prophase, and are arrested in the infant ovary. Then, with the onset of adolescence, they mature to second meiotic metaphase and are arrested again. Some of them are released by ovulation and complete meiosis by the entry of a sperm [27]. Similar criteria for oogenesis and oocyte maturation also apply in other kinds of vertebrates, including frog and fish [28, 29]. Testicular sperm look morphologically mature, but they are immotile. Therefore, after sperm leave the testis, they require a further maturation process to acquire the functions for fertilizing an oocyte during transmission through the epididymis [30].

The sperm pass through the caput, corpus, and cauda epididymides sequentially. Then, they are stored at the cauda epididymis until ejaculation. While transiting through the epididymis, they undergo biochemical and physiological modifications, resulting in the acquisition of basal motility and the ability to fertilize an oocyte. These modifications include changes in the glycosylation of acrosomal proteins [31, 32] and in the lipid composition of sperm [33], as well as elevations of cyclic adenosine monophosphate (cAMP) [34, 35] and negative charge on the sperm surface [36]. The other difference between caput and cauda epididymal sperm is the pattern of protein tyrosine phosphorylation [37].

Mammalian sperm need to change their status further to acquire the ability to become competent to bind and fuse with an oocyte after release into the female reproductive tract [38, 39]. This change is termed "capacitation" and confers hyperactivated motility (hyperactivation) and an ability to undergo acrosomal exocytosis (AE) or acrosome reaction to the sperm [8]. To be capacitated, sperm require a period of incubation and interaction in the female reproductive tract. However, this can be induced in vitro in an appropriate experimental medium [40]. Capacitation promotes changes in cholesterol content, plasma membrane fluidity, and intracellular ion concentrations [41]. Another good hallmark for capacitation is an increase in protein tyrosine phosphorylation [42]. Chemotaxis is a phenomenon that guides cells to undergo correct movement toward or away from certain chemicals. This is also known to be important for sperm to interact with an oocyte in the female reproductive tract [43], maybe because sperm are extremely small compared with oocytes. Chemotaxis for sperm guidance was discovered first in marine invertebrate species [44], then in amphibians and mammals [45]. In eutherian mammals, AE releases proteolytic enzymes from the acrosome stored in sperm head [8]. It was believed that these enzymes assist in sperm penetration through the zona pellucida (ZP), the glycoprotein coating on the surface of oocytes, and fusion with an oocyte. However, a recent observation from in vitro fertilization suggests that most sperm undergo AE before contact with the ZP [46], showing the need to reconsider the timing and biological significance of AE during a series of sperm events.

Fertilization-related phenomena include gamete interaction and fusion, egg activation, polyspermy block, and nuclear fusion, all of which culminates in initiation of embryonic development. To date, the sperm membrane protein Izumo1 [47] and the oocyte surface protein CD9 [48–50] are reported to be indispensable for the fusion between sperm and the oocyte plasma membrane in mouse. The gamete fusion triggers repeated increases (e.g., mouse) or a transient elevation (e.g., frog) in intracellular calcium ($[Ca^{2+}]_i$) in oocyte, so-called Ca^{2+} oscillation or Ca^{2+} wave, which serves as an initiator of egg activation [17, 51, 52]. It is still debatable how sperm can act as a trigger for egg activation [19]. One possibility is receptor-mediated activator, while another is diffusible activator, "sperm factor." Recent findings suggest that inositol trisphosphate (IP$_3$) acts as a second messenger for the Ca^{2+} release reactions and that the egg-associated Src-phospholipase Cγ (PLCγ) (e.g., sea urchin, frog) [14, 16] or the sperm-derived components such as PLCζ (e.g., mouse) [53] and citrate synthase (newt) [54]

mediate the gamete interaction/fusion and the activation of IP$_3$-dependent Ca^{2+} release. After a sperm enters an oocyte, the nucleus has to be decondensed as a pronucleus for nuclear fusion. Then, the fertilized egg starts DNA synthesis for the following early embryogenesis.

Recently, using proteomics approaches, a number of sperm proteins in mouse and rat have been identified as those that are phosphorylated on tyrosine residues during epididymal maturation and capacitation [55–57]. Our group has also reported important roles of Src family PTKs (SFKs) in the sperm-induced egg activation during gamete interaction and fusion by using the African clawed frog, *Xenopus laevis*. The following sections are an overview of the recent progress to understand the correlations between PTKs and various sperm events.

3. Involvement of PTKs in Spermatogenesis

PTKs play various biological roles in many types of somatic cell, so it is not surprising that they act on spermatogenic cells and their supporting cells, that is, Sertoli cells, in the testis. Actually, it has been demonstrated that several families of PTKs including Src kinase are correlated with most spermatogenic events (Figure 2). In adult mouse testis, the protein expression of Src, Lyn, and Hck were observed, while the expressions of eight members of the SFK were detected by quantitative polymerase chain reaction. For instance, Src protein localizes weakly to the cytoplasm in spermatocytes and strongly in round and elongated spermatids, leading to strong accumulation in acrosome of cauda epididymal sperm with entire flagellum detection [58]. In humans, Src protein was detected strongly around the acrosomal region in round and elongated spermatids [59].

c-Kit is a transmembrane tyrosine kinase receptor that binds to stem cell factor (SCF). SCF induces dimerization of c-Kit that activates the tyrosine kinase residues by autophosphorylation [60], leading to the downstream signaling through phospho-tyrosine-binding adaptor proteins such as PLCγ1. During mouse early development, c-Kit is essential for the migration of PGCs to the genital ridges in the embryo and then functions in the maintenance of PGCs [61]. Src kinase is also involved in this process [62]. In adult mouse testis, the expression of c-Kit is detected in differentiating spermatogonia, whereas the expression of SCF is detected in Sertoli cells; therefore, c-Kit/SCF is important for maintaining differentiating type A spermatogonia [63]. On the other hand, to maintain the property of self-renewal in mouse SSCs, c-Ret tyrosine kinase receptor mediates between glial cell line-derived neurotrophic factor (GDNF) and Src family kinase signaling [64]. Recently, it has also been suggested that c-Kit plays a pivotal role in regulating the ratio between differentiation and self-renewal during maintenance of the SSC population [65].

There are a few reports about tyrosine phosphorylation in meiosis during spermatogenesis (Figure 2). Mouse has Fes-related proteins (Fer) of two different size, which correspond to 94 kDa or 51 kDa tyrosine kinase. The latter accumulates in primary spermatocytes where the cell cycle is

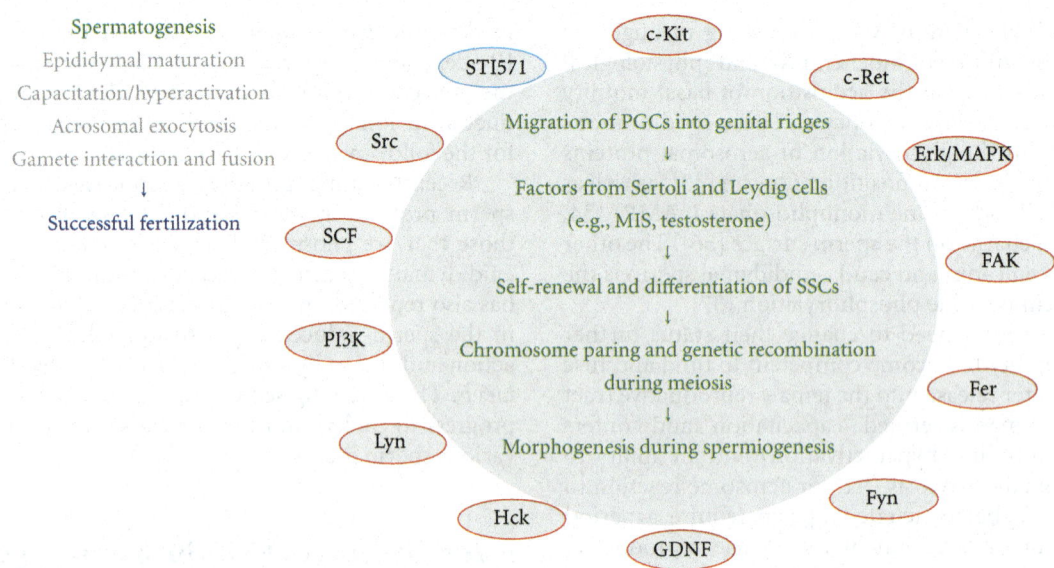

FIGURE 2: Protein-tyrosine phosphorylation and a sequence of events associated with spermatogenesis. For details of spermatogenesis and its associated signaling molecules (the full spelling of all abbreviations as well), see text. Note that MIS, Mullerian-inhibiting substance, is a testicular-differentiating factor that is produced in Sertoli cells and Leydig cells, whose differentiation is promoted by the actions of Sry and other sex-determining gene products. Also note that MIS acts in concert with testosterone. Note that positive regulators for protein-tyrosine phosphorylation are indicated in red circles

in the first meiotic prophase, and the role of phosphorylation for the timing of meiosis entry is suggested in mammals as well as in yeast [66]. c-Kit/SCF system is also required for transition when mouse spermatogonia undergo cell division to enter meiosis [67]. This was also examined using a specific inhibitor to c-Kit (STI571), resulting in reduction of the number of mouse meiotic cells under the control of retinoic acid [68].

Interestingly, some of the truncated forms of PTK seem to have roles in the process of sperm morphogenesis: spermiogenesis. At least three examples of nonreceptor tyrosine kinase, Fyn as well as Fer and Hck [69], have been reported. Truncated Fer was detected in the Golgi, acroplaxome, and manchette of rat spermatid [70], while truncated Hck was observed mainly at the acrosome of bovine sperm [71]. They are also suggested to regulate actin assembly via phosphorylation. Therefore, these observations suggest that truncated forms of Fer kinase and Hck may participate in sperm head shaping. Similarly, Golgi membrane in spermatids contains truncated Fyn that is missing the kinase domain, and this protein may be required for acrosome biogenesis [70]. A truncated isoform of c-Kit has also been detected in mouse round spermatids [72]. This protein lacks SCF-binding and dimerization domains, but retains a part of the kinase domain that would facilitate activation of PLCγ1 [73, 74]. It is suggested that truncated c-Kit is related to DNA integrity in human sperm [75]; however, its role is still unclear.

Another correlation of PTKs with spermatogenesis is in the regulation of Sertoli cell tight junction, including at the blood-testis barrier (BTB). Male germ cells need to contact with Sertoli cells during most spermatogenic processes.

Spermatogonia differentiate to preleptotene/leptotene spermatocytes in the basal compartment of the seminiferous epithelium. In addition, these spermatocytes have to translocate to the adluminal compartment of the seminiferous epithelium for further differentiation. However, there is the BTB, which acts as the immunological barrier between basal and adluminal compartments. Recently, it has been demonstrated that focal adhesion kinase (FAK), a nonreceptor tyrosine kinase, plays a key role in this process. FAK regulates the opening and/or closing of BTB by modulating the phosphorylation status of integral membrane proteins [76]. Besides, traditionally, FAK has been suggested to be involved in adherens junctions (AJ) between Sertoli and germ cells by the interactions with β1-integrin and other associated proteins including Src [76]. Moreover, Fer kinase has been shown to participate in the regulation of rat AJ [77]. Fyn functions in the basal ectoplasmic specialization (ES) of actin filaments: at the junction between Sertoli cells as well as apical ES and at the junction between spermatids and Sertoli cells [78]. Apical ES also contains many lipids and protein kinases such as phosphatidylinositol 3-kinase (PI3K) and extracellular signal-regulated kinase/mitogen-activated protein kinase (Erk/MAPK), which are associated with Src [79].

The major problem for research on mammalian spermatogenesis was the lack of a stable in vitro culture system, despite the efforts of many investigators [80, 81]. However, recently, an improved organ culture system using neonatal testis has been established, which can make SSCs differentiate to mature sperm in mouse [82]. This method for in vitro spermatogenesis should greatly facilitate the identification and characterization of more factors and genes correlated

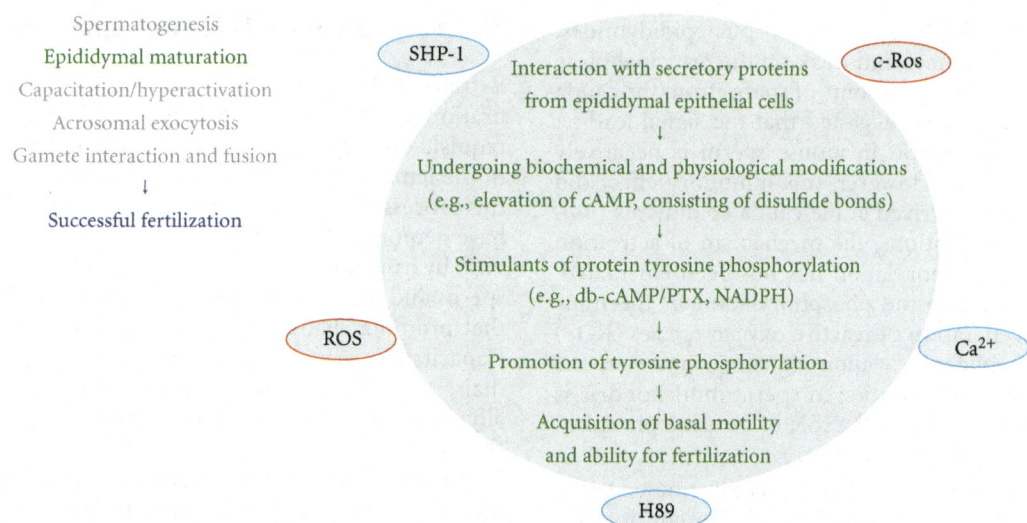

FIGURE 3: Protein-tyrosine phosphorylation and a sequence of events associated with epididymal maturation of sperm. For details of the epididymal maturation and its associated signaling molecules (the full spelling of all abbreviations as well), see text. Note that positive regulators for protein-tyrosine phosphorylation are indicated in red circles.

with PTKs for self-renewal and differentiation in spermatogonia, meiosis in spermatocytes, and morphogenesis in spermatids.

4. Involvement of PTKs in Epididymal Maturation

Like other cells, sperm need adenosine trisphosphate (ATP) as an energy resource for their functions, for example, motility. The dominant pathway for ATP production in mouse sperm is glycolysis, while spermatocytes and spermatids prefer oxidative phosphorylation [83–85]. It is suggested that this switching to glycolysis occurs during epididymal maturation in rabbit [86]. During epididymal maturation, sperm proteins contain a greater number of disulfide bonds, leading to the stabilization of sperm structures and promotion of tyrosine phosphorylation of sperm proteins (Figure 3) [87–89].

To investigate the importance of protein tyrosine phosphorylation during epididymal maturation, most analyses were performed with the antiphosphotyrosine antibody. Using western blotting, the contents of plasma membranes were compared between hamster caput and cauda epididymal sperm, resulting in a differential phosphorylation pattern: the proteins with sizes of 94, 52, and 47 kDa looked more intense in cauda epididymal sperm while the 67 kDa band had more intensity in caput epididymal sperm [90]. However, western blotting detected caput epididymal sperm-specific phosphotyrosine expression in 93, 66, and 45 kDa bands in boar [91]; in addition, rat sperm from caput epididymis tended to show a stronger total band pattern of tyrosine phosphorylation than that of cauda epididymal sperm [37]. Immunofluorescence analyses with the antiphosphotyrosine antibody were performed to visualize the distribution of tyrosine phosphorylation in sperm. After

permeabilization with methanol, boar sperm from proximal caput epididymis had strong labeling on the midacrosome as well as a faint signal on the whole tail. After transit through distal caput and corpus epididymides, this signal was detected only as a triangular shape on the posterior region of the midacrosome [91]. In mouse and rat, caput epididymal sperm, permeabilized with Nonidet P-40, resulted in fluorescence over the whole equatorial segment; however, the signal became restricted to a small region in the posterior equatorial segment after sperm moved to the cauda epididymis [92]. It is suggested that the equatorial segment plasma membrane works as a site of fusion with an oocyte membrane during fertilization; therefore, the accumulation of tyrosine phosphorylation may be connected to the later fusion process.

Lewis and Aitken have investigated the tyrosine phosphorylation pattern of sperm proteins after stimulation with cAMP by adding dibutyryl cAMP (db-cAMP) and pentoxifylline (PTX) [37]. By western blotting with the antiphosphotyrosine antibody in rat, the increase of cAMP resulted in more intense tyrosine phosphorylation bands in caput epididymal sperm proteins and much more intensity for cauda epididymal sperm proteins. However, this induction of tyrosine phosphorylation was inhibited by a protein kinase A (PKA)-inhibitor, H89 [37]. Immunofluorescence using the sperm fixed with methanol increased the signal in the tail region after db-cAMP/PTX stimulation [37]. Similar results were observed when the reduced form of NADPH (nicotinamide adenine dinucleotide phosphate) was added instead of db-cAMP, suggesting that this cAMP-dependent tyrosine phosphorylation is regulated by the redox system during epididymal maturation [93]. Furthermore, db-cAMP/PTX stimulation showed drastic change of the phosphotyrosine pattern in mouse sperm permeabilized with Triton X-100 as follows: staining on the acrosome and the principal piece of sperm from the proximal caput epididymis, strong on the midpiece as well as the acrosome and the principal piece of sperm from the distal caput and corpus epididymides, still strong on the midpiece and weak on the principal piece without any signal on the acrosome of sperm from the cauda epididymis [94]. It is also suggested that the signal leading to tyrosine phosphorylation in mouse sperm is negatively regulated by Ca^{2+} [95]. However, this inhibitory effect did not work when sperm arrived at the cauda epididymis [94]. Even with these observations, the mechanism of activation for this tyrosine phosphorylation has not been elucidated. One explanation of tyrosine phosphorylation in the midpiece is that the generation of reactive oxygen species (ROS) activates tyrosine phosphorylation signaling; however, the role of oxidative phosphorylation in sperm mitochondria is still controversial. At present, the role of tyrosine phosphorylation in the acrosome is unknown.

The progress of proteomic analysis has contributed to the identification of sperm proteins that are important for epididymal maturation, including the protein phosphorylation process. Using two-dimensional fluorescence difference gel electrophoresis, eight rat sperm proteins were identified as candidates that undergo posttranslational modifications during epididymal maturation, and one of them, β-subunit of mitochondrial F_1-ATPase, was serine-phosphorylated [96]. Recently, new methods using titanium dioxide have been developed to identify phosphopeptides, suggesting that 77 titanium-dioxide-enriched peptides (corresponding to 53 proteins) showed significant modifications during rat epididymal maturation [97].

Here, if we focus on PTKs in epididymal epithelium, the receptor tyrosine kinase Ros and Src homology-2 (SH2-) domain-containing protein tyrosine phosphatase SHP-1 are expressed there. The mutant mice for Ros or for SHP-1 showed defects in the differentiation of the epididymis [98, 99]. Moreover, the sperm interact with various secretory proteins from epithelial cells of epididymides during epididymal transit, and some of them are proposed to be involved in sperm maturation [100, 101]. Therefore, it will be necessary to study the epididymal luminal environment as well as sperm proteins to obtain a deeper understanding of the role of PTKs in the sperm maturation process.

Note. During the processes of galley proof, one paper about Src and epididymal development and sperm functions was published [102]. As highlighted in our manuscript, Src has been identified as a PTK involved in capacitation-associated tyrosine phosphorylation downstream of PKA pathway. Added to this aspect, in this newly published paper, Visconti and colleagues reported that the details about the male reproductive phenotypes of Src knockout (KO) mice and Src localization in epididymis as well as in sperm. Src is not detected in caput epididymal sperm but in the midpiece and the postacrosomal region of cauda epididymal sperm. Src is also detected strongly in clear cells and weakly in principle cells of cauda epididymis and is shown to transfer into cauda epididymal sperm via epididymosomes during epididymal transit. Src KO mice have smaller size of cauda epididymis and reduced sperm motility, leading to unsuccessful in vitro fertilization.

5. Involvement of PTKs in Capacitation

Extratesticular sperm that has completed epididymal maturation must undergo a process called capacitation, a prerequisite for hyperactivated motility and acrosome reaction, in the female reproductive tract. Two researchers discovered this process independently in the 1950s [38, 39]. Later studies have demonstrated that capacitation can be reconstituted in vitro by using cauda (but not caput) epididymal or ejaculated sperm and artificial media supplemented with components that promote changes associated with in vivo capacitation. Capacitation seems to be a phenomenon specific to mammals, and accumulating evidence indicates that it generally involves a burst of protein-tyrosine phosphorylation (Figure 4).

In mice, treatment of sperm with capacitation-inducing media promotes cAMP-dependent (i.e., PKA-dependent) tyrosine phosphorylation of several sperm proteins with molecular sizes of 116, 105, 95, 86, 76, and 54 kDa [103]. In particular, it is suggested that the 95 kDa phosphotyrosine-containing protein is identical to one that has been identified as a ZP3-dependent PTK substrate, namely, p95/zona receptor kinase (ZRK)/hexokinase (see below). Further studies by Visconti and colleagues have demonstrated that the sperm media should include bovine serum albumin (BSA), $CaCl_2$, and $NaHCO_3$ to induce capacitation and its associated tyrosine phosphorylation (proteins of 40–120 kDa) [104]. Interestingly, caput epididymal sperm, which lack an ability to undergo capacitation in vivo, cannot induce the tyrosine phosphorylation event in response to the treatment with capacitation media, indicating that epididymal maturation is required for the sperm response. In addition, it has also been shown that the requirement for BSA, $CaCl_2$, and $NaHCO_3$ in capacitation and associated PTK signaling is completely overcome by the addition of cAMP or its active analogs and that chemical inhibitors for PKAs (H-89, a substance that blocks ATP binding, and Rp-cAMPS, a nonhydrolysable AMP analog) interfere with the aforementioned processes [105]. These results clearly demonstrate that capacitation involves sequential activation of cAMP production and PKA-PTK pathway in response to the capacitation-inducing substances.

A similar system has also been demonstrated in other species including human [106] and mice of both domestic and wild-field species [107, 108]. Unlike mouse sperm, however, human sperm do not contain the 95 kDa phosphotyrosine-containing protein (p95/ZRK/hexokinase). Instead, the fibrous sheath proteins, AKAP82 (A-kinase/PKA anchoring protein 82: now referred as AKAP4), its precursor pro-AKAP82, and FSP95, a structural homolog of AKAP82, have been identified as prominently tyrosine-phosphorylated proteins in the capacitated sperm [109, 110]. Artificial Ca^{2+} signals, which promote the occurrence of acrosome reaction, lead to dephosphorylation of a subset of these phosphotyrosine-containing proteins. AKAP82 has also been identified as the major protein of the fibrous sheath of the mouse sperm flagellum, and its possible function to compartmentalize inactive PKA (before capacitation) to the cytoskeleton has been suggested [111]. Immunocytochemical and/or

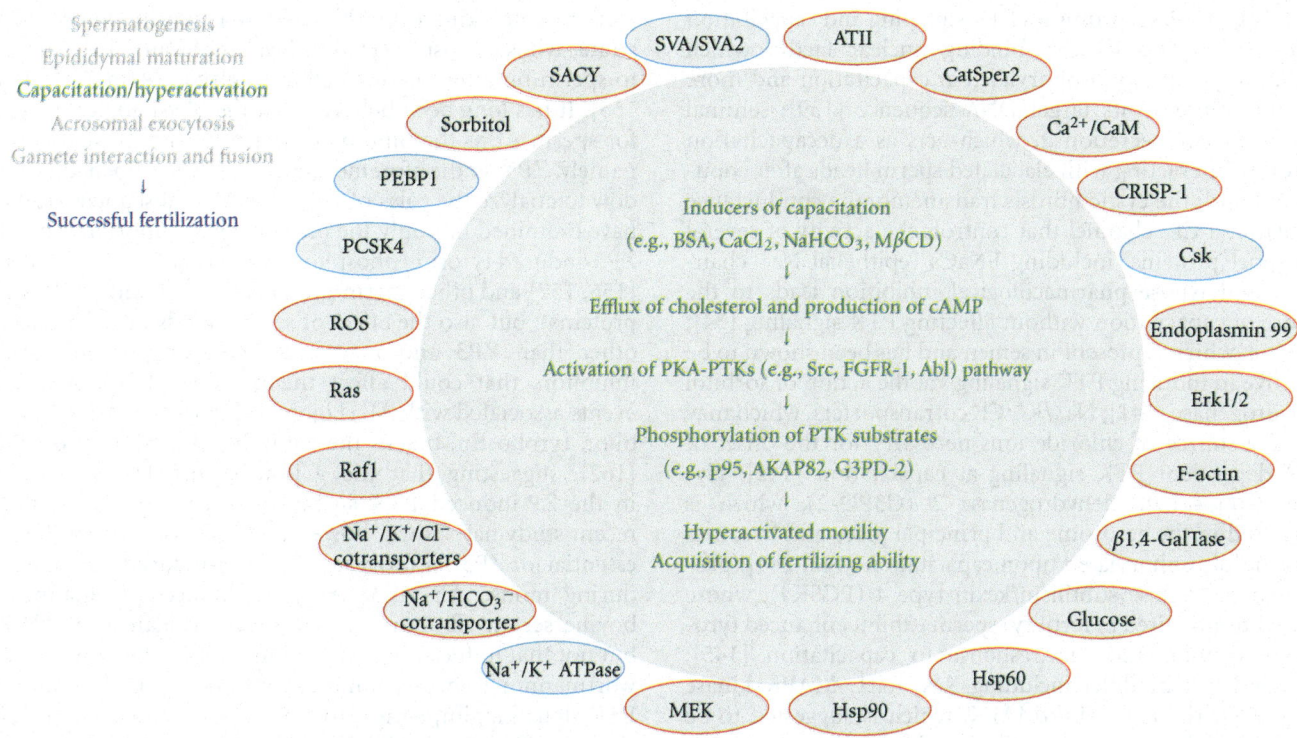

FIGURE 4: Protein-tyrosine phosphorylation and a sequence of events associated with capacitation and/or hyperactivation of sperm. For details of the capacitation/hyperactivation and its associated signaling molecules (the full spelling of all abbreviations as well), see text. Note that positive regulators for protein-tyrosine phosphorylation are indicated in red circles, whereas the negative regulators are indicated in blue circles.

biochemical experiments also demonstrate that the tyrosine-phosphorylated forms of c-Abl tyrosine kinase are present in the capacitated human sperm [112].

It has been shown that the cholesterol-binding heptasaccharides, methyl-β-cyclodextrin (MβCD) and OH-propyl-β-cyclodextrin, primarily promote release of cholesterol from the sperm plasma membrane and induce PTK signaling and capacitation in the absence of BSA [113, 114]. The MβCD's effects, like the BSA's effects, depend on both NaHCO$_3$ and PKA activity, suggesting that they resemble those under physiological capacitation. In fact, BSA has also been shown to promote the release of cholesterol, and the addition of exogenous cholesterol interferes with the BSA-induced PTK signaling and capacitation [113]. These and other results suggest that efflux of cholesterol plays a pivotal role in up-regulation of the cAMP-PKA-PTK pathway leading to capacitation [115].

Other important factors that promote or suppress the onset of PTK signaling and/or capacitation include calmodulin, which may act as a positive regulator for the production of cAMP [116, 117]; seminal vesicle autoantigen, which has been shown to block BSA-induced capacitation [118, 119]; fertilization-promoting peptide or adenosine, which stimulates and inhibits PTK signaling in uncapacitated and capacitated sperm, respectively [120, 121]; extracellular glucose, whose shortage has been shown to delay the appearance of protein tyrosine phosphorylation [122]; Na$^+$/HCO$_3^-$ cotransporter in the sperm, which provides Na$^+$ ions as a positive regulator of PTK signaling and capacitation [123]; F-actin, whose generation and breakdown is required for capacitation and AE, respectively [124, 125]; endogenous redox activity, which is up-regulated under the control of the actions of HCO$_3^-$ [126, 127]; molecular chaperones such as hsp90, endoplasmin 99, and hsp60, which become tyrosine-phosphorylated upon capacitation and some of them may be involved in sperm-ZP recognition (in mouse, but not human) [128–130]; sperm-specific voltage-gated cation channel, CatSper2, whose gene knockout significantly alters sperm production; PTK signaling, which is associated with capacitation and induction of the AE [131]; extracellular Ca^{2+} ions, which may suppress tyrosine phosphorylation by decreasing the availability of intracellular ATP [132]; β 1,4-galactosyltransferase I, a possible ZP3-interacting protein whose gene knockout leads to precocious capacitation, which may be involved because of spontaneous elevation of cAMP [133]; angiotensin II, which is found in seminal plasma and has been shown to induce PTK signaling and capacitation via stimulation of adenylyl cyclase-dependent accumulation of cAMP [134]; HCO$_3^-$- and Ca^{2+}-responsive soluble adenylyl cyclase (SACY), which has been identified as the dominant source of cAMP production [135, 136]; phosphatidylethanolamine-binding protein 1, a possible decapacitation factor, whose acquisition on the sperm surface during epididymal maturation and release before the onset of capacitation have been identified [137]; Na$^+$/K$^+$ ATPase, whose interaction with ouabain, a specific inhibitor of Na^+/K^+ ATPase, promotes PTK signaling and capacitation [138]; a 130 kDa CCCTC-binding nuclear factor, which becomes tyrosine-phosphorylated at capacitation and more potently binds to its target DNA sequence [139]; seminal vesicle protein secretion 2, which acts as a decapacitation factor by interacting with ejaculated sperm heads after copulation [140]; the cystic fibrosis transmembrane conductance regulator, a Cl^- channel that controls the activity of several transport proteins, including ENaCs (epithelial Na^+ channels), and whose pharmacological inhibition leads to the failure of capacitation without affecting PTK signaling [34]; sorbitol, which is present in semen and has been shown to be effective in inducing PTK signaling via the action of sorbitol dehydrogenase [141]; $Na^+/K^+/Cl^-$ cotransporters, which may act as a source of chloride ions necessary for the onset of PKA-dependent PTK signaling at capacitation [142]; glycerol-3-phosphate dehydrogenase 2 (G3PD-2), which is expressed in the acrosome and principal piece and becomes tyrosine-phosphorylated upon capacitation [143, 144]; proprotein convertase subtilisin/kexin type 4 (PCSK4), whose null (thus impaired in fertility) sperm exhibit enhanced tyrosine phosphorylation in response to capacitation [145]; so-called Erk module, including Ras, Raf1, MAPK kinase (MAPKK/MEK), and Erk/MAPK, which is suggested to be involved in the presentation of phosphotyrosine-containing proteins on the sperm surface at capacitation [146].

Recent proteomics analysis has revealed more identities of tyrosine-phosphorylated proteins in response to capacitation: they include voltage-dependent anion channel, tubulin, pyruvate dehydrogenase E1 β chain, glutathione-S-transferase, NADH dehydrogenase (ubiquinone) Fe-S protein 6, acrosin-binding protein precursor (sp32), proteasome subunit αtype 6b, and cytochrome b-c1 complex [42], although their functions remain to be elucidated. A more recent study has shown that Toll-like receptors 2 and 4 present on cumulus cells were activated by coculture with sperm in a hyaluronan fragment-dependent manner and that chemokines secreted from cumulus-oocyte complexes induced sperm PTK signaling and capacitation [147], providing evidence for the association of chemotaxis with capacitation. In addition, study of the knockout mouse suggests that an epididymal secretory protein CRISP-1 contributes to PTK signaling during capacitation [148].

Candidate PTKs related to capacitation include Src, whose interaction with PKA and enzymatic activation are seen in capacitated sperm [149, 150]; C-terminal Src kinase (Csk), whose negative regulatory function toward Src is canceled by serine phosphorylation (maybe by PKA) at capacitation [149, 151]; fibroblast growth factor receptor-1, whose dominant-negative mutant leads to the failure of PTK signaling and capacitation [152]; Abl tyrosine kinase, which is activated in response to capacitation in a PKA-dependent manner [153].

6. Involvement of PTKs in Acrosomal Exocytosis

Early reports by Saling and colleagues have demonstrated that a 95 kDa mouse sperm protein, termed p95/ZRK (for zona receptor kinase)/hexokinase, is a tyrosine kinase substrate, whose phosphorylation level is elevated in response to sperm binding to zona pellucida glycoprotein ZP3 [154, 155]. It has long been believed that the physiological trigger for sperm AE is the binding of sperm to the ZP structures, namely, ZP3; so the aforementioned study has opened a window to analyze the roles of PTKs for AE. Subsequent studies have examined not only the physiological importance of the ZP3-induced tyrosine phosphorylation of the 95 kDa protein [156, 157] and other sperm proteins (e.g., 51 and 14–18 kDa proteins), but also the effect of several kinds of AE inducers other than ZP3 and/or various PTK or protein kinase inhibitors that could affect the tyrosine phosphorylation events associated with AE (Figure 5) [158–161]. A PTK inhibitor, tyrphostin, blocks the ZP-induced activation of PLC [162], suggesting that the γ isoform of PLC is involved in the ZP-induced PTK signaling leading to AE. A more recent study has shown, however, that $\delta4$-isoform of PLC is essential for ZP3- or progesterone (PG)-induced Ca^{2+} release during mouse AE [163, 164]. AE induced by mannose-bovine serum albumin and an antibody against p95/ZRK, but not that induced by Ca^{2+} ionophore, can be inhibited by wortmannin, a specific inhibitor of PI3K, without inhibiting PTK signaling, implying a role of PI3K downstream of PTK signaling [165, 166]. AE induced by PG or platelet-activating factor has also been shown to involve an increase in protein-tyrosine phosphorylation of 75 and 97 kDa proteins, and PTK inhibitors (erbstatin, genistein) interfere with the induction of AE [167]. The PG-induced tyrosine phosphorylation is involved in the generation of the plateau phase of Ca^{2+} influx [168] and modulation of sperm GABAA-like receptor/chloride channel (chloride efflux) [169]. Study of domestic cat sperm has shown that ZP-induced AE, but not Ca^{2+} ionophore- or spontaneously induced AE, is inhibited by PTK inhibitors (genistein, tyrphostin), indicating that PTK signaling acts upstream of the Ca^{2+} increase during AE [170]. The involvement of PTK signaling mediated by Src has also been suggested for the promotion of capacitative Ca^{2+} entry, as reconstituted by thapsigargin treatment of sperm, during AE [171].

Tyrosine-phosphorylated proteins during AE also include p52[shc], an isoform of the Shc adaptor proteins [172], a 107 kDa protein, whose phospholevel correlates well with the extent of AE (induced by Ca^{2+} ionophore) [173], and a heparin-binding sperm membrane protein (during AE induced by heparin) [174]. On the other hand, recent studies suggest the importance of proteintyrosine dephosphorylation in AE [175]. In support of this, tyrosine dephosphorylation of N-ethylmaleimide-sensitive factor, which undergoes SNARE complex disassembly, by protein-tyrosine phosphatase 1B has been shown to be required for the Ca^{2+} ionophore-induced AE [176], and gelsolin, an actin-severing protein that becomes tyrosinephosphorylated and inactivated during capacitation, has been shown to be dephosphorylated during AE, allowing its activation leading to actin depolymerization [177].

Another line of evidence demonstrates the identity of PTKs working during AE. An early report by Lax et al. showed that epidermal growth factor (EGF) can induce AE in

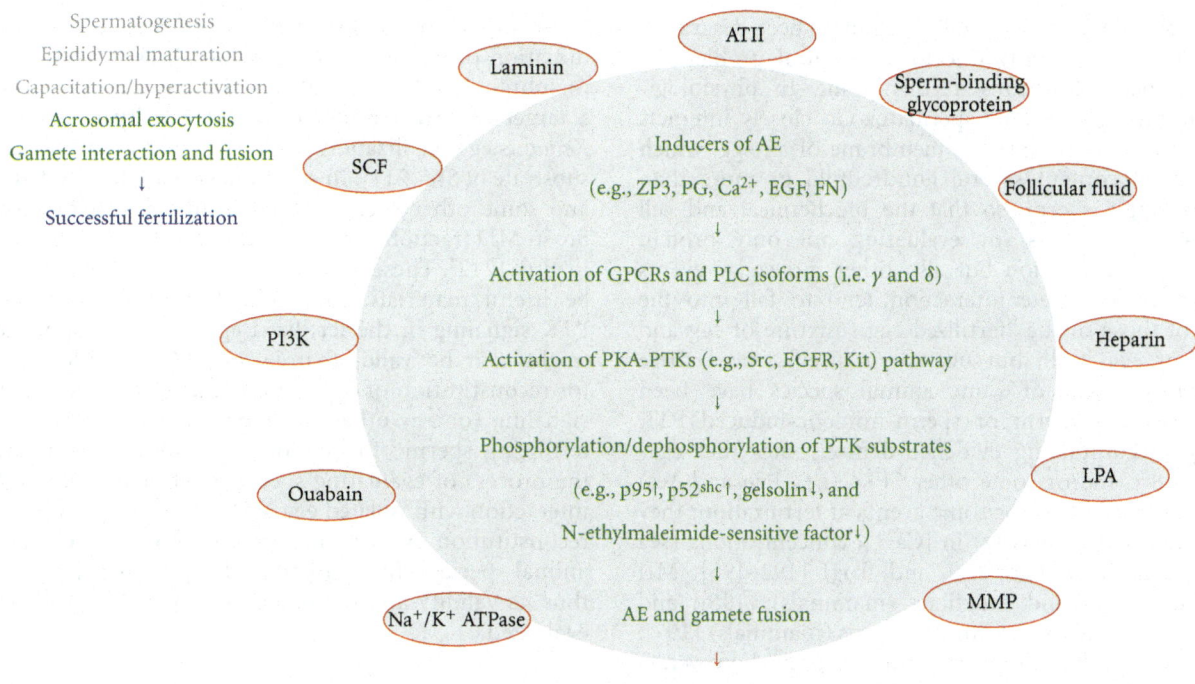

FIGURE 5: Protein-tyrosine phosphorylation and a sequence of events associated with acrosomal exocytosis. For details of the acrosomal exocytosis and its associated signaling molecules (the full spelling of all abbreviations as well), see text.

bovine sperm [178], suggesting that EGF receptor (EGFR)/ kinase is involved in this process. Further studies using this species have demonstrated that AE primarily involving activation of G protein-coupled receptors by lysophosphatidic acid or angiotensin II or AE induced by ouabain-Na$^+$/K$^+$ ATPase system promotes transactivation of EGFR/kinase via PKA-Src-matrixmetalloproteinase (MMP) or PKA-Src pathway [179, 180]. In the former system, G-protein-mediated production of AMP promotes PKA activation, PKA up-regulates Src (as seen in capacitated sperm), Src activates the secretion of heparin-binding EGF-like growth factor via MMP activation, thereby activating EGFR/kinase, and Src also affects the activity of EGFR/kinase through direct phosphorylation on tyrosine 845 [179], an Src-dependent phosphorylation site, whose phosphorylation has been implicated in some types of cancer cells [181–183]. Src activation and its importance for AE have also been demonstrated in humans [184, 185]. Another line of evidence suggests that SCF is involved in the promotion of mouse sperm AE through the activation of its cognate receptor/PTK c-Kit, PLCγ1, and phosphatidylinositol 3-kinase (PI3K) [186].

While many studies using mammals have shown the importance of PTK signaling in sperm AE, only limited findings have been described on the same subject in non-mammalian species. One potentially interesting finding reported recently demonstrates that egg components are capable of promoting protein-tyrosine phosphorylation and capacitation-like changes in sperm of the amphibian *Bufo arenarum* [187], implying its subsequent functions in AE.

A recent report by Hirohashi and colleagues has shown that most fertilizing mouse sperm have undergone AE before contact with ZP during in vitro fertilization [46]. Furthermore, it has been shown that sperm binding to the zona pellucida is not sufficient to induce AE and that some mechanical process is important for physiological AE [188]. These results lead us to reconsider where and how sperm AE is initiated under physiological conditions and when and how PTK signaling contributes to the "real" AE. As described above, not only ZP3, but also other reagents or experimental conditions (e.g., PG) are reportedly inducible for AE in vitro. Additionally, possible oviductal substances such as sperm-binding glycoprotein [189], laminin [185], fibronectin [190], and follicular fluid [191] have been shown to induce AE accompanied by PTK signaling. Taking these findings together, further analysis focusing on the roles of the sperm microenvironment during capacitation and AE (before reaching the egg plasma membrane) in vivo should enable greater understanding of the physiological impact of PTK signaling.

7. Involvement of PTKs in Gamete Interaction Fusion

Compared with the aforementioned categories of sperm biology, the relationship between sperm's PTK signaling and gamete interaction, especially at the level of plasma membranes (i.e., adhesion and fusion of gametes), has not yet been fully investigated. Immunocytochemical study demonstrates that sperm tail displays a time-dependent increase in tyrosine phosphorylation in response to ZP-free oocyte-sperm interactions [122], although its physiological importance and molecular detail have not yet been described. This seems to be mainly due to a technical problem in analyzing sperm functions at this point. In physiological conditions, a fertilizing spermatozoon closely interacts with or fuses with the plasma membrane of an egg, which has a protein content several hundredfold or more than that of a single sperm, so that the biochemical and cell biological experiments for evaluating not only protein tyrosine phosphorylation but also other molecular events associated with gamete interaction tend to fall into the analysis of those of the "fertilized egg (mixture of egg and sperm)" or egg itself, but not sperm itself. Under these circumstances, eggs of some animal species have been analyzed for the sperm or sperm-mimetic-induced PTK signaling. Accumulating evidence demonstrates that egg-associated Src and/or some other SFKs (i.e., Fyn and Yes) may play a crucial role for some events at fertilization: they include transient increase(s) in $[Ca^{2+}]_i$ concentrations (sea urchin, starfish, ascidian, fish, and frog) [192–195], MII spindle structures and functions (mammals) [196], and cleavage furrow ingression during mitosis (mammals) [197]. Roles played by the SFKs vary among species; however, it is worth noting that a wide range of animal species (from sea invertebrates to mammals) employ egg-associated SFKs as a sperm-induced trigger for activation of development. In this connection, it has been demonstrated that the sperm acrosomal or perinuclear theca-associated proteins may act as a trigger of signal transduction for initiation of development inside fertilized egg: so-called "sperm factors" (see "General View of Sperm Biology"). Among these are truncated c-Kit protein [198–200] and a WW domain-binding protein PAWP [201], both of which are specific proteins that may contribute to the modulation of the PTK signaling in eggs.

Egg analysis often involves parthenogenetic experiments, in which one or more of sperm's function-mimetic substances (e.g., Ca^{2+} ionophore) are used to reconstitute signaling events of fertilization, allowing easier functional evaluation of the egg-associated proteins. On the other hand, an absence of substitutes for sperm analysis has remained a problem. Ideally, some egg- or egg plasma membrane-mimetic substances, if applicable, would be helpful for solving this technical problem. In this regard, we suggest that egg membrane microdomains (MDs) could serve as excellent model materials of physiological value. As mentioned earlier, MDs or alternatively lipid/membrane "rafts" have been generally recognized as cholesterol-dependent micron- or nanometer-scaled membrane structures of cells, where a specific subset of glycosphingolipids, membrane-spanning and cytoplasmic proteins, and some other membrane components are assembled [202, 203]. Detailed analysis of egg MDs and fertilization signaling was first reported in sea urchin [204] and frog [205, 206], and thereafter, eggs or early embryos of mouse have also been documented to some extent [207, 208].

In *Xenopus laevis*, the egg MDs are suggested to serve as a platform for sperm-induced Src PTK signaling. Namely, Src has been shown to be concentrated in the MDs of unfertilized eggs, and it is activated upon fertilization. MβCD treat-ment impairs the ability of eggs to undergo sperm induced initiation of development [205]. An MD-associated, trans-membrane protein, uroplakin III, has been identified as a target of sperm protease, whose activity is required for *Xenopus* egg fertilization [209, 210], and as an intracellular substrate of Src [211]. In addition, we have found that sperm and some other sperm mimetics are capable of activating Src in MD fractions isolated from unfertilized *Xenopus* eggs, in vitro [212]. These results demonstrate that egg MDs would be useful materials for reconstitution of sperm-induced PTK signaling in the fertilized egg. If so, an opposite idea might also be valid, that is, egg MDs would be useful for reconstitution of egg (plasma membrane)-induced PTK signaling (or any other signaling event if it occurs) in the fertilizing sperm. To develop these ideas, we are now in the process of evaluating sperm functions before and after interaction with isolated egg MDs. It seems that this kind of reconstitution experiment can also be carried out in other animal species where isolation of egg MDs is possible, and thus its validity and physiological importance will soon be evaluated.

8. Conclusion and Perspectives

Among all the cells constituting multicellular organisms, egg and sperm are unique in terms of their history of production (i.e., gametogenesis, maturation, and/or differentiation), final structures, and physiological functions. In spite of enormous research efforts in recent years, many questions remain about how egg and sperm are produced and how they acquire their gamete-specific functions; in addition, new questions are continuously arising. Recent studies using pluripotent stem cells (e.g., embryonic or induced pluripotent stem cells) and/or molecular genetic approaches (e.g., gene knockout/KO and transgenic animals) have begun to disclose the genetic as well as cell biological background of gametogenesis, fertilization, and subsequent early embryogenesis. Moreover, study on the gametogenesis and fertilization in nonanimal species (e.g., plants, algae), which is not highlighted in this paper, and that in animal species have begun to merge, enabling researchers to learn more about the general scheme of sexual reproduction. Taking this background into account, it is certain that study on the signal transduction system involving protein-tyrosine phosphorylation in egg, sperm, and fertilized egg/zygote/early embryo will continue to be at the cutting edge of this research field.

Abbreviations

PTK: Protein-tyrosine kinase
PGC: Primordial germ cell
SSC: Spermatogonial stem cell
cAMP: Cyclic adenosine monophosphate
AE: Acrosomal exocytosis
ZP: Zona pellucida
$[Ca^{2+}]_i$: Intracellular calcium

IP$_3$:   Inositol trisphosphate
PLC: Phospholipase C
SFK: Src family protein-tyrosine kinase
SCF: Stem cell factor
GDNF: Glial cell-derived neurotropic factor
BTB: Blood-testis barrier
FAK: Focal adhesion kinase
AJ: Adherence junction
ES: Ectoplasmic specialization
PI3K: Phosphatidylinositol 3-kinase
Erk: Extracellular signal-regulated kinase
MAPK: Mitogen-activated protein kinase
ATP: Adenosine trisphosphate
db-cAMP: Dibutyryl cAMP
PTX: Pentoxifylline
PKA: Protein kinase A
NADPH: Nicotinamide adenine dinucleotide
                phosphate
ROS: Reactive oxygen species
SH2:   Src homology 2
SHP: SH2 domain-containing protein-tyrosine
                phosphatase
ZRK: Zona receptor kinase
BSA: Bovine serum albumin
AKAP: A-kinase/PKA-anchoring protein
MβCD: Methyl-β-cyclodextrin
SACY: Soluble adenylyl cyclase
ENaC: Epithelial Na$^+$ channel
G3PD-2:   Glycerol-3-phosphate dehydrogenase 2
PCSK4:   Pro-protein convertase subtilisin/kexin type
                4
MAPKK: MAPK kinase

Csk: C-terminal Src kinase
PG: Progesterone
EGF: Epidermal growth factor
MMP: Matrix metalloproteinase
MD: Membrane microdomain

Acknowledgments

The authors apologize to those whose work was not cited or insufficiently cited. This work is supported by a grant for the collaboration research from the Asahi Kasei Corporation, a Grant-in-Aid on Innovative Areas (22112522, 24112714), and a grant for Private University Strategic Research Foundation Support Program (S0801060) from the Ministry of Education, Culture, Sports, Science and Technology, Japan to K.-i. Sato.

References

[1] T. Hunter, "Tyrosine phosphorylation: thirty years and counting," Current Opinion in Cell Biology, vol. 21, no. 2, pp. 140–146, 2009.

[2] T. Hunter and B. M. Sefton, "Transforming gene product of Rous sarcoma virus phosphorylates tyrosine," Proceedings of the National Academy of Sciences of the United States of America, vol. 77, no. 3 I, pp. 1311–1315, 1980.

[3] W. Eckhart, M. A. Hutchinson, and T. Hunter, "An activity phosphorylating tyrosine in polyoma T antigen immunoprecipitates," Cell, vol. 18, no. 4, pp. 925–933, 1979.

[4] J. M. Bishop, "Molecular themes in oncogenesis," Cell, vol. 64, no. 2, pp. 235–248, 1991.

[5] C. Grangeasse, A. J. Cozzone, J. Deutscher, and I. Mijakovic, "Tyrosine phosphorylation: an emerging regulatory device of bacterial physiology," Trends in Biochemical Sciences, vol. 32, no. 2, pp. 86–94, 2007.

[6] D. Pincus, I. Letunic, P. Bork, and W. A. Lim, "Evolution of the phospho-tyrosine signaling machinery in premetazoan lineages," Proceedings of the National Academy of Sciences of the United States of America, vol. 105, no. 28, pp. 9680–9684, 2008.

[7] S. M. Thomas and J. S. Brugge, "Cellular functions regulated by SRC family kinases," Annual Review of Cell and Developmental Biology, vol. 13, pp. 513–609, 1997.

[8] R. Yanagimachi, "Mammalian fertilization," in The Physiology of Reproduction, E. Knobil and J. D. Neil, Eds., pp. 189–317, Raven Press, New York, NY, USA, 1994.

[9] G. Wei and A. P. Mahowald, "The germline: familiar and newly uncovered properties," Annual Review of Genetics, vol. 28, pp. 309–324, 1994.

[10] A. Darszon, T. Nishigaki, C. Beltran, and C. L. Treviño, "Calcium channels in the development, maturation, and function of spermatozoa," Physiological Reviews, vol. 91, no. 4, pp. 1305–1355, 2011.

[11] K. Toshimori, "Dynamics of the mammalian sperm head: modifications and maturation events from spermatogenesis to egg activation," Advances in Anatomy, Embryology, and Cell Biology, vol. 204, pp. 5–94, 2009.

[12] E. Voronina and G. M. Wessel, "The regulation of oocyte maturation," Current Topics in Developmental Biology, vol. 58, pp. 53–110, 2003.

[13] B. Ciapa and S. Chiri, "Egg activation: upstream of the fertilization calcium signal," Biology of the Cell, vol. 92, no. 3-4, pp. 215–233, 2000.

[14] A. M. Hasan, Y. Fukami, and K. I. Sato, "Gamete membrane microdomains and their associated molecules in fertilization signaling," Molecular Reproduction and Development, vol. 78, no. 10-11, pp. 814–830, 2011.

[15] W. H. Kinsey, "Tyrosine kinase signaling at fertilization," Biochemical and Biophysical Research Communications, vol. 240, no. 3, pp. 519–522, 1997.

[16] L. K. Mcginnis, D. J. Carroll, and W. H. Kinsey, "Protein tyrosine kinase signaling during oocyte maturation and fertilization," Molecular Reproduction and Development, vol. 78, no. 10-11, pp. 831–845, 2011.

[17] L. L. Runft, L. A. Jaffe, and L. M. Mehlmann, "Egg activation at fertilization: where it all begins," Developmental Biology, vol. 245, no. 2, pp. 237–254, 2002.

[18] K. I. Sato, T. Iwasaki, S. Hirahara, Y. Nishihira, and Y. Fukami, "Molecular dissection of egg fertilization signaling with the aid of tyrosine kinase-specific inhibitor and activator strategies," Biochimica et Biophysica Acta, vol. 1697, no. 1-2, pp. 103–121, 2004.

[19] M. Whitaker, "Calcium at fertilization and in early development," Physiological Reviews, vol. 86, no. 1, pp. 25–88, 2006.

[20] M. A. Handel, "Genetic control of spermatogenesis in mice," Results and Problems in Cell Differentiation, vol. 15, pp. 1–62, 1987.

[21] D. G. de Rooij, "Stem cells in the testis," International Journal of Experimental Pathology, vol. 79, no. 2, pp. 67–80, 1998.

[22] G. S. Roeder, "Meiotic chromosomes: it takes two to tango," *Genes and Development*, vol. 11, no. 20, pp. 2600–2621, 1997.

[23] K. Toshimori, "Biology of spermatozoa maturation: an overview with an introduction to this issue," *Microscopy Research and Technique*, vol. 61, no. 1, pp. 1–6, 2003.

[24] E. M. Eddy, K. Toshimori, and D. A. O'Brien, "Fibrous sheath of mammalian spermatozoa," *Microscopy Research and Technique*, vol. 61, no. 1, pp. 103–115, 2003.

[25] K. Steger, "Transcriptional and translational regulation of gene expression in haploid spermatids," *Anatomy and Embryology*, vol. 199, no. 6, pp. 471–487, 1999.

[26] E. M. Eddy, "Male germ cell gene expression," *Recent Progress in Hormone Research*, vol. 57, pp. 103–128, 2002.

[27] B. Senthilkumaran, "Recent advances in meiotic maturation and ovulation: comparing mammals and pisces," *Frontiers in Bioscience*, vol. 16, no. 5, pp. 1898–1914, 2011.

[28] M. Yamashita, "Molecular mechanisms of meiotic maturation and arrest in fish and amphibian oocytes," *Seminars in Cell and Developmental Biology*, vol. 9, no. 5, pp. 569–579, 1998.

[29] J. Deng, L. Carbajal, K. Evaul, M. Rasar, M. Jamnongjit, and S. R. Hammes, "Nongenomic steroid-triggered oocyte maturation: of mice and frogs," *Steroids*, vol. 74, no. 7, pp. 595–601, 2009.

[30] G. A. Cornwall, "New insights into epididymal biology and function," *Human Reproduction Update*, vol. 15, no. 2, pp. 213–227, 2009.

[31] X. Deng, K. Czymmek, and P. A. Martin-DeLeon, "Biochemical maturation of Spam1 (PH-20) during epididymal transit of mouse sperm involves modifications of N-linked oligosaccharides," *Molecular Reproduction and Development*, vol. 52, no. 2, pp. 196–206, 1999.

[32] G. Morin, C. Lalancette, R. Sullivan, and P. Leclerc, "Identification of the bull sperm p80 protein as a PH-20 ortholog and its modification during the epididymal transit," *Molecular Reproduction and Development*, vol. 71, no. 4, pp. 523–534, 2005.

[33] M. Nikolopoulou, D. A. Soucek, and J. C. Vary, "Changes in the lipid content of boar sperm plasma membranes during epididymal maturation," *Biochimica et Biophysica Acta*, vol. 815, no. 3, pp. 486–498, 1985.

[34] E. O. Hernández-González, C. L. Treviño, L. E. Castellano et al., "Involvement of cystic fibrosis transmembrane conductance regulator in mouse sperm capacitation," *Journal of Biological Chemistry*, vol. 282, no. 33, pp. 24397–24406, 2007.

[35] D. R. White and R. J. Aitken, "Influence of epididymal maturation on cyclic AMP levels in hamster spermatozoa," *International Journal of Andrology*, vol. 12, no. 1, pp. 29–43, 1989.

[36] R. Yanagimachi, Y. D. Noda, M. Fujimoto, and G. L. Nicolson, "The distribution of negative surface charges on mammalian spermatozoa," *American Journal of Anatomy*, vol. 135, no. 4, pp. 497–519, 1972.

[37] B. Lewis and R. J. Aitken, "Impact of epididymal maturation on the tyrosine phosphorylation patterns exhibited by rat spermatozoa," *Biology of Reproduction*, vol. 64, no. 5, pp. 1545–1556, 2001.

[38] C. R. Austin, "Observations on the penetration of the sperm in the mammalian egg," *Australian Journal of Scientific Research B*, vol. 4, no. 4, pp. 581–596, 1951.

[39] M. C. Chang, "Fertilizing capacity of spermatozoa deposited into the fallopian tubes," *Nature*, vol. 168, no. 4277, pp. 697–698, 1951.

[40] R. Yanagimachi and M. C. Chang, "Fertilization of hamster eggs in vitro," *Nature*, vol. 200, no. 4903, pp. 281–282, 1963.

[41] E. O. Hernández-González, J. Sosnik, J. Edwards et al., "Sodium and epithelial sodium channels participate in the regulation of the capacitation-associated hyperpolarization in mouse sperm," *Journal of Biological Chemistry*, vol. 281, no. 9, pp. 5623–5633, 2006.

[42] E. Arcelay, A. M. Salicioni, E. Wertheimer, and P. E. Visconti, "Identification of proteins undergoing tyrosine phosphorylation during mouse sperm capacitation," *International Journal of Developmental Biology*, vol. 52, no. 5-6, pp. 463–472, 2008.

[43] M. Eisenbach and L. C. Giojalas, "Sperm guidance in mammals—an unpaved road to the egg," *Nature Reviews Molecular Cell Biology*, vol. 7, no. 4, pp. 276–285, 2006.

[44] M. Yoshida, N. Kawano, and K. Yoshida, "Control of sperm motility and fertility: diverse factors and common mechanisms," *Cellular and Molecular Life Sciences*, vol. 65, no. 21, pp. 3446–3457, 2008.

[45] L. A. Burnett, X. Xiang, A. L. Bieber, and D. E. Chandler, "Crisp proteins and sperm chemotaxis: discovery in amphibians and explorations in mammals," *International Journal of Developmental Biology*, vol. 52, no. 5-6, pp. 489–501, 2008.

[46] M. Jin, E. Fujiwara, Y. Kakiuchi et al., "Most fertilizing mouse spermatozoa begin their acrosome reaction before contact with the zona pellucida during in vitro fertilization," *Proceedings of the National Academy of Sciences of the United States of America*, vol. 108, no. 12, pp. 4892–4896, 2011.

[47] N. Inoue, M. Ikawa, A. Isotani, and M. Okabe, "The immunoglobulin superfamily protein Izumo is required for sperm to fuse with eggs," *Nature*, vol. 434, no. 7030, pp. 234–238, 2005.

[48] K. Kaji, S. Oda, T. Shikano et al., "The gamete fusion process is defective in eggs of Cd9-deficient mice," *Nature Genetics*, vol. 24, no. 3, pp. 279–282, 2000.

[49] C. Boucheix, "Severely reduced female fertility in CD9-deficient mice," *Science*, vol. 287, no. 5451, pp. 319–321, 2000.

[50] K. Miyado, G. Yamada, S. Yamada et al., "Requirement of CD9 on the egg plasma membrane for fertilization," *Science*, vol. 287, no. 5451, pp. 321–324, 2000.

[51] T. Ducibella and R. Fissore, "The roles of Ca^{2+}, downstream protein kinases, and oscillatory signaling in regulating fertilization and the activation of development," *Developmental Biology*, vol. 315, no. 2, pp. 257–279, 2008.

[52] S. A. Stricker, "Comparative biology of calcium signaling during fertilization and egg activation in animals," *Developmental Biology*, vol. 211, no. 2, pp. 157–176, 1999.

[53] M. Nomikos, K. Swann, and F. A. Lai, "Starting a new life: sperm PLC-zeta mobilizes the Ca^{2+} signal that induces egg activation and embryo development: an essential phospholipase C with implications for male infertility," *BioEssays*, vol. 34, no. 2, pp. 126–134, 2012.

[54] Y. Harada, T. Matsumoto, S. Hirahara et al., "Characterization of a sperm factor for egg activation at fertilization of the newt *Cynops pyrrhogaster*," *Developmental Biology*, vol. 306, no. 2, pp. 797–808, 2007.

[55] M. A. Baker, N. D. Smith, L. Hetherington et al., "Label-free quantitation of phosphopeptide changes during rat sperm capacitation," *Journal of Proteome Research*, vol. 9, no. 2, pp. 718–729, 2010.

[56] M. A. Baker, G. Reeves, L. Hetherington, and R. J. Aitken, "Analysis of proteomic changes associated with sperm capacitation through the combined use of IPG-strip prefractionation followed by RP chromatography LC-MS/ MS analysis," *Proteomics*, vol. 10, no. 3, pp. 482–495, 2010.

[57] M. D. Piatt, A. M. Salicioni, D. F. Hunt, and P. E. Visconti, "Use of differential isotopic labeling and mass spectrometry

to analyze capacitation-associated changes in the phosphorylation status of mouse sperm proteins," *Journal of Proteome Research*, vol. 8, no. 3, pp. 1431–1440, 2009.

[58] S. Goupil, S. La Salle, J. M. Trasler, L. J. Bordeleau, and P. Leclerc, "Developmental expression of Src-related tyrosine kinases in the mouse testis," *Journal of Andrology*, vol. 32, no. 1, pp. 95–110, 2011.

[59] C. Lawson, S. Goupil, and P. Leclerc, "Increased activity of the human sperm tyrosine kinase SRC by the cAMP-dependent pathway in the presence of calcium," *Biology of Reproduction*, vol. 79, no. 4, pp. 657–666, 2008.

[60] S. Lev, Y. Yarden, and D. Givol, "Dimerization and activation of the kit receptor by monovalent and bivalent binding of the stem cell factor," *Journal of Biological Chemistry*, vol. 267, no. 22, pp. 15970–15977, 1992.

[61] I. Godin, R. Deed, J. Cooke, K. Zsebo, M. Dexter, and C. C. Wylie, "Effects of the steel gene product on mouse primordial germ cells in culture," *Nature*, vol. 352, no. 6338, pp. 807–809, 1991.

[62] D. Farini, G. La Sala, M. Tedesco, and M. De Felici, "Chemoattractant action and molecular signaling pathways of Kit ligand on mouse primordial germ cells," *Developmental Biology*, vol. 306, no. 2, pp. 572–583, 2007.

[63] K. Yoshinaga, S. Nishikawa, M. Ogawa et al., "Role of c-kit in mouse spermatogenesis: identification of spermatogonia as a specific site of c-kit expression and function," *Development*, vol. 113, no. 2, pp. 689–699, 1991.

[64] J. M. Oatley, M. R. Avarbock, and R. L. Brinster, "Glial cell line-derived neurotrophic factor regulation of genes essential for self-renewal of mouse spermatogonial stem cells is dependent on Src family kinase signaling," *Journal of Biological Chemistry*, vol. 282, no. 35, pp. 25842–25851, 2007.

[65] H. Morimoto, M. Kanatsu-Shinohara, S. Takashima et al., "Phenotypic plasticity of mouse spermatogonial stem cells," *PLoS ONE*, vol. 4, no. 11, Article ID e7909, 2009.

[66] A. Navon, Y. Schwarz, B. Hazan, Y. Kassir, and U. Nir, "Meiosis-dependent tyrosine phosphorylation of a yeast protein related to the mouse p51(ferT)," *Molecular and General Genetics*, vol. 244, no. 2, pp. 160–167, 1994.

[67] S. Vincent, D. Segretain, S. Nishikawa et al., "Stage-specific expression of the Kit receptor and its ligand (KL) during male gametogenesis in the mouse: a Kit-KL interaction critical for meiosis," *Development*, vol. 125, no. 22, pp. 4585–4593, 1998.

[68] M. Pellegrini, D. Filipponi, M. Gori et al., "ATRA and KL promote differentiation toward the meiotic program of male germ cells," *Cell Cycle*, vol. 7, no. 24, pp. 3878–3888, 2008.

[69] C. Lalancette, L. J. Bordeleau, R. L. Faure, and P. Leclerc, "Bull testicular haploid germ cells express a messenger encoding for a truncated form of the protein tyrosine kinase HCK," *Molecular Reproduction and Development*, vol. 73, no. 4, pp. 520–530, 2006.

[70] A. L. Kierszenbaum, E. Rivkin, A. Talmor-Cohen, R. Shalgi, and L. L. Tres, "Expression of full-length and truncated fyn tyrosine kinase transcripts and encoded proteins during spermatogenesis and localization during acrosome biogenesis and fertilization," *Molecular Reproduction and Development*, vol. 76, no. 9, pp. 832–843, 2009.

[71] L. J. Bordeleau and P. Leclerc, "Expression of hck-tr, a truncated form of the src-related tyrosine kinase hck, in bovine spermatozoa and testis," *Molecular Reproduction and Development*, vol. 75, no. 5, pp. 828–837, 2008.

[72] C. Albanesi, R. Geremia, M. Giorgio, S. Dolci, C. Sette, and P. Rossi, "A cell- and developmental stage-specific promoter drives the expression of a truncated c-kit protein during mouse spermatid elongation," *Development*, vol. 122, no. 4, pp. 1291–1302, 1996.

[73] P. Rossi, G. Marziali, C. Albanesi, A. Charlesworth, R. Geremia, and V. Sorrentino, "A novel c-kit transcript, potentially encoding a truncated receptor, originates within a kit gene intron in mouse spermatids," *Developmental Biology*, vol. 152, no. 1, pp. 203–207, 1992.

[74] M. P. Paronetto, J. P. Venables, D. J. Elliott, R. Geremia, P. Rossi, and C. Sette, "Tr-kit promotes the formation of a multimolecular complex composed by Fyn, PLCγ1 and Sam68," *Oncogene*, vol. 22, no. 54, pp. 8707–8715, 2003.

[75] B. Muciaccia, C. Sette, M. P. Paronetto et al., "Expression of a truncated form of KIT tyrosine kinase in human spermatozoa correlates with sperm DNA integrity," *Human Reproduction*, vol. 25, no. 9, pp. 2188–2202, 2010.

[76] M. K. Y. Siu, D. D. Mruk, W. M. Lee, and C. Y. Cheng, "Adhering junction dynamics in the testis are regulated by an interplay of β1-integrin and focal adhesion complex-associated proteins," *Endocrinology*, vol. 144, no. 5, pp. 2141–2163, 2003.

[77] Y. M. Chen, N. P. Y. Lee, D. D. Mruk, W. M. Lee, and C. Y. Cheng, "Fer kinase/FerT and adherens junction dynamics in the testis: an in vitro and in vivo study," *Biology of Reproduction*, vol. 69, no. 2, pp. 656–672, 2003.

[78] M. Maekawa, Y. Toyama, M. Yasuda, T. Yagi, and S. Yuasa, "Fyn tyrosine kinase in sertoli cells is involved in mouse spermatogenesis," *Biology of Reproduction*, vol. 66, no. 1, pp. 211–221, 2002.

[79] M. K. Y. Siu, C. H. Wong, W. M. Lee, and C. Y. Cheng, "Sertoli-germ cell anchoring junction dynamics in the testis are regulated by an interplay of lipid and protein kinases," *Journal of Biological Chemistry*, vol. 280, no. 26, pp. 25029–25047, 2005.

[80] M. Rassoulzadegan, V. Paquis-Flucklinger, B. Bertino et al., "Transmeiotic differentiation of male germ cells in culture," *Cell*, vol. 75, no. 5, pp. 997–1006, 1993.

[81] M. C. Hofmann, R. A. Hess, E. Goldberg, and J. L. Millán, "Immortalized germ cells undergo meiosis in vitro," *Proceedings of the National Academy of Sciences of the United States of America*, vol. 91, no. 12, pp. 5533–5537, 1994.

[82] T. Sato, K. Katagiri, A. Gohbara et al., "In vitro production of functional sperm in cultured neonatal mouse testes," *Nature*, vol. 471, no. 7339, pp. 504–507, 2011.

[83] K. Miki, W. Qu, E. H. Goulding et al., "Glyceraldehyde 3-phosphate dehydrogenase-S, a sperm-specific glycolytic enzyme, is required for sperm motility and male fertility," *Proceedings of the National Academy of Sciences of the United States of America*, vol. 101, no. 47, pp. 16501–16506, 2004.

[84] M. Nakamura, S. Okinaga, and K. Arai, "Metabolism of round spermatids: evidence that lactate is preferred substrate," *The American journal of physiology*, vol. 247, no. 2, pp. E234–E242, 1984.

[85] M. Nakamura, S. Okinaga, and K. Arai, "Metabolism of pachytene primary spermatocytes from rat testes: pyruvate maintenance of adenosine triphosphate level," *Biology of Reproduction*, vol. 30, no. 5, pp. 1187–1197, 1984.

[86] B. T. Storey and F. J. Kayne, "Energy metabolism of spermatozoa. V. The Embden Myerhof pathway of glycolysis: activities of pathway enzymes in hypotonically treated rabbit epididymal spermatozoa," *Fertility and Sterility*, vol. 26, no. 12, pp. 1257–1265, 1975.

[87] H. I. Calvin and J. M. Bedford, "Formation of disulphide bonds in the nucleus and accessory structures of mammalian spermatozoa during maturation in the epididymis," *Journal*

of reproduction and fertility. Supplement, vol. 13, supplement 13, pp. 65–75, 1971.

[88] G. A. Cornwall, D. Vindivich, S. Tillman, and T. S. Chang, "The effect of sulfhydryl oxidation on the morphology of immature hamster epididymal spermatozoa induced to acquire motility in vitro," *Biology of Reproduction*, vol. 39, no. 1, pp. 141–155, 1988.

[89] J. Seligman, Y. Zipser, and N. S. Kosower, "Tyrosine phosphorylation, thiol status, and protein tyrosine phosphatase in rat epididymal spermatozoa," *Biology of Reproduction*, vol. 71, no. 3, pp. 1009–1015, 2004.

[90] K. U. Devi, M. B. Ahmad, and S. Shivaji, "A maturation-related differential phosphorylation of the plasma membrane proteins of the epididymal spermatozoa of the hamster by endogenous protein kinases," *Molecular Reproduction and Development*, vol. 47, no. 3, pp. 341–350, 1997.

[91] A. Fàbrega, M. Puigmulé, M. Yeste, I. Casas, S. Bonet, and E. Pinart, "Impact of epididymal maturation, ejaculation and in vitro capacitation on tyrosine phosphorylation patterns exhibited of boar (*Sus domesticus*) spermatozoa," *Theriogenology*, vol. 76, no. 7, pp. 1356–1366, 2011.

[92] R. Jones, P. S. James, D. Oxley, J. Coadwell, F. Suzuki-Toyota, and E. A. Howes, "The equatorial subsegment in mammalian spermatozoa is enriched in tyrosine phosphorylated proteins," *Biology of Reproduction*, vol. 79, no. 3, pp. 421–431, 2008.

[93] B. Lewis and R. J. Aitken, "A redox-regulated tyrosine phosphorylation cascade in rat spermatozoa," *Journal of Andrology*, vol. 22, no. 4, pp. 611–622, 2001.

[94] M. Lin, H. L. Yun, W. Xu, M. A. Baker, and R. J. Aitken, "Ontogeny of tyrosine phosphorylation-signaling pathways during spermatogenesis and epididymal maturation in the mouse," *Biology of Reproduction*, vol. 75, no. 4, pp. 588–597, 2006.

[95] H. Ecroyd, K. L. Asquith, R. C. Jones, and R. J. Aitken, "The development of signal transduction pathways during epididymal maturation is calcium dependent," *Developmental Biology*, vol. 268, no. 1, pp. 53–63, 2004.

[96] M. A. Baker, R. Witherdin, L. Hetherington, K. Cunningham-Smith, and R. J. Aitken, "Identification of post-translational modifications that occur during sperm maturation using difference in two-dimensional gel electrophoresis," *Proteomics*, vol. 5, no. 4, pp. 1003–1012, 2005.

[97] M. A. Baker, N. D. Smith, L. Hetherington, M. Pelzing, M. R. Condina, and R. J. Aitken, "Use of titanium dioxide to find phosphopeptide and total protein changes during epididymal sperm maturation," *Journal of Proteome Research*, vol. 10, no. 3, pp. 1004–1017, 2011.

[98] E. Sonnenberg-Riethmacher, B. Walter, D. Riethmacher, S. Gödecke, and C. Birchmeier, "The c-ros tyrosine kinase receptor controls regionalization and differentiation of epithelial cells in the epididymis," *Genes and Development*, vol. 10, no. 10, pp. 1184–1193, 1996.

[99] H. Keilhack, M. Müller, S. A. Böhmer et al., "Negative regulation of Ros receptor tyrosine kinase signaling: an epithelial function of the SH2 domain protein tyrosine phosphatase SHP-1," *Journal of Cell Biology*, vol. 152, no. 2, pp. 325–334, 2001.

[100] P. Syntin, F. Dacheux, X. Druart, J. L. Gatti, N. Okamura, and J. L. Dacheux, "Characterization and identification of proteins secreted in the various regions of the adult boar epididymis," *Biology of Reproduction*, vol. 55, no. 5, pp. 956–974, 1996.

[101] J. L. Dacheux, M. Belghazi, Y. Lanson, and F. Dacheux, "Human epididymal secretome and proteome," *Molecular and Cellular Endocrinology*, vol. 250, no. 1-2, pp. 36–42, 2006.

[102] D. Krapf, Y. Chun Ruan, E. V. Wertheimer et al., "cSrc is necessary for epididymal development and is incorporated into sperm during epididymal transit," *Developmental Biology*, vol. 369, no. 1, pp. 43–53, 2012.

[103] A. E. Duncan and L. R. Fraser, "Cyclic AMP-dependent phosphorylation of epididymal mouse sperm proteins during capacitation in vitro: identification of an M(r) 95, 000 phosphotyrosine-containing protein," *Journal of Reproduction and Fertility*, vol. 97, no. 1, pp. 287–299, 1993.

[104] P. E. Visconti, J. L. Bailey, G. D. Moore, D. Pan, P. Olds-Clarke, and G. S. Kopf, "Capacitation of mouse spermatozoa. 1. Correlation between the capacitation state and protein tyrosine phosphorylation," *Development*, vol. 121, no. 4, pp. 1129–1137, 1995.

[105] P. E. Visconti, G. D. Moore, J. L. Bailey et al., "Capacitation of mouse spermatozoa. II. Protein tyrosine phosphorylation and capacitation are regulated by a cAMP-dependent pathway," *Development*, vol. 121, no. 4, pp. 1139–1150, 1995.

[106] E. Baldi, M. Luconi, L. Bonaccorsi, C. Krausz, and G. Forti, "Human sperm activation during capacitation and acrosome reaction: role of calcium, protein phosphorylation and lipid remodelling pathways," *Frontiers in Bioscience*, vol. 1, pp. d189–d205, 1996.

[107] B. S. Pukazhenthi, D. E. Wildt, M. A. Ottinger, and J. Howard, "Compromised sperm protein phosphorylation after capacitation, swim-up, and zona pellucida exposure in teratospermic domestic cats," *Journal of Andrology*, vol. 17, no. 4, pp. 409–419, 1996.

[108] B. S. Pukazhenthi, J. A. Long, D. E. Wildt, M. A. Ottinger, D. L. Armstrong, and J. Howard, "Regulation of sperm function by protein tyrosine phosphorylation in diverse wild felid species," *Journal of Andrology*, vol. 19, no. 6, pp. 675–685, 1998.

[109] A. Carrera, J. Moos, X. P. Ning et al., "Regulation of protein tyrosine phosphorylation in human sperm by a calcium/calmodulin-dependent mechanism: identification of A kinase anchor proteins as major substrates for tyrosine phosphorylation," *Developmental Biology*, vol. 180, no. 1, pp. 284–296, 1996.

[110] A. Mandal, S. Naaby-Hansen, M. J. Wolkowicz et al., "FSP95, a testis-specific 95-kilodalton fibrous sheath antigen that undergoes tyrosine phosphorylation in capacitated human spermatozoa," *Biology of Reproduction*, vol. 61, no. 5, pp. 1184–1197, 1999.

[111] P. E. Visconti, L. R. Johnson, M. Oyaski et al., "Regulation, localization, and anchoring of protein kinase a subunits during mouse sperm capacitation," *Developmental Biology*, vol. 192, no. 2, pp. 351–363, 1997.

[112] R. K. Naz, "c-abl proto-oncoprotein is expressed and tyrosine phosphorylated in human sperm cell," *Molecular Reproduction and Development*, vol. 51, no. 2, pp. 210–217, 1998.

[113] P. E. Visconti, X. Ning, M. W. Fornés et al., "Cholesterol efflux-mediated signal transduction in mammalian sperm: cholesterol release signals an increase in protein tyrosine phosphorylation during mouse sperm capacitation," *Developmental Biology*, vol. 214, no. 2, pp. 429–443, 1999.

[114] P. E. Visconti, H. Galantino-Homer, X. Ning et al., "Cholesterol efflux-mediated signal transduction in mammalian sperm: β-cyclodextrins initiate transmembrane signaling leading to an increase in protein tyrosine phosphorylation

and capacitation," *Journal of Biological Chemistry*, vol. 274, no. 5, pp. 3235–3242, 1999.

[115] J. E. Osheroff, P. E. Visconti, J. P. Valenzuela, A. J. Travis, J. Alvarez, and G. S. Kopf, "Regulation of human sperm capacitation by a cholesterol efflux-stimulated signal transduction pathway leading to protein kinase A-mediated upregulation of protein tyrosine phosphorylation," *Molecular Human Reproduction*, vol. 5, no. 11, pp. 1017–1026, 1999.

[116] Y. Si and P. Olds-Clarke, "Evidence for the involvement of calmodulin in mouse sperm capacitation," *Biology of Reproduction*, vol. 62, no. 5, pp. 1231–1239, 2000.

[117] H. T. Zeng and D. R. P. Tulsiani, "Calmodulin antagonists differentially affect capacitation-associated protein tyrosine phosphorylation of mouse sperm components," *Journal of Cell Science*, vol. 116, no. 10, pp. 1981–1989, 2003.

[118] Y. H. Huang, S. T. Chu, and Y. H. Chen, "A seminal vesicle autoantigen of mouse is able to suppress sperm capacitation-related events stimulated by serum albumin," *Biology of Reproduction*, vol. 63, no. 5, pp. 1562–1566, 2000.

[119] Y. H. Huang, S. P. Kuo, M. H. Lin et al., "Signals of seminal vesicle autoantigen suppresses bovine serum albumin-induced capacitation in mouse sperm," *Biochemical and Biophysical Research Communications*, vol. 338, no. 3, pp. 1564–1571, 2005.

[120] S. A. Adeoya-Osiguwa and L. R. Fraser, "Fertilization promoting peptide and adenosine, acting as first messengers, regulate cAMP production and consequent protein tyrosine phosphorylation in a capacitation-dependent manner," *Molecular Reproduction and Development*, vol. 57, no. 4, pp. 384–392, 2000.

[121] H. Funahashi, A. Asano, T. Fujiwara, T. Nagai, K. Niwa, and L. R. Fraser, "Both fertilization promoting peptide and adenosine stimulate capacitation but inhibit spontaneous acrosome loss in ejaculated boar spermatozoa in vitro," *Molecular Reproduction and Development*, vol. 55, no. 1, pp. 117–124, 2000.

[122] F. Urner, G. Leppens-Luisier, and D. Sakkas, "Protein tyrosine phosphorylation in sperm during gamete interaction in the mouse: the influence of glucose," *Biology of Reproduction*, vol. 64, no. 5, pp. 1350–1357, 2001.

[123] I. A. Demarco, F. Espinosa, J. Edwards et al., "Involvement of a Na^+/HCO_3^- cotransporter in mouse sperm capacitation," *Journal of Biological Chemistry*, vol. 278, no. 9, pp. 7001–7009, 2003.

[124] E. Brener, S. Rubinstein, G. Cohen, K. Shternall, J. Rivlin, and H. Breitbart, "Remodeling of the actin cytoskeleton during mammalian sperm capacitation and acrosome reaction," *Biology of Reproduction*, vol. 68, no. 3, pp. 837–845, 2003.

[125] M. G. Buffone, T. W. Ijiri, W. Cao, T. Merdiushev, H. K. Aghajanian, and G. L. Gerton, "Heads or tails? Structural events and molecular mechanisms that promote mammalian sperm acrosomal exocytosis and motility," *Molecular Reproduction and Development*, vol. 79, no. 1, pp. 4–18, 2012.

[126] H. W. Ecroyd, R. C. Jones, and R. J. Aitken, "Endogenous redox activity in mouse spermatozoa and its role in regulating the tyrosine phosphorylation events associated with sperm capacitation," *Biology of Reproduction*, vol. 69, no. 1, pp. 347–354, 2003.

[127] R. J. Aitken and M. A. Baker, "Oxidative stress and male reproductive biology," *Reproduction, Fertility and Development*, vol. 16, no. 5, pp. 581–588, 2004.

[128] H. Ecroyd, R. C. Jones, and R. J. Aitken, "Tyrosine phosphorylation of HSP-90 during mammalian sperm capacitation," *Biology of Reproduction*, vol. 69, no. 6, pp. 1801–1807, 2003.

[129] K. L. Asquith, R. M. Baleato, E. A. McLaughlin, B. Nixon, and R. J. Aitken, "Tyrosine phosphorylation activates surface chaperones facilitating sperm-zona recognition," *Journal of Cell Science*, vol. 117, pp. 3645–3657, 2004.

[130] L. A. Mitchell, B. Nixon, and R. J. Aitken, "Analysis of chaperone proteins associated with human spermatozoa during capacitation," *Molecular Human Reproduction*, vol. 13, no. 9, pp. 605–613, 2007.

[131] T. A. Quill, S. A. Sugden, K. L. Rossi, L. K. Doolittle, R. E. Hammer, and D. L. Garbers, "Hyperactivated sperm motility driven by CatSper2 is required for fertilization," *Proceedings of the National Academy of Sciences of the United States of America*, vol. 100, no. 25, pp. 14869–14874, 2003.

[132] M. A. Baker, L. Hetherington, H. Ecroyd, S. D. Roman, and R. J. Aitken, "Analysis of the mechanism by which calcium negatively regulates the tyrosine phosphorylation cascade associated with sperm capacitation," *Journal of Cell Science*, vol. 117, pp. 211–222, 2004.

[133] C. Rodeheffer and B. D. Shur, "Sperm from β1,4-galactosyltransferase l-null mice exhibit precocious capacitation," *Development*, vol. 131, no. 3, pp. 491–501, 2004.

[134] S. Mededovic and L. R. Fraser, "Angiotensin II stimulates cAMP production and protein tyrosine phosphorylation in mouse spermatozoa," *Reproduction*, vol. 127, no. 5, pp. 601–612, 2004.

[135] K. C. Hess, B. H. Jones, B. Marquez et al., "The "soluble" adenylyl cyclase in sperm mediates multiple signaling events required for fertilization," *Developmental Cell*, vol. 9, no. 2, pp. 249–259, 2005.

[136] F. Xie, M. A. Garcia, A. E. Carlson et al., "Soluble adenylyl cyclase (sAC) is indispensable for sperm function and fertilization," *Developmental Biology*, vol. 296, no. 2, pp. 353–362, 2006.

[137] B. Nixon, D. A. MacIntyre, L. A. Mitchell, G. M. Gibbs, M. O'Bryan, and R. J. Aitken, "The identification of mouse sperm-surface-associated proteins and characterization of their ability to act as decapacitation factors," *Biology of Reproduction*, vol. 74, no. 2, pp. 275–287, 2006.

[138] J. C. Thundathil, M. Anzar, and M. M. Buhr, "Na^+/K^+ ATPase as a signaling molecule during bovine sperm capacitation," *Biology of Reproduction*, vol. 75, no. 3, pp. 308–317, 2006.

[139] J. B. Tang and Y. H. Chen, "Identification of a tyrosine-phosphorylated CCCTC-binding nuclear factor in capacitated mouse spermatozoa," *Proteomics*, vol. 6, no. 17, pp. 4800–4807, 2006.

[140] N. Kawano and M. Yoshida, "Semen-coagulating protein, SVS2, in mouse seminal plasma controls sperm fertility," *Biology of Reproduction*, vol. 76, no. 3, pp. 353–361, 2007.

[141] W. Cao, H. K. Aghajanian, L. A. Haig-Ladewig, and G. L. Gerton, "Sorbitol can fuel mouse sperm motility and protein tyrosine phosphorylation via sorbitol dehydrogenase," *Biology of Reproduction*, vol. 80, no. 1, pp. 124–133, 2009.

[142] E. V. Wertheimer, A. M. Salicioni, W. Liu et al., "Chloride is essential for capacitation and for the capacitation-associated increase in tyrosine phosphorylation," *Journal of Biological Chemistry*, vol. 283, no. 51, pp. 35539–35550, 2008.

[143] V. Kota, V. M. Dhople, and S. Shivaji, "Tyrosine phosphoproteome of hamster spermatozoa: role of glycerol-3-phosphate dehydrogenase 2 in sperm capacitation," *Proteomics*, vol. 9, no. 7, pp. 1809–1826, 2009.

[144] V. Kota, P. Rai, J. M. Weitzel, R. Middendorff, S. S. Bhande, and S. Shivaji, "Role of glycerol-3-phosphate dehydrogenase 2 in mouse sperm capacitation," *Molecular Reproduction and Development*, vol. 77, no. 9, pp. 773–783, 2010.

[145] C. Gyamera-Acheampong, J. Vasilescu, D. Figeys, and M. Mbikay, "PCSK4-null sperm display enhanced protein tyrosine phosphorylation and ADAM2 proteolytic processing during in vitro capacitation," *Fertility and Sterility*, vol. 93, no. 4, pp. 1112–1123, 2010.

[146] B. Nixon, A. Bielanowicz, A. L. Anderson et al., "Elucidation of the signaling pathways that underpin capacitation-associated surface phosphotyrosine expression in mouse spermatozoa," *Journal of Cellular Physiology*, vol. 224, no. 1, pp. 71–83, 2010.

[147] M. Shimada, Y. Yanai, T. Okazaki et al., "Hyaluronan fragments generated by sperm-secreted hyaluronidase stimulate cytokine/chemokine production via the TLR2 and TLR4 pathway in cumulus cells of ovulated COCs, which may enhance fertilization," *Development*, vol. 135, no. 11, pp. 2001–2011, 2008.

[148] V. G. Da Ros, J. A. Maldera, W. D. Willis et al., "Impaired sperm fertilizing ability in mice lacking Cysteine-RIch Secretory Protein 1 (CRISP1)," *Developmental Biology*, vol. 320, no. 1, pp. 12–18, 2008.

[149] M. A. Baker, L. Hetherington, and R. J. Aitken, "Identification of SRC as a key PKA-stimulated tyrosine kinase involved in the capacitation-associated hyperactivation of murine spermatozoa," *Journal of Cell Science*, vol. 119, pp. 3182–3192, 2006.

[150] L. A. Mitchel, B. Nixon, M. A. Baker, and R. J. Aitken, "Investigation of the role of SRC in capacitation-associated tyrosine phosphorylation of human spermatozoa," *Molecular Human Reproduction*, vol. 14, no. 4, pp. 235–243, 2008.

[151] D. Krapf, E. Arcelay, E. V. Wertheimer et al., "Inhibition of Ser/Thr phosphatases induces capacitation-associated signaling in the presence of Src kinase inhibitors," *Journal of Biological Chemistry*, vol. 285, no. 11, pp. 7977–7985, 2010.

[152] L. Cotton, G. M. Gibbs, L. G. Sanchez-Partida, J. R. Morrison, D. M. de Kretser, and M. K. O'Bryan, "Erratum: FGFR-1 signaling is involved in spermiogenesis and sperm capacitation," *Journal of Cell Science*, vol. 119, pp. 75–84, 2006.

[153] M. A. Baker, L. Hetherington, B. Curry, and R. J. Aitken, "Phosphorylation and consequent stimulation of the tyrosine kinase c-Abl by PKA in mouse spermatozoa; its implications during capacitation," *Developmental Biology*, vol. 333, no. 1, pp. 57–66, 2009.

[154] L. Leyton and P. Saling, "95 kd sperm protein binds ZP3 and serve as tyrosine kinase substrates in response to zona binding," *Cell*, vol. 57, no. 7, pp. 1123–1130, 1989.

[155] L. Leyton, P. LeGuen, D. Bunch, and P. M. Saling, "Regulation of mouse gamete interaction by a sperm tyrosine kinase," *Proceedings of the National Academy of Sciences of the United States of America*, vol. 89, no. 24, pp. 11692–11695, 1992.

[156] R. K. Naz, C. Morte, K. Ahmad, and P. Martinez, "Hexokinase present in human sperm is not tyrosine phosphorylated but its antibodies affect fertilizing capacity," *Journal of Andrology*, vol. 17, no. 2, pp. 143–150, 1996.

[157] A. J. Travis, J. A. Foster, N. A. Rosenbaum et al., "Targeting of a germ cell-specific type 1 hexokinase lacking a porin-binding domain to the mitochondria as well as to the head and fibrous sheath of murine spermatozoa," *Molecular Biology of the Cell*, vol. 9, no. 2, pp. 263–276, 1998.

[158] S. Benoff, "Modelling human sperm-egg interactions in vitro: signal transduction pathways regulating the acrosome reaction," *Molecular Human Reproduction*, vol. 4, no. 5, pp. 453–471, 1998.

[159] G. Berruti and E. Martegani, "Identification of proteins cross-reactive to phosphotyrosine antibodies and of a tyrosine kinase activity in boar spermatozoa," *Journal of Cell Science*, vol. 93, pp. 667–674, 1989.

[160] R. K. Naz, "Protein tyrosine phosphorylation and signal transduction during capacitation-acrosome reaction and zona pellucida binding in human sperm," *Systems Biology in Reproductive Medicine*, vol. 37, no. 1, pp. 47–55, 1996.

[161] R. K. Naz and P. B. Rajesh, "Role of tyrosine phosphorylation in sperm capacitation/acrosome reaction," *Reproductive Biology and Endocrinology*, vol. 2, article 75, 2004.

[162] C. N. Tomes, C. R. Mcmaster, and P. M. Saling, "Activation of mouse sperm phosphatidylinositol-4,5 bisphosphate-phospholipase C by zona pellucida is modulated by tyrosine phosphorylation," *Molecular Reproduction and Development*, vol. 43, no. 2, pp. 196–204, 1996.

[163] K. Fukami, M. Yoshida, T. Inoue et al., "Phospholipase Cδ4 is required for Ca^{2+} mobilization essential for acrosome reaction in sperm," *Journal of Cell Biology*, vol. 161, no. 1, pp. 79–88, 2003.

[164] K. Fukami, K. Nakao, T. Inoue et al., "Requirement of phospholipase Cδ4 for the zona pellucida-induced acrosome reaction," *Science*, vol. 292, no. 5518, pp. 920–923, 2001.

[165] H. M. Fisher, I. A. Brewis, C. L. R. Barratt, I. D. Cooke, and H. D. M. Moore, "Phosphoinositide 3-kinase is involved in the induction of the human sperm acrosome reaction downstream of tyrosine phosphorylation," *Molecular Human Reproduction*, vol. 4, no. 9, pp. 849–855, 1998.

[166] H. Breitbart, T. Rotman, S. Rubinstein, and N. Etkovitz, "Role and regulation of PI3K in sperm capacitation and the acrosome reaction," *Molecular and Cellular Endocrinology*, vol. 314, no. 2, pp. 234–238, 2010.

[167] M. Luconi, L. Bonaccorsi, C. Krausz, G. Gervasi, G. Forti, and E. Baldi, "Stimulation of protein tyrosine phosphorylation by platelet-activating factor and progesterone in human spermatozoa," *Molecular and Cellular Endocrinology*, vol. 108, no. 1-2, pp. 35–42, 1995.

[168] L. Bonaccorsi, M. Luconi, G. Forti, and E. Baldi, "Tyrosine kinase inhibition reduces the plateau phase of the calcium increase in response to progesterone in human sperm," *FEBS Letters*, vol. 364, no. 1, pp. 83–86, 1995.

[169] S. Meizel and K. O. Turner, "Chloride efflux during the progesterone-initiated human sperm acrosome reaction is inhibited by lavendustin A, a tyrosine kinase inhibitor," *Journal of Andrology*, vol. 17, no. 4, pp. 327–330, 1996.

[170] B. S. Pukazhenthi, D. E. Wildt, M. A. Ottinger, and J. Howard, "Inhibition of domestic cat spermatozoa acrosome reaction and zona pellucida penetration by tyrosine kinase inhibitors," *Molecular Reproduction and Development*, vol. 49, no. 1, pp. 48–57, 1998.

[171] V. Dorval, M. Dufour, and P. Leclerc, "Role of protein tyrosine phosphorylation in the thapsigargin-induced intracellular Ca^{2+} store depletion during human sperm acrosome reaction," *Molecular Human Reproduction*, vol. 9, no. 3, pp. 125–131, 2003.

[172] C. Morte, A. Iborra, and P. Martínez, "Phosphorylation of Shc proteins in human sperm in response to capacitation and progesterone treatment," *Molecular Reproduction and Development*, vol. 50, no. 1, pp. 113–120, 1998.

[173] C. Picherit-Marchenay, S. Bréchard, D. Boucher, and G. Grizard, "Correlation between tyrosine phosphorylation intensity of a 107 kDa protein band and A23187-induced acrosome reaction in human spermatozoa," *Andrologia*, vol. 36, no. 6, pp. 370–377, 2004.

[174] V. Mor, T. Das, M. Bhattacharjee, and T. Chatterjee, "Protein tyrosine phosphorylation of a heparin-binding sperm membrane mitogen (HBSM) is associated with capacitation and acrosome reaction," *Biochemical and Biophysical Research Communications*, vol. 352, no. 2, pp. 404–409, 2007.

[175] C. N. Tomes, C. M. Roggero, G. De Blas, P. M. Saling, and L. S. Mayorga, "Requirement of protein tyrosine kinase and phosphatase activities for human sperm exocytosis," *Developmental Biology*, vol. 265, no. 2, pp. 399–415, 2004.

[176] V. E. P. Zarelli, M. C. Ruete, C. M. Roggero, L. S. Mayorga, and C. N. Tomes, "PTP1B dephosphorylates N-ethylmaleimide-sensitive factor and elicits SNARE complex disassembly during human sperm exocytosis," *Journal of Biological Chemistry*, vol. 284, no. 16, pp. 10491–10503, 2009.

[177] M. Finkelstein, N. Etkovitz, and H. Breitbart, "Role and regulation of sperm gelsolin prior to fertilization," *Journal of Biological Chemistry*, vol. 285, no. 51, pp. 39702–39709, 2010.

[178] Y. Lax, S. Rubinstein, and H. Breitbart, "Epidermal growth factor induces acrosomal exocytosis in bovine sperm," *FEBS Letters*, vol. 339, no. 3, pp. 234–238, 1994.

[179] N. Etkovitz, Y. Tirosh, R. Chazan et al., "Bovine sperm acrosome reaction induced by G protein-coupled receptor agonists is mediated by epidermal growth factor receptor transactivation," *Developmental Biology*, vol. 334, no. 2, pp. 447–457, 2009.

[180] L. Daniel, N. Etkovitz, S. R. Weiss, S. Rubinstein, D. Ickowicz, and H. Breitbart, "Regulation of the sperm EGF receptor by ouabain leads to initiation of the acrosome reaction," *Developmental Biology*, vol. 344, no. 2, pp. 650–657, 2010.

[181] K. I. Sato, A. Sato, M. Aoto, and Y. Fukami, "C-SRC phosphorylates epidermal growth factor receptor on tyrosine 845," *Biochemical and Biophysical Research Communications*, vol. 215, no. 3, pp. 1078–1087, 1995.

[182] D. A. Tice, J. S. Biscardi, A. L. Nickles, and S. J. Parsons, "Mechanism of biological synergy between cellular Src and epidermal growth factor receptor," *Proceedings of the National Academy of Sciences of the United States of America*, vol. 96, no. 4, pp. 1415–1420, 1999.

[183] J. S. Biscardi, M. C. Maa, D. A. Tice, M. E. Cox, T. H. Leu, and S. J. Parsons, "C-Src-mediated phosphorylation of the epidermal growth factor receptor on Tyr845 and Tyr1101 is associated with modulation of receptor function," *Journal of Biological Chemistry*, vol. 274, no. 12, pp. 8335–8343, 1999.

[184] G. Varano, A. Lombardi, G. Cantini, G. Forti, E. Baldi, and M. Luconi, "Src activation triggers capacitation and acrosome reaction but not motility in human spermatozoa," *Human Reproduction*, vol. 23, no. 12, pp. 2652–2662, 2008.

[185] S. Tapia, M. Rojas, P. Morales, M. A. Ramirez, and E. S. Diaz, "The laminin-induced acrosome reaction in human sperm is mediated by src kinases and the proteasome," *Biology of Reproduction*, vol. 85, no. 2, pp. 357–366, 2011.

[186] H. Feng, J. I. Sandlow, and A. Sandra, "The c-kit receptor and its possible signaling transduction pathway in mouse spermatozoa," *Molecular Reproduction and Development*, vol. 49, no. 3, pp. 317–326, 1998.

[187] D. Krapf, P. E. Visconti, S. E. Arranz, and M. O. Cabada, "Egg water from the amphibian *Bufo arenarum* induces capacitation-like changes in homologous spermatozoa," *Developmental Biology*, vol. 306, no. 2, pp. 516–524, 2007.

[188] B. Baibakov, L. Gauthier, P. Talbot, T. L. Rankin, and J. Dean, "Sperm binding to the zona pellucida is not sufficient to induce acrosome exocytosis," *Development*, vol. 134, no. 5, pp. 933–943, 2007.

[189] J. M. Teijeiro, M. O. Cabada, and P. E. Marini, "Sperm binding glycoprotein (SBG) produces calcium and bicarbonate dependent alteration of acrosome morphology and protein tyrosine phosphorylation on boar sperm," *Journal of Cellular Biochemistry*, vol. 103, no. 5, pp. 1413–1423, 2008.

[190] E. S. Diaz, M. Kong, and P. Morales, "Effect of fibronectin on proteasome activity, acrosome reaction, tyrosine phosphorylation and intracellular calcium concentrations of human sperm," *Human Reproduction*, vol. 22, no. 5, pp. 1420–1430, 2007.

[191] M. C. Gye, "Changes in sperm phosphotyrosine proteins by human follicular fluid in mice," *Archives of Andrology*, vol. 49, no. 6, pp. 417–422, 2003.

[192] I. K. Townley, E. Schuyler, M. Parker-Gür, and K. R. Foltz, "Expression of multiple Src family kinases in sea urchin eggs and their function in Ca^{2+} release at fertilization," *Developmental Biology*, vol. 327, no. 2, pp. 465–477, 2009.

[193] A. F. Giusti, D. J. Carroll, Y. A. Abassi, M. Terasaki, K. R. Foltz, and L. A. Jaffef, "Requirement of a Src family kinase for initiating calcium release at fertilization in starfish eggs," *Journal of Biological Chemistry*, vol. 274, no. 41, pp. 29318–29322, 1999.

[194] L. L. Runft and L. A. Jaffe, "Sperm extract injection into ascidian eggs signals Ca^{2+} release by the same pathway as fertilization," *Development*, vol. 127, no. 15, pp. 3227–3236, 2000.

[195] K. I. Sato, A. A. Tokmakov, T. Iwasaki, and Y. Fukami, "Tyrosine kinase-dependent activation of phospholipase Cγ is required for calcium transient in *Xenopus* egg fertilization," *Developmental Biology*, vol. 224, no. 2, pp. 453–469, 2000.

[196] L. K. McGinnis, D. F. Albertini, and W. H. Kinsey, "Localized activation of Src-family protein kinases in the mouse egg," *Developmental Biology*, vol. 306, no. 1, pp. 241–254, 2007.

[197] M. Levi, B. Maro, and R. Shalgi, "Fyn kinase is involved in cleavage furrow ingression during meiosis and mitosis," *Reproduction*, vol. 140, no. 6, pp. 827–834, 2010.

[198] C. Sette, A. Bevilacqua, A. Bianchini, F. Mangia, R. Geremia, and P. Rossi, "Parthenogenetic activation of mouse eggs by microinjection of a truncated c-kit tyrosine kinase present in spermatozoa," *Development*, vol. 124, no. 11, pp. 2267–2274, 1997.

[199] C. Sette, A. Bevilacqua, R. Geremia, and P. Rossi, "Involvement of phospholipase Cγ1 in mouse egg activation induced by a truncated form of the c-kit tyrosine kinase present in spermatozoa," *Journal of Cell Biology*, vol. 142, no. 4, pp. 1063–1074, 1998.

[200] C. Sette, M. P. Paronetto, M. Barchi, A. Bevilacqua, R. Geremia, and P. Rossi, "Tr-kit-induced resumption of the cell cycle in mouse eggs requires activation of a Src-like kinase," *The EMBO Journal*, vol. 21, no. 20, pp. 5386–5395, 2002.

[201] A. T. H. Wu, P. Sutovsky, G. Manandhar et al., "PAWP, a sperm-specific WW domain-binding protein, promotes meiotic resumption and pronuclear development during fertilization," *Journal of Biological Chemistry*, vol. 282, no. 16, pp. 12164–12175, 2007.

[202] K. Simons and D. Toomre, "Lipid rafts and signal transduction," *Nature Reviews Molecular Cell Biology*, vol. 1, no. 1, pp. 31–39, 2000.

[203] L. J. Pike, "Rafts defined: a report on the Keystone symposium on lipid rafts and cell function," *Journal of Lipid Research*, vol. 47, no. 7, pp. 1597–1598, 2006.

[204] R. J. Belton Jr., N. L. Adams, and K. R. Foltz, "Isolation and characterization of sea urchin egg lipid rafts and their

possible function during fertilization," *Molecular Reproduction and Development*, vol. 59, no. 3, pp. 294–305, 2001.

[205] K. I. Sato, T. Iwasaki, K. Ogawa, M. Konishi, A. A. Tokmakov, and Y. Fukami, "Low density detergent-insoluble membrane of *Xenopus* eggs: subcellular microdomain for tyrosine kinase signaling in fertilization," *Development*, vol. 129, no. 4, pp. 885–896, 2002.

[206] A. Luria, V. Vegelyte-Avery, B. Stith et al., "Detergent-free domain isolated from *Xenopus* egg plasma membrane with properties similar to those of detergent-resistant membranes," *Biochemistry*, vol. 41, no. 44, pp. 13189–13197, 2002.

[207] M. Comiskey and C. M. Warner, "Spatio-temporal localization of membrane lipid rafts in mouse oocytes and cleaving preimplantation embryos," *Developmental Biology*, vol. 303, no. 2, pp. 727–739, 2007.

[208] B. Sato, Y. U. Katagiri, K. Miyado et al., "Lipid rafts enriched in monosialylGb5Cer carrying the stage-specific embryonic antigen-4 epitope are involved in development of mouse preimplantation embryos at cleavage stage," *BMC Developmental Biology*, vol. 11, article 22, 2011.

[209] A. K. M. Hasan, Z. Ou, K. Sakakibara et al., "Characterization of *Xenopus* egg membrane microdomains containing uroplakin Ib/III complex: roles of their molecular interactions for subcellular localization and signal transduction," *Genes to Cells*, vol. 12, no. 2, pp. 251–267, 2007.

[210] A. K. M. Hasan, K. I. Sato, K. Sakakibara et al., "Uroplakin III, a novel Src substrate in *Xenopus* egg rafts, is a target for sperm protease essential for fertilization," *Developmental Biology*, vol. 286, no. 2, pp. 483–492, 2005.

[211] K. Sakakibara, K. I. Sato, K. I. Yoshino et al., "Molecular identification and characterization of *Xenopus* egg uroplakin III, an egg raft-associated transmembrane protein that is tyrosine-phosphorylated upon fertilization," *Journal of Biological Chemistry*, vol. 280, no. 15, pp. 15029–15037, 2005.

[212] K. I. Sato, A. A. Tokmakov, C. L. He et al., "Reconstitution of Src-dependent phospholipase Cγ phosphorylation and transient calcium release by using membrane rafts and cell-free extracts from *Xenopus* eggs," *Journal of Biological Chemistry*, vol. 278, no. 40, pp. 38413–38420, 2003.

6

Prolactin and Dexamethasone Regulate Second Messenger-Stimulated Cl⁻ Secretion in Mammary Epithelia

Utchariya Anantamongkol,[1,2] Mei Ao,[1] Jayashree Sarathy nee Venkatasubramanian,[1,3] Y. Sangeeta Devi,[1,4] Nateetip Krishnamra,[2] and Mrinalini C. Rao[1]

[1] *Department of Physiology and Biophysics, University of Illinois at Chicago, Chicago, IL 60612, USA*
[2] *Department of Physiology, Faculty of Science, Mahidol University, Bangkok 10400, Thailand*
[3] *Department of Biological Sciences, Benedictine University, Lisle, IL 60532, USA*
[4] *Obstetrics, Gynecology and Reproductive Biology, Michigan State University, Grand Rapids, MI 49503, USA*

Correspondence should be addressed to Mrinalini C. Rao, meenarao@uic.edu

Academic Editor: Jesus Garcia

Mammary gland ion transport is essential for lactation and is regulated by prolactin and glucocorticoids. This study delineates the roles of prolactin receptors (PRLR) and long-term prolactin and dexamethasone (P-D)-mediation of $[Ca^{2+}]_i$ and Cl⁻ transport in HC-11 cells. P-D (24 h) suppressed ATP-induced $[Ca^{2+}]_i$. This may be due to decreased Ca^{2+} entry since P-D decreased transient receptor potential channel 3 (TRPC3) but not secretory pathway Ca^{2+}-ATPase 2 (SPCA2) mRNA. ATP increased Cl⁻ transport, measured by iodide (I⁻) efflux, in control and P-D-treated cells. P-D enhanced I⁻ efflux response to cAMP secretagogues without altering Cl⁻ channels or NKCC cotransporter expression. HC-11 cells contain only the long form of PRLR (PRLR-L). Since the short isoform, PRLR-S, is mammopoietic, we determined if transfecting PRLR-S (rs) altered PRLR-L-mediated Ca^{2+} and Cl⁻ transport. Untreated rs cells showed an attenuated $[Ca^{2+}]_i$ response to ATP with no further response to P-D, in contrast to vector-transfected (vtc) controls. P-D inhibited TRPC3 in rs and vtc cells but increased SPCA2 only in rs cells. As in wild-type, cAMP-stimulated Cl⁻ transport, in P-D-treated vtc and rs cells. In summary, 24 h P-D acts via PRLR-L to attenuate ATP-induced $[Ca^{2+}]_i$ and increase cAMP-activated Cl⁻ transport. PRLR-S fine-tunes these responses underscoring its mammopoietic action.

1. Introduction

Prolactin is critical for the development of the mammary gland into a secretory type gland during lactation. Either acting alone or in concert with other hormones, prolactin has a plethora of effects on mammary epithelial function during lactation. Amongst other functions prolactin stimulates the production and/or secretion of casein, lipid [1], amino acids [2], and lactose [3] and activates ion transport processes such as those of sodium (Na^+), chloride (Cl⁻), iodide (I⁻), and calcium (Ca^{2+}) [4–6]. An increase in intracellular Ca^{2+} ($[Ca^{2+}]_i$) in the mammary epithelium can serve two functions—it can contribute to the increased Ca^{2+} content of milk seen during lactation and it can serve as a signaling molecule to stimulate cell function, including fluid, that is, Cl⁻ secretion, necessary for milk production. Although many studies describe the effect of prolactin on Ca^{2+} or on fluid transport, there are few studies linking these effects to the two roles of Ca^{2+}. Furthermore the studies are often performed in different animal or cell model systems making inferences difficult. The present study attempts to delineate interplay between hormonal mediation of Ca^{2+} transporters and fluid secretion, in a single model system, the nontransformed mouse mammary epithelial cell line, HC-11.

Prolactin exerts its pleiotropic effects by acting via the transmembrane receptor, PRLR, a member of the cytokine receptor superfamily [7]. Alternative splicing of the PRLR gene results in isoforms of varying lengths [8]. Most prominent are the long (PRLR-L) and short (PRLR-S) isoforms whose expression is both species and organ specific [9, 10]. They may also differ in their C-terminal sequences as seen in the mouse receptors where PRLR-S has a a stretch of

23 aminoacids not seen in PRLR-L. The downstream signaling mechanisms associated with the long form of PRLR have been well studied and implicate many kinases including Janus-, Src-, MAP- and Phosphoinositide 3-kinases [7]. While, not much is known about how prolactin acts via the PRLR-S, it is clear that it is a pathway distinct from that used by the long form of PRLR [11, 12]. Recent studies demonstrate that prolactin may be utilizing the complementary functions of the two isoforms to elicit its final biological effect. For example, PRLR-L alone is not sufficient to maintain progesterone production and fertility despite the activation of Jak2/STAT5 signaling and both PRLR-L and PRLR-S are required for normal female fertility [13]. Secretion of nutrients and electrolytes to form milk involves transcellular and paracellular mechanisms. Movement of glucose, water, and ions such as Na^+ and Cl^- occur transcellularly across the apical and basolateral membranes resulting in a large gradient for Na^+, K^+, and Cl^- between the plasma and milk and promoting paracellular movement of water. Further, Ca^{2+}, lactose, casein and whey proteins are transported from the Golgi apparatus and secreted into the lumen of the mammary glands via exocytosis.

A picture of the molecular mechanisms underlying transepithelial Ca^{2+} transport to increase the Ca^{2+} content of milk during lactation is beginning to emerge [14]. The current view, based on localization and functional data, is that Ca^{2+} is transported from plasma into mammary epithelial cells via Ca^{2+} channels of the transient receptor potential ion channel (TRP) family. The mRNA and protein of various isoforms of the classical TRP (TRPC) were found in the human mammary cancerous cell lines, MCF-7 and MDA-MB-231 [14]. In rat mammary gland, mRNA expression of TRPC 1, 3, 5, and 6 is increased during lactation [14]. Based on inhibitor studies, it is proposed that either TRPC1 and/or TRPC6 may be responsible for the Ca^{2+}-sensitive current triggered by activation of the Ca^{2+}-sensing receptor [15, 16]. The exit of Ca^{2+} via the apical membrane was initially thought to occur solely via vesicular exocytosis via casein bound Ca^{2+}. Secretory-pathway Ca^{2+}-ATPases (SPCAs) localized to the Golgi membrane sequester Ca^{2+} for this exocytotic route [15, 16]. More recently, apical plasma membrane Ca^{2+}-ATPases (PMCAs), specifically PMCA2, are suggested to extrude Ca^{2+} into the lumen although the underlying mechanisms in view of low $[Ca^{2+}]_i$ remain to be elucidated [2]. Reinhardt and colleagues demonstrated that there is a 60% reduction in milk $[Ca^{2+}]$ [17], and a modest 6–8 fold increase in SPCA1 expression in mice deficient in PMCA2 [16]. Both PMCA and SPCA protein expression are increased during lactation in rat mammary glands [15, 16]. In addition the Ca^{2+} sensitive receptor appears to regulate PMCA2 expression [18]. In contrast, PMCA2 is not detected in the human MCF-7 cells and prolactin promotes sequestration by increasing SPCA2 mRNA expression, and thereby suppresses ATP-induced increases in $[Ca^{2+}]_i$ [4].

The second function of Ca^{2+} as a signaling molecule regulating ion transport has been less well-studied. In contrast the long-term effects of prolactin and glucocorticoids on ion transport processes in tissue explants and in cell lines have been documented. Thus, these hormones have been implicated in the gradual drop of Na^+ and Cl^- concentrations in milk after the onset of parturition due to the closure of tight junctions [19, 20]. Rillema et al. [6, 21] showed that prolactin elevates Na^+-I^- symporter (NIS) protein and increases I^- accumulation in cultured mammary tissues of pregnant mice. In HC-11 cells, 48 h of prolactin and cortisol with additional 1–24 h prolactin exposure increases zinc uptake and the expression of its transporter, Zip3 [22]. In many models, including HC-11 cells, the synthetic glucocorticoid, dexamethasone, potentiates the effect of prolactin. For example, in the induction of casein production in HC-11 and in 31EG4 cells [23] and in tight junction formation in HC-11 cells and in rabbit mammary glands [19, 20].

The secretion of fluid by the mammary epithelium is important in milk production and as in other secretory epithelia, it is most likely dependent on transepithelial ion transport. It has been well established that lactating mammary epithelia contain a functional Na^+/K^+ pump in the basolateral membrane. In addition mammary epithelia possess a furosemide-sensitive Na^+-K^+-$2Cl^-$ cotransporter (NKCC). Thus mammary epithelia possess the necessary machinery—Na^+/K^+ pump, NKCC, and Cl^- channels for Cl^- secretion. In terms of hormonal regulation, we previously showed that 10 min exposure to prolactin activated Cl^- transport through the phosphorylation of JAK2/STAT5 in HC-11 cells. This in turn increases phosphorylation of NKCC-1, the transporter responsible for Cl^- entry into the cell [24]. The HC-11 cells also possess channels needed for Cl^- exit, namely, the cystic fibrosis transmembrane conductance regulator (CFTR) and Ca^{2+}-dependent Cl^- channels (ClCa) [25, 26]. Though our microarray study in pregnant rats showed that lactation induced a transient increase in the expression of chloride intracellular channel 6 (Clic6) [27], these studies did not examine function. However, the effects of long term exposure to prolactin on Cl^- transport are not known.

Since the prolactin receptor has multiple isoforms, it is conceivable that it elicits its effects on ion transport via different receptors. For example, the mouse mammary gland possesses one long and three short isoforms of PRLR [9]. Mice with the homozygous PRLR knockout become sterile and therefore cannot be used to study mammary development [28]. The heterozygous PRLR knockout mice (PRLR±) are fertile but do not exhibit lobulo-alveolar development and milk secretion in young females and fail to lactate after the first pregnancy [29]. Since PRLR-S lacks the cytoplasmic regulatory domain, it was postulated that PRLR-L was responsible for PRL signaling and that PRLR-S was a dominant negative of PRLR-L. However, studies from one of us (Y. S. Devi) and colleagues have demonstrated that mice expressing PRL-RS showed early follicular recruitment and premature ovarian failure [12], and overexpression of short-form PRLR (PRLR-S) into PRLR± mice rescued mammopoiesis and functional development of the mammary gland [30]. The expression of PRLR-S in HC-11 cells is controversial; while Wu et al. [31] reported its presence, we were able to detect only PRLR-L and not PRLR-S in our earlier studies in HC-11 cells [24].

Therefore, in the present study, we aimed to elucidate the long-term effects of prolactin treatment, via PRLR-L, on intracellular Ca^{2+} and Cl^- transport in HC-11 cells. By transfecting HC-11 with PRLR-S we further examined if coexpression of both PRLR-L and PRLR-S isoforms altered the response to prolactin.

2. Materials and Methods

2.1. Reagents. Ovine prolactin was obtained from Dr. Arieh Gertler, the Faculty of Agricultural, Food and Environmental Quality Sciences, the Hebrew University of Jerusalem, Rehovot, Israel. Fluo-3/AM (molecular probes), lipofectamine 2000 transfection reagent and SuperScript II Reverse Transcriptase were from Invitrogen, Carlsbad, CA, USA. RNAeasy Mini Kit was purchased from Qiagen, Valencia, CA, USA. Glass bottom dishes were obtained from MatTek Corporation, Ashland, MA, USA. RPMI1640 containing 1% Nutridoma-SP serum-free media supplement was from Roche Applied Science, Indianapolis, IN, USA. SYBR Green PCR Master Mix was purchased from Applied Biosystems, Carlsbad, CA, USA. GenEluteTM High Perfomance Plasmid Maxiprep Kit was from Sigma-Aldrich, St. Louis, MO, USA. All other reagents were obtained from Sigma-Aldrich or Fischer Scientific, Hannover Park, IL, USA and were of analytical grade.

2.2. Cell Culture. The HC-11 cells were grown in RPMI1640 containing $5 \mu g/mL$ insulin, $10 ng/mL$ EGF, and 10% fetal-bovine serum. The medium was changed every two days. Cells were plated in 10-cm^2 dish for RNA preparation, 4-cm^2 dish for iodide efflux assay, and 2 cm^2 glass bottom dish for $[Ca^{2+}]_i$ measurement. During hormone treatment, the medium was changed to RPMI1640 containing 1% Nutridoma-SP serum-free media supplement. Cells were treated with $1 \mu g/mL$ dexamethasone for 24 h for dexamethasone-treated cells, $1 \mu g/mL$ prolactin for 24 h for prolactin-treated cells, and $1 \mu g/mL$ dexamethasone for 24 h, washed, followed by exposure to $1 \mu g/mL$ prolactin for another 24 h for prolactin + dexamethasone-treated cells.

2.3. PRLR-S Transfection. Expression plasmid for rat PRLR-S [32] was prepared using GenEluteTM High Perfomance Plasmid Maxiprep Kit. After cells reached 70% confluency, PRLR-S plasmid was transfected into cells for 4.5 h using Lipofectamine 2000 transfection reagent and washed with PBS. Cells were subsequently treated with or without prolactin $(1 \mu g/mL)$ + dexamethasone $(1 \mu g/mL)$ before performing Ca^{2+} imaging, iodide efflux assays, or RNA extraction procedures.

2.4. [Ca^{2+}]$_i$ Measurement. Cells were loaded with $5 \mu M$ Fluo-3/AM in serum-free RPMI1640 for 30 min and washed twice with Krebs-Ringer-Hepes medium (KRH) containing 120 mM NaCl, 5.4 mM KCl, 0.8 mM $MgCl_2$, 1 mM $CaCl_2$, 11.1 mM glucose, and 20 mM HEPES (pH 7.4). Ca^{2+} signals were captured using a Zeiss LSM510 confocal laser scanning microscope (New York, NY, USA). An Ar/Kr laser was used to excite the Fluo-3 at 488 nm and emission signals were

detected at 515 nm. Imaging for $[Ca^{2+}]_i$ was conducted with a 40X objective for wild-type cells or 10X objective for transfected cells. The fluorescence intensity obtained from individual cells were normalized as a relative ratio from the background and averaged. On the average 70–80% of wild-type cells in a culture dish respond to ATP with a robust signal. In wild-type cells, 10–15 cells that responded to $100 \mu M$ ATP were selected in each dish. Dishes of transfected cells were viewed in low magnification so 60–80 cells could be randomly selected to obtain a larger sampling. This is to avoid biasing our selection of ATP-responsive cells since there is always a certain amount of cell to cell variability in the efficiency of transient transfections. Among these, only cells that showed the changes in the relative fluorescence ratio were used for calculating area under the curve. To compare effectively the data of the various transfected cells, the relative fluorescence in response to ATP in vector transfected controls is set at 100% (Figure 2(b)). Average data was collected from 4–6 dishes of each treatment. The area under curve of individual cells was determined by using the following formula (obtained from http://www.duncanwil.co.uk/areacurv.html): $[(f_1 + f_2)/2 \times (t_2 - t_1)] - [(b_1 + b_2)/2 \times (t_2 - t_1)]$, where f = fluorescent intensity changes at each time point, t = time (s), b = fluorescent intensity of the baseline.

2.5. Iodide Efflux Assay. The iodide efflux assay was performed as we had previously described [33], based on the original method of Venglarik et al. [34]. Briefly, attached HC-11 cells were washed twice with iodide-free buffer (136 mM $NaNO_3$, 3 mM KNO_3, 2 mM $Ca(NO_3)_2$, 11 mM glucose, and 20 mM HEPES, pH 7.4) and incubated with iodide-loading buffer (136 mM NaI, 3 mM KNO_3, 2 mM $Ca(NO_3)_2$, 11 mM glucose and 20 mM HEPES, pH 7.4) for 1 h at room temperature. Cells were washed 3 times rapidly with iodide-free buffer, and then samples were collected every 1 min in iodide free buffer. Iodide content was measured by an iodide-sensitive electrode (Orion 96-53, Fisher Scientific) and a pH/mV meter. The iodide concentrations were determined according to the calibration curve. Results were expressed as fold increase of cumulative iodide efflux as described previously [33]. Iodide efflux was measured in the presence and absence of the following reagents: a cAMP cocktail to elevate intracellular cAMP (containing $10 \mu M$ 8-Br-cAMP, $10 \mu M$ forskolin and $10 \mu M$ 3-isobutyl-1-methylxanthine (IBMX)); $100 \mu M$ ATP; $10 \mu M$ diphenylamine-2-carboxylic acid (DPC); or $10 \mu M$ furosemide.

2.6. RT-PCR and Real-Time PCR. RNA was extracted by RNAeasy Mini Kit and reverse transcribed by SuperScript II Reverse Transcriptase. The expression of PRLR-L and PRLR-S in HC-11 cells were analyzed by RT-PCR as described previously [35]. Total mRNA from whole ovary of normal cycling mouse was used as control to detect PRLR-S.

Realtime PCR was done using SYBR Green PCR Master Mix in an ABI 7900HT using the System Software (Applied Biosystems, USA), 200 nM sense and antisense primers (sequences shown in Table 1), and cDNA equivalent to $0.5 \mu g$ RNA. The reactions were performed in triplicate and run as follows: 50°C 2 min, 95°C 10 min, and 45 cycles of 95°C

TABLE 1: Primer sequences for studying the gene expressions in HC-11 cells.

Genes	Size (bp)	Forward	Backward
mPRLR-L	442	ATACTGGAGTAGATGGGGCCAGGAGAAATC	CTTCCATGACCAGAGTCACTGTCAGGATCT
mPRLR-S	332	ATACTGGAGTAGATGGGGCCAGGAGAAATC	ATATTTGAGTCTGCTGCTTCAGTAGTCAAG
rPRLR-S	332	ATACTGGAGTAGATGGAGCCAGGAGAGTTC	CTATTTGAGTCTGCAGCTTCAGTAGTCA
SPCA2	215	GAAGCCCTTTCTCAGCATGT	TTTCGTTGGCTGTCAGAGTG
TRPC3	153	TAGCACAACGTGGGCAATAA	GGTCAACTGCTGGAACCATT
CFTR	234	ATCAACGGAATCGTCCTACG	AAATCCCTCCTCCCAAAATG
CLCA	425	ACTCGAAGACACGGCTGTATGAAC	CTGTCAAATGTGACTAATCCAAC
ClC1	179	CGAGCTGATCCTGTGAACAA	AATTCTTCCCTGCCCAAGAT
ClC2	221	TGCCTGTCTTTGTCATTGGA	AGGCAGAATGTGAGCGATCT
NKCC1	199	GGCTGGATCAAGGGTGTATTA	ATCGGGCCCAAAGTTCTCATT
L19	194	AGCGCCTCCAGGCCAAGAAGG	CCAGGCCGCTATGTACAGACACGA

15 s and 60°C 1 min. Data were analyzed using the Relative Quantification (RQ) Manager software and presented as relative expression to L-19 used as an internal control.

2.7. Western Blotting. Vector- or prolactin receptor short form-tranfected HC-11 cells were treated $\pm 1\,\mu$g/mL prolactin and dexamethasone for 24 h. Cells were then sonicated ($\sim$20–25 sec pulses) in homogenization buffer (HB: 1 mM EDTA, 2 mM $MgCl_2$, 5 mM ß-mercaptoethanol, 25 mM Tris-HCl, pH 7.4, 1 mM DTT, and protease inhibitor cocktail). The homogenate was centrifuged at 3,000 xg for 1 min to remove cell debris. The protein concentrations were quantified via the Bradford method (BioRad, Hercules, CA, USA) and the proteins analyzed by Western blotting procedures as described previously [36]. Briefly, equal amounts of protein (15 μg) from each lysate were subjected to 4–12% SDS-PAGE and transferred onto PVDF membrane at 250 mAmps for 1.5 h, in transfer buffer (25 mM Tris, pH 8.1 192 mM glycine, 20% methanol, and 0.1% SDS). The membrane was washed in TBS-T (tris-buffered saline: 50 mM tris-HCl, pH 7.4, 150 mM NaCl, and 0.1% tween-20) 3 × 5 min each and blocked in blotto (5% carnation nonfat dry milk in TBS-T) for 1 h at room temperature. The membrane was then incubated with a rabbit polyclonal anti-CFTR antibody (Santa Cruz, CA, USA; 1 : 1000 dilution in TBS-T containing 1% nonfat milk) overnight at 4°C on a shaker. The blots were next washed 3 × 5 min each in TBS-T and incubated with a horseradish peroxidase-conjugated secondary antibody (Santa Cruz, CA; 1 : 10,000 dilution in TBS-T containing 1% nonfat milk) for 1 h at room temperature. The blots were washed 3 × 5 min in TBS-T and then visualized using a SuperSignal West Pico Chemiluminescent Substrate kit (Pierce, Rockford, IL, USA).

2.8. Statistical Analysis. Data were expressed as mean ± standard error of mean (SEM) and compared by using one-way ANOVA and Student's *t*-test. $P < 0.05$ is considered significant for all statistical tests.

3. Results

3.1. Effect of Prolactin on Ca^{2+} Transport. We had previously demonstrated that short-term exposure to prolactin did not alter $[Ca^{2+}]_i$ in HC-11 cells [24] but suppressed ATP-dependent Ca^{2+} increases in MCF-7 cells [4]. The response of MCF-7 cells could be a property of transformed cells. HC-11 cells are a useful in vitro model of mammary cell differentiation; for example, when treated with dexamethasone and prolactin these cells synthesize the milk protein ß-casein. Many studies on milk production and secretion have utilized dexamethasone for its stability and potency. To parallel these models we also utilized dexamethasone in the present study, with the recognition that in the future these results will need to be confirmed with a more nuanced investigation on the efficacy of endogenous glucocorticoids. Therefore we examined if prolactin (1 μg/mL) and dexamethasone (1 μg/mL), either alone or in combination, affects ATP mediated Ca^{2+} release and resequestration in HC-11 cells. Cells were treated with these hormonal regimens for 24 h and changes in $[Ca^{2+}]_i$ were determined using Fluo-3 and confocal imaging. Figure 1(a1) shows representative tracings of the changes in $[Ca^{2+}]_i$ after the addition of 100 μM ATP in control (C) and prolactin + dexamethasone-treated cells. The effects on the magnitude and duration of the Ca^{2+} transient were quantitated by determining the area under the curve as described in Section 2. As shown in Figure 1(a2), prolactin alone or prolactin + dexamethasone decreased the ATP-dependent elevation of $[Ca^{2+}]_i$ compared to control or cells treated with dexamethasone alone.

The effects of prolactin alone or prolactin + dexamethasone on $[Ca^{2+}]_i$ could be due to either increased sequestration or decreased entry. Therefore, using mouse-specific primers and real-time PCR, the effects of dexamethasone, prolactin, and prolactin + dexamethasone on the secretory pathway Ca-ATPase, SPCA2 mRNA, an index of altered sequestration, was determined. As shown in Figure 1(b1) prolactin and dexamethasone, either alone or in combination, did not cause any significant change in SPCA2 mRNA

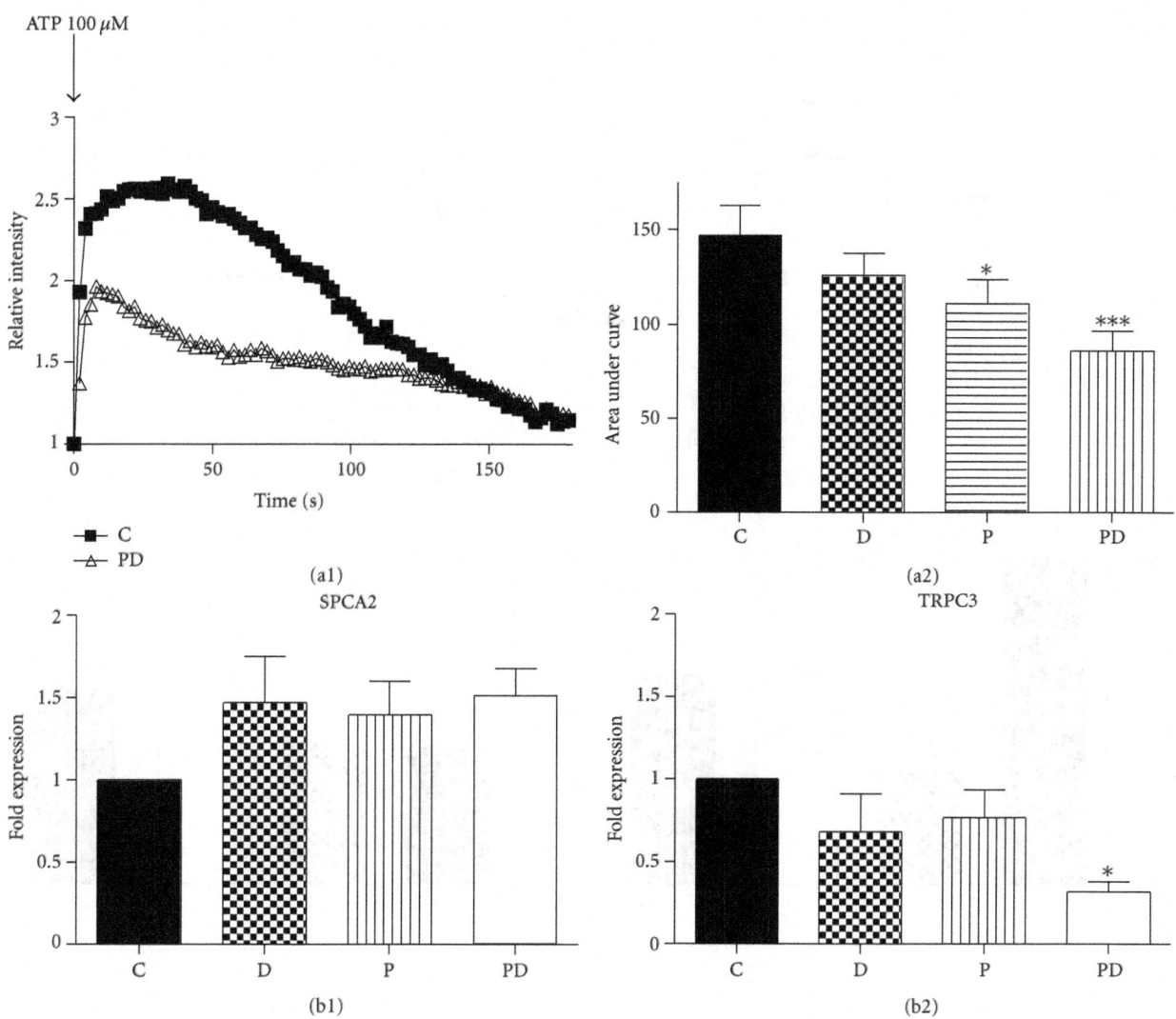

FIGURE 1: ((a1) and (a2)) effect of ATP on $[Ca^{2+}]_i$ in control and prolactin and/or dexamethasone-treated HC-11 cells. (a1) Representative tracing shows changes of $100\,\mu M$ ATP-evoked $[Ca^{2+}]_i$ in control (C) and 24 h $1\,\mu g/mL$ prolactin + dexamethasone-treated ($1\,\mu g/mL$) (P-D) cells. $[Ca^{2+}]_i$ changes were detected from fluorescent intensity of Fluo-3 under confocal microscopy. Data are presented relative to the pretreatment, baseline level. (a2) $[Ca^{2+}]_i$ changes were calculated as area under curve for (C), prolactin alone (P $1\,\mu g/mL$), dexamethasone alone ($1\,\mu g/mL$) or P-D cells as described in Section 2. Data are mean ± SEM, $n = 4$, where each n value represents the mean of 39–44 cells from one dish. ((b1) and (b2)) effect of prolactin and/or dexamethasone treatment on SPCA2 (b1) and TRPC3 (b2) mRNA expression. HC-11 cells were pre-treated with $1\,\mu g/mL$ prolactin (P) and/or $1\,\mu g/mL$ dexamethasone (D) for 24 h. Total RNA was extracted, and realtime PCR was performed. L19 was used as internal control. C = control. Data are mean ± SEM, $n = 3$ for SPCA and $n = 4$ for TRPC3. *$P < 0.05$ and ***$P < 0.001$ versus control.

expression in HC-11 cells. Therefore we examined if prolactin was attenuating the Ca^{2+} response to ATP by decreasing Ca^{2+} entry via pathways such as the store-operated Ca^{2+} channels, TRPCs. We found that untreated HC-11 cells express TRPC isoforms 1–7, with TRPC3 mRNA exhibiting the highest level of expression (Anantamongkol, Krishnamra, and Rao, data not shown). We next compared the effect of dexamethasone, prolactin, and prolactin + dexamethasone treatment on TRPC3 mRNA expression by real-time PCR. As shown in Figure 1(b2), only prolactin + dexamethasone suppressed TRPC3 mRNA expression, to 30% of the control group. Collectively, these results suggest

that prolactin and dexamethasone lower the $[Ca^{2+}]_i$ response to ATP, by decreasing TRPC3 expression and thereby Ca^{2+} entry. The effects of dexamethasone on enhancing prolactin action are in keeping with published reports and therefore we focused our remaining studies on the actions of prolactin + dexamethasone.

3.2. Influence of Prolactin Receptor Isoforms on $[Ca^{2+}]_i$ Response. We had reported detecting only the long form of the PRLR in HC-11 cells [24]. However, Wu et al. [31] documented both PRLR-L and PRLR-S in these cells and suggested a role for PRLR-S in modulating casein

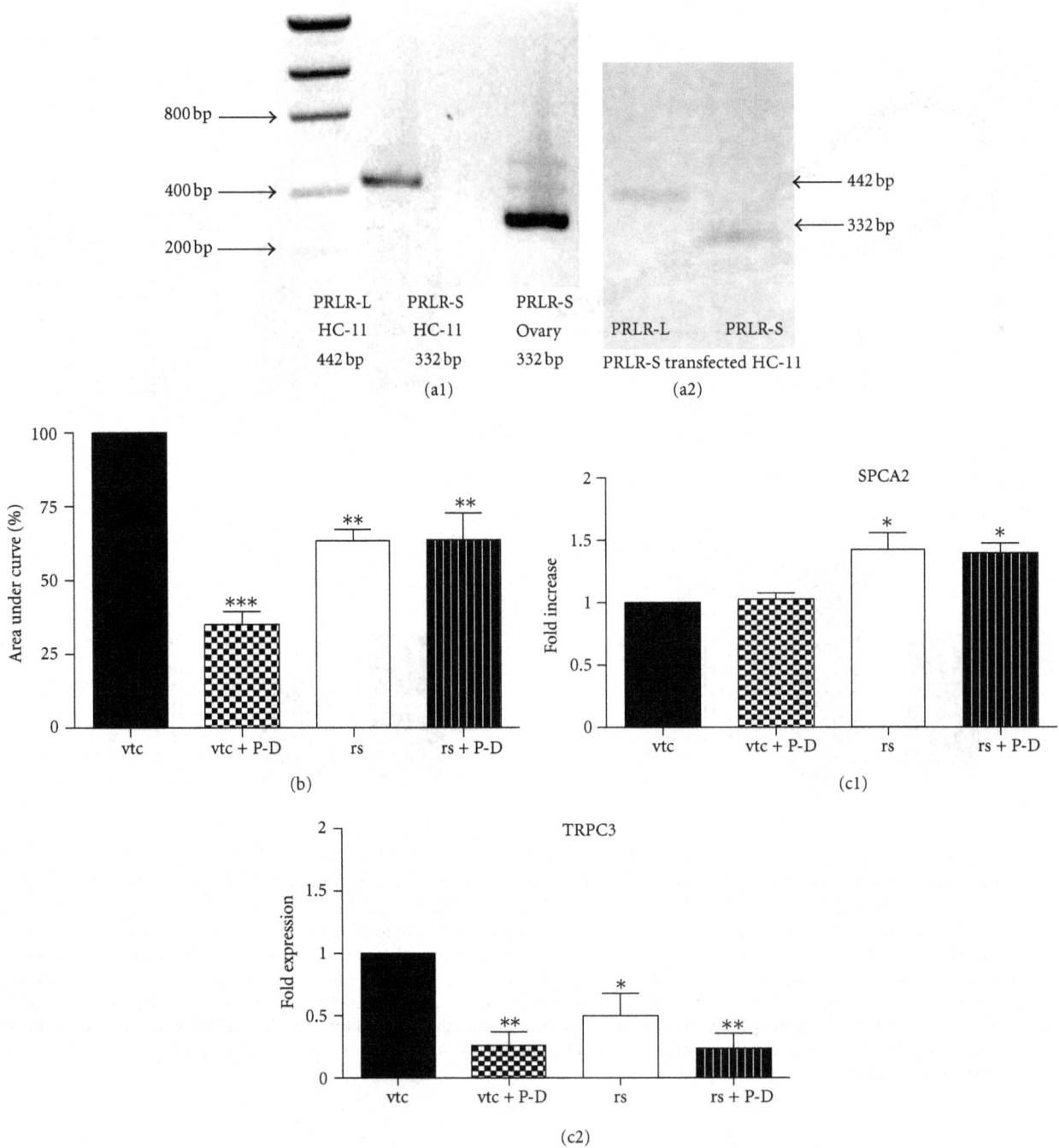

FIGURE 2: ((a1) and (a2)) messenger RNA expression of prolactin receptor long form (PRLR-L) and short form (PRLR-S) in HC-11 and mouse ovary (a1) and PRLR-S-transfected HC-11 cells (a2). (a1) PRLR-L (442 bp), but not PRLR-S (332 bp), is found in HC-11 cells. PRLR-S is present in the ovary cells. (a2) HC-11 cells were transfected with PRLR-S, and both PRLR-L and PRLR-S can be detected in transfected HC-11 cells. ((b) and (c)) vector-transfected HC-11 cells (vtc) or prolactin receptor short form (PRLR-S)-transfected cells (rs) were pretreated with or without 1 μg/mL prolactin and dexamethasone (P-D) for 24 h. (b) Effect of ATP on $[Ca^{2+}]_i$ in vector-transfected or PRLR-S tranfected cells with or without prolactin and dexamethasone treatment. 100 μM ATP-evoked $[Ca^{2+}]_i$ changes are calculated as area under curve as described in Section 2. Data are mean ± SEM, and are normalized to vtc, $n = 4$. ((c1) and (c2)) expression of mRNA of SPCA2 (c1) and TRPC3 (c2) in vector-transfected (vtc) or PRLR-S-tranfected (rs) cells ± prolactin and dexamethasone treatment. Total RNA was extracted, and realtime PCR was performed. The mRNA of ribosomal protein L19 was used as an internal control. Data represent mean ± SEM, and are normalized to vtc, $n = 4$. *$P < 0.05$, **$P < 0.01$, and ***$P < 0.001$ versus vtc.

production. Therefore, we first reevaluated the types of PRLR expressed in our cultures of HC-11 cells. As shown in Figure 2(a1), we were still able to detect only mRNA of the long-form of PRLR (PRLR-L) in HC-11 cells whereas the short-form PRLR-S was detected only in the ovary of the normal cycling mouse. This implies that the above described observations, of prolactin action on ATP-induced $[Ca^{2+}]_i$ changes are mediated by PRLR-L in HC-11 cells.

To determine if PRLR-S could play a role in the long-term effects of prolactin, HC-11 cells were transiently transfected with PRLR-S. As shown in Figure 2(a2), transfection of PRLR-S ($2 \mu g$) into HC-11 cells resulted in the mRNA expression of PRLR-S and these cells also contain PRLR-L (Figure 2(a2)). The changes of $[Ca^{2+}]_i$ in response to $100 \mu M$ ATP in the cells transfected with vector alone (vtc) and the PRLR-S (rs) transfected cells were compared. As in untransfected cells, prolactin + dexamethasone treatment in vector-transfected cells (vtc) showed a greater than 50% reduction in $[Ca^{2+}]_i$ (Figure 2(b)). PRLR-S transfection, even in the absence of prolactin + dexamethasone showed a 33% reduction in $[Ca^{2+}]_i$ compared to vector transfected cells. However, these rs cells did not show any further alterations in $[Ca^{2+}]_i$ in response to ATP after prolactin + dexamethasone treatment (rs+P-D).

As shown in Figure 2(c1), as in the wild-type cells, empty vector transfected cells (vtc) did not show an alteration in SPCA2 mRNA expression. In marked contrast, PRLR-S (rs) transfected cells, either in the presence or absence of 24 h prolactin + dexamethasone treatment showed increases in SPCA2 mRNA expression as compared to control vtc cells (Figure 2(c1)). Transfection of PRLR-S decreased TRPC3 mRNA expression by 50%, and this effect was further suppressed by treatment with prolactin + dexamethasone (Figure 2(c2)). As in the case of wild type cells (compare Figure 2(c2) and Figure 1(b2)), treatment with prolactin + dexamethasone, suppressed TRPC3 expression in vtc cells by about 75%. Thus, transfection of PRLR-S, even in the absence of prolactin + dexamethasone, attenuates the Ca^{2+} signal in response to ATP, presumably by decreasing TRPC3 mRNA and increasing SPCA2 mRNA.

3.3. Effect of Prolactin on Cl⁻ Secretion in HC-11 Cells. While short-term (10 min) incubation with prolactin stimulates Cl⁻ transport in HC-11 cells but does not alter $[Ca^{2+}]_i$ [24], results in Figure 1 suggest that 24 h treatment of these cells with prolactin or prolactin + dexamethasone resulted in a diminution of ATP-induced $[Ca^{2+}]_i$ elevation. Therefore we probed whether this effect of long-term prolactin action on Ca^{2+} sequestration influences its action on Cl⁻ transport in HC-11 cells. Cl⁻ transport was assessed by the iodide (I⁻) efflux method [34]. As shown in Figure 3, 24 h treatment with prolactin, dexamethasone, and prolactin + dexamethasone did not alter basal I⁻ efflux in HC-11 cells. I⁻ efflux in all these treatments are sensitive to $10 \mu M$ DPC, but not to $10 \mu M$ of furosemide (as examples, data for control and prolactin + dexamethasone are shown in Figures 3(b) and 3(c), resp.). At these concentrations DPC largely inhibits CFTR and furosemide affects NKCC.

Next, we examined the effects of the hormone regimen on secretagogue-stimulated Cl⁻ transport. ATP is known to stimulate Cl⁻ secretion in 31EG4 mouse mammary epithelial cells by triggering Ca^{2+} release [37]. In HC-11 cells, ATP ($100 \mu M$) caused a rapid and transient (1–3 min) increase in I⁻ efflux of control cells (Figure 4(a1)). Prolactin + dexamethasone-treated cells also show a similar rapid and transient increase in I⁻ efflux at early time point (Figure 4(a2)). However, there was a late decrease in I⁻ efflux in prolactin + dexamethasone-treated cells at 8–10 minutes (Figure 4(a2)). When control, and prolactin + dexamethasone cells were exposed to a cocktail to elevate intracellular cAMP {forskolin to activate adenylyl cyclase, IBMX to inhibit phosphodiesterase and 8-Br-cAMP}, I⁻ efflux was significantly increased only in prolactin + dexamethasone-treated cells (Figures 4(b2) versus 4(b1)).

To determine if the increase in responsiveness to cAMP was related to the expression of transporters associated with Cl⁻ transport, mRNA expression of key Cl⁻ transporters were assessed by RT-PCR. As previously reported, HC-11 cells contain CFTR (Figure 5(a1)) and NKCC1 [24]. In contrast to the report of Elble et al. [25], ClCa mRNA could not be detected (data not shown). However, we report for the first time that these cells possess ClC-1 and ClC-2 (Figure 5(a2)), members of the ClC family known to be present on the plasma membrane. In addition, ClC-2 is associated with transepithelial Cl⁻ transport [38, 39]. Realtime PCR was used to assess the mRNA expression of these transporters in response to the different hormonal regimens. Twenty-four hour treatment with any of the treatments, prolactin alone, dexamethasone alone or prolactin + dexamethasone, did not alter the mRNA expression of CFTR and NKCC1 (Figures 5(b1) and 5(b2), resp.). Interestingly, in HC-11 cells, prolactin and dexamethasone, suppress the expression of CLC-2 when treated individually while prolactin + dexamethasone did not cause a significant change (Figure 5(b3)).

Both vector-transfected cells (Figure 6(a)) and cells transfected with PRLR-S (rs) (Figure 6(b)), showed an increase in I⁻ efflux in response to the cAMP cocktail. Response in the former was slightly faster than in the latter cells. Neither vector-transfected nor PRLR-S transfected cells, exhibited changes in CFTR or NKCC mRNA expression in the presence or absence of prolactin + dexamethasone-treatment (Figures 7(a) and 7(c)). These results are qualitatively similar to those exhibited by wild type cells (Figures 5(b1) and 5(b2)). Finally Western blotting, confirmed that the protein expression of CFTR was not altered by either PRLR-S transfection or hormonal treatment (Figure 7(b)).

4. Discussion

The actions of prolactin on mammary epithelial function are complex and occur via at least two major receptor isoforms and can involve varied signaling pathways. In addition, prolactin's actions can be further modulated by other hormones, specifically glucocorticoids. Dissecting the molecular basis of these actions is compounded by nuances

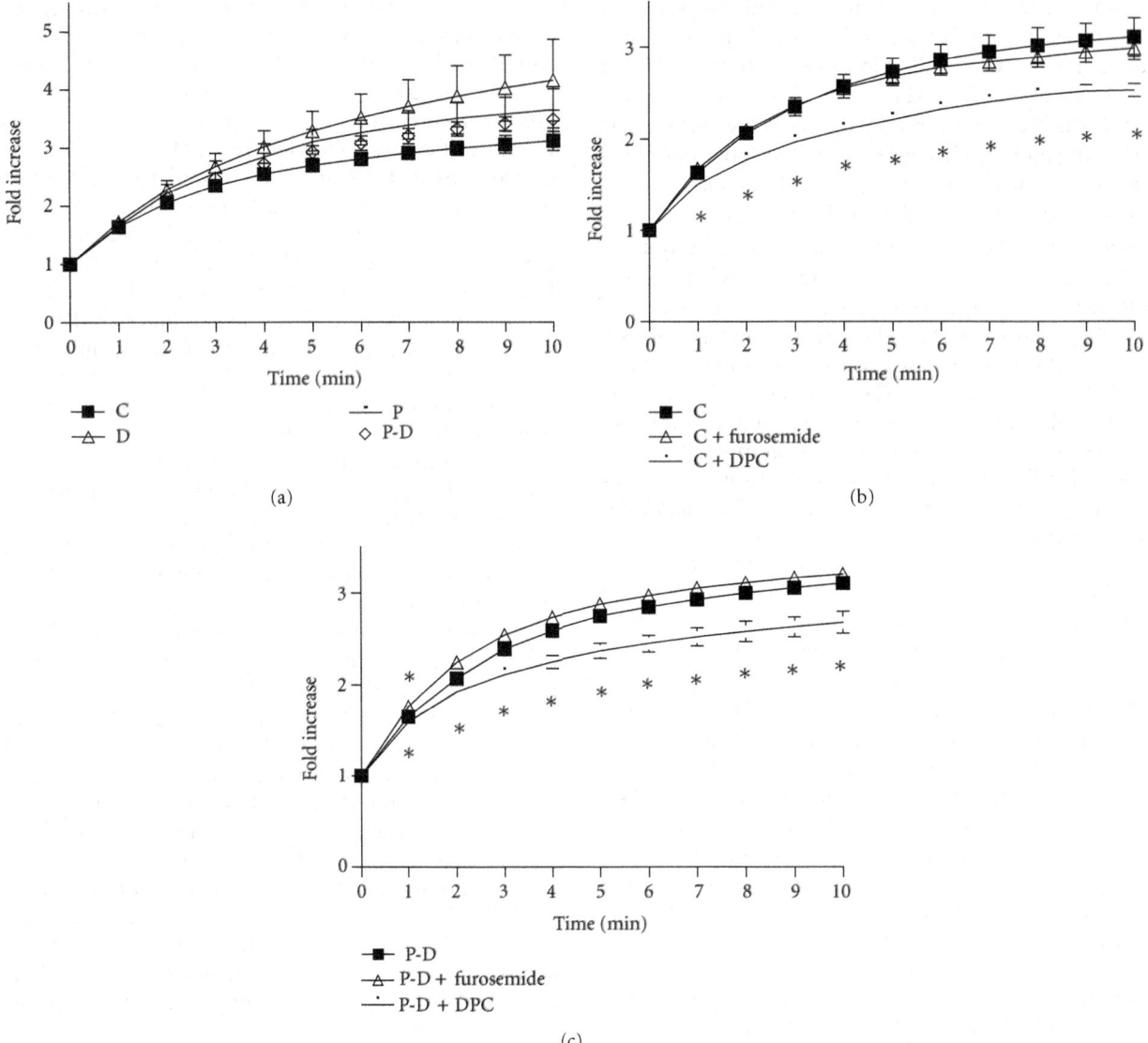

FIGURE 3: Effect of prolactin and/or dexamethasone (a) DPC and furosemide ((b) and (c)) treatment on cumulative iodide efflux. (a) HC-11 cells were pretreated with 1 μg/mL prolactin (P) and/or 1 μg/mL dexamethasone (D) for 24 h prior to iodide efflux assay ((b) and (c)) effect of 10 μM DPC (a CFTR inhibitor) and 10 μM furosemide (a NKCC1 inhibitor) on iodide efflux in control (b) and 24 h P-D-treated cells (c). Data represent mean $\pm$ SEM relative to value at starting point. $n \geq 3$. *$P < 0.05$ versus non-inhibitor treated groups.

in times of exposure to prolactin, and variability in the models used including species and in the case of cell lines, differences in transformed and nontransformed cells. For example, prolactin is known to alter mammary epithelial Ca^{2+} transport and Cl^- transport, and yet there are no systematic studies examining these two actions in the same model system. Equally important, in addition to augmenting milk Ca^{2+} content, an increase in $[Ca^{2+}]_i$ can serve as a second messenger stimulus of cell function, including Cl^- secretion. This regulation clearly is physiologically relevant during lactation. Therefore, this study focused on examining the long-term effect of prolactin on Ca^{2+} responsiveness and Cl^- transport in the normal mouse mammary epithelial cell line, HC-11.

The HC-11 cell line was selected as it offered some useful features. The HC-11 cells available to us contain only the long form of PRLR ([24] and Figure 2(a1)). Second, against this backdrop these cells serve as a good model in which to transfect and examine the effects of short form-PRLR. Finally, this cell line has previously been characterized with respect to Cl^- transport [24]. Therefore studies were conducted both in nontransfected HC-11 cells containing only PRLR-L and in cells transfected with PRLR-S and therefore containing both PRLR-L and PRLR-S.

A physiologically relevant tool to examine Ca^{2+} and Cl^- signaling is ATP. ATP is released upon mechanical stimulation in mammary epithelial cells [40], most likely with relation to myoepithelial contraction facilitating milk

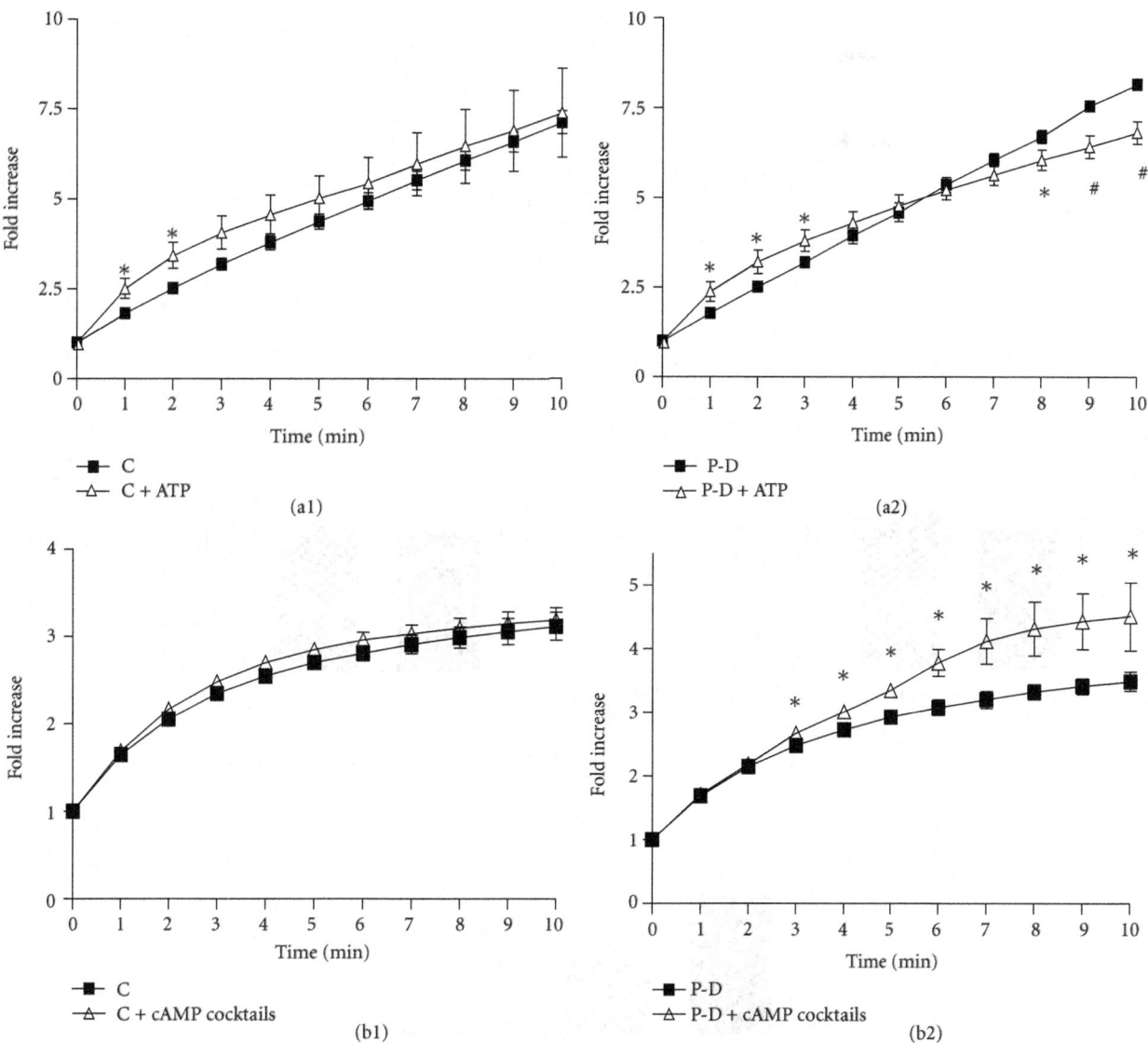

FIGURE 4: ((a1) and (a2)) Effect of ATP on iodide efflux in control (a1) and prolactin and dexamethasone-treated (a2) HC-11 cells. (a1) Iodide efflux assays were performed in the absence or presence of $100\,\mu M$ ATP. (a2) HC-11 cells were pretreated with $1\,\mu g/mL$ prolactin and dexamethasone (P-D) for 24 h prior to iodide efflux assay. $n \geq 3$. *$P < 0.05$ and #$P < 0.01$ versus non-ATP treated groups. ((b1) and (b2)) effect of cAMP cocktails on iodide efflux in control (b1) and prolactin and dexamethasone-treated (b2) HC-11 cells. (b1): Iodide efflux assays were performed in the absence or presence of cAMP cocktails ($100\,\mu M$ cAMP, $10\,\mu M$ forskolin, and $100\,\mu M$ IBMX). (b2) HC-11 cells were pretreated with $1\,\mu g/mL$ prolactin and dexamethasone (P-D) for 24 h prior to iodide efflux assay. Data represent mean ± SEM relative to value at starting point. $n \geq 3$. *$P < 0.05$ versus non-cAMP treated groups.

secretion. In many cell types, ATP activates plasma membrane P2Y receptors which stimulate a PLCγ cascade to signal Ca^{2+} release from intracellular stores. In another mouse mammary epithelial cell line, 31EG4, ATP increased Cl⁻ secretion was suggested to be Ca^{2+} dependent but the effects of prolactin were not examined [41].

As shown in Figure 1, wild type HC-11 cells, show an increase in $[Ca^{2+}]_i$ in response to $100\,\mu M$ ATP. However, this response is attenuated when the cells are exposed to prolactin alone for 24 h or prolactin in the presence of dexamethasone, but not when exposed to dexamethasone alone (Figure 1(a2)). A decrease in $[Ca^{2+}]_i$ could be due

to increased sequestration, decreased entry, or both. HC-11 cells treated with prolactin + dexamethasone but not in those treated with prolactin or dexamethasone alone, showed a significant decrease in the mRNA expression of TRPC3, the Ca^{2+} channel protein (Figure 1(b2)). Prolactin is presumably affecting these changes through the long form of its receptor, PRLR-L, the only form detectable in wild-type HC-11 cells (Figure 2(a1)). None of these treatment regimens had an effect on mRNA expression of SPCA2, the secretory pathway Ca^{2+} ATPase, involved in Ca^{2+} sequestration into cellular compartments. These results differ from the effects of prolonged prolactin exposure in the MCF-7, cancerous human

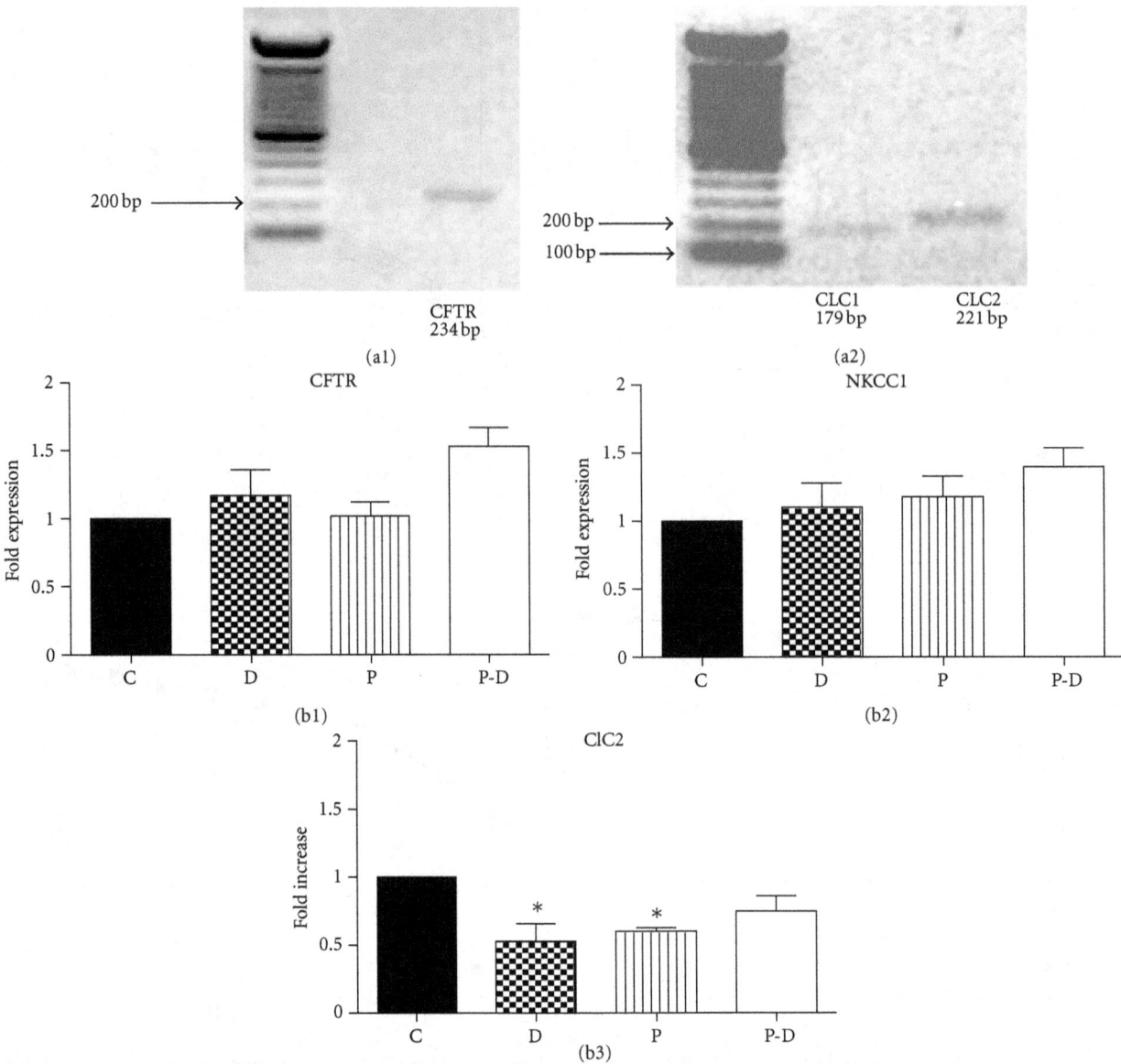

FIGURE 5: ((a1) and (a2)) mRNA expression of CFTR (234 bp) (a1), and ClC1 (179 bp), ClC2 (221 bp) (a2) in HC-11 cells. Representative agarose gel image shows ethidium bromide-stained PCR products. (b1)–(b3) effect of prolactin and/or dexamethasone treatment on CFTR (b1), NKCC1 (b2), and ClC2 (b3) mRNA expression in HC-11 cells. HC-11 cells were treated with or without 1 μg/mL prolactin (P) and/or dexamethasone (D) for 24 h. Total RNA was extracted, and realtime PCR was performed. Ribosomal protein L19 mRNA was used as internal control. C = control. Data represent mean ± SEM relative to control, $n = 4$ for CFTR and NKCC1, and $n = 3$ for ClC2. *$P < 0.05$ versus control.

mammary epithelial cell line in two respects. First, in MCF-7 cells, the prolactin-induced decreases in $[Ca^{2+}]_i$ responses to ATP are linked to an increase in SPCA2 mRNA [4], with no change in TRPC3 mRNA expression (Anantamongkol and Krishnamra, unpublished observations). Second, the effects of prolactin on MCF-7 cells are not enhanced by dexamethasone treatment. It remains to be established if these differences reflect either species or cell line (normal versus cancerous) variations and the functional relationship of the secretory pathway Ca^{2+} ATPases, (SPCAs), the plasma membrane calcium ATPase (PMCAs) and the store operated Ca^{2+} channels (TRPCs) remains to be established. Although

not evident in MCF-7 cells, the synergistic actions of prolactin and dexamethasone, has been well documented. For example, in HC-11 cells, both hormones are needed to enhance casein production [23, 32, 42–44], and in the mice, at the end of pregnancy, increases in prolactin and cortisol increase tight junction formation [41].

Fluid secretion across the epithelium requires secretion of ions, in particular, Cl^-. We had demonstrated earlier that short term (10 minute) incubation of HC-11 cells with prolactin increased Cl^- transport via a JAK2/STAT5 pathway involving tyrosine phosphorylation of NKCC1 [24]. This effect was transient and exposure of prolactin up to 1 h

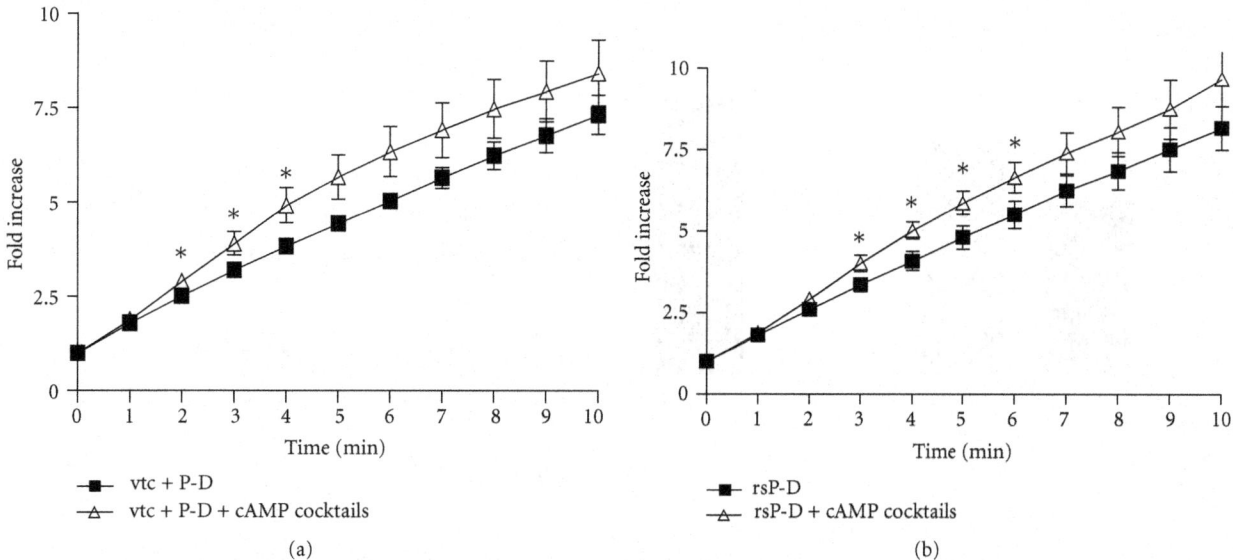

FIGURE 6: Effect of cAMP cocktail on iodide efflux in prolactin and dexamethasone treated, vector- (a) or PRLR-S-transfected (b) HC-11 cells. Vector transfected HC-11 cells (vtc, (a)) and PRLR-S-transfected cells (rs, (b)) were treated with 1 μg/mL prolactin and dexamethasone (P-D) for 24 h prior to the iodide efflux assays. Iodide efflux assays were performed in the absence or presence of the cAMP cocktail (100 μM cAMP, 10 μM forskolin, 100 μM IBMX). Data represent mean ± SEM relative to value at starting point. $n \geq 3$. *$P < 0.05$ versus non-cAMP treated groups.

did not lead to any further increases in Cl⁻ transport. The present study extended these studies to examining the effects of 24 hr prolactin (± dexamethasone) treatment and of ATP on Cl⁻ transport in HC-11 cells. Chloride transport was assessed using the iodide efflux assay. In all treatment groups (data shown for control and prolactin + dexamethasone, Figures 3(b) and 3(c)), this efflux was diminished by the Cl⁻ channel blocker, DPC, but not by the NKCC cotransporter inhibitor, furosemide. This is not surprising since NKCC is halide-selective and transports only Cl⁻ and Br⁻, but not I⁻ and F⁻ [45], and suggests that I⁻ efflux is occurring via Cl⁻ channels. Similarly, radioactive I⁻ efflux in *Xenopus* oocytes was inhibited by DPC but not by by the NKCC inhibitor bumetanide [46]. As in the case of an 1 h exposure, prolonging the exposure to prolactin to 24 h, did not cause an increase in cumulative I⁻ efflux, (Figure 3(a)); neither did overnight treatment with dexamethasone alone or prolactin + dexamethasone (Figure 3(a)).

As reported for 31EG4 and other cells, ATP acts via a Ca²⁺-signaling system to stimulate Cl⁻ secretion in HC-11 cells. The transient increase in I⁻ efflux (Figure 4(a1)) is characteristic of Ca²⁺-dependent secretagogues in Cl⁻ secretory epithelia [37, 47] and is generally reflective of the transient increase in [Ca²⁺]ᵢ induced by ATP (cf. Figure 1). In prolactin + dexamethasone-treated cells ATP likewise caused a transient early increase in I⁻ efflux (Figure 4(a2)). In addition, there was a late decrease in I⁻ efflux and it is reasonable to postulate that this is due to the suppressing effect of prolactin + dexamethasone on [Ca²⁺]ᵢ (Figure 4(a2)). Thus, while prolactin + dexamethasone attenuate ATP-induced [Ca²⁺]ᵢ increases, they do not suppress the initial transient stimulation of Cl⁻ transport, a characteristic of ATP-stimulation in secretory epithelia.

Another potent stimulator of Cl⁻ secretion is cAMP and the effects of prolonged prolactin treatment on cAMP-mediated Cl⁻ transport was examined. Addition of a cAMP cocktail to 24 h prolactin + dexamethasone treated cells (Figure 4(b2)), but not to control (Figure 4(b1)) cells or cells treated with prolactin or dexamethasone alone (data not shown), stimulated I⁻ efflux. In addition, long-term incubation with prolactin + dexamethasone did not alter the mRNA expression of Cl⁻ transporters (Figures 5(b1)–5(b3)). Thus, increased Cl⁻ transport seen in the prolactin + dexamethasone-treated cells in response to cAMP cocktail (Figure 4(b2)) are most likely due to alterations in transporter function and not expression.

In the present study both ATP and long-term prolactin + dexamethasone treatment result in activation of Cl⁻ transport as measured by iodide efflux. The three "candidate" routes for this transport are CFTR, Ca²⁺-dependent Cl⁻ channels (ClCa1 and ClCa2), and members of the ClC family (ClC-1 and ClC-2). Although ClCa1 and ClCa2 were previously reported in HC-11 cells [25], we could not detect them by RT-PCR in the present study. While HC-11 cells express ClC-2 mRNA, we posit that it may not be the transporter responsible for I⁻ efflux, for three reasons. It is uncertain whether I⁻ efflux can measure ClC-2 activity as I⁻ has been shown to be a permanent blocker of ClC [48]. Second, the ClC-2 mRNA expression was suppressed by prolactin or dexamethasone treatment alone (Figure 5(b3)). Finally, there is controversy in the literature whether ClC-2 functions as an apical Cl⁻ channel [49], a lateral membrane channel [26, 50], or a basolateral channel [51]. In contrast CFTR localizes at the apical membrane in several epithelia such as airway, intestine, pancreas, and sweat gland [52]. HC-11 cells express CFTR, demonstrate DPC-sensitive halide

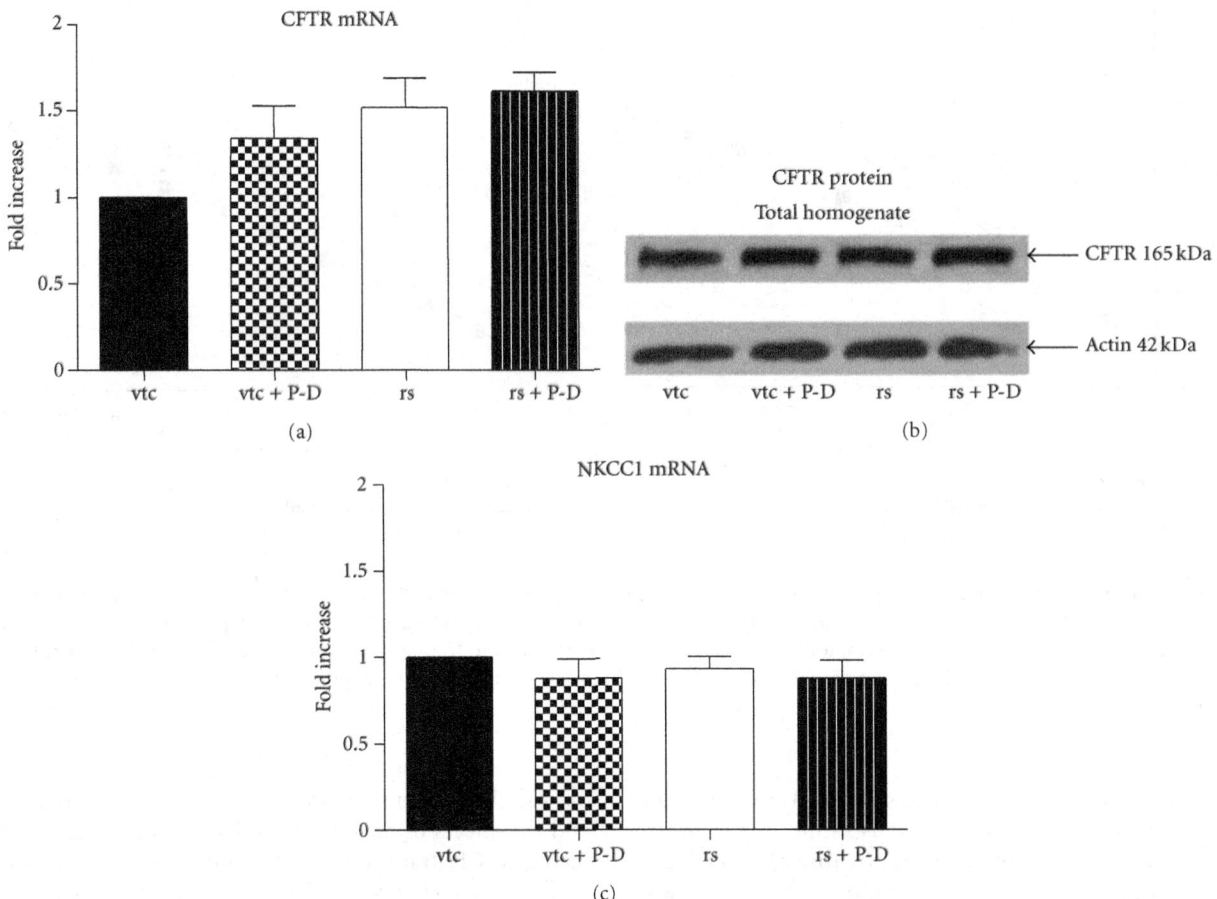

FIGURE 7: Expression of CFTR mRNA (a), protein (b) and of NKCC1 mRNA (c) in vector-transfected control or PRLR-S-tranfected (rs) HC-11 cells. HC-11 cells were transfected with vector (vtc) or PRLR-S. Transfected cells were treated with or without 1 μg/mL prolactin and dexamethasone (P-D) for 24 h. ((a) and (c)) Total RNA was extracted, and realtime PCR was performed using ribosomal L19 as internal control. (b) Total homogenate of cells were subjected to SDS-PAGE and immunoblotting and probed with a polyclonal CFTR antibody. The blot is representative of 3 experiments. Data represent mean ± SEM relative to vtc, $n = 3$ for CFTR and $n = 4$ for NKCC1.

efflux, and we propose that it is the most likely route for Cl$^-$ secretion in these cells. The molecular mechanisms underlying these actions remain to be determined and are clearly posttranscriptional.

All of the above actions of prolactin are through the PRLR-L receptor, since HC-11 cells do not possess PRLR-S. While PRLR-L has been extensively studied [9], the physiological function of PRLR-S is less well characterized and controversial. Both a dominant negative effect and other distinct functions of this receptor have been reported [12, 32, 42–44]. However, it is clear that introduction of PRLR-S in the PRLR ± mice brings a distinct change in the development of mammary alveolar glands and compensates for the haploinsufficiency of PRLR-L [30]. Therefore it is not surprising, that in this study, the presence of both PRLR-L and PRLR-S (rs) elicited some distinct responses from wild-type HC-11 cells, with respect to ATP-induced changes in [Ca^{2+}]$_i$. First, introduction of PRLR-S (rs cells) appears to attenuate the response to ATP even in the absence of additional prolactin + dexamethasone (Figure 2(b)). Second, addition of prolactin + dexamethasone to rs cells

did not cause a further decrease in [Ca^{2+}]$_i$. Third, the attenuation in rs cells is accompanied both by an increase in SPCA2 expression (Figure 2(c1)) and a decrease in TRPC3 expression (Figure 2(c2)). These effects cannot be due to transfection per se as vector-transfected controls showed responses similar to the nontransfected controls in terms of changes in [Ca^{2+}]$_i$ (Figure 2(b)), lack of change in SPCA2 (Figure 2(c1)) and a decrease in TRPC (Figure 2(c2)). It remains to be determined if in the rs cells, prolactin acts through PRLR-S to increase SPCA2 and through PRLR-L to decrease TRPC3 or if both receptor isoforms are involved in both effects. Regardless, introducing PRLR-S into the cells appears to trigger pathways similar to those evoked by prolactin + dexamethasone treatment with respect to Ca^{2+}-signaling. PRLR-S has been shown to physically associate with signaling molecules in the absence of ligand binding [53, 54]. An intriguing possibility may be that PRLR-S associates with molecules that can modulate [Ca^{2+}]$_i$ such as chemokine receptor family allowing regulation of Ca^{2+}-signaling via this receptor independent of prolactin treatment.

The influences of PRLR-S on Cl^- transport are more nuanced. First, transfection with vector alone (Figure 6(a)) or with PRLR-S (Figure 6(b)) showed a smaller response to cAMP cocktails as compared to nontransfected cells (Figures 4(b1) and 4(b2)). Second, the time course of stimulation in vector-transfected and PRLR-S transfected cells are slightly different (Figures 6(a) and 6(b)). It remains to be determined if these are due to transfection per se or the presence of PRLR-S. The interplay of PRLR-L and PRLR-S and their signaling pathways in mammary epithelial function is intriguing. The purpose of PRL signaling via different receptors and transduction pathways could be that one isoform serves as a "complementary" or "braking" mechanism for the action of the other, thereby fine tuning the response. As mentioned in the introduction, this notion is supported by recent studies performed on transgenic mice expressing the short or the long form of PRLR selectively [11–13]. For example, the deleterious effect of PRLR-S in the ovary is prevented by the presence of PRLR-L. Ultimately regardless of the differences in receptor isoform consensus domains and signaling pathways the 3D structure will determine the final function. To our best knowledge, no crystal structure or 3D model has been analyzed for the C-terminal domain of either form of the prolactin receptor.

In summary, these results demonstrate that in HC-11 cells, long term prolactin + dexamethasone, act via PRLR-L to modulate the ability of the cell to respond to ATP and to cAMP-dependent secretagogues. In the former case it is due to a dampening of the Ca^{2+} signaling by decreasing Ca^{2+} entry via TRPC3 channels and in the latter by an increase in Cl^- secretion, most likely stimulating CFTR function. This modulation is further fine-tuned by the presence of PRLR-S, which appears to obviate the need for exposure to prolactin + dexamethasone by causing a decrease in $[Ca^{2+}]_i$, both by increasing sequestration via SPCA2 and decreasing entry via TRPC3. These fine-tuning mechanisms may explain the ability of PRLR-S to rescue mammopoiesis in PRLR± mice [30].

Acknowledgments

This work was supported by a grant from the National Institute of Diabetes and Digestive and Kidney Diseases (1 P01 DK067887 Project 3) (to M. C. Rao and R. V. Benya), grants from the National Institutes of Health HD11119 and HD 12356 (P. I.: Professor Geula Gibori; Trainee: Y. S. Devi).

References

[1] J. A. Rillema, R. N. Etindi, and C. M. Cameron, "Prolactin actions on casein and lipid biosynthesis in mouse and rabbit mammary gland explants are abolished by p-bromphenacyl bromide and quinacrine, phospholipase A2 inhibitors," *Hormone and Metabolic Research*, vol. 18, no. 10, pp. 672–674, 1986.

[2] J. L. McManaman and M. C. Neville, "Mammary physiology and milk secretion," *Advanced Drug Delivery Reviews*, vol. 55, no. 5, pp. 629–641, 2003.

[3] D. J. Flint and M. Gardner, "Evidence that growth hormone stimulates milk synthesis by direct action on the mammary gland and that prolactin exerts effects on milk secretion by maintenance of mammary deoxyribonucleic acid content and tight junction status," *Endocrinology*, vol. 135, no. 3, pp. 1119–1124, 1994.

[4] U. Anantamongkol, H. Takemura, T. Suthiphongchai, N. Krishnamra, and Y. Horio, "Regulation of Ca^{2+} mobilization by prolactin in mammary gland cells: possible role of secretory pathway Ca^{2+}-ATPase type 2," *Biochemical and Biophysical Research Communications*, vol. 352, no. 2, pp. 537–542, 2007.

[5] F. Arturi, E. Ferretti, I. Presta et al., "Regulation of iodide uptake and sodium/iodide symporter expression in the MCF-7 human breast cancer cell line," *Journal of Clinical Endocrinology and Metabolism*, vol. 90, no. 4, pp. 2321–2326, 2005.

[6] J. A. Rillema, S. Collins, and C. H. Williams, "Prolactin stimulation of iodide uptake and incorporation into protein is polyamine-dependent in mouse mammary gland explants (44512)," *Experimental Biology and Medicine*, vol. 224, no. 1, pp. 41–44, 2000.

[7] J. Bouilly, C. Sonigo, J. Auffret, G. Gibori, and N. Binart, "Prolactin signaling mechanisms in ovary," *Molecular and Cellular Endocrinology*, vol. 356, no. 1-2, pp. 80–87, 2012.

[8] J. F. Trott, R. C. Hovey, S. Koduri, and B. K. Vonderhaar, "Multiple new isoforms of the human prolactin receptor gene," *Advances in Experimental Medicine and Biology*, vol. 554, pp. 495–499, 2004.

[9] C. Bole-Feysot, V. Goffin, M. Edery, N. Binart, and P. A. Kelly, "Prolactin (PRL) and its receptor: actions, signal transduction pathways and phenotypes observed in PRL receptor knockout mice," *Endocrine Reviews*, vol. 19, no. 3, pp. 225–268, 1998.

[10] M. E. Freeman, B. Kanyicska, A. Lerant, and G. Nagy, "Prolactin: structure, function, and regulation of secretion," *Physiological Reviews*, vol. 80, no. 4, pp. 1523–1631, 2000.

[11] Y. S. Devi, A. Shehu, C. Stocco et al., "Regulation of transcription factors and repression of Sp1 by prolactin signaling through the short isoform of its cognate receptor," *Endocrinology*, vol. 150, no. 7, pp. 3327–3335, 2009.

[12] J. Halperin, S. Y. Devi, S. Elizur et al., "Prolactin signaling through the short form of its receptor represses forkhead transcription factor FOXO3 and its target gene Galt causing a severe ovarian defect," *Molecular Endocrinology*, vol. 22, no. 2, pp. 513–522, 2008.

[13] J. A. Le, H. M. Wilson, A. Shehu et al., "Generation of mice expressing only the long form of the prolactin receptor reveals that both isoforms of the receptor are required for normal ovarian function," *Biology of Reproduction*, vol. 86, no. 3, Article ID 86, 2012.

[14] D. B. Shennan, "Calcium transport by mammary secretory cells: mechanisms underlying transepithelial movement," *Cellular and Molecular Biology Letters*, vol. 13, no. 4, pp. 514–525, 2008.

[15] T. A. Reinhardt and R. L. Horst, "Ca^{2+}-ATPases and their expression in the mammary gland of pregnant and lactating rats," *American Journal of Physiology, Cell Physiology*, vol. 276, no. 4, pp. C796–C802, 1999.

[16] T. A. Reinhardt, A. G. Filoteo, J. T. Penniston, and R. L. Horst, "Ca^{2+}-ATPase protein expression in mammary tissue," *American Journal of Physiology, Cell Physiology*, vol. 279, no. 5, pp. C1595–C1602, 2000.

[17] T. A. Reinhardt, J. D. Lippolis, G. E. Shulland, and R. L. Horst, "Null mutation in the gene encoding plasma membrane Ca^{2+}-ATPase isoform 2 impairs calcium transport into milk," *Journal of Biological Chemistry*, vol. 279, no. 41, pp. 42369–42373, 2004.

[18] J. N. Van Houten, M. C. Neville, and J. J. Wysolmerski, "The calcium-sensing receptor regulates plasma membrane calcium adenosine triphosphatase isoform 2 activity in mammary epithelial cells: a mechanism for calcium-regulated calcium transport into milk," *Endocrinology*, vol. 148, no. 12, pp. 5943–5954, 2007.

[19] K. Stelwagen, H. A. McFadden, and J. Demmer, "Prolactin, alone or in combination with glucocorticoids, enhances tight junction formation and expression of the tight junction protein occludin in mammary cells," *Molecular and Cellular Endocrinology*, vol. 156, no. 1-2, pp. 55–61, 1999.

[20] K. S. Zettl, M. D. Sjaastad, P. M. Riskin, G. Parry, T. E. Machen, and G. L. Firestone, "Glucocorticoid-induced formation of tight junctions in mouse mammary epithelial cells in vitro," *Proceedings of the National Academy of Sciences of the United States of America*, vol. 89, no. 19, pp. 9069–9073, 1992.

[21] J. A. Rillema, T. X. Yu, and S. M. Jhiang, "Effect of prolactin on sodium iodide symporter expression in mouse mammary gland explants," *American Journal of Physiology, Endocrinology and Metabolism*, vol. 279, no. 4, pp. E769–E772, 2000.

[22] S. L. Kelleher and B. Lönnerdal, "Zip3 plays a major role in zinc uptake into mammary epithelial cells and is regulated by prolactin," *American Journal of Physiology, Cell Physiology*, vol. 288, no. 5, pp. C1042–C1047, 2005.

[23] W. Doppler, B. Gorner, and R. K. Ball, "Prolactin and glucocorticoid hormones synergistically induce expression of transfected rat β-casein gene promoter constructs in a mammary epithelial cell line," *Proceedings of the National Academy of Sciences of the United States of America*, vol. 86, no. 1, pp. 104–108, 1989.

[24] N. G. Selvaraj, E. Omi, G. Gibori, and M. C. Rao, "Janus kinase 2 (JAK2) regulates prolactin-mediated chloride transport in mouse mammary epithelial cells through tyrosine phosphorylation of Na^+-K^+-$2Cl^-$ cotransporter," *Molecular Endocrinology*, vol. 14, no. 12, pp. 2054–2065, 2000.

[25] R. C. Elble and B. U. Pauli, "Tumor suppression by a proapoptotic calcium-activated chloride channel in mammary epithelium," *Journal of Biological Chemistry*, vol. 276, no. 44, pp. 40510–40517, 2001.

[26] K. Gyömörey, H. Yeger, C. Ackerley, E. Garami, and C. E. Bear, "Expression of the chloride channel ClC-2 in the murine small intestine epithelium," *American Journal of Physiology, Cell Physiology*, vol. 279, no. 6, pp. C1787–C1794, 2000.

[27] U. Anantamongkol, N. Charoenphandhu, K. Wongdee et al., "Transcriptome analysis of mammary tissues reveals complex patterns of transporter gene expression during pregnancy and lactation," *Cell Biology International*, vol. 34, no. 1, pp. 67–74, 2010.

[28] C. J. Ormandy, A. Camus, J. Barra et al., "Null mutation of the prolactin receptor gene produces multiple reproductive defects in the mouse," *Genes and Development*, vol. 11, no. 2, pp. 167–178, 1997.

[29] C. Brisken, S. Kaur, T. E. Chavarria et al., "Prolactin controls mammary gland development via direct and indirect mechanisms," *Developmental Biology*, vol. 210, no. 1, pp. 96–106, 1999.

[30] N. Binart, P. Imbert-Bolloré, N. Baran, C. Viglietta, and P. A. Kelly, "A short form of the prolactin (PRL) receptor is able to rescue mammopoiesis in heterozygous PRL receptor mice," *Molecular Endocrinology*, vol. 17, no. 6, pp. 1066–1074, 2003.

[31] W. Wu, D. Coss, M. Y. Lorenson, C. B. Kuo, X. Xu, and A. M. Walker, "Different biological effects of unmodified prolactin and a molecular mimic of phosphorylated prolactin involve different signaling pathways," *Biochemistry*, vol. 42, no. 24, pp. 7561–7570, 2003.

[32] M. Perrot-Applanat, O. Gualillo, A. Pezet, V. Vincent, M. Edery, and P. A. Kelly, "Dominant negative and cooperative effects of mutant forms of prolactin receptor," *Molecular Endocrinology*, vol. 11, no. 8, pp. 1020–1032, 1997.

[33] C. Boonkaewwan, M. Ao, C. Toskulkao, and M. C. Rao, "Specific immunomodulatory and secretory activities of stevioside and steviol in intestinal cells," *Journal of Agricultural and Food Chemistry*, vol. 56, no. 10, pp. 3777–3784, 2008.

[34] C. J. Venglarik, R. J. Bridges, and R. A. Frizzell, "A simple assay for agonist-regulated Cl and K conductances in salt-secreting epithelial cells," *American Journal of Physiology, Cell Physiology*, vol. 259, no. 2, pp. C358–C364, 1990.

[35] C. Stocco, J. Djiane, and G. Gibori, "Prostaglandin $F_{2\alpha}$ ($PGF_{2\alpha}$) and prolactin signaling: $PGF_{2\alpha}$-mediated inhibition of prolactin receptor expression in the corpus luteum," *Endocrinology*, vol. 144, no. 8, pp. 3301–3305, 2003.

[36] J. Venkatasubramanian, N. Selvaraj, M. Carlos, S. Skaluba, M. M. Rasenick, and M. C. Rao, "Differences in Ca^{2+} signaling underlie age-specific effects of secretagogues on colonic Cl^- transport," *American Journal of Physiology, Cell Physiology*, vol. 280, no. 3, pp. C646–C658, 2001.

[37] S. Blaug, J. Rymer, S. Jalickee, and S. S. Miller, "P2 purinoceptors regulate calcium-activated chloride and fluid transport in 31EG4 mammary epithelia," *American Journal of Physiology, Cell Physiology*, vol. 284, no. 4, pp. C897–C909, 2003.

[38] T. J. Jentsch, I. Neagoe, and O. Scheel, "CLC chloride channels and transporters," *Current Opinion in Neurobiology*, vol. 15, no. 3, pp. 319–325, 2005.

[39] T. J. Jentsch, M. Poët, J. C. Fuhrmann, and A. A. Zdebik, "Physiological functions of CLC Cl^- channels gleaned from human genetic disease and mouse models," *Annual Review of Physiology*, vol. 67, pp. 779–807, 2005.

[40] K. Enomoto, K. Furuya, S. Yamagishi, T. Oka, and T. Maeno, "The increase in the intracellular Ca^{2+} concentration induced by mechanical stimulation is propagated via release of pyrophosphorylated nucleotides in mammary epithelial cells," *Pflugers Archiv European Journal of Physiology*, vol. 427, no. 5-6, pp. 533–542, 1994.

[41] M. C. Neville, T. B. McFadden, and I. Forsyth, "Hormonal regulation of mammary differentiation and milk secretion," *Journal of Mammary Gland Biology and Neoplasia*, vol. 7, no. 1, pp. 49–66, 2002.

[42] L. Lesueur, M. Edery, S. Ali, J. Paly, P. A. Kelly, and J. Djiane, "Comparison of long and short forms of the prolactin receptor on prolactin-induced milk protein gene transcription," *Proceedings of the National Academy of Sciences of the United States of America*, vol. 88, no. 3, pp. 824–828, 1991.

[43] J. J. Berlanga, J. P. Garcia-Ruiz, M. Perrot-Applanat, P. A. Kelly, and M. Edery, "The short form of the prolactin (PRL) receptor silences PRL induction of the β-casein gene promoter," *Molecular Endocrinology*, vol. 11, no. 10, pp. 1449–1457, 1997.

[44] K. Huang, E. Ueda, Y. Chen, and A. M. Walker, "Paradigm-shifters: phosphorylated prolactin and short prolactin receptors," *Journal of Mammary Gland Biology and Neoplasia*, vol. 13, no. 1, pp. 69–79, 2008.

[45] J. M. Russell, "Sodium-potassium-chloride cotransport," *Physiological Reviews*, vol. 80, no. 1, pp. 211–276, 2000.

[46] A. C. Chao and Y. Katayama, "Regulation of endogenous chloride conductance in xenopus oocytes," *Biochemical and Biophysical Research Communications*, vol. 180, no. 3, pp. 1377–1382, 1991.

[47] K. E. Barrett and S. J. Keely, "Chloride secretion by the intestinal epithelium: molecular basis and regulatory aspects," *Annual Review of Physiology*, vol. 62, pp. 535–572, 2000.

[48] C. Miller, "ClC chloride channels viewed through a transporter lens," *Nature*, vol. 440, no. 7083, pp. 484–489, 2006.

[49] J. Cuppoletti, D. H. Malinowska, K. P. Tewari et al., "SPI⁻0211 activates T84 cell chloride transport and recombinant human ClC-2 chloride currents," *American Journal of Physiology, Cell Physiology*, vol. 287, no. 5, pp. C1173–C1183, 2004.

[50] R. Mohammad-Panah, K. Gyomorey, J. Rommens et al., "ClC-2 Contributes to Native Chloride Secretion by a Human Intestinal Cell Line, Caco-2," *Journal of Biological Chemistry*, vol. 276, no. 11, pp. 8306–8313, 2001.

[51] G. Peña-Münzenmayer, M. Catálan, I. Cornejo et al., "Basolateral localization of native ClC-2 chloride channels in absorptive intestinal epithelial cells and basolateral sorting encoded by a CBS-2 domain di-leucine motif," *Journal of Cell Science*, vol. 118, no. 18, pp. 4243–4252, 2005.

[52] C. Li and A. P. Naren, "CFTR chloride channel in the apical compartments: spatiotemporal coupling to its interacting partners," *Integrative Biology*, vol. 2, no. 4, pp. 161–177, 2010.

[53] Y. S. Devi, A. M. Seibold, A. Shehu et al., "Inhibition of MAPK by prolactin signaling through the short form of its receptor in the ovary and decidua: involvement of a novel phosphatase," *Journal of Biological Chemistry*, vol. 286, no. 9, pp. 7609–7618, 2011.

[54] W. Rachel Duan, D. I. Linzer, and G. Gibori, "Cloning and characterization of an ovarian-specific protein that associates with the short form of the prolactin receptor," *Journal of Biological Chemistry*, vol. 271, no. 26, pp. 15602–15607, 1996.

Extracellular Signal-Regulated Kinase (ERK) Activation and Mitogen-Activated Protein Kinase Phosphatase 1 Induction by Pulsatile Gonadotropin-Releasing Hormone in Pituitary Gonadotrophs

Haruhiko Kanasaki, Indri Purwana, Aki Oride, Tselmeg Mijiddorj, and Kohji Miyazaki

*Department of Obstetrics and Gynecology, Faculty of Medicine, Shimane University,
Izumo 693-8501, Japan*

Correspondence should be addressed to Haruhiko Kanasaki, kanasaki@med.shimane-u.ac.jp

Academic Editor: J. Adolfo García-Sáinz

The frequency of gonadotropin-releasing hormone (GnRH) pulse secreted from the hypothalamus differently regulates the expressions of gonadotropin subunit genes, luteinizing hormone β (LHβ) and follicle-stimulating hormone β (FSHβ), in the pituitary gonadotrophs. FSHβ is preferentially stimulated at slower GnRH pulse frequencies, whereas LHβ is preferentially stimulated at more rapid pulse frequencies. Several signaling pathways are activated, including mitogen-activated protein kinase (MAPK), protein kinase C, calcium influx, and calcium-calmodulin kinases, and these may be preferentially regulated under certain conditions. Previous studies demonstrated that MAPK pathways, especially the extracellular signal-regulated kinase (ERK), play an essential role for induction of gonadotropin subunit gene expression by GnRH, whereas, MAPK phosphatases (MKPs) inactivate MAPKs through dephosphorylation of threonine and/or tyrosine residues. MKPs are also induced by GnRH, and potential feedback regulation between MAPK signaling and MKPs within the GnRH signaling pathway is evident in gonadotrophs. In this paper, we reviewed and mainly focused on our observations of the pattern of ERK activation and the induction of MKP by different frequencies of GnRH stimulation.

1. Introduction

Reproductive functions in mammalians are regulated largely by the gonadotropins, luteinizing hormone (LH) and follicle-stimulating hormone (FSH), from anterior pituitary gonadotrophs, which are also involved in sex steroid hormone synthesis, follicular growth, and oocyte maturation [1]. Gonadotropins LH and FSH contain α and β subunits, and the α subunit is common to both gonadotropin hormones, whereas the β subunits differ from each other and confer specificity to the gonadotropin hormones [2]. Gonadotropins LH and FSH are mainly under the control of the hypothalamic peptide, gonadotropin-releasing hormone (GnRH), which is released into the hypophyseal portal vascular system [3].

GnRH is released from hypothalamus in a pulsatile manner, in which the pulse pattern varies physiologically as a function of hormonal status and reproductive cycle stage [4, 5]. In a study using primate model, Knobil demonstrated that pulsatile secretion of GnRH, but not continuous, was essential to maintain normal LH and FSH secretion. Continuous GnRH stimulation resulted in a decrease of LH and FSH due to the downregulation of the gonadotrophs [6]. Moreover, the frequency of GnRH pulses plays a critical role in determining the output of LH and FSH from the pituitary; that is, more rapid frequencies of GnRH pulses increase the secretion of LH, whereas slower frequencies result in a decrease in LH secretion but a rise in FSH secretion [7]. In addition, changes in the frequency of GnRH pulse signals have been shown to differently regulate gonadotropin

Extracellular Signal-Regulated Kinase (ERK) Activation and Mitogen-Activated Protein Kinase Phosphatase 1 Induction by
Pulsatile Gonadotropin-Releasing Hormone in Pituitary Gonadotrophs

85

subunit gene expression. LHβ gene expression is maximally stimulated by a GnRH pulse of 30 min interval, whereas FSHβ gene expression is optimally stimulated by a slower GnRH pulse frequency every 2 h [8–11]. GnRH specifically controls LH and FSH secretion and also regulates LHβ and FSHβ subunit gene expression by changing its pattern of secretion to gonadotrophs. However, at present, how GnRH pulse frequency determines the specificity of gonadotropin subunit expression still remains unclear.

2. Intracellular Signal Transduction by GnRH Stimulation

The GnRH receptor is a member of seven-transmembrane G-protein-coupled receptor family. The initial phase of GnRH action involves Gq-protein-mediated stimulation of phospholipase C, leading to the formation of 1,4,5-triphosphate (IP3) and diacylglycerol (DG). Subsequently, IP3 induces the release of intracellular calcium from the endoplasmic reticulum and DG activates protein kinase C (PKC), which ultimately activates extracellular signal-regulated kinase (ERK), a member of mitogen-activated protein kinase (MAPK) family, by the activation of Raf. This activation is supported by a pathway that involves dynamin, c-Src, and Ras and a pathway that involves calcium-signaling and possibly other signaling components [12–14]. Activation of MAPK family proteins such as ERK, c-Jun N-terminal kinase (JNK), p38 MAPK, and ERK5 has been reported to mediate GnRH-induced gonadotropin subunit expression [15–19]. The JNK cascade utilizes MKK4/7 to activate transcription factors such as c-Jun, ATF2, and Elk 1 [20]. The p38 MAPK utilizes many MKK3/6 to activate Elk, AtF2, CHOP, and MEF [21]. Calcium- and calmodulin-dependent protein kinase are also activated by GnRH [22, 23]. Interestingly, the MAPK pathways are activated by the downstream of calmodulin [24]. In addition, GnRH also couples with Gs protein to increase cAMP accumulation [25]. The signal transduction systems through GnRH receptor were shown in Figure 1.

3. LβT2 Cells as a Model for Pituitary Gonadotrophs

Different types of hormone-producing cells exist in the anterior pituitary. Approximately 50% of the adenohypophysis consist of growth-hormone-producing somatotrophs and 15% are considered to be lactotrophs which produce prolactin. These cell types are acidophilic and are also believed to be derived from the same origin. Somatolactotrophs, which produce both growth hormone and prolactin, are candidate cells for the origin of lactotrophs and exist in a small population [27]. Corticotrophs, which secrete ACTH, make up approximately 15–20% and TSH-producing thyrotrophs are approximately 5% of the total adenohypophysial cell populations. Pituitary LH and FSH are secreted from gonadotrophs, and these cells likely represent up to 10% of the cell population. Although it is difficult to isolate a single colony of hormone-secreting cells, clonal strains of pituitary tumor cells have been widely used as models for the study

of distinct hormone-secreting cell types. Development of the immortalized murine pituitary-gonadotroph-derived cell model, LβT2, has facilitated the study of signal transduction pathways activated by the GnRH receptor [28]. This cell line expresses the gonadotropin α-, LHβ-, and FSHβ-subunits as well as the GnRH receptor, and they synthesize and release LH and FSH in response to GnRH stimulation. Studies of the regulation of pituitary gonadotropin gene expression have also been performed using αT3-1 cells, a gonadotropin α-subunit-producing cell line of gonadotroph lineage [28]. Our studies were conducted using LβT2 cells as a model to determine the cellular response to pulsatile GnRH.

4. Activation of ERK by GnRH (Continuous and Pulsatile Condition) in LβT2 Cells

Generally, to study the intracellular signaling using cell culture, experiments were conducted in static condition. Cells were prepared and plated in the culture dishes and then stimulated by test reagent followed by an assay of the targets. As described above, GnRH is released in pulsatile manner in vivo, which exposes the pituitary gonadotrophs intermittently to GnRH. We examined the pattern of ERK activation induced by GnRH in static or perifused pulsatile conditions in LβT2 cells. In static GnRH stimulation (under which GnRH was added directly to the cell culture dish before harvesting), ERK activation was significantly increased after 10 min of GnRH stimulation and the increased ERK phosphorylation was sustained and gradually decreased to the basal level within 4–20 h [29, 30]. When cells were exposed to continuous GnRH for similar time intervals in a perifused, not static, condition, ERK phosphorylation was increased to a similar degree with maximal peak as in static culture; however, the ERK activation was more sustained and remained increased [29]. On the other hand, the ERK activation in response to pulsatile GnRH in perifused gonadotrophs was totally different compared to those observed in response to continuous GnRH. After a pulse of GnRH, ERK phosphorylation were rapidly increased, but was not sustained, returning to baseline levels within 60 min [29]. A similar pattern of ERK activation was observed in subsequent pulse of GnRH. Interestingly, the pattern of ERK phosphorylation in response to pulsatile GnRH administered at high and low frequencies were distinct. After exposures to pulsatile GnRH at high frequency (one pulse every 30 min), ERK phosphorylation increased to a maximum level at 10 min and then rapidly decreased, returning to baseline levels within 20–30 min. A similar pattern of ERK phosphorylation was observed following the next pulse of GnRH. The pattern of ERK phosphorylation in response to pulsatile GnRH at low frequency (one pulse every 2 h) was contrastingly different. By a single GnRH pulse at lower frequency, ERK was more rapidly phosphorylated, reaching a maximum level by 5 min after the pulse and remaining elevated until 20 min time point and then slowly decreasing, returning to the basal levels by 40–50 min. In light of the pattern of ERK phosphorylation during pulsatile treatment, we could speculate that ERK is activated in response to GnRH occupation of its receptor

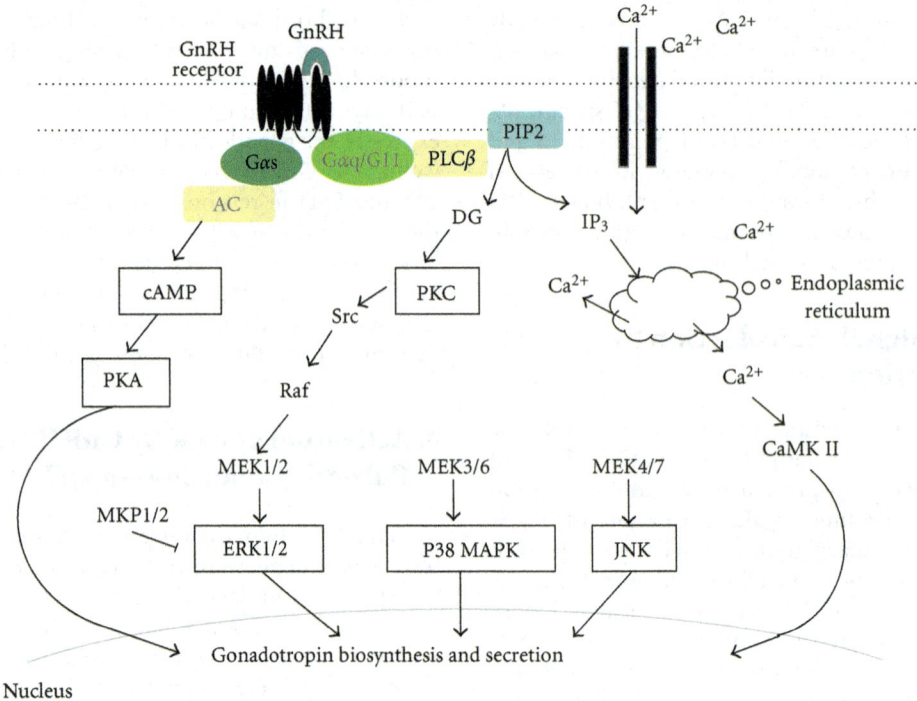

FIGURE 1: Schematic summary of intracellular signaling by GnRH. The initial phase of GnRH action involves Gq-protein-mediated stimulation of phospholipase Cβ (PLCβ), leading to the formation of 1,4,5-triphosphate (IP3) and diacylglycerol (DG). IP3 induces the release of intracellular calcium from endoplasmic reticulum, and DG activates protein kinase C (PKC), which ultimately activates extracellular signal-regulated kinase (ERK). P38 MAPK, c-Jun N-terminal kinase (JNK), and calcium-calmodulin kinase II (CaMK II) are also activated by GnRH. Not predominant, but GnRH also couples to Gs protein which are linked with adenylate cyclase and induces rapid cAMP production, which ultimately activates protein kinase A (PKA). MAP kinase phosphatase 1/2 (MKP1/2) inactivates ERK by dephosphorylation.

and this receptor signaling is not prolonged. It is likely that GnRH binding to its receptor has only transient effects on the downstream signaling events, which result in the unsustained ERK phosphorylation in pulsatile condition compared to the sustained pattern after continuous stimulation. In addition, the pattern of ERK phosphorylation in response to low and high GnRH pulse frequencies was distinct from each other, suggesting the role of the ERK dephosphorylation enzyme that works differently in each condition (Figure 2).

5. Induction of MAP Kinase Phosphatase 1 by GnRH Stimulation (Continuous and Pulsatile Condition) in LβT2 Cells

MAP kinase phosphatases (MKPs) are a family of protein phosphatases that inactivated MAPKs through dephosphorylation of threonine and/or tyrosine residues. MKP1 belongs to a group comprised of type I dual-specificity phosphatases (DUSPs) that inactivates ERK through dephosphorylation [31]. MKP1 is localized in the nuclear compartment, and the activation of ERK cascade is also known to promote induction of MKP1 activity, which then attenuates ERK-dependent events [32]. Therefore, MKP1 is thought to play an important role in the feedback control of ERK in the nucleus, where it attenuates the stimuli [33]. MKP1 effectively inactivates p38 MAPK and JNK [34]. With regard to

the pituitary gonadotrophs, MKPs are increased in association with ERK and JNK [35, 36]. The potential feedback of regulation between MAPK signaling and MKPs with GnRH signaling pathways is also evident in gonadotrophs. In LβT2 cell, the induction of MKP1 occurred 60 min after GnRH stimulation and continued to be expressed in static culture, with a concomitant decrease of ERK phosphorylation [30]. MKP1 induction also occurred by pulsatile GnRH, but the expression patterns following high or low frequencies of GnRH pulse stimulation are distinct.

In LβT2 cells, after 16 h of exposure to GnRH pulse, MKP1 expression was increased predominantly following high- (5 min GnRH pulse, every 30 min) rather than low-frequency (every 120 min) GnRH pulse stimulation. Under the high-frequency GnRH pulse stimulation, MKP1 protein expression was observed clearly at 2 h after the start of pulse stimulation (four GnRH pulses) (Figure 3). Even when greater concentration (100 nM GnRH) was applied for each pulse in low-frequency GnRH stimulation, MKP1 protein was not observed after the cells received 4 GnRH pulses [26]. These results suggest that the number of pulse and the high frequency with which they were delivered are more important than the GnRH concentration in terms of MKP1 expression induction. As described in the previous section, ERK phosphorylation occurs more rapidly, is sustained for a longer time period, and decreases more slowly in lower frequency of GnRH pulse, whereas, with high-frequency GnRH

Extracellular Signal-Regulated Kinase (ERK) Activation and Mitogen-Activated Protein Kinase Phosphatase 1 Induction by
Pulsatile Gonadotropin-Releasing Hormone in Pituitary Gonadotrophs

87

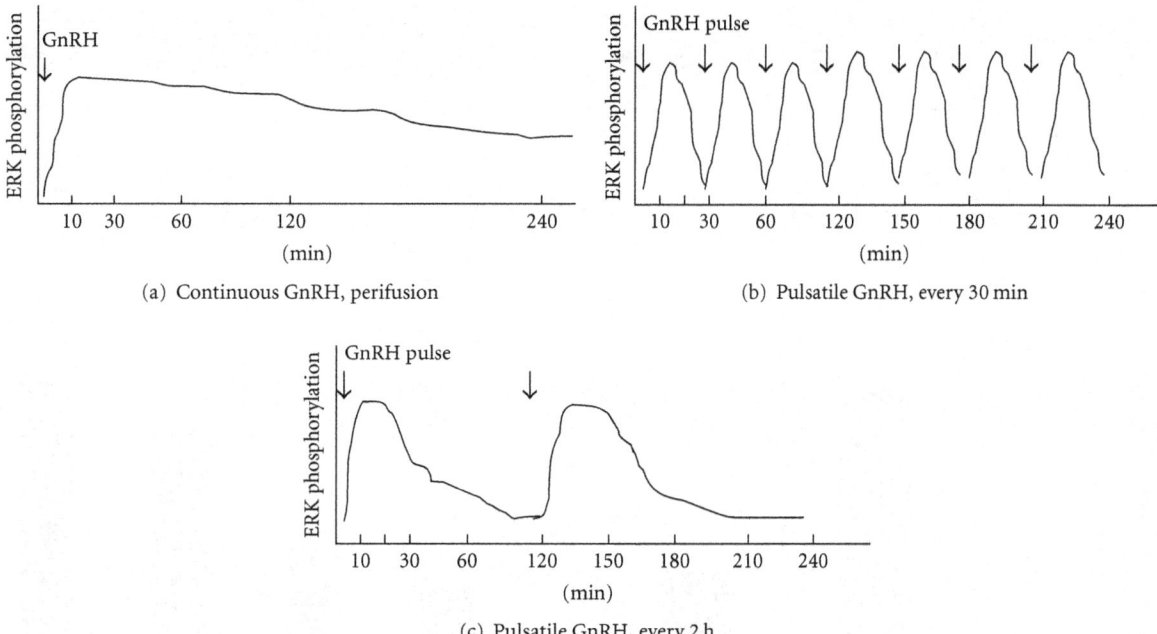

(a) Continuous GnRH, perifusion

(b) Pulsatile GnRH, every 30 min

(c) Pulsatile GnRH, every 2 h

FIGURE 2: Schematic pattern of ERK activation by perifused GnRH stimulation. (a) When cells were exposed to continuous GnRH in perifused conditions, ERK activation was significantly increased, after 10 min, and increased ERK phosphorylation was sustained and gradually decreased to the basal. (b) At high frequency of GnRH pulse stimulation (one pulse very 30 min), ERK phosphorylation increased to a maximum at 10 min, and then levels rapidly decreased to bas line levels within 30 min. A similar pattern of ERK phosphorylation was observed in response to subsequent pulse of GnRH. (c) At a slower frequency of GnRH pulse stimulation (one pulse every 2 h), ERK was more rapidly phosphorylated by GnRH pulse, and increase was more sustained, remaining elevated, and then slowly decreased to the baseline levels. A similar pattern of ERK phosphorylation was observed in response to subsequent pulse of GnRH.

pulses, ERK phosphorylation induced by each single pulse returns to the basal level more rapidly. Another study has also shown the role of MKP1 feedback activity in modulating ERK activation and transcriptional response to GnRH [37]. These differences in the pattern of ERK phosphorylation between the various GnRH pulse stimulations might be associated with the differential regulation of MKP1 expression by pulsatile GnRH stimulation. A study by Armstrong et al. showed that the MKP had no or little effect on the rapid and transient translocation responses of ERK within nuclear level in HeLa cells, which argues against the role of MKPs or ERK-mediated feedback in shaping ERK activation during pulsatile GnRH stimulation [38].

6. ERK Activation and Gene Expression of Gonadotropin Subunits

The involvement of ERK pathways in GnRH-induced gonadotropin α-subunit [19, 39, 40], LHβ [16, 41, 42], and FSHβ [43] gene expressions in pituitary cells has been described in previous reports. Indeed, inhibition of ERK phosphorylation by a specific inhibitor prevented both LHβ and FSHβ subunit expressions dose dependently in LβT2 cells [30]. Overexpression of MEKK, an upstream activator of ERK, increased gonadotropin promoters without GnRH stimulation [44]. In addition, overexpression of MKPs downregulated gonadotropin promoter expression in gonadotroph cell line [30, 39]. These observations suggested that ERK

pathways are strongly involved in gonadotropin subunit gene expressions.

The pattern of ERK activation and the induction pattern of MKP1 protein were distinct in gonadotrophs stimulated by different frequencies of GnRH pulse. At present, we have not found an exact evidence on how these differences in ERK activation and induction of MKP1 contribute to the differential regulation of gonadotropin LHβ and FSHβ subunit gene expressions. Previously, Haisenleder et al. have reported that GnRH-stimulated FSHβ gene expression in rat pituitary, as well as α-subunit and GnRH receptor, was MAPK pathway dependent, while the LHβ gene relied on different intracellular pathways [45]. Based on these observations, we could speculate that MKP1 expression induced after high-frequency GnRH pulse might prevent FSHβ transcription via decreased ERK activity and would affect LHβ to a lesser extent. On the other hand, however, other studies have suggested that MAPK pathway might play a role in the GnRH regulation of LHβ expression [46], as the transcription of LHβ was affected to a greater extent than that of FSHβ when ERK was inhibited [30].

7. Conclusion

High-frequency GnRH pulse signal from the hypothalamus stimulates the gonadotrophs to predominantly produce LHβ subunit, whereas low-frequency GnRH pulse signal preferentially produces FSHβ subunit. Herein, we have described

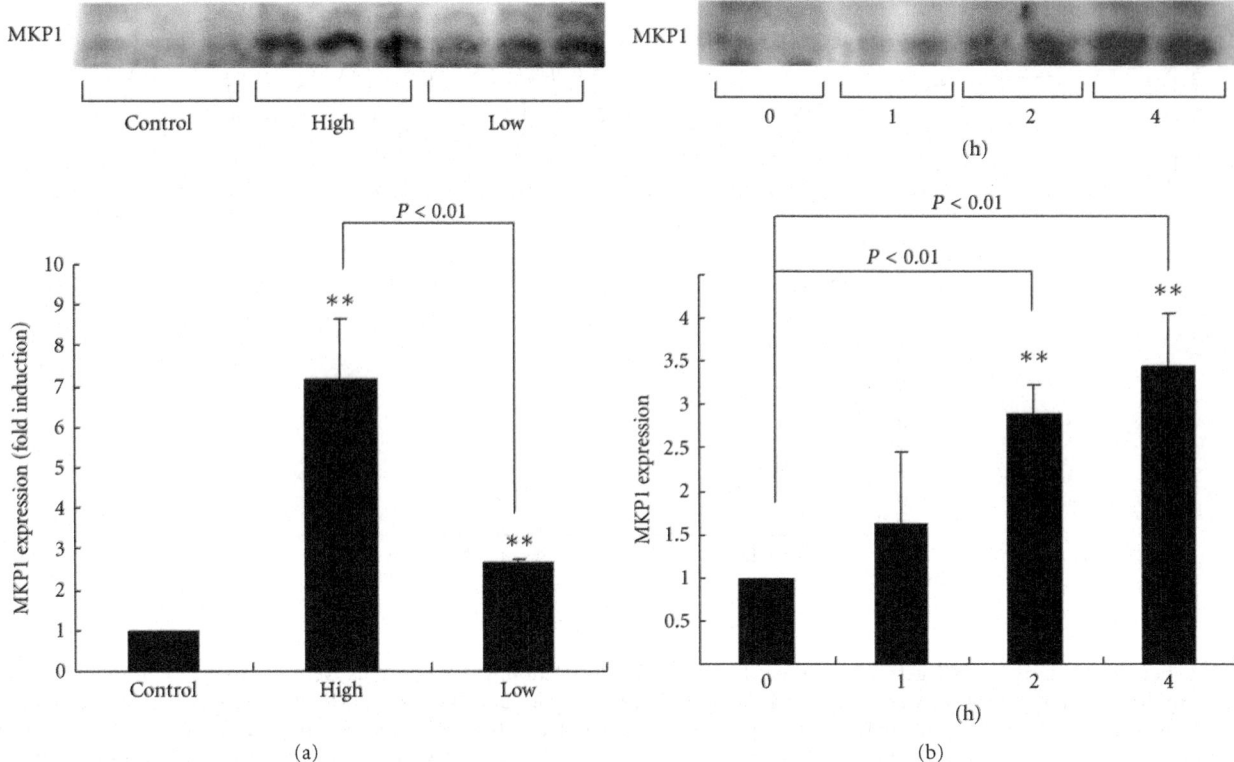

(a)   (b)

FIGURE 3: Induction of MKP1 by high frequency of GnRH pulse stimulation. (a) LbT2 cells were stimulated with vehicle (control) or pulsatile GnRH (10 nM, 5 min pulse flow per each pulse) at a frequency of one pulse every 30 min (high) or one pulse every 2 h (low). After 16 h stimulation, MKP1 protein expression was determined by Western blotting. MKP1 expression was increased predominantly following high rather than low-frequency GnRH pulse stimulation. (b) Time course of MKP1 expression following high-frequency GnRH pulse. Under the high frequency GnRH pulse stimulation, MKP1 protein expression was observed clearly at 2 h after the start of pulse stimulation (four GnRH pulses). **$P < 0.01$ versus control [26].

the possible contribution of MAPK pathways in this regulation. There are several potential mechanisms for differential regulation of the gonadotropins LH and FSH gene. Signaling pathways stimulated by different frequencies of GnRH pulse may induce transcription factor or coactivator synthesis, cause posttranslational modifications of transcription factors, or modify the chromatin to allow transcription factors to bind, as described in a previous review [47]. In addition, other factors such as activin, follistatin, and PACAP should be considered in order to understand the mechanisms responsible for the differential regulation of LHβ and FSHβ by pulsatile GnRH [48–53].

References

[1] L. C. Layman, "Genetics of human hypogonadotropic hypogonadism," *American Journal of Medical Genetics*, vol. 89, no. 4, pp. 240–248, 1999.

[2] J. G. Pierce and T. F. Parsons, "Glycoprotein hormones: structure and function," *Annual Review of Biochemistry*, vol. 50, pp. 465–495, 1981.

[3] S. D. Gharib, M. E. Wierman, M. A. Shupnik, and W. W. Chin, "Molecular biology of the pituitary gonadotropins," *Endocrine Reviews*, vol. 11, no. 1, pp. 177–199, 1990.

[4] W. F. Crowley Jr., M. Filicori, D. I. Spratt, and N. F. Santoro, "The physiology of gonadotropin-releasing hormone (GnRH) secretion in men and women," *Recent Progress in Hormone Research*, vol. 41, pp. 473–531, 1985.

[5] J. E. Levine and V. D. Ramirez, "Luteinizing hormone-releasing hormone release during the rat estrous cycle and after ovariectomy, as estimated with push-pull cannulae," *Endocrinology*, vol. 111, no. 5, pp. 1439–1448, 1982.

[6] E. Knobil, "The neuroendocrine control of the menstrual cycle," *Recent Progress in Hormone Research*, vol. 36, pp. 53–88, 1980.

[7] L. Wildt, A. Hausler, G. Marshall et al., "Frequency and amplitude of gonadotropin-releasing hormone stimulation and gonadotropin secretion in the rhesus monkey," *Endocrinology*, vol. 109, no. 2, pp. 376–385, 1981.

[8] A. C. Dalkin, D. J. Haisenleder, G. A. Ortolano, T. R. Ellis, and J. C. Marshall, "The frequency of gonadotropin-releasing hormone stimulation differentially regulates gonadotropin subunit messenger ribonucleic acid expression," *Endocrinology*, vol. 125, no. 2, pp. 917–924, 1989.

[9] D. J. Haisenleder, A. C. Dalkin, G. A. Ortolano, J. C. Marshall, and M. A. Shupnik, "A pulsatile gonadotropin-releasing hormone stimulus is required to increase transcription of the gonadotropin subunit genes: evidence for differential regulation of transcription by pulse frequency in vivo," *Endocrinology*, vol. 128, no. 1, pp. 509–517, 1991.

Extracellular Signal-Regulated Kinase (ERK) Activation and Mitogen-Activated Protein Kinase Phosphatase 1 Induction by
Pulsatile Gonadotropin-Releasing Hormone in Pituitary Gonadotrophs

89

[10] U. B. Kaiser, A. Jakubowiak, A. Steinberger, and W. W. Chin, "Differential effects of gonadotropin-releasing hormone (GnRH) pulse frequency on gonadotropin subunit and GnRH receptor messenger ribonucleic acid levels in vitro," *Endocrinology*, vol. 138, no. 3, pp. 1224–1231, 1997.

[11] D. J. Haisenleder, S. Khoury, S. M. Zmeili et al., "The frequency of gonadotropin-releasing hormone secretion regulates expression of α and luteinizing hormone β-subunit messenger ribonucleic acids in male rats," *Molecular Endocrinology*, vol. 1, no. 11, pp. 834–838, 1987.

[12] P. M. Conn, W. R. Huckle, W. V. Andrews, and C. A. McArdle, "The molecular mechanism of action of gonadotropin releasing hormone (GnRH) in the pituitary," *Recent Progress in Hormone Research*, vol. 43, pp. 29–68, 1987.

[13] S. Sundaresan, I. M. Colin, R. G. Pestell, and J. L. Jameson, "Stimulation of mitogen-activated protein kinase by gonadotropin-releasing hormone: evidence for the involvement of protein kinase C," *Endocrinology*, vol. 137, no. 1, pp. 304–311, 1996.

[14] S. Kraus, Z. Naor, and R. Seger, "Intracellular signaling pathways mediated by the gonadotropin-releasing hormone (GnRH) receptor," *Archives of Medical Research*, vol. 32, no. 6, pp. 499–509, 2001.

[15] D. Bonfil, D. Chuderland, S. Kraus et al., "Extracellular signal-regulated kinase, Jun N-terminal kinase, p38, and c-Src are involved in gonadotropin-releasing hormone-stimulated activity of the glycoprotein hormone follicle-stimulating hormone β-subunit promoter," *Endocrinology*, vol. 145, no. 5, pp. 2228–2244, 2004.

[16] G. B. Call and M. W. Wolfe, "Gonadotropin-releasing hormone activates the equine luteinizing hormone β promoter through a protein kinase C/mitogen-activated protein kinase pathway," *Biology of Reproduction*, vol. 61, no. 3, pp. 715–723, 1999.

[17] L. M. Halvorson, U. B. Kaiser, and W. W. Chin, "The protein kinase C system acts through the early growth response protein 1 to increase LHβ gene expression in synergy with steroidogenic factor-1," *Molecular Endocrinology*, vol. 13, no. 1, pp. 106–116, 1999.

[18] C. Klausen, M. Booth, H. R. Habibi, and J. P. Chang, "Extracellular signal-regulated kinase mediates gonadotropin subunit gene expression and LH release responses to endogenous gonadotropin-releasing hormones in goldfish," *General and Comparative Endocrinology*, vol. 158, no. 1, pp. 36–46, 2008.

[19] J. Weck, P. C. Fallest, L. K. Pitt, and M. A. Shupnik, "Differential gonadotropin-releasing hormone stimulation of rat luteinizing hormone subunit gene transcription by calcium influx and mitogen-activated protein kinase-signaling pathways," *Molecular Endocrinology*, vol. 12, no. 3, pp. 451–457, 1998.

[20] R. J. Davis, "Signal transduction by the JNK group of MAP kinases," *Cell*, vol. 103, no. 2, pp. 239–252, 2000.

[21] J. Raingeaud, A. J. Whitmarsh, T. Barrett, B. Dérijard, and R. J. Davis, "MKK3- and MKK6-regulated gene expression is mediated by the p38 mitogen-activated protein kinase signal transduction pathway," *Molecular and Cellular Biology*, vol. 16, no. 3, pp. 1247–1255, 1996.

[22] D. J. Haisenleder, L. L. Burger, K. W. Aylor, A. C. Dalkin, and J. C. Marshall, "Gonadotropin-releasing hormone stimulation of gonadotropin subunit transcription: evidence for the involvement of calcium/calmodulin-dependent kinase II (Ca/CAMK II) activation in rat pituitaries," *Endocrinology*, vol. 144, no. 7, pp. 2768–2774, 2003.

[23] D. J. Haisenleder, H. A. Ferris, and M. A. Shupnik, "The calcium component of gonadotropin-releasing hormone-stimulated luteinizing hormone subunit gene transcription is mediated by calcium/calmodulin-dependent protein kinase type II," *Endocrinology*, vol. 144, no. 6, pp. 2409–2416, 2003.

[24] M. S. Roberson, S. P. Bliss, J. Xie et al., "Gonadotropin-releasing hormone induction of extracellular signal-regulated kinase is blocked by inhibition of calmodulin," *Molecular Endocrinology*, vol. 19, no. 9, pp. 2412–2423, 2005.

[25] F. Liu, I. Usui, L. G. Evans et al., "Involvement of both Gq/11 and Gs proteins in gonadotropin-releasing hormone receptor-mediated signaling in LβT2 cells," *Journal of Biological Chemistry*, vol. 277, no. 35, pp. 32099–32108, 2002.

[26] I. N. Purwana, H. Kanasaki, T. Mijiddorj, A. Oride, and K. Miyazaki, "Induction of dual-specificity phosphatase 1 (DUSP1) by pulsatile gonadotropin-releasing hormone stimulation: role for gonadotropin subunit expression in mouse pituitary LbetaT2 Cells1," *Biology of Reproduction*, vol. 84, no. 5, pp. 996–1004, 2011.

[27] S. L. Asa, K. Kovacs, E. Horvath et al., "Human fetal adenohypophysis. Electron microscopic and ultrastructural immunocytochemical analysis," *Neuroendocrinology*, vol. 48, no. 4, pp. 423–431, 1988.

[28] J. J. Windle, R. I. Weiner, and P. L. Mellon, "Cell lines of the pituitary gonadotrope lineage derived by targeted oncogenesis in transgenic mice," *Molecular Endocrinology*, vol. 4, no. 4, pp. 597–603, 1990.

[29] H. Kanasaki, G. Y. Bedecarrats, K. Y. Kam, S. Xu, and U. B. Kaiser, "Gonadotropin-releasing hormone pulse frequency-dependent activation of extracellular signal-regulated kinase pathways in perifused LβT2 Cells," *Endocrinology*, vol. 146, no. 12, pp. 5503–5513, 2005.

[30] I. N. Purwana, H. Kanasaki, A. Oride, and K. Miyazaki, "Induction of dual specificity phosphatase 1 (DUSP1) by gonadotropin-releasing hormone (GnRH) and the role for gonadotropin subunit gene expression in mouse pituitary gonadotroph L beta T2 cells," *Biology of Reproduction*, vol. 82, no. 2, pp. 352–362, 2010.

[31] S. M. Keyse, "Protein phosphatases and the regulation of MAP kinase activity," *Seminars in Cell and Developmental Biology*, vol. 9, no. 2, pp. 143–152, 1998.

[32] J. M. Brondello, A. Brunet, J. Pouysségur, and F. R. McKenzie, "The dual specificity mitogen-activated protein kinase phosphatase-1 and -2 are induced by the p42/p44(MAPK) cascade," *Journal of Biological Chemistry*, vol. 272, no. 2, pp. 1368–1376, 1997.

[33] K. Kondoh and E. Nishida, "Regulation of MAP kinases by MAP kinase phosphatases," *Biochimica et Biophysica Acta—Molecular Cell Research*, vol. 1773, no. 8, pp. 1227–1237, 2007.

[34] C. C. Franklin and A. S. Kraft, "Conditional expression of the mitogen-activated protein kinase (MAPK) phosphatase MKP-1 preferentially inhibits p38 MAPK and stress-activated protein kinase in U937 cells," *Journal of Biological Chemistry*, vol. 272, no. 27, pp. 16917–16923, 1997.

[35] T. Zhang, J. M. Mulvaney, and M. S. Roberson, "Activation of mitogen-activated protein kinase phosphatase 2 by gonadotropin-releasing hormone," *Molecular and Cellular Endocrinology*, vol. 172, no. 1-2, pp. 79–89, 2001.

[36] T. Zhang and M. S. Roberson, "Role of MAP kinase phosphatases in GnRH-dependent activation of MAP kinases," *Journal of Molecular Endocrinology*, vol. 36, no. 1, pp. 41–50, 2006.

[37] K. A. Nguyen, R. E. Intriago, H. C. Upadhyay, S. J. Santos, N. J. G. Webster, and M. A. Lawson, "Modulation of gonadotropin-releasing hormone-induced extracellular signal-regulated kinase activation by dual-specificity protein phosphatase 1 in LβT2 gonadotropes," *Endocrinology*, vol. 151, no. 10, pp. 4882–4893, 2010.

[38] S. P. Armstrong, C. J. Caunt, R. C. Fowkes, K. Tsaneva-Atanasova, and C. A. McArdle, "Pulsatile and sustained gonadotropin-releasing hormone (GnRH) receptor signaling: does the ERK signaling pathway decode GnRH pulse frequency?" *Journal of Biological Chemistry*, vol. 285, no. 32, pp. 24360–24371, 2010.

[39] M. S. Roberson, A. Misra-Press, M. E. Laurance, P. J. S. Stork, and R. A. Maurer, "A role for mitogen-activated protein kinase in mediating activation of the glycoprotein hormone α-subunit promoter by gonadotropin-releasing hormone," *Molecular and Cellular Biology*, vol. 15, no. 7, pp. 3531–3539, 1995.

[40] D. Harris, D. Chuderland, D. Bonfil, S. Kraus, R. Seger, and Z. Naor, "Extracellular signal-regulated kinase and c-Src, but not Jun N-terminal kinase, are involved in basal and gonadotropin-releasing hormone-stimulated activity of the glycoprotein hormone α-subunit promoter," *Endocrinology*, vol. 144, no. 2, pp. 612–622, 2003.

[41] F. Liu, D. A. Austin, P. L. Mellon, J. M. Olefsky, and N. J. G. Webster, "GnRH activates ERK1/2 leading to the induction of c-fos and LHβ protein expression in LβT2 cells," *Molecular Endocrinology*, vol. 16, no. 3, pp. 419–434, 2002.

[42] D. Harris, D. Bonfil, D. Chuderland, S. Kraus, R. Seger, and Z. Naor, "Activation of MAPK cascades by GnRH: ERK and Jun N-terminal kinase are involved in basal and Gnrh-stimulated activity of the glycoprotein hormone LHβ-subunit promoter," *Endocrinology*, vol. 143, no. 3, pp. 1018–1025, 2002.

[43] V. V. Vasilyev, F. Pernasetti, S. B. Rosenberg et al., "Transcriptional activation of the ovine follicle-stimulating hormone-β gene by gonadotropin-releasing hormone involves multiple signal transduction pathways," *Endocrinology*, vol. 143, no. 5, pp. 1651–1659, 2002.

[44] Y. Yamada, H. Yamamoto, T. Yonehara et al., "Differential activation of the luteinizing hormone β-subunit promoter by activin and gonadotropin-releasing hormone: a role for the mitogen-activated protein kinase signaling pathway in LβT2 gonadotrophs," *Biology of Reproduction*, vol. 70, no. 1, pp. 236–243, 2004.

[45] D. J. Haisenleder, M. E. Cox, S. J. Parsons, and J. C. Marshall, "Gonadotropin-releasing hormone pulses are required to maintain activation of mitogen-activated protein kinase: role in stimulation of gonadotrope gene expression," *Endocrinology*, vol. 139, no. 7, pp. 3104–3111, 1998.

[46] R. Mitchell, P. J. Sim, M. S. Johnson, and F. J. Thomson, "Activation of MAP kinase associated with the priming effect of LHRH," *Journal of Endocrinology*, vol. 140, no. 2, pp. R15–R18, 1994.

[47] H. A. Ferris and M. A. Shupnik, "Mechanisms for pulsatile regulation of the gonadotropin subunit genes by GNRH1," *Biology of Reproduction*, vol. 74, no. 6, pp. 993–998, 2006.

[48] J. Weiss, M. J. Guendner, L. M. Halvorson, and J. L. Jameson, "Transcriptional activation of the follicle-stimulating hormone β-subunit gene by activin," *Endocrinology*, vol. 136, no. 5, pp. 1885–1891, 1995.

[49] M. Shimonaka, S. Inouye, S. Shimasaki, and N. Ling, "Follistatin binds both activin and inhibin through the common beta-subunit," *Endocrinology*, vol. 128, no. 6, pp. 3313–3315, 1991.

[50] L. L. Burger, A. C. Dalkin, K. W. Aylor, D. J. Haisenleder, and J. C. Marshall, "GnRH pulse frequency modulation of gonadotropin subunit gene transcription in normal gonadotropes—Assessment by primary transcript assay provides evidence for roles of GnRH and follistatin," *Endocrinology*, vol. 143, no. 9, pp. 3243–3249, 2002.

[51] S. Mutiara, H. Kanasaki, A. Oride et al., "Follistatin gene expression by gonadotropin-releasing hormone: a role for cyclic AMP and mitogen-activated protein kinase signaling pathways in clonal gonadotroph LβT2 cells," *Molecular and Cellular Endocrinology*, vol. 307, no. 1-2, pp. 125–132, 2009.

[52] H. Kanasaki, I. N. Purwana, T. Mijiddorj, A. Oride, and K. Miyazaki, "Possible involvement of PACAP and PACAP type 1 receptor in GnRH-induced FSH β-subunit gene expression," *Regulatory Peptides*, vol. 167, no. 2-3, pp. 227–232, 2011.

[53] I. N. Purwana, H. Kanasaki, A. Oride et al., "GnRH-induced PACAP and PAC1 receptor expression in pituitary gonadotrophs: a possible role in the regulation of gonadotropin subunit gene expression," *Peptides*, vol. 31, no. 9, pp. 1748–1755, 2010.

8

Estrogen Regulates MAPK-Related Genes through Genomic and Nongenomic Interactions between IGF-I Receptor Tyrosine Kinase and Estrogen Receptor-Alpha Signaling Pathways in Human Uterine Leiomyoma Cells

Linda Yu,[1] Alicia B. Moore,[1] Lysandra Castro,[1] Xiaohua Gao,[1] Hoang-Long C. Huynh,[1] Michelle Klippel,[1] Norris D. Flagler,[2] Yi Lu,[3] Grace E. Kissling,[3] and Darlene Dixon[1]

[1] *Molecular Pathogenesis Group, National Toxicology Program (NTP) Laboratory, NTP, Department of Health and Human Services (DHHS), National Institute of Environmental Health Sciences (NIEHS), National Institutes of Health (NIH), Research Triangle Park, NC 27709, USA*
[2] *Cellular and Molecular Pathology Branch, NTP, Department of Health and Human Services (DHHS), National Institute of Environmental Health Sciences (NIEHS), National Institutes of Health (NIH), Research Triangle Park, NC 27709, USA*
[3] *Biostatistics Branch, Department of Health and Human Services (DHHS), National Institute of Environmental Health Sciences (NIEHS), National Institutes of Health (NIH), Research Triangle Park, NC 27709, USA*

Correspondence should be addressed to Darlene Dixon, dixon@niehs.nih.gov

Academic Editor: Bertrand Jean-Claude

Estrogen and growth factors play a major role in uterine leiomyoma (UtLM) growth possibly through interactions of receptor tyrosine kinases (RTKs) and estrogen receptor-alpha (ERα) signaling. We determined the genomic and nongenomic effects of 17β-estradiol (E$_2$) on IGF-IR/MAPKp44/42 signaling and gene expression in human UtLM cells with intact or silenced IGF-IR. Analysis by RT^2 Profiler PCR-array showed genes involved in IGF-IR/MAPK signaling were upregulated in UtLM cells by E$_2$ including cyclin D kinases, MAPKs, and MAPK kinases; RTK signaling mediator, GRB2; transcriptional factors ELK1 and E2F1; CCNB2 involved in cell cycle progression, proliferation, and survival; and COL1A1 associated with collagen synthesis. Silencing (si)IGF-IR attenuated the above effects and resulted in upregulation of different genes, such as transcriptional factor ETS2; the tyrosine kinase receptor, EGFR; and DLK1 involved in fibrosis. E$_2$ rapidly activated IGF-IR/MAPKp44/42 signaling nongenomically and induced phosphorylation of ERα at ser118 in cells with a functional IGF-IR versus those without. E$_2$ also upregulated IGF-I gene and protein expression through a prolonged genomic event. These results suggest a pivotal role of IGF-IR and possibly other RTKs in mediating genomic and nongenomic hormone receptor interactions and signaling in fibroids and provide novel genes and targets for future intervention and prevention strategies.

1. Introduction

Although the exact etiology of uterine leiomyomas (fibroids) is unknown, the fact that they develop during the reproductive years and regress after menopause indicates that they are hormonally regulated [1–3]. The important role of estrogen in the promotion of uterine leiomyoma growth has been well supported through clinical and biological studies [4–6]. However, the overexpression of growth factors and their receptors, such as the type I insulin-like growth factor (IGF-I) and IGF-I receptor (IGF-IR), shows that sex steroids are not the only modulators of leiomyoma cell proliferation and exuberant extracellular matrix formation observed in many fibroids [2, 7–9]. Studies have revealed that IGF-I expression is most abundant in leiomyomas during the proliferative phase of the menstrual cycle [10, 11]. The expression of IGF-I mRNA increases in leiomyomas, and estrogen receptor alpha (ERα) mRNA is positively correlated with IGF-I mRNA levels, which implies as we and others have shown that estrogen upregulates the gene encoding IGF-I through ERα in leiomyoma tissue and cells [10–13].

The accumulated data from extensive studies of breast cancer, another disease that is often hormonally regulated, have shown that the interactions of estrogen/ERα with IGF-IR/MAPK signaling can occur at different molecular levels [14, 15]. It is known that 17β-estradiol (E$_2$) primarily acts through cognate nuclear ERα leading to regulation of gene expression, which has traditionally been defined as genomic estrogen activity. It has also been reported that many of the E$_2$-responsive genes are key signaling molecules that participate in IGF-IR signaling [16]. Alternatively, a cell membrane-associated form of ERα has been reported to couple with and activate IGF-IR through phosphorylated Shc [17, 18], thereby triggering rapid nongenomic effects through transactivation of the IGF-IR. More recently, our and other studies have shown that E$_2$ and environmental phytoestrogens (genistein) can induce E$_2$-dependent signals prompting major biological responses such as gene expression and human uterine leiomyoma (UtLM) cell proliferation [12, 13, 19]. In addition, E$_2$ is able to upregulate IGF-I gene expression [12, 16, 20] and increases IGF-I synthesis, which leads to activation of IGF-IRβ and MAPKp44/42 [19, 21]. Increased activated MAPKp44/42 with enhanced phosphorylation of ERα-phospho-ser118 has been observed in uterine leiomyomas, but not in uterine smooth muscle tissue [22].

All of these studies suggest that the effect of growth promoter IGF-I and its receptor IGF-IR and downstream target MAPK-related genes may be regulated by estrogen at genomic and nongenomic levels, and the interaction of ERα and IGF-IR/MAPKp44/42 may play a pivotal role in fibroid tumorigenesis, but the exact mechanism(s) of how this all occurs is unknown. There are several questions that need to be addressed such as (1) how does estrogen regulate MAPK related gene expression through IGF-I and the IGF-IR/MAPKp44/42 pathway; (2) what is the role of E$_2$ in the activation of IGF-IR leading to MAPKp44/42 phosphorylation of ERα at the serine 118 site; (3) which specific mediators of the signaling pathways are involved in the interactions of IGF-I/IGF-IR and ERα in uterine leiomyomas. In this study, we explored the regulatory effects of E$_2$ on intermediates of the IGF-IR/MAPK signaling cascade and related gene expression in UtLM cells and identified new genomic mediators involved in fibroid growth and development by genomic array profiling. We also determined if the effects of E$_2$ were through genomic and nongenomic interactions of IGF-I, IGF-IR, ERαser118, and MAPKp44/42 by silencing IGF-IR followed by western blotting, immunoprecipitation, and immunofluorescence microscopy. To our knowledge, this is the first study in human leiomyoma research focusing on determining the profile of E$_2$-mediated IGF-IR/MAPK-related genes and exploring the genomic and nongenomic interactions of ERα/IGF-IR/MAPKp44/42 pathways.

2. Material and Methods

2.1. Cell and Cell Culture. UtLM cells (GM10964) were purchased from Coriell Institute for Medical Research (Camden, NJ, USA) and maintained in MEM (Gibco Life Technologies, Grand Island, NY, USA) with supplements at 37°C, with 95%

humidity, and 5% carbon dioxide as previously described [9].

2.2. siIGF-IR and Real-Time Profiler PCR Array. The RT^2 Profiler PCR Array System (MAP Kinase Signaling Pathway PCR Array, PAHS-061) from SABiosciences (Frederick, MD, USA) was used to analyze gene expression related to the MAPK signaling pathway in UtLM cells in response to E$_2$ (Sigma, St. Louis, MO, USA) treatment, with and without IGF-IR silencing (siIGF-IR). The transfection of siIGF-IR oligo targeting human IGF-IR gene (5' to 3' CGUCUUCCAUAGAAAGAGAtt) and a control scrambled siRNA (siScr) with a nonsense sequence designed to have no significant sequence similarity to mouse, rat, or human transcript sequences (Ambion, Foster City, CA, USA) into cells was done using Lipofectamine (Invitrogen, Carlsbad, CA, USA) as a transfection agent following the manufacturer's protocol. UtLM cells were incubated in serum-free medium containing 0.001% of vehicle (ethanol) for 24 h after siIGF-IR, then treated with E$_2$ (10^{-8} M), and harvested at 24 h using Trizol Reagent (Invitrogen). Total cellular RNA was extracted from the cells using Qiagen RNeasy Mini Kit (SABiosciences) followed by the RT^2 First Strand C-03 Kit (SABiosciences) to remove any residual contamination from the RNA samples with 2 μg purified RNA per treatment condition. The template combined with the RT^2 SYBR green/ROX qPCR mix (25 μL/well) was loaded into a 96-well array plate coated with 84 predispensed MAPK-related gene-specific primer sets (SABiosciences) with each treatment condition per plate and processed on a TaqMan ABI Prism 7900 Sequence Detector System (Applied Biosystems, Foster City, CA, USA) according to the RT^2 Profiler PCR Array (SABiosciences) manufacturer's protocol. The data analysis was based on the $\Delta\Delta C_t$ method with normalization to GAPDH and HPRT (SABiosciences), (http://www.sabiosciences.com/pcrarraydataanalysis.php).

2.3. Real-Time PCR. Real-time (RT) PCR was performed to detect estrogen responsive gene, IGF-I mRNA expression levels following E$_2$ treatment at 0 min, 10 min, 60 min, 24 h, and 48 h in UtLM cells. Starvation of cells with serum-free medium was the same as described for RT^2 Profiler PCR Array and occurred 24 h prior to E$_2$ (10^{-8} M) treatment. Cells were harvested with Trizol Reagent, and total cellular RNA was extracted from the cells using a Trizol Plus RNA Purification Kit (Qiagen, Valencia, CA, USA). One microgram total RNA was used to prepare cDNA and reverse-transcribed with Superscript II (Invitrogen). RT-PCR was performed using IGF-I and GAPDH primers [19] with Applied Biosystems Power SYBR Green PCR Mix on an AB cycler. The results were expressed as fold changes compared to untreated groups and normalized with GAPDH.

2.4. Immunofluorescence Staining (Confocal Microscopy). Immunofluorescence staining was performed to detect IGF-I peptide expression at 0 min, 10 min, 60 min, 24 h, and 48 h, and phospho-ERαser118 and phospho-MAPKp44/42 colocalization at 0 min, 10 min, and 60 min in UtLM cells following E$_2$ treatment. The cells were starved the same as described for the real-time RT^2 Profiler PCR Array for 24 h prior to E$_2$ treatment at 10^{-8} M. The cells were fixed with 4% paraformaldehyde (Electron Microscopy Sciences, Hatfield, PA, USA), permeabilized with 0.2% Triton X-100 (Sigma), and blocked with 5% BSA (Sigma) and 0.1% gelatin (Sigma) in PBS. The cells were incubated overnight with primary IGF-I goat polyclonal antibody (sc-1422, 1 : 200 dilution; Santa Cruz Biotechnology, Santa Cruz, CA, USA), phospho-ERαser118 mouse monoclonal antibody (number 2511, 1 : 50 dilution; Cell Signaling, Danvers, MA) and phosho-MAPKp44/42 rabbit monoclonal antibody (number 9101, 1 : 100 dilution, Cell Signaling). Alexa Fluor (Invitrogen) 488 goat anti-rabbit for phospho-MAPKp44/42, Alexa Fluor (Invitrogen) 594 donkey anti-mouse for phospho-ERαser118, and 594 donkey anti-goat for IGF-I (1 : 3000 dilution) were used as secondary antibodies and DAPI (Invitrogen) for nuclear staining. Normal rabbit, normal mouse, or normal goat serum (Jackson Immunoresearch, West Grove, PA, USA) served as negative controls. Confocal images were taken on a Zeiss LSM510-UV meta (Carl Zeiss Inc, Oberkochen, Germany) using a C-Apochromat 40x/1.2 ∞/0.14–0.19 Korr UV-VIS-IR objective. The 488 nm laser line from a Krypton/Argon laser was used for excitation of the Alexa 488. A 505–550 nm bandpass emission filter was used to collect this image with a pinhole setting of 1.09 airy unit. For the second channel, the 543 nm laser line from a Helium Neon laser was used for excitation of the Alexa 594. A 560 nm longpass emission filter was used to collect the images with a pinhole setting of 1 airy unit.

2.5. Western Blot Analysis.

Western blot analysis was performed using a standard procedure as described previously [9] to assess rapid effects of E$_2$ on target protein expression in UtLM cells. The siIGF-IR and siScr transfection procedure were the same as described in siIGF-IR and real-time RT^2 Profiler PCR Array. The serum-starved cells were treated with E$_2$ (10^{-8} M) at 0, 10, and 60 min. The protein was extracted with a lysis buffer as previously described [9]. Primary antibodies used for the western blotting were as follows: rabbit polyclonal anti-phospho-IGF-1RβTyr1131/IR-βTyr1146 (number 3021, Cell Signaling), rabbit polyclonal anti-IGF-IRβ (sc-713, Santa Cruz Biotechnology), rabbit polyclonal anti-phospho-Shc (number 2434, Cell Signaling), rabbit polyclonal anti-Shc (sc-288, Santa Cruz), rabbit polyclonal anti-ERα (sc-7207, Santa Cruz), mouse monoclonal anti-phospho-ERαSer118 (number 2511, Cell Signaling), rabbit polyclonal anti-MAPKp44/42, and rabbit polyclonal anti-phospho-MAPKp44/42 (number 9201 and number 9101, Cell Signaling). The rabbit anti-ERα, rabbit anti-IGF-IRβ, and rabbit anti-Shc antibodies used in the western blotting studies were used for immunoprecipitation samples. Primary antibodies were detected with horseradish peroxidase-conjugated secondary anti-mouse or anti-rabbit antibodies (GE Healthcare, Buchinghamshire, UK).

2.6. Immunoprecipitation.

A Seize Primary Immunoprecipitation Kit (Pierce Biotechnology, Rockford, IL, USA) was used to detect the association of ERα, IGF-IRβ, and Shc in the cells treated with E$_2$. The kit was used because IgG of anti-ERα, which was used to pull down Shc, and IGF-IRβ, has the same molecular weight as the target protein Shc and this kit allows the immunoglobulin to remain adherent to Aminolink Plus Gel following elution. The procedures were done according to the manufacturer's protocol [9]. Briefly, 200 µg of ERα rabbit polyclonal antibody (Santa Cruz) were coupled to 50 µL of 50% of Aminolink Plus Gel Slurry in coupling buffer overnight at 4°C. The coupled gel and antibody complex was incubated with 300 µg of the total protein harvested from the cells treated with E$_2$ at 0, 10, and 60 min same as described in western blotting procedures in binding buffer overnight at 4°C. The gel was washed three times with washing buffer. Only the antigens (Shc and IGF-IR) in the antigen-antibody complexes were eluted by the elution buffer (all buffers were supplied in the kit) and stored for western blot analysis.

2.7. Statistics.

The experiments for RT-PCR of IGF-I mRNA expression, immunoprecipitation, and western blot analysis were repeated at least three times independently. The data obtained from RT-PCR were expressed as mean ± SEM, and the two-tailed Student's t-test was used to compare statistical significance between different groups and between various time points. Most data obtained from immunoprecipitation and western blot analyses were not normally distributed, hence, nonparametric statistical methods and Mann-Whitney tests [23] were used to determine statistically significant differences between silenced and nonsilenced IGF-IR groups at various time points after E$_2$ treatment in UtLM cells with respect to ratio of band intensity of phosphorylated/total protein (mean ± SEM) of IGF-IR, Shc, MAPKp44/42, and ERαser118 expression. The statistical significance was defined as one-sided $P < 0.05$.

For the RT^2 Profiler PCR Array data, the receptor tyrosine kinase IGF-IR, MAPK signaling pathway, and fibrosis-related genes were chosen to be analyzed. The fold changes in response to E$_2$ treatment were calculated separately for silenced and non-silenced IGF-IR groups (<-2 or >2 for either groups) and examined with scatter plots.

3. Results

3.1. Differential Expression of IGF-IR/MAPK-Related Genes Mediated by E$_2$ with and without IGF-IR Gene Knockdown in UtLM Cells.

In order to explore signaling intermediates of the IGF-IR/MAPK cascade and related genes regulated by E$_2$ and find new genomic mediators of fibroid growth and development, we performed genomic arrays to determine MAPK-related gene profiles mediated by E$_2$ with and without IGF-IR gene knockdown. We found 35 genes related to the IGF-IR/MAPK signaling pathway and fibrosis that were differentially expressed between the groups with or without E$_2$ treatment at 24 h with a functional IGF-IR (scrambled siRNA; siScr), compared to those groups under siIGF-IR conditions (Table 1, Figure 1) within a total of 62 differentially expressed MAPK-related genes (see supplementary material available online at doi:10.1155/2012/204236, Table 1). The PCR array showed that E$_2$ exposure in UtLM cells with a functional IGF-IR (siScr) resulted in >2-fold

TABLE 1: Differential MAPK-related gene expression in uterine leiomyoma (UtLM) cells with scrambled siRNA (siScr) or IFG-IR silencing (siIGF-IR) followed by E_2 treatment.

Heat map position	Symbol	Accession number	Description	siScr $+E_2/-E_2$	siIGF-IR $+E_2/-E_2$
A01	ARAF	NM_001654	V-raf murine sarcoma viral oncogene homolog, transduction of mitogenic signal to nucleus	23.3	−1.2
A07	CCNB2	NM_004701	Cyclin B2, related to transforming growth factor beta-mediated cell cycle control	94.0	1.3
A08	CCND1	NM_053056	Cyclin D1, cell cycle regulation, G1-S transition	2.4	−3.7
A09	CCND2	NM_001759	Cyclin D2, cell cycle regulation, G1-S transition	1.4	29.7
A10	CCND3	NM_001760	Cyclin D3, cell cycle regulation, G1-S transition	2.3	1652.0
B02	CDK4	NM_000075	Cyclin-dependent kinase 4, A subunit of protein kinases complex in cell cycle G1 phase	2148.2	2.5
B06	CDKN1C	NM_000076	Cyclin-dependent kinase inhibitor 1C (p57, Kip2)	37.6	1.3
B08	CDKN2B	NM_004936	Cyclin-dependent kinase inhibitor 2B (p15, inhibits CDK4)	198.8	1.1
B12	COL1A1	NM_000088	Collagen, type I, alpha 1	7.3	−15.8
C03	DLK1	NM_003836	Delta-like 1 homolog (Drosophila), contains EGF-like repeat, related to fibrosis	−2.5	604.7
C04	E2F1	NM_005225	E2F transcription factor 1	3.1	−1.9
C05	EGFR	NM_005228	Epidermal growth factor receptor	1.5	67.2
C06	EGR1	NM_001964	Early growth response 1, a zinc finger protein, and nuclear transcriptional regulator	55.5	166.6
C07	ELK1	NM_005229	Transcription factor, a nuclear target of ras-raf-MAPK signaling cascade	4.4	1.3
C09	ETS2	NM_005239	V-Ets erythroblastosis virus E26 oncogene homolog 2 (avian), a transcriptional factor	−1.4	>5000
C10	FOS	NM_005252	Leucine-zip-protein, dimerizes with Jun, involved in AP-1 complex	32.8	1.1
C11	GRB2	NM_002086	Growth factor receptor-bound protein 2	12.4	−3.0
D01	HSPA5	NM_005347	Heat shock 70 kDa protein 5 (glucose-regulated protein, 78 kDa), related to protein transport in cells	−4.0	>5000
D03	JUN	NM_002228	Jun oncogene, interacts with target DNA sequence to regulate gene expression	14.7	−1.7
D05	KSR1	NM_014238	A scaffold protein connecting MEK to RAF	12.1	−1.3
D06	MAP2K1	NM_002755	Mitogen-activated protein kinase kinase 1	470.9	−2.7
D08	MAP2K2	NM_030662	A MAP kinase kinase, activates MAPK1/ ERK2 cascade	84.2	−6.2
D10	MAP2K4	NM_003010	A MAP kinase kinase, activates MAPK8/JUK cascade	411.0	3.0
D11	MAP2K5	NM_002757	A MAP kinase kinase, activates MAPK7/ERK5 cascade	253.7	−1.1
E02	MAP3K1	NM_005921	A MAP kinase kinase, activates ERK/JUK cascade	1.5	53.1
E05	MAP3K4	NM_005922	A MAP kinase kinase, activates JUK/MAPK cascade	475.8	1951.0
E06	MAP4K1	NM_007181	A MAP kinase kinase, acts upstream of JUN-N terminal pathway	1.0	>5000
E07	MAPK1	NM_002745	Mitogen-activated protein kinase, encoding of MAPKp42, activates Elk-1	1101.7	1.3
E09	MAPK11	NM_002751	A MAP kinase kinase related to p38	111.1	2.4
E11	MAPK13	NM_002754	A MAP kinase kinase related to p38	107.8	3.2
F01	MAPK3	NM_002746	Mitogen-activated protein kinase 3, encoding of MAPKp44, activates Elk-1	19.9	1.6
F03	MAPK7	NM_002749	Mitogen-activated protein kinase 7, encoding of ERK4/5	−495.9	1.3
F09	MAX	NM_002382	MYC-associated factor X, a transcription factor	3.0	28.1
G02	MYC	NM_002467	V-myc myelocytomatosis viral oncogene homolog (avian), a transcription factor	11.4	51.3
G07	RAC1	NM_006908	Ras-related C3 botulinum toxin substratel (Rho family), GTPase of Ras family of small GTP-binding proteins	4552.5	3.1

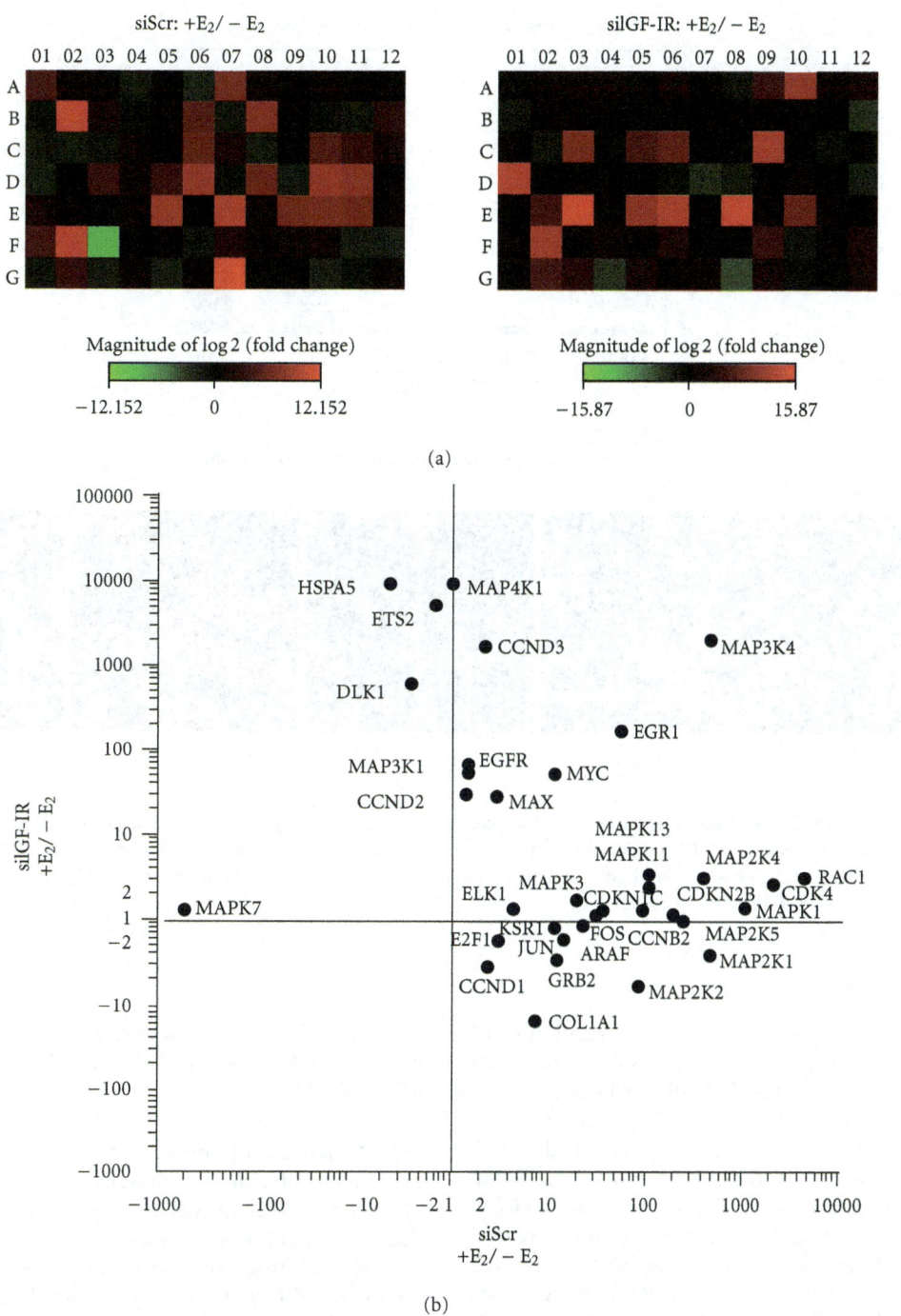

FIGURE 1: Differential MAPK pathway-related gene expression in UtLM cells mediated by 17β-estradiol (E$_2$) in the presence of scrambled siRNA (siScr) or IGF-IR silencing (siIGF-IR). (a) Heat maps of real-time RT^2 Profiler PCR Array of MAPK-related genes. The red areas represent the genes that are upregulated, and the green areas represent the genes that are downregulated by E$_2$ treatment. (b) Plot of fold changes of MAPK-related genes in response to E$_2$ treatment in UtLM cells with siScr or siIGF-IR.

upregulation of 27 genes and <−2-fold downregulation of 3 genes involved in the IGF-IR/MAPK signaling cascade at 24 h as shown in a heat map (Figure 1(a)) and by fold changes (Figure 1(b)); the other 5 genes were unchanged (<2-fold and > −2-fold). Those genes upregulated >2-fold in the presence of an intact IGF-IR included several D-type cyclins and other cyclin-dependent kinases involved

in cell cycle progression, growth factor receptor-bound protein (GRB2), and ARAF associated with IGF-IR signaling through MAPK, MAPKs, and MAPK kinases involved in proliferation, differentiation, and survival. Collagen type I alpha I (COL1A1) which is involved in collagen synthesis and fibrosis, a prominent feature of fibroids, and transcriptional factors ELK1, E2F1, and EGR1 were upregulated as well.

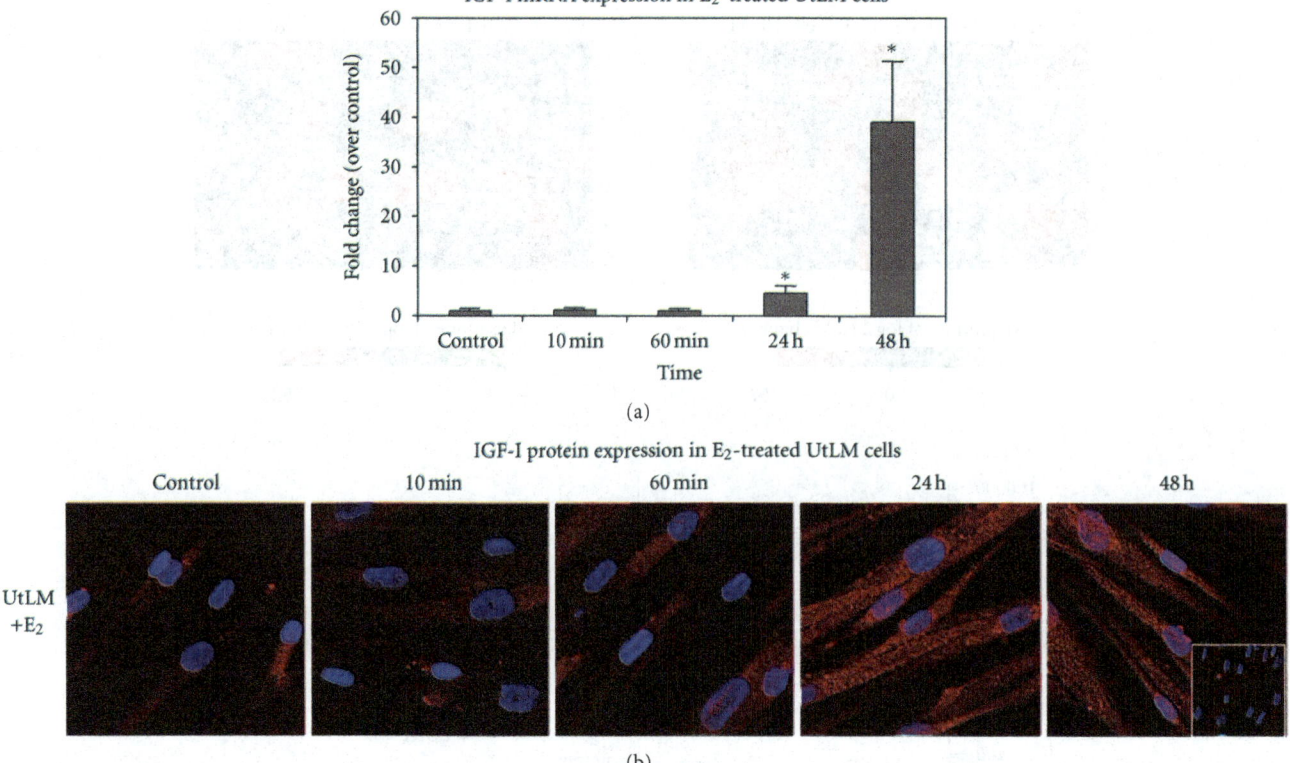

FIGURE 2: IGF-I mRNA and IGF-I peptide expression levels induced by 17β-estradiol (E_2) in UtLM cells. (a) IGF-I gene expression in UtLM cells following E_2 treatment at 0 (control), 10 and 60 min, and 24 h and 48 h. (b) IGF-I protein expression in UtLM cells following E_2 exposure at 0 (control), 10 and 60 min, and 24 h and 48 h. Inset: Negative control with normal mouse IgG. Representative of mean $\pm$ SEM from three independent experiments. $^{*}P \leq 0.05$ versus control.

Also, RAC1, a Rho GTPase, involved in the regulation of several cellular processes and often activated following stimulation of RTKs [24], such as IGF-IR was increased.

The upregulated genes induced by E_2 in the presence of an intact IGF-IR were mostly abrogated, and the 5 unchanged genes observed in the presence of a functional IGF-IR were upregulated after IGF-IR was silenced in UtLM cells. The E_2 treatment with siIGF-IR resulted in differential expression of >2-fold upregulation of additional genes such as epidermal growth factor receptor (EGFR) involved in cell growth and survival, cyclin D2 (CCND2) and D3 (CCND3) involved in cell cycle progression, v-Ets erythroblastosis virus E26 oncogene homolog 2 (ETS2), a transcriptional factor involved in cell development and tumorigenesis, delta-like 1 homolog (DLK1) involved in fibrosis, and the glucose-regulated protein 78 kDa (HSPA5) associated with monitoring protein transport (Table 1, Figures 1(a) and 1(b)). Alternatively, COL1A1 and GRB2, typically increased in the presence of a functional IGF-IR, showed decreased expression with silenced IGF-IR. However, the transcriptional factor EGR1 showed further upregulation when IGF-IR was silenced.

The differences in gene expression in response to E_2 treatment with and without IGF-IR silencing indicate the important role of IGF-IR and its signaling molecules in E_2-mediated activation of MAPK and MAPK-related pathways in UtLM cells.

3.2. 17β-Estradiol Upregulates IGF-I Gene and Protein Expression in UtLM Cells.
To determine if the regulatory effects of E_2 on MAPK-related gene expression could also occur through the genomic action of E_2 on the expression of one of its early response genes and a MAPK and IGF-IR activating peptide, IGF-I, we assessed IGF-I mRNA and protein levels in UtLM cells. We performed real-time RT PCR at 0, 10, 60 min, 24 h, and 48 h after E_2 treatment and found that E_2 at 10^{-8} M induced a time-dependent increase in IGF-I gene expression. A prolonged response started at 24 h and reached maximum levels by 48 h in UtLM cells ($P < 0.05$, Figure 2(a)).

Confocal microscopy of immunofluorescence staining for IGF-I protein in UtLM cells further revealed that IGF-I peptide expression was increased by E_2 and mostly localized in the cytoplasm, but appeared to translocate to the nucleus at 24 h and 48 h (Figure 2(b)). Interestingly, to date, IGF-I protein expression has only been reported to occur in the cytoplasm of uterine leiomyoma cells, although there has been one report of its localization in the nucleus of kidney cells [25].

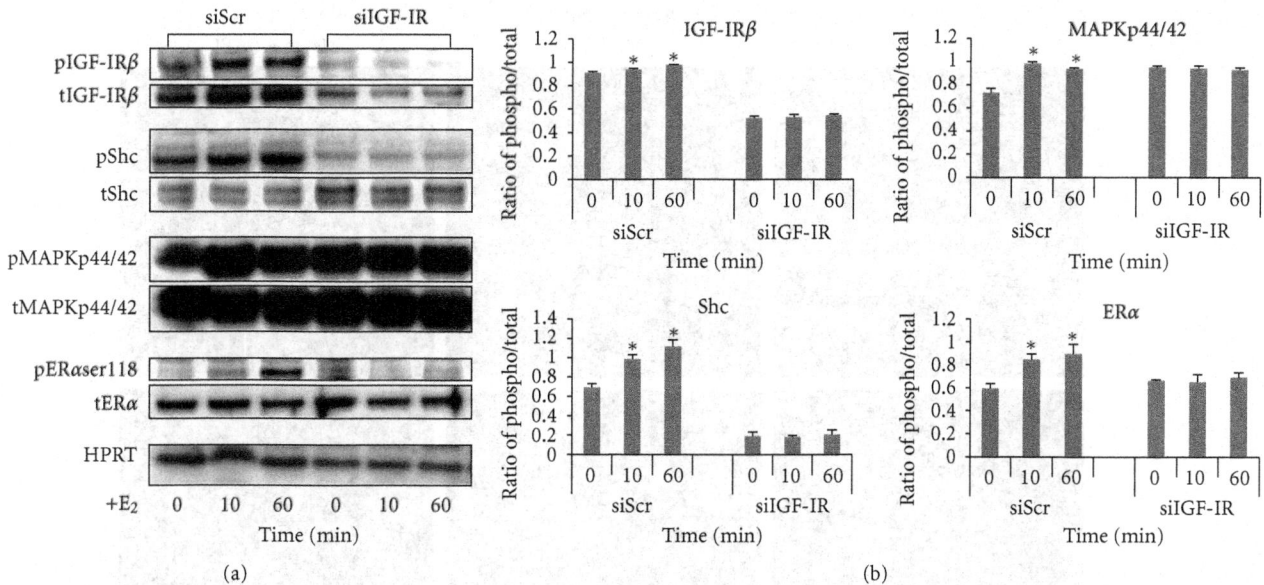

FIGURE 3: Differential expression of phosphorylated (p)IGF-IR, pMAPKp44/42, and pERαser118 in UtLM cells with scrambled siRNA (siScr) or IGF-IR silencing (siIGF-IR) followed by 17β-estradiol (E$_2$) treatment. (a) Western blot of IGF-IR/ERα pathway proteins in UtLM cells. (b) Comparison of ratio of densitometric band intensities of phosphorylated (phospho)/total proteins in UtLM cells with siScr or siIGF-IR followed by E$_2$ treatment. Bars represent mean ± SEM of three independent experiments. *$P < 0.05$ versus 0 min.

3.3. Increased Phosphorylation of IGF-IRβ by E$_2$ Leads to MAPKp44/42 Activation and ERα Phosphorylation at serine118 in UtLM Cells. To determine the rapid nongenomic actions of E$_2$, we treated UtLM cells with a functional IGF-IR with E$_2$ at 10^{-8} M for 0, 10, and 60 min and measured phosphorylated IGF-IRβ, Shc, and MAPKp44/42 using western blot analysis. We found that there was a quick phosphorylation of IGF-Rβ, Shc, and MAPKp44/42 at 10 min until 60 min in UtLM cells when treated with E$_2$ (Figure 3). It has been previously shown that estrogen treatment can cause an increase in MAPKp44/42 activation and phosphorylation of ERα at serine118 site in estrogen-responsive breast cancer cell lines [26]. It has also been shown that the IGF-IR downstream protein Shc can act as a transporter for the ER leading to activation of the MAPK signaling cascade [27]. Additionally, in earlier studies, we found that fibroid tissue samples from women in the proliferative phase expressed more phosphorylated ERαser118 and had more nuclear colocalization and immunoprecipitation of phospho-MAPKp44/42 and ERαser118 compared to patient-matched myometrial controls [22]. We therefore examined whether administration of estrogen could produce similar effects in human uterine leiomyoma cells *in vitro*. As shown in Figures 3(a) and 3(b), the phosphorylation level of ERα at serine 118 rapidly increased at 10 min and continued until 60 min in UtLM cells following E$_2$ treatment. These effects were not present with siIGF-IR. Confocal microscopy further revealed that there was increased colocalization of phosphorylated ERαser118 and MAPKp44/42 in E$_2$ treated UtLM cells at 10 min (Figure 4).

3.4. IGF-IR Is Required to Modulate the ERα and MAPK Interaction in UtLM Cells Exposed to E$_2$. Immunoprecipitation

studies (Figure 5) further revealed that ERα is associated with both IGF-IRβ and Shc proteins following E$_2$ treatment, and the amounts of both proteins were decreased when the IGF-IR gene was knocked down, which indicates that there is an association between IGF-IR and ERα and between Shc and ERα in UtLM cells exposed to E$_2$.

4. Discussion

The collective view of extranuclear ERα signaling suggests that its transduction pathways and its interaction with IGF-IR/MAPK pathways may connect the nongenomic actions of estrogen to genomic responses, since many of them interact and regulate the phosphorylation status and activities of multiple transcription factors, which affect gene expression [14, 27–30]. Therefore, in this study we first investigated the gene profile involved in the MAPK pathway to explore the effects of E$_2$ treatment on IGF-IR/MAPK pathway related gene expression using siIGF-IR and real-time PCR array technology. As shown in Table 1 and Figure 1, UtLM cells treated with E$_2$ in the presence of an intact IGF-IR had a high induction of 27 genes including genes encoding Cyclins, Cyclin Kinases, MAPKs, MAPK kinases, and transcription factors all involved in the cell proliferation, differentiation and survival. However, by silencing the IGF-IR the effects induced by E$_2$ were diminished in UtLM cells and further indicated that E$_2$-mediated MAPK pathway activation requires the presence of the IGF-IR in UtLM cells.

A cascade of MAPKs can be induced by a variety of signaling molecules [31, 32]. Transduction of the signals is achieved by a sequential series of phosphorylation reactions, wherein each downstream kinase serves as a substrate for the upstream activator. For example, in the mitogenic

Colocalization of pERαser118 and pMAPKp44/42 in UtLM cells treated with E₂

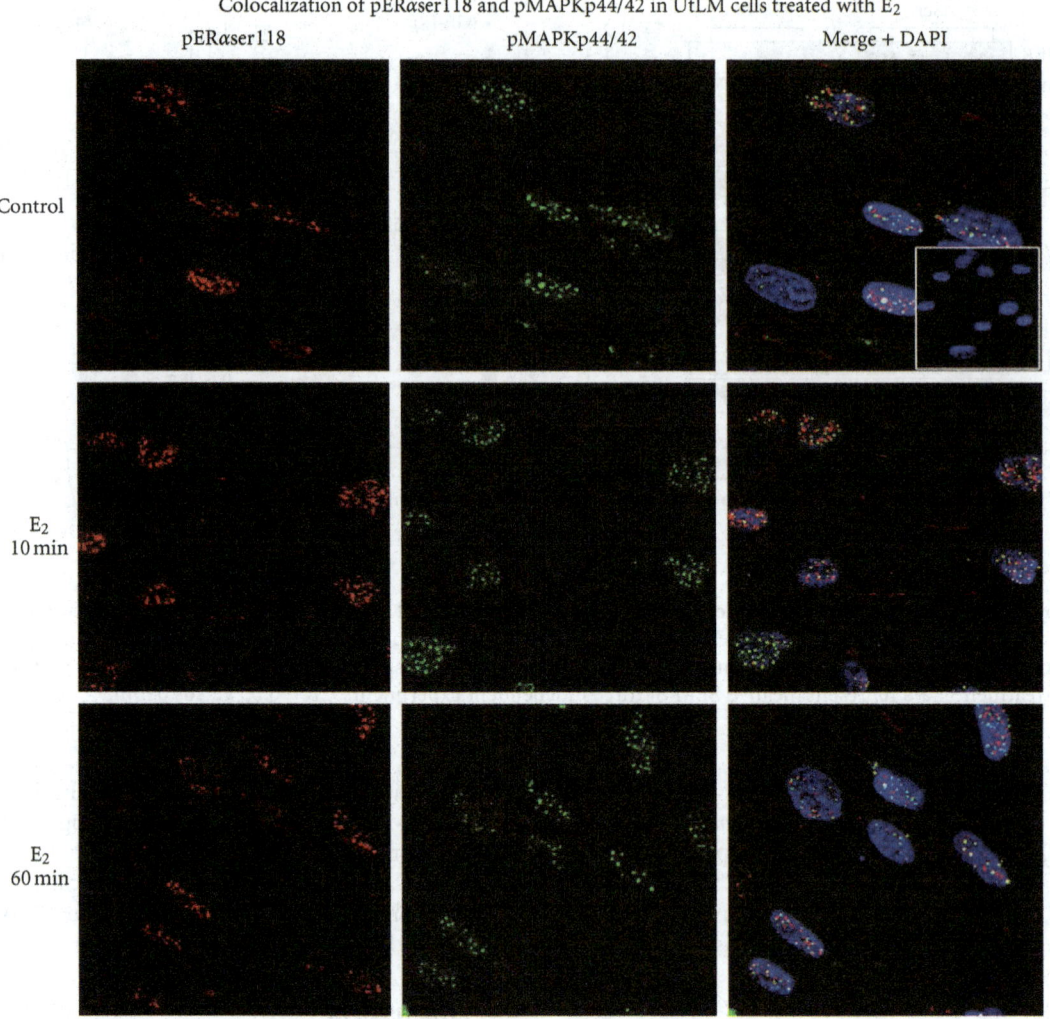

FIGURE 4: Increased colocalization of phosphorylated (p)MAPKp44/42 and pERαser118 in UtLM cells exposed to 17β-estradiol (E₂). Localization of pERαser118 expression (red), pMAPKp44/42 (green) and colocalization of both (yellow) in UtLM cells following E₂ treatment. The staining was primarily localized to the nucleus. Inset: Negative control with normal mouse and rabbit IgG. Representative of three independent experiments.

extracellular signal regulated kinase (ERK1/2) cascade, the two related mammalian MAPKs, ERK1 and ERK2 (p44mapk and p42mapk), are phosphorylated by MAP kinase/ERK kinase (MEK), which is activated primarily by the protein kinase Raf-1 after having been recruited to the plasma membrane by Ras [33, 34]. In our previous studies, the MAPKp44/42 cascade, preferentially regulating cell growth and differentiation, was upregulated in leiomyomas [9, 22]. The MAPK-related gene profiling RT-PCR array applied in this study further proves that the expression of genes involved in MAPK pathway, such as MAPK1, MAPK3, and GRB2, and the genes encoding transcriptional factors, ELK1, E2F1, MYC, and MAX are mediated by E₂, and their expression levels are elevated when UtLM cells are exposed to E₂ in the presence of a functional IGF-IR.

In the highly conserved cyclin family, whose members are characterized by a dramatic periodicity in protein abundance throughout the cell cycle, cyclin D1 can complex with and function as a regulatory subunit of CDK4 or CDK6, which is required for cell cycle G1/S progression [35]. In this study, cyclin D1 and CDK4 expression levels were increased, which further indicates that E₂ not only upregulates the MAPK/ERK1/2 pathway, but can also induce cyclin family proteins leading to cell cycle progression from G1 to S phase, thereby increasing cell proliferation. It was interesting to note that some genes encoding cyclin kinase inhibitors, such as CDKN2B, were also increased following E₂ exposure and may have been increased to counterbalance the extremely high expression of CDK4. These findings are consistent with the concept of different cyclins and their kinases exhibiting distinct expression and degradation patterns which contribute to the temporal coordination of each mitotic event [35].

The abrogation of upregulation of genes by E₂ in the presence of siIGF-IR in UtLM cells further strengthened our hypothesis that IGF-IR plays an important role in the

Estrogen Regulates MAPK-Related Genes through Genomic and Nongenomic Interactions between IGF-I Receptor Tyrosine Kinase and Estrogen Receptor-Alpha Signaling Pathways in Human Uterine Leiomyoma Cells

99

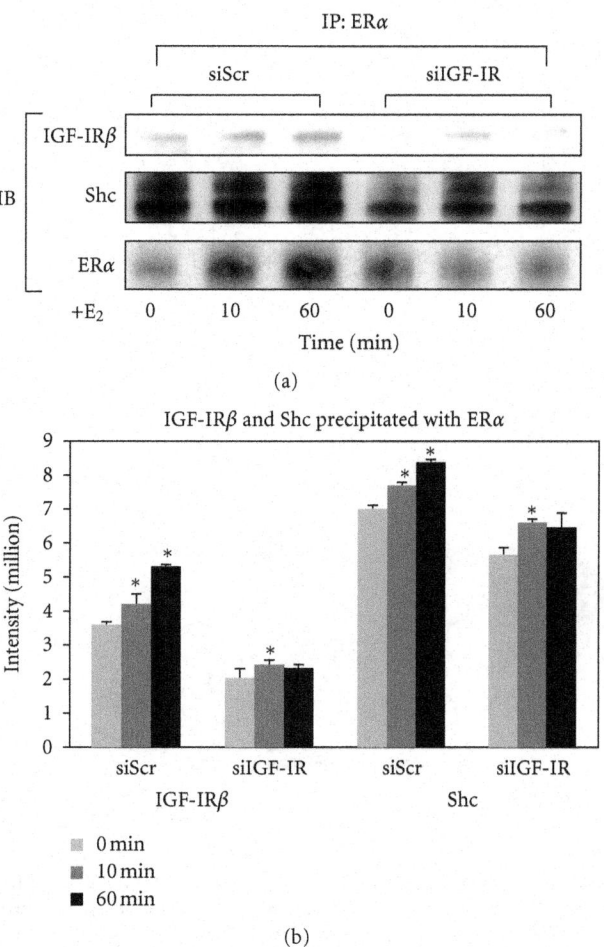

FIGURE 5: Increased immunoprecipitation of IGF-IR and Shc with ERα in cells exposed to 17β-estradiol (E_2). (a) Interactions between IGF-IRβ and Shc with ERα in UtLM cells were determined by immunoprecipitation (IP). (b) Comparison of densitometric band intensity of immunoblots (IB) in UtLM cells with siScr or siIGF-IR followed by E_2 treatment. Representative of three independent experiments. Bars represent mean intensities ± SEM. *$P < 0.05$ versus 0 min.

crosstalk between the estrogen/ERα and IGF-I/MAPKp44/42 pathways. However, other genes were differentially expressed by E_2 treatment in UtLM cells with and without siIGF-IR, which indicates that with silencing of the IGF-IR, other mechanisms compensated in response to E_2 exposure, resulting in differential gene expression. The increased EGFR, EGR1, CCND2, and CCND3 gene expression pattern with siIGF-IR suggests that E_2 treatment promotes alternative pathways for growth and survival when IGF-IR levels are decreased in UtLM cells. In other genes, such as DLK-1, involved in fibrosis [36], the expression level was increased, and COL1A1, a gene involved in collagen synthesis and fibrosis, which is typically increased in the presence of a functional IGF-IR [37, 38], was decreased after siIGF-IR further indicating that IGF-IR may play an important role in fibrosis in uterine leiomyomas.

We next investigated whether E_2 upregulates IGF-I and IGF-IR, and their target proteins in leiomyoma cells, and what mechanisms are involved in the interaction between E_2/ERα and IGF-I/IGF-IR pathways. We found that IGF-I gene and protein expression levels increased during the

course of E_2 exposure with a peak fold-change at 48 hours in UtLM cells; this prolonged response indicates a possible mechanism of IGF-I gene expression mediated by E_2 at a genomic level. We also found that phosphorylated ERαser118, IGF-IRβ, and their target protein MAPKp44/42 were all increased within minutes after E_2 treatment. The rapid activation of IGF-IR and its target downstream proteins indicates that the interaction between E_2 and IGF-IR is mediated by nongenotropic signaling, that is, by kinase-initiated events that do not involve estrogen receptor binding to canonical steroid response elements on DNA [18, 28]. Furthermore, increased colocalization of phospho-MAPKp44/42 and ERαser118 occurred in UtLM cells 10 minutes after E_2 treatment. These results are consistent with the findings that several mechanisms are associated with E_2 exposure, including rapid activation of IGF-IR and MAP kinase, a nongenomic process observed in estrogen-responsive breast cancer cell lines [39], which could lead to ERα activation at serine 118 [14, 28].

The molecules involved in the nongenomic signaling process have been identified. More recently, it has been

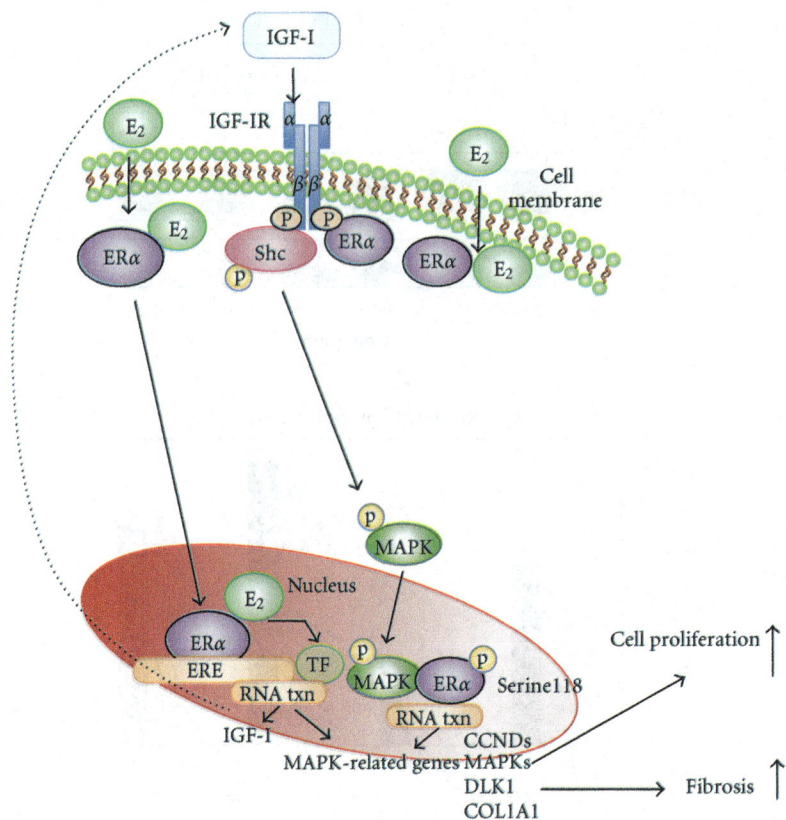

FIGURE 6: Schematic illustration of genomic and nongenomic actions of ERα on target gene transcription. Genomic actions involve the translocation of cytoplasmic E_2-ERα complexes to the nucleus which can then bind directly to estrogen response elements (EREs) in target gene promoters or nuclear E_2-ERα complexes. These complexes are tethered through protein-protein interactions to a transcription factor complex (TF) that contacts the target gene promoter to induce transcription of IGF-I and MAPK related genes. Nongenomically, E_2 can bind to membrane associated ERα which then binds to the adaptor protein, Src collagen homologue (Shc) to form a protein complex consisting of ERα and Shc and/or ERα and IGF-IR. E_2 signals through the IGF-IR and activates MAPKp44/42, which can then phosphorylate ERα at the serine118 site to initiate transcription (txn) of MAPK related genes. CCNDs = Cyclin Ds; MAPKs = mitogen-activated protein kinases; DLK1 = delta-like 1 homolog; COL1A1 = collagen type I alpha 1.

shown that a pool of ERs resides in or is associated with the plasma membrane. These ERs utilize the membrane IGF-IR to rapidly signal through various kinase cascades that influence both transcriptional and nontranscriptional actions of estrogen [28]. In this study, UtLM cells treated with E_2, showed upregulation of RAC1, a Rho GTPase involved in the regulation of several cellular processes that is often activated following stimulation of RTKs [24]. This gene expression of RAC1 was decreased upon IGF-IR silencing. These data indicate that E_2 can directly, or through the involvement of the ERα, activate IGF-IR and MAPK signaling. The IGF-IR may serve as an anchor for the plasma membrane-associated ERα. Estradiol causes rapid phosphorylation of IGF-IR and Shc. It has been reported that activated Shc, after binding to ERα, serves as a transporter, which carries ERα to Shc-binding sites on the activated IGF-I receptors [39], which subsequently signals to MAPKs and other pathways. Our immunoprecipitation results also show that these three proteins, ERα, IGF-IR, and Shc, are associated with each other

when UtLM cells are treated with E_2. Therefore, we proposed that IGF-IR should be a key mediator in this interaction, and applied siIGF-IR methodology to knockdown the IGF-IR gene to block the E_2 effect on the interaction of these two pathways through their respective receptors. We found that siIGF-IR decreased the phosphorylation of IGF-IRβ and the activation of MAPKp44/42 induced by E_2. At same time, ERα phosphorylation at the serine118 site was also attenuated. These findings indicate that IGF-IRβ activation is required in the rapid nongenomic response of ERα following E_2 exposure in UtLM cells. Silencing of IGF-IR abrogated the ERα activity at the serine118 site induced by E_2 confirming a potential relationship between membrane-related signals and intracellular ERα, in agreement with the findings that E_2 binds to cell membrane-associated ERα, which physically associates with the adaptor protein Shc through IGF-IR activation and induces its phosphorylation [39]. In turn, Shc binds GRB2 and Sos, which also results in the rapid activation of MAP kinase, and we have shown an association

Estrogen Regulates MAPK-Related Genes through Genomic and Nongenomic Interactions between IGF-I Receptor Tyrosine
Kinase and Estrogen Receptor-Alpha Signaling Pathways in Human Uterine Leiomyoma Cells

101

between IGF-IR and Grb2 and MAP kinase activation in fibroid tissue samples taken from women in the proliferative phase of the menstrual cycle [9, 40].

Therefore, the possible convergence of distinct ERα-mediated genomic and/or nongenomic actions at multiple response elements provides an extremely fine control system in the regulation of target gene transcript [14] leading to the alternation of gene expression profiles found in this study. In conclusion, the results obtained in this study indicate that the two growth regulatory pathways, E_2/ERα and IGF-I/IGF-IR, are tightly linked in UtLM cells. The E_2 effects can occur through both genomic and nongenomic events, which involve IGF-IR activation of MAP kinase cascades mediated by the association between ERαser118 and MAPKp44/42 (Figure 6). The observations that: (1) IGF-IR is required for the interaction and the differential expression of MAPK pathway-related genes mediated by E_2; (2) IGF-I gene expression is responsive to E_2; (3) the activation of alternative pathways induced by E_2 when IGF-IR is silenced enhances our understanding of IGF-I/IGF-IR and E_2/ERα interactions and may suggest a multipronged or cocktail approach to fibroid treatment. Considering that the pure antiestrogen or anti-IGF-IR agents may only be partially effective in antagonizing E_2-induced IGF-I/MAPK pathway activation and because other alternative pathways (EGFR) could compensate, it suggests that inhibitors of small downstream molecules, such as Src and ERKs, or transcription factors may better block these effects and could possibly serve as noninvasive adjuvant therapies for fibroids.

Conflict of Interests

No conflict of interests, financial or otherwise, is declared by the authors.

Disclaimer

This paper may be the work product of an employee or group of employees of the NIEHS, NTP, and NIH, however, the statements, opinions, or conclusions contained therein do not necessarily represent the statements, opinions, or conclusions of NIEHS, NTP, NIH, or the United States government.

Acknowledgments

The authors would like to thank Dr. Kyathanahalli Janardhan and Ms. Retha R. Newbold for their critical review of this paper. This research was supported, in part, by the National Toxicology Program (NTP) and the Intramural Research Program of the National Institutes of Health (NIH), National Institute of Environmental Health Sciences (NIEHS).

References

[1] T. Maruo, N. Ohara, J. Wang, and H. Matsuo, "Sex steroidal regulation of uterine leiomyoma growth and apoptosis," Human Reproduction Update, vol. 10, no. 3, pp. 207–220, 2004.

[2] C. L. Walker and E. A. Stewart, "Uterine fibroids: the elephant in the room," Science, vol. 308, no. 5728, pp. 1589–1592, 2005.

[3] X. Luo and N. Chegini, "The expression and potential regulatory function of MicroRNAs in the pathogenesis of leiomyoma," Seminars in Reproductive Medicine, vol. 26, no. 6, pp. 500–514, 2008.

[4] A. J. Jakimiuk, M. Bogusiewicz, R. Tarkowski et al., "Estrogen receptor α and β expression in uterine leiomyomas from premenopausal women," Fertility and Sterility, vol. 82, no. 3, supplement, pp. 1244–1249, 2004.

[5] P. Bakas, A. Liapis, S. Vlahopoulos et al., "Estrogen receptor α and β in uterine fibroids: a basis for altered estrogen responsiveness," Fertility and Sterility, vol. 90, no. 5, pp. 1878–1885, 2008.

[6] H. Asada, Y. Yamagata, T. Taketani et al., "Potential link between estrogen receptor-α gene hypomethylation and uterine fibroid formation," Molecular Human Reproduction, vol. 14, no. 9, pp. 539–545, 2008.

[7] J. Huang, J. Zou, B. Xu, Y. Zhang, X. Chen, and D. Liu, "Affect of insulin-like growth factor I and estradiol on the growth of uterine leiomyoma," Hunan Yi Ke da Xue Xue Bao, vol. 24, no. 1, pp. 29–32, 1999.

[8] G. P. Flake, J. Andersen, and D. Dixon, "Etiology and pathogenesis of uterine leiomyomas: a review," Environmental Health Perspectives, vol. 111, no. 8, pp. 1037–1054, 2003.

[9] L. Yu, K. Saile, C. D. Swartz et al., "Differential expression of receptor tyrosine kinases (RTKs) and IGF-I pathway activation in human uterine leiomyomas," Molecular Medicine, vol. 14, no. 5-6, pp. 264–275, 2008.

[10] K. Englund, B. Lindblom, K. Carlström, I. Gustavsson, P. Sjöblom, and A. Blanck, "Gene expression and tissue concentrations of IGF-I in human myometrium and fibroids under different hormonal conditions," Molecular Human Reproduction, vol. 6, no. 10, pp. 915–920, 2000.

[11] Y. Zhao, W. Zhang, and S. Wang, "The expression of estrogen receptor isoforms α, β and insulin-like growth factor-I in uterine leiomyoma," Gynecological Endocrinology, vol. 24, no. 10, pp. 549–554, 2008.

[12] C. D. Swartz, C. A. Afshari, L. Yu, K. E. Hall, and D. Dixon, "Estrogen-induced changes in IGF-I, Myb family and MAP kinase pathway genes in human uterine leiomyoma and normal uterine smooth muscle cell lines," Molecular Human Reproduction, vol. 11, no. 6, pp. 441–450, 2005.

[13] S. Li and J. A. McLachlan, "Estrogen-associated genes in uterine leiomyoma," Annals of the New York Academy of Sciences, vol. 948, pp. 112–120, 2001.

[14] M. Lanzino, C. Morelli, C. Garofalo et al., "Interaction between estrogen receptor alpha and insulin/IGF signaling in breast cancer," Current Cancer Drug Targets, vol. 8, no. 7, pp. 597–610, 2008.

[15] M. A. Shupnik, "Crosstalk between steroid receptors and the c-Src-receptor tyrosine kinase pathways: implications for cell proliferation," Oncogene, vol. 23, no. 48, pp. 7979–7989, 2004.

[16] R. Suter and J. A. Marcum, "The molecular genetics of breast cancer and targeted therapy," Biologics, vol. 1, no. 3, pp. 241–258, 2007.

[17] R. X. D. Song, Z. Zhang, and R. J. Santen, "Estrogen rapid action via protein complex formation involving ERα and Src," Trends in Endocrinology and Metabolism, vol. 16, no. 8, pp. 347–353, 2005.

[18] Z. Zhang, R. Kumar, R. J. Santen, and R. X. D. Song, "The role of adapter protein Shc in estrogen non-genomic action," Steroids, vol. 69, no. 8-9, pp. 523–529, 2004.

[19] X. Di, L. Yu, A. B. Moore et al., "A low concentration of genistein induces estrogen receptor-alpha and insulin-like growth factor-I receptor interactions and proliferation in

uterine leiomyoma cells," *Human Reproduction*, vol. 23, no. 8, pp. 1873–1883, 2008.

[20] K. B. Reddy and S. Glaros, "Inhibition of the MAP kinase activity suppresses estrogen-induced breast tumor growth both in vitro and in vivo," *International Journal of Oncology*, vol. 30, no. 4, pp. 971–975, 2007.

[21] E. N. Nierth-Simpson, M. M. Martin, T. C. Chiang et al., "Human uterine smooth muscle and leiomyoma cells differ in their rapid 17/J-estradiol signaling: implications for proliferation," *Endocrinology*, vol. 150, no. 5, pp. 2436–2445, 2009.

[22] T. L. Hermon, A. B. Moore, L. Yu, G. E. Kissling, F. J. Castora, and D. Dixon, "Estrogen receptor alpha (ERα) phospho-serine-118 is highly expressed in human uterine leiomyomas compared to matched myometrium," *Virchows Archiv*, vol. 453, no. 6, pp. 557–569, 2008.

[23] W. J. Conover and R. L. Iman, "Analysis of covariance using the rank transformation," *Biometrics*, vol. 38, no. 3, pp. 715–724, 1982.

[24] M. R. Schiller, "Coupling receptor tyrosine kinases to Rho GTPases-GEFs what's the link," *Cellular Signalling*, vol. 18, no. 11, pp. 1834–1843, 2006.

[25] W. Li, J. Fawcett, H. R. Widmer, P. J. Fielder, R. Rabkin, and G. A. Keller, "Nuclear transport of insulin-like growth factor-I and insulin-like growth factor binding protein-3 in opossum kidney cells," *Endocrinology*, vol. 138, no. 4, pp. 1763–1766, 1997.

[26] H. Yamashita, M. Nishio, T. Toyama et al., "Low phosphorylation of estrogen receptor α (ERα) serine 118 and high phosphorylation of ERα serine 167 improve survival in ER-positive breast cancer," *Endocrine-Related Cancer*, vol. 15, no. 3, pp. 755–763, 2008.

[27] L. Björnström and M. Sjöberg, "Mechanisms of estrogen receptor signaling: convergence of genomic and nongenomic actions on target genes," *Molecular Endocrinology*, vol. 19, no. 4, pp. 833–842, 2005.

[28] E. R. Levin, "Integration of the extranuclear and nuclear actions of estrogen," *Molecular Endocrinology*, vol. 19, no. 8, pp. 1951–1959, 2005.

[29] Z. Madak-Erdogan, K. J. Kieser, H. K. Sung, B. Komm, J. A. Katzenellenbogen, and B. S. Katzenellenbogen, "Nuclear and extranuclear pathway inputs in the regulation of global gene expression by estrogen receptors," *Molecular Endocrinology*, vol. 22, no. 9, pp. 2116–2127, 2008.

[30] M. Marino, P. Galluzzo, and P. Ascenzi, "Estrogen signaling multiple pathways to impact gene transcription," *Current Genomics*, vol. 7, no. 8, pp. 497–508, 2006.

[31] T. P. Garrington and G. L. Johnson, "Organization and regulation of mitogen-activated protein kinase signaling pathways," *Current Opinion in Cell Biology*, vol. 11, no. 2, pp. 211–218, 1999.

[32] C. Widmann, S. Gibson, M. B. Jarpe, and G. L. Johnson, "Mitogen-activated protein kinase: conservation of a three-kinase module from yeast to human," *Physiological Reviews*, vol. 79, no. 1, pp. 143–180, 1999.

[33] A. Brunet, D. Roux, P. Lenormand, S. Dowd, S. Keyse, and J. Pouysségur, "Nuclear translocation of p42/p44 mitogen-activated protein kinase is required for growth factor-induced gene expression and cell cycle entry," *EMBO Journal*, vol. 18, no. 3, pp. 664–674, 1999.

[34] A. V. Khokhlatchev, B. Canagarajah, J. Wilsbacher et al., "Phosphorylation of the MAP kinase ERK2 promotes its homodimerization and nuclear translocation," *Cell*, vol. 93, no. 4, pp. 605–615, 1998.

[35] P. G. Ganchevska, A. P. Uchikov, V. S. Ishev, I. A. Batashki, V. N. Nizamov, and E. H. Uchikova, "Estrogen receptors–known and unknown biological functions," *Folia medica*, vol. 48, no. 2, pp. 5–10, 2006.

[36] J. C. M. Tsibris, J. Segars, D. Coppola et al., "Insights from gene arrays on the development and growth regulation of uterine leiomyomata," *Fertility and Sterility*, vol. 78, no. 1, pp. 114–121, 2002.

[37] P. C. Leppert, W. H. Catherino, and J. H. Segars, "A new hypothesis about the origin of uterine fibroids based on gene expression profiling with microarrays," *American Journal of Obstetrics and Gynecology*, vol. 195, no. 2, pp. 415–420, 2006.

[38] M. M. Grudzien, P. S. Low, P. C. Manning, M. Arredondo, R. J. Belton, and R. A. Nowak, "The antifibrotic drug halofuginone inhibits proliferation and collagen production by human leiomyoma and myometrial smooth muscle cells," *Fertility and Sterility*, vol. 93, no. 4, pp. 1290–1298, 2010.

[39] R. J. Santen, R. X. Song, Z. Zhang et al., "Long-term estradiol deprivation in breast cancer cells up-regulates growth factor signaling and enhances estrogen sensitivity," *Endocrine-Related Cancer*, vol. 12, no. 1, supplement, pp. S61–S73, 2005.

[40] Y. Mebratu and Y. Tesfaigzi, "How ERK1/2 activation controls cell proliferation and cell death is subcellular localization the answer?" *Cell Cycle*, vol. 8, no. 8, pp. 1168–1175, 2009.

9

Nuclear Transport: A Switch for the Oxidative Stress—Signaling Circuit?

Mohamed Kodiha and Ursula Stochaj

Department of Physiology, McGill University, Montreal, QC, Canada H3G 1Y6

Correspondence should be addressed to Ursula Stochaj, ursula.stochaj@mcgill.ca

Academic Editor: Paola Chiarugi

Imbalances in the formation and clearance of reactive oxygen species (ROS) can lead to oxidative stress and subsequent changes that affect all aspects of physiology. To limit and repair the damage generated by ROS, cells have developed a multitude of responses. A hallmark of these responses is the activation of signaling pathways that modulate the function of downstream targets in different cellular locations. To this end, critical steps of the stress response that occur in the nucleus and cytoplasm have to be coordinated, which makes the proper communication between both compartments mandatory. Here, we discuss the interdependence of ROS-mediated signaling and the transport of macromolecules across the nuclear envelope. We highlight examples of oxidant-dependent nuclear trafficking and describe the impact of oxidative stress on the transport apparatus. Our paper concludes by proposing a cellular circuit of ROS-induced signaling, nuclear transport and repair.

1. Introduction

1.1. Reactive Oxygen Species. Oxidative stress is generated by an increase in reactive oxygen species (ROS), either in the form of free radicals or nonradical oxidants [1, 2]. Although elevated levels of ROS can damage a wide variety of molecules, ROS production is essential to normal cell physiology [3–12]. As such, ROS participate in cell-signaling events and can function as second messengers. Moreover, ROS are generated at sites of inflammation, where they fend off microbial infections [13–16]. On the other hand, ROS are believed to contribute to aging [3–9, 12]; they are also produced in response to environmental insults, such as X-rays, UV light, ultrasound, or microwave radiation [17–19]. At the cellular level, ROS are generated as metabolic byproducts of normal biological processes, with oxidative phosphorylation in mitochondria as the primary source in eukaryotic cells [20]. Aside from the mitochondrial electron transport chain, NADPH oxidases, cyclooxygenases, lipoxygenases, xanthine oxidase, and other cellular enzymes make also important contributions to cellular ROS production [21–25].

The different types of ROS and their mode of action have been discussed in detail [1, 11, 26–30]. ROS that are particularly important to cell physiology include the hydroxyl radical $\bullet OH$, superoxide anion $\bullet O_2^-$, the nonradical hydrogen peroxide (H_2O_2), alkoxy and peroxy radicals, hypochlorous acid or peroxynitrite, and reactive sulfur species [1, 29, 31, 32]. Here, we recapitulate the properties of those ROS only that are relevant to the experiments discussed in this review.

The hydroxyl radical $\bullet OH$ is highly reactive and causes damage to nucleic acids and proteins, this radical also promotes lipid peroxidation [2, 12, 33]. Due to their high reactivity, hydroxyl radicals are especially harmful and considered a major cause of oxidant-induced damage [34]. The superoxide free radical $\bullet O_2^-$ can interfere with the proper function of enzymes by damaging their active sites, with cysteine residues being particularly susceptible [32]. In an experimental setting, superoxide radicals can be generated by providing xanthine oxidase with the appropriate substrates [35].

There is some debate about the impact of H_2O_2 on the cellular redox homeostasis. On one hand, H_2O_2 is not deemed a major direct threat for the cellular redox homeostasis due to its poor reactivity towards biomolecules [36]. However, H_2O_2 rapidly translocates through lipid bilayers and is a potential precursor for •OH radicals [32, 37]. Thus, high concentrations of H_2O_2 can release iron from heme proteins and catalyze the conversion of H_2O_2 to hydroxyl radicals [37]. It was also proposed that the nonradical oxidant H_2O_2 may have profound effects on redox signaling in living cells, where it alters the function of redox circuits that are composed of redox-sensitive building blocks [1]. Despite these different views on how H_2O_2 contributes to oxidant-induced damage, we and others [38–42] have used this compound extensively to examine the impact of oxidative stress on nuclear transport (see below).

1.2. Oxidative Stress and Cellular Defense Mechanisms. The appropriate response to stress is fundamental to cell survival and the recovery from disease-related or environmental damage [3, 5, 6, 9, 11]. Thus, in order to maintain redox homeostasis, the balance between production and clearance of ROS is essential. Imbalances in ROS concentration, if left without proper intervention, can interfere with a wide variety of cellular processes, leading to serious injuries and possibly cell death, either by apoptosis or necrosis [28, 43].

Upon accumulation, ROS can interact inappropriately with a large number of biomolecules, including lipids, proteins, and DNA, thereby interfering with numerous cellular functions [28, 37]. For instance, ROS may induce damage to various enzymes, leading to the partial or complete loss of their function. Notably, ROS-damaged proteins can form toxic aggregates that cause cell injury and ultimately cell death [16]. Furthermore, ROS-induced lipid peroxidation may alter the permeability of cellular membranes, potentially destroying the membrane integrity and triggering cell death [33, 44]. In addition, ROS-induced modifications of DNA can be mutagenic, possibly initiating cell transformation and promoting cancer [45].

In line with the complex pattern of damage triggered by oxidative stress, ROS accumulation contributes to the pathophysiologies of many human diseases and syndromes. In particular, oxidative stress plays a critical role in the onset and the progression of neurodegenerative disorders, diabetes, cardiovascular diseases, and nephropathy [27, 46–58].

To counteract the potential damage of elevated ROS concentrations, cells have developed different strategies that limit the action of reactive compounds and prevent their accumulation. To this end, eukaryotic cells are equipped with multiple defense mechanisms that promote the removal and inactivation of ROS in different cellular compartments [59–62]. These mechanisms rely on the coordinated action of several enzymatic systems that are able to react with and neutralize different ROS. For example, the superoxide dismutase (SOD) system is essential to redox homeostasis [11, 63–65], as it catalyzes the conversion of $•O_2^-$ to H_2O_2. H_2O_2 produced by SOD can then be eliminated by the enzymatic action of catalases.

The glutathione/glutathione disulfide system (GSH/GSSG) is one of the major contributors to redox homeostasis and of particular importance to the intracellular redox state. Accordingly, glutathione is believed to be the primary defense when cells are injured by oxidative stress during

ischemia/reperfusion [66, 67]. Moreover, changes in the GSH/GSSG ratio affect the intracellular redox state, and depletion of intracellular glutathione generates oxidative stress [61]. Owing to its pivotal importance to redox homeostasis, imbalance of the GSH/GSSG system has been linked to many human diseases, pathologies, and aging [11, 66, 68]. The GSH/GSSG system can be modulated experimentally, and diethyl maleate is one of compounds that deplete glutathione, thereby causing oxidative stress [38, 69]. Furthermore, the cellular redox homeostasis can also be altered by changing the activity of glutathione peroxidase, glutathione, or thioredoxin reductase.

2. Oxidative Stress and Nucleocytoplasmic Transport

2.1. Nuclear Transport of Macromolecules. Nucleocytoplasmic transport is central to the cellular homeostasis, as the proper and timely response to endogenous and environmental stimuli relies on the communication between the nucleus and cytoplasm. This applies in particular to kinases and phosphatases, many of which move in and out of the nucleus in response to oxidants or other stressors (see below). The nuclear envelope provides the barrier between these two compartments [70, 71], and macromolecules traverse the nuclear envelope via nuclear pore complexes (NPCs). Trafficking in and out of the nucleus controls signal transduction, gene expression, cell-cycle progression, and apoptosis; regulated nuclear transport is also essential for development and required for the proper response to stress [72–75]. The separation of nucleus and cytoplasm is ideal to divide signaling and other events. However, this compartmentalization can impede the intracellular communication if components of the nuclear transport apparatus are affected by ROS. This is indeed the case, as nuclear transport factors are primary cellular targets for oxidants. Before describing the impact of oxidative stress on nuclear transport, we briefly summarize those mechanisms of nuclear trafficking that are relevant to our review (Figure 1).

Although diffusion across the NPC is not simply a function of the molecular mass, most proteins that are larger than 40 kD do not efficiently diffuse across the nuclear envelope. Nevertheless, molecules exceeding the diffusion channel of the NPC can move in or out of the nucleus if they carry specialized transport signals. Nuclear localization (NLS), nuclear export (NES), or shuttling sequences serve as permanent signals that mediate targeting to the proper location. Classical NLSs are characterized by clusters of basic amino acid residues, whereas NESs are frequently enriched for leucine or isoleucine residues. However, the final destination of a macromolecule not only depends on such transport signals; the steady-state distribution is also controlled by its retention in the nuclear or cytoplasmic compartment.

Nuclear Carriers. Nuclear transport of most proteins depends on transporters of the importin-β group (also called karyopherin-β). Importin-β family members interact with their cargo either directly or through an adaptor. The latter

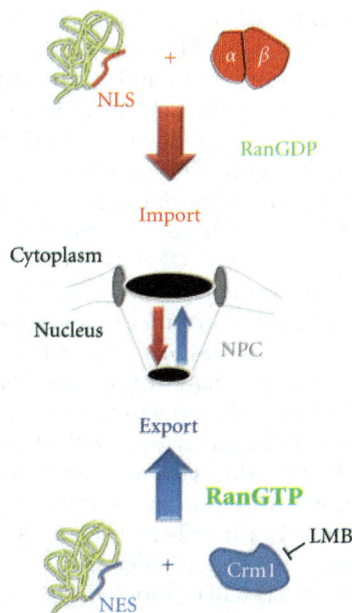

FIGURE 1: Simplified model for classical nuclear import and Crm1-mediated export, two essential transport pathways. Classical nuclear import depends on the carrier importin-β and the adaptor protein importin-α. Together, importin-α/β move NLS-containing cargos to the nucleus. The absence of RanGTP from the cytoplasm permits the assembly of import complexes in the cytoplasm. Conversely, the high RanGTP concentration in the nucleus promotes the dissociation of classical import complexes after they translocate across the NPC. RanGTP in the nucleus is also necessary to generate export complexes that contain Crm1 and NES-containing cargo. The function of Crm1 is inhibited by leptomycin B (LMB).

applies to classical nuclear import, which relies on the carrier importin-β1 and its adaptor importin-α (Figure 1). Multiple isoforms of importin-α exist in higher eukaryotes, where they recognize classical NLSs in endogenous and fluorescent cargos such as NLS-mCherry (Figure 2(a)). Crm1/exportin-1 [76], another importin-β family member, moves NES-containing proteins like mCit-NES to the cytoplasm (Figure 2(b)). This transport route can be inhibited specifically with leptomycin B, a compound that covalently modifies a cysteine residue of Crm1 [77].

The RanGTPase System. Carriers of the importin-β family require the small GTPase Ran and factors that modulate Ran activity. These factors include in the cytoplasm RanBP1 (Ran-binding protein 1) and the GTPase activating protein RanGAP1, with RanGAP1 binding to Nup358 at the cytoplasmic side of the NPC. By contrast, the RanGTP-binding protein RanBP3 and the guanine nucleotide exchange factor RCC1 (RanGEF) are located in the nucleus, where RCC1 binds to chromatin. The asymmetric distribution of Ran modulators generates a gradient across the nuclear envelope, with RanGTP in nuclei and RanGDP in the cytoplasm (Figure 1). This gradient provides the driving force for all importin-β dependent transport [70, 71].

Regulation of Nuclear Transport. Control of nuclear trafficking is crucial under normal, stress, and disease conditions, and it occurs on multiple levels [72, 73]. For instance, phosphorylation and other posttranslational modifications can change the transport of individual cargos [73, 78]. A more general regulation that affects multiple transport cargos is achieved by targeting components of the nuclear transport machinery. This can be accomplished by altering the localization or posttranslational modification of transport factors, and such changes are observed in response to oxidative stress [72].

The following sections summarize the effects of oxidative stress on specific cargos that are relevant to human health, the nucleocytoplasmic transport apparatus, and important signaling components. We will then build on this information to propose that the interdependence of oxidative stress, nucleocytoplasmic transport, and signaling provides a circuit that controls cell survival.

2.2. Oxidative Stress Impinges on Multiple Nuclear Cargos. As discussed above, oxidative stress causes the modification of targets in the nucleus and cytoplasm. Together, ROS-dependent modifications of cargos and the nuclear transport apparatus regulate the intracellular distribution of many of these targets. Among the oxidant-sensitive targets that translocate through NPCs are transcription factors, some of which are also implicated in the stress response. Prominent examples of transcription factors that relocate in response to oxidative stress are NF-κB and Nrf2 (NF-E2-related factor 2). The ROS-mediated redistribution of NF-κB and Nrf2 has been described extensively [80–83] and the relevant data will only be summarized here. Our discussion will focus on high-mobility group box 1 protein (HMGB1) and glycerolaldehyde-3-phosphate dehydrogenase (GAPDH) to illustrate the link between ROS, nuclear trafficking and signalling.

The role of NF-κB in immunity and inflammation is well established; however, this transcription factor is also critical for the synthesis of antioxidant proteins [80, 81]. The genes upregulated by NF-κB include MnSOD, Cu,ZnSOD, and HO-1 (heme oxygenase 1), all of which participate in antioxidant defense processes. ROS and numerous other stimuli control the intracellular distribution of NF-κB. In the absence of these stimuli, NF-κB is retained in the cytoplasm due to its association with I-κB. ROS trigger the degradation of I-κB, thereby promoting the nuclear accumulation of NF-κB and the subsequent transcription of genes that contain NF-κB response elements [81].

Nrf2 is another key player in the antioxidant response that relocates upon oxidant exposure. Under nonstress conditions, concentrations of the transcription factor Nrf2 are low, and the protein is retained in the cytoplasm owing to its association with Keap1 [82, 83]. In response to oxidative stress, a complex series of events leads to the stabilization of Nrf2 and its translocation into the nucleus. In the nucleus, Nrf2 upregulates the expression of several genes that are implicated in the antioxidant response [84]. The oxidant-induced nuclear accumulation of Nrf2 can be mediated by

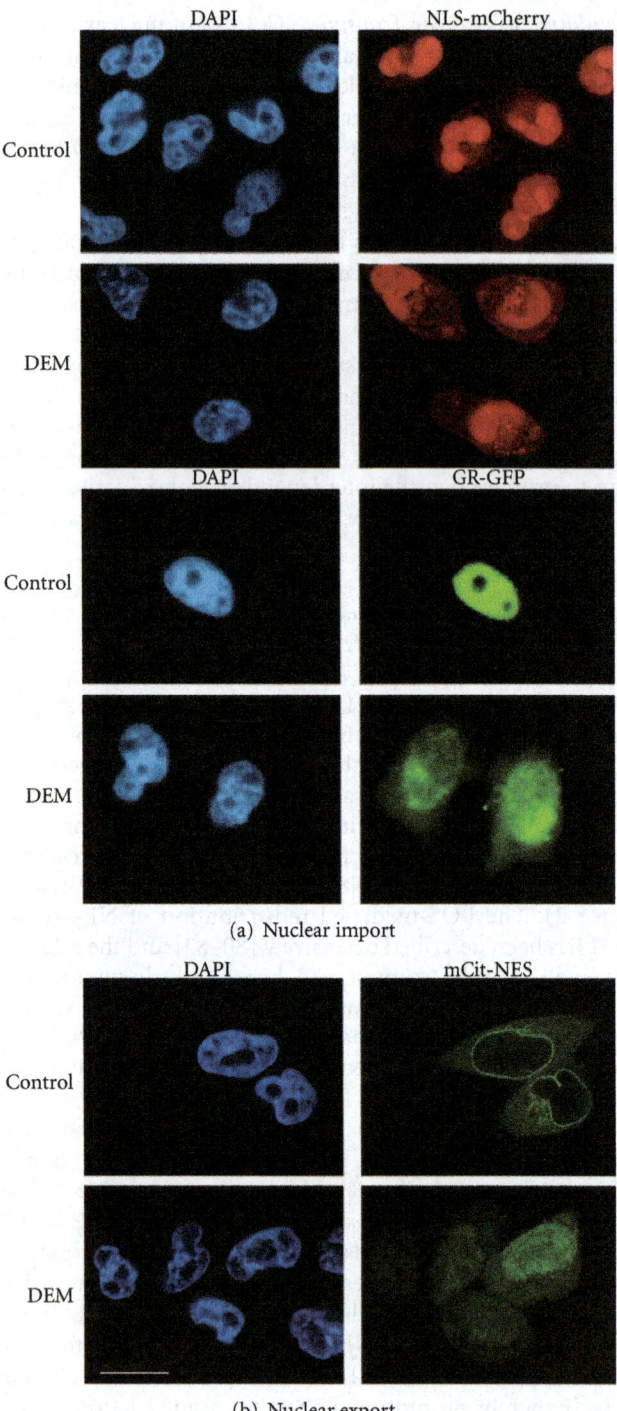

(a) Nuclear import

(b) Nuclear export

FIGURE 2: Oxidative stress inhibits classical nuclear import and Crm1-mediated export. (a) Nuclear import. HeLa cells transiently synthesizing the import substrates NLS-mCherry or GFP-tagged glucocorticoid receptor (GR-GFP) were incubated under nonstress conditions (control) or with DEM as described [69]. Note that a significant amount of the reporter proteins relocated to the cytoplasm upon oxidant treatment, indicating that classical nuclear import was inhibited. (b) Nuclear export. HeLa cells synthesizing the fluorescent reporter protein mCit-NES, a Crm1 cargo, were exposed to DEM and processed as in part a. The Crm1 export cargo was excluded from the nucleus under control conditions, but relocated to nuclei upon oxidative stress. Size bar is 20 μm.

importin-α5/importin-β1 [85], whereas Nrf2 nuclear export is promoted by Crm1 [86]. Phosphorylation of Nrf2 likely plays a role in its nuclear import and export, with PI3 kinase possibly stimulating Nrf2 nuclear accumulation [83, 84].

More recent studies identified HMGB1 and GAPDH as redox sensitive proteins whose nucleocytoplasmic distribution is regulated by ROS and signaling [87, 88]. Like Keap1/Nrf2, HMGB1 functions as a redox sensor [87]. In nuclei, HMGB1 serves as a DNA chaperone and participates in replication, transcription, as well as DNA repair. However, HMGB1 also contributes to a variety of signaling processes, which involve HMGB1 export to the cytoplasm and its subsequent secretion. At steady-state HMGB1 shuttles between the nucleus and cytoplasm, but hyperacetylation triggers its relocation to the cytosol [89]. It was speculated that lysine acetylation reduces the number of positive charges and thus interferes with nuclear import of the protein [89]. Karyopherin-α1, a member of the importin-α family, was identified as a binding partner that supports *in vitro* nuclear import of HMGB1, most likely in conjunction with importin-β1 [90]. The interaction of HMGB1 with karyopherin-α1 can be abrogated by phosphorylation, and modification of two NLS segments is necessary to relocate HMGB1 to the cytoplasm [90]. Taken together, a combination of acetylation and phosphorylation controls HMBG1 nuclear accumulation. These posttranslational modifications likely prevent the recognition of HMBG1 by the classical import apparatus.

Nuclear export of HMGB1 is at least in part mediated by Crm1, as leptomycin B drastically reduced HMGB1 exit from the nucleus [89]. Treatment with H_2O_2 upregulated the interaction Crm1/HMBG1 and relocated HMBG1 to the cytoplasm for secretion [91]. This oxidant-dependent secretion was sensitive to JNK and MEK inhibitors, in line with the idea that several members of the MAP kinase families control HMBG1 movement from the nucleus to the cytoplasm and its subsequent release. In other studies, IL-1β-dependent ERK1/2 activation increased the concentration of Crm1 and led to HMBG1 accumulation in the cytoplasm [92]. Whether H_2O_2 treatment, which activates ERK1/2, has the same effect on Crm1 levels is an exciting question that has to be answered in the future.

In recent years GAPDH has emerged as an enzyme that is involved in diverse cellular processes [88, 93]. Thus, GAPDH not only functions in glycolysis in the cytoplasm, but also plays additional important roles in other compartments of the cell, including the nucleus [88, 94–101]. The nuclear accumulation of GAPDH is controlled by posttranslational modifications and the interaction with different binding partners in the cytoplasm and nucleus. In response to oxidative stress, GAPDH undergoes S-nitrosylation and subsequent association with Siah. The GAPDH-Siah complex then moves into the nucleus, where it participates in the regulation of gene expression and apoptosis [88]. GAPDH nuclear accumulation depends on the acetylation of three lysine residues by the acetyltransferase p300 [101]. Furthermore, O-GlcNAc glycosylation of GAPDH occurs close to the Siah-binding site, and this modification promotes GAPDH nuclear accumulation [100]. Although not tested by the authors, O-GlcNAc modifications rise in response to oxidative stress [102] and could therefore assist in the stress-induced nuclear accumulation of GAPDH. Interestingly, the nucleocytoplasmic trafficking of GAPDH has been linked to several signaling pathways. In particular, activation of AMPK promoted the nuclear accumulation of GAPDH, whereas signaling through the PI3 kinase → Akt module is required for Crm1-dependent nuclear export [96].

The intracellular location of GAPDH is directly relevant to human health (see below). For example, when in the nucleus GAPDH might contribute to the initiation of apoptosis in brain cells. Moreover, the oxidant-induced changes in GAPDH subcellular localization probably play a role in the pathology of Alzheimer disease [93]. GAPDH is also critical to the development of diabetic complications, and changes in its nuclear accumulation might aggravate diabetic retinopathy [97].

Taken together, there is a growing list of proteins whose nucleocytoplasmic distribution is controlled by the intracellular redox homeostasis. This regulation frequently relies on posttranslational modifications, which can alter the interaction of a particular cargo with its carrier or the retention in nuclear and cytoplasmic compartments.

2.3. Oxidative Stress as a Key Player in Human Health. The cellular damage caused by oxidative stress promotes the onset as well as progression of several diseases and pathophysiologies. Thus, oxidative stress plays a critical role in neurodegenerative disorders, cardiovascular and metabolic diseases, as well as the complications associated with diabetes. Here, we focus on some examples that highlight the adverse effects of oxidative stress on human health.

Oxidative Stress and Neurodegenerative Diseases. The human brain is particularly vulnerable to oxidant-induced damage owing to high oxygen consumption, lipids rich in polyunsaturated fatty acids, high amounts of redox-active transition metals, and relatively poor defense against oxidative stress [30, 48, 103]. Several lines of evidence implicate oxidative stress in the neuronal damage that accompanies neurodegenerative disorders [25, 30, 34, 103, 104]. For instance, analysis of cerebrospinal fluid, plasma, and urine samples or postmortem brain specimens demonstrated the increase in oxidative damage in patients suffering from amyotrophic lateral sclerosis [105], Friedreich ataxia, Parkinson, Alzheimer, and Huntington diseases [30, 48, 103]. Oxidant-induced injury is elevated in the brain at early stages of these diseases, supporting the model that oxidative stress contributes to the etiology of neurodegeneration. In line with this hypothesis, mitochondrial dysfunction and oxidative damage to mitochondrial proteins are shared features of different neurodegenerative diseases [25, 30, 34, 103]. Animal models further support this idea, as inhibitors of mitochondrial function can induce some of the pathologies associated with Parkinson disease [34]. In addition, proteomics identified a large number of proteins that show increased oxidative damage in patients suffering from various forms of neurodegeneration. These proteins

include several enzymes that are critical to oxidative phosphorylation and glycolysis. Notably, when compared to control subjects GAPDH oxidation was increased in Alzheimer and Parkinson patients; GAPDH was also affected in ALS mouse models [103]. This is significant, because GAPDH and its subcellular trafficking are of particular importance to human metabolism and the pathologies associated with neurodegenerative diseases. As such, oxidative damage not only reduces the enzymatic activity of GAPDH in Alzheimer disease, but also supports the association with Siah and the subsequent translocation of the GAPDH-Siah complex to the nucleus (see above). In Alzheimer disease, both GAPDH expression and nitrosylation are increased, probably leading to elevated concentrations of GAPDH-Siah in the nucleus, which in turn promotes apoptosis [93]. Taken together, the oxidant-induced changes in GAPDH enzyme activity and intracellular distribution will reduce the energy supply and advance apoptosis in the brain of Alzheimer patients. Since GAPDH is an established target of oxidative damage in several neurodegenerative diseases [103], it is possible that its oxidant-dependent change in nuclear transport and the subsequent increase in cell death are common to multiple forms of neurodegeneration. Interestingly, GAPDH also plays a critical role in the development of diabetic complications.

Oxidative Stress and Diabetes. Oxidative stress is crucial to the etiology of diabetes mellitus and the ensuing damage to different tissues and organs [27, 49, 55, 106, 107]. Thus, oxidative stress can alter insulin signaling by targeting insulin receptor and insulin receptor substrates or through the activation of ser/thr kinases that regulate insulin signaling [55]. In this scenario, the ROS-induced changes to the insulin signaling pathway will advance insulin resistance and the subsequent development of diabetes. PI3 kinase and the MAP kinases ERK1/2 are major components of insulin-mediated signaling. Interestingly, signaling through these kinases is also modulated by oxidative stress and regulates nuclear trafficking (see below).

Oxidative stress not only promotes the development of diabetes, but diabetes also triggers the increase in oxidative stress due to elevated blood glucose and free fatty acids. Such disease-induced ROS production further exacerbates cellular damage and contributes to diabetic complications. In the following, we discuss some of the routes that generate oxidative stress in the diabetic patient [49, 55, 106–108].

Hyperglycemia rises intracellular glucose concentrations and the subsequent production of pyruvate, which is ultimately metabolized via the tricarboxylic acid cycle. As a result of the high abundance of pyruvate, increased amounts of NADH and $FADH_2$ are generated by the tricarboxylic acid cycle. Both NADH and $FADH_2$ enter into the mitochondrial electron transport chain, but their excess interferes eventually with the proper transfer of electrons. As a consequence of this overload, superoxide production by mitochondria increases and promotes cellular damage, especially in the diabetic vasculature [109, 110]. The importance of mitochondria in hyperglycemia-induced injuries was demonstrated experimentally, as inhibitors of

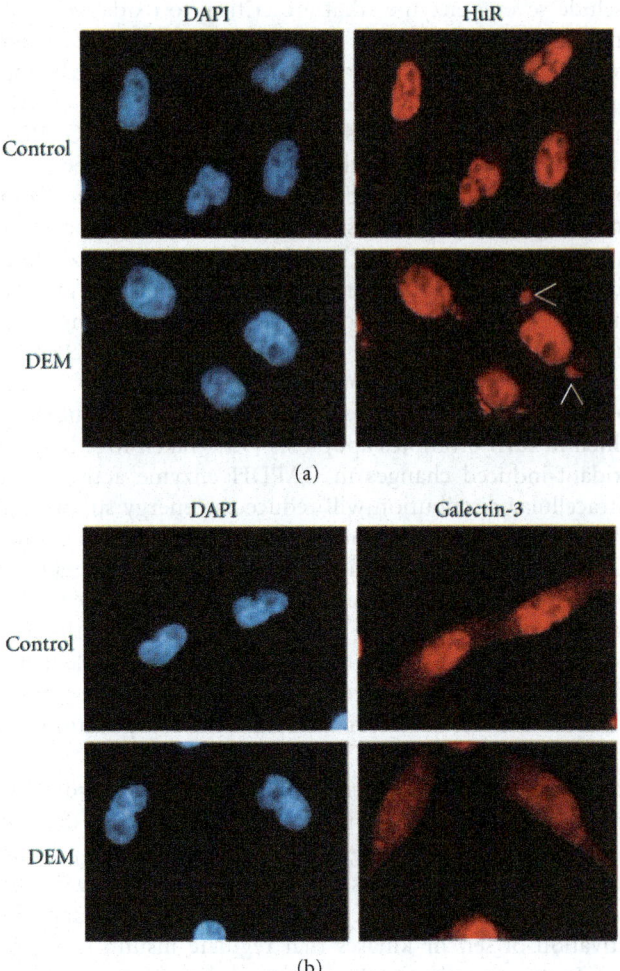

FIGURE 3: Oxidative stress interferes with importin-α1-dependent import of endogenous cargos. The import of two endogenous proteins, the RNA-binding protein HuR and galectin-3, was monitored in HeLa cells under the conditions described for Figure 2(a). Importin-α1 promotes nuclear import of both proteins. HuR and galectin-3 were visualized by indirect immunofluorescence and nuclei were stained with DAPI [69]. HuR was nuclear in control cells and redistributed to the cytoplasm of stressed cells, where it accumulated in stress granules (SGs). Similarly, galectin-3 was more concentrated in the nuclei of control cells and relocated to the cytoplasm upon DEM treatment. Arrows indicate the position of some of the SGs.

the electron transport chain, upregulation of the uncoupling protein UCP1, or mitochondrial SOD ameliorated some of the damage [49, 106].

The excess of mitochondrial superoxide, combined with other hyperglycemia-induced changes, culminates in secondary diabetic complications. In particular, diabetic nephropathy, retinopathy, neuropathy, and cardiomyopathy arise from the modulation of multiple biochemical pathways, some of which alter the cellular redox homeostasis [27, 49, 107]. For example, upon diabetes, the abundance of intracellular glucose and glycolytic metabolites leads to the increased production of sorbitol and other sugar alcohols by the polyol pathway. This generation of sugar alcohols

mediated by members of the aldo-keto reductase family relies on the conversion of NADPH to NADP+ [49]. Since NADPH is necessary to generate GSH from GSSG, excessive NADPH consumption will compromise the antioxidant defense and promote ROS-induced damage.

Moreover, ROS concentrations can also be elevated by hyperglycemia-dependent changes in cell signaling. As described above, GAPDH is sensitive to oxidative stress, and the inhibition of GAPDH by ROS increases intracellular concentrations of triose phosphate, a precursor of the PKC activator diacylglycerol. Hence, hyperglycemia triggers PKC activation, thereby changing the signaling events in the diabetic retina, heart, and endothelial cells [49, 106]. Moreover, this hyperglycemia-induced PKC activation is particularly detrimental to the kidney, as it stimulates ROS production by NAD(P)H oxidases and advances diabetic nephropathy [106, 111].

Like other forms of stress, diabetes modulates the nucleo-cytoplasmic distribution of transcription factors, with NF-κB as a prominent example [112]. Similarly, high glucose concentrations accumulated GAPDH in the nucleus of bovine retinal endothelial cells [97], where it could contribute to the progression of diabetic retinopathy.

The downstream effects of hyperglycemia further include changes in the posttranslational modification of proteins. Thus, elevated glucose concentrations raise the amount of fructose-6-phosphate that enters the hexosamine pathway [27, 106], which in turn increases the production of UDP-N-Acetylglucosamine and the subsequent O-GlcNAc modification of proteins. These changes are important to nuclear transport, because nucleoporins are well established targets for O-GlcNAc-glycosylation.

In summary, oxidative stress is implicated in different pathophysiological conditions, some of which alter the proper coordination of nuclear and cytoplasmic events. As discussed in the following section, ROS impinge on the nuclear transport apparatus and thereby modify the communication between nucleus and cytoplasm.

2.4. Nuclear Transport and Redox Homeostasis. Changes in cell physiology affect nucleocytoplasmic trafficking in a wide variety of eukaryotes, and the effects of oxidative stress on the nuclear transport apparatus have been analyzed during the past years. We have shown for the yeast *S. cerevisiae* and mammalian culture cells that different forms of stress, including oxidants, heat, and nutrient deprivation inhibit classical nuclear import and export [38, 39, 69, 72, 79, 113–121]. Our previous studies examined the impact of severe and mild oxidative stress. While severe oxidative stress was produced with high concentrations of H_2O_2 [39], mild oxidative stress was generated by the oxidant diethyl maleate, DEM [69]. Under severe stress conditions, cells underwent apoptosis, but a large fraction of cells survived the milder stress inflicted with DEM [69]. Nevertheless, Figures 2 and 3 show that DEM treatment diminished nuclear transport of both fluorescent reporter proteins and endogenous cargos [69, 79, 117]. This is not simply a consequence of stress-induced permeabilization of nuclear envelopes, because the barrier function of nuclear membranes was preserved under

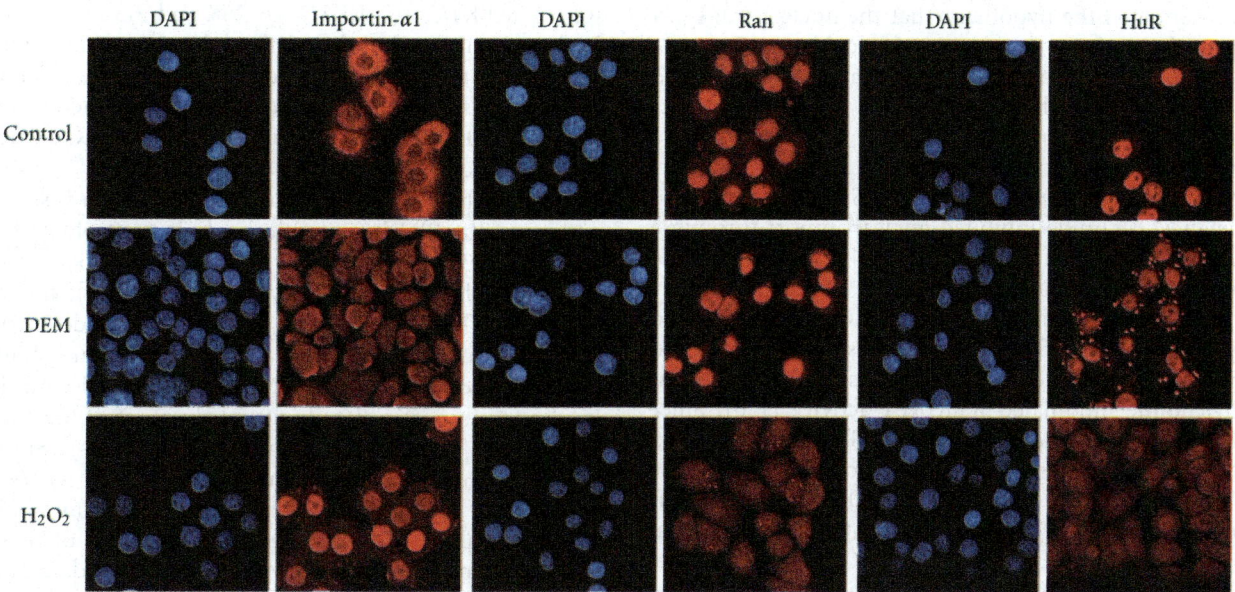

FIGURE 4: Mild and severe oxidative stress have different effects on nuclear transport factors. The effects of mild (2 mM DEM) and severe oxidative stress (10 mM H_2O_2) on the subcellular distribution of importin-α1, Ran, and HuR were analyzed in HeLa cells. Proteins were located by indirect immunofluorescence [39, 69, 79]. DEM treatment accumulated importin-α1 in nuclei but did not drastically affect the distribution of Ran. By contrast, severe oxidative stress induced by H_2O_2 caused a pronounced nuclear accumulation of importin-α1 and collapsed the nucleocytoplasmic Ran gradient. Both treatments relocated HuR to the cytoplasm. However, DEM triggered the assembly of HuR-containing SGs, which were rare or absent upon incubation with H_2O_2.

these conditions [122]. Since fluorescent reporter proteins like NLS-mCherry or mCit-NES do not contain nuclear or cytoplasmic retention signals, it was reasonable to assume that their stress-induced redistribution reflected changes to the transport apparatus. As described below, such changes were indeed reported by different laboratories, both for severe and mild forms of oxidative stress.

A common consequence of H_2O_2-induced severe oxidative stress is the collapse of the nucleocytoplasmic Ran GTPase gradient in growing cells (Figure 4); this collapse contributes to classical import inhibition [35, 38, 39, 121]. In addition, three key components of the transport apparatus, nucleoporin Nup153, the carrier importin-β1, and importin-α1 (Figure 4), redistributed when cells were treated with H_2O_2 [39]. Aside from transport factor redistribution, H_2O_2 also caused the degradation of Ran, Nup153 and importin-β1, both by proteasome and caspase-dependent mechanisms. In addition to growing cells, the consequences of H_2O_2 incubation were also examined in vitro. In these experiments, oxidant treatment led to a significant reduction of the docking step of nuclear import, as it diminished the binding of importin-α1/β1/cargo complexes at the nuclear envelope [39].

Our more recent studies investigated how nonlethal oxidative stress affects the transport apparatus. To this end, intracellular glutathione concentrations were depleted with DEM. Unlike severe oxidative stress, DEM incubation caused neither a dissipation of the Ran gradient (Figure 4) nor the degradation of transport receptors. However, DEM treatment mislocalized several transport components, including importin-α1, its nuclear exporter CAS as well

as nucleoporins Nup153, Nup88, and Nup50 [69]. Nuclear retention was one of the mechanisms that contributed to the oxidant-induced nuclear accumulation of these proteins. Concomitant with nuclear retention, high molecular mass complexes were formed in nuclei that contained importin-α1, Nup153, and Nup88. A second mechanism promoting the redistribution of transport factors was the increase in nuclear import for importin-α1 and CAS [69]. Notably, the subcellular redistribution of importin-α1, CAS, Nup153, and Nup88 was accompanied by changes in their posttranslational modification. For example, DEM augmented the phosphorylation for each factor and increased the O-GlcNAc modification of Nup153 [117]. All of these events are possibly linked to oxidant-induced signaling, as the relocation of importin-α1, CAS, Nup153 and Nup88 was modulated by MEK $\rightarrow$ ERK1/2 and PI3K $\rightarrow$ Akt pathways [117].

Oxidative stress not only inhibits nuclear import, the Crm1 export pathway is sensitive to oxidants as well [79], and our group demonstrated that Crm1-mediated export was inhibited by DEM. Consequently, mCit-NES, a Crm1 cargo predominantly in the cytoplasm of unstressed cells, relocated to nuclei in DEM-treated samples (Figure 2). Several mechanisms participated in the oxidant-induced inhibition of Crm1-dependent export [79]. First, oxidative stress changed the association of Nup358, Nup214, Nup62, and Crm1 with the nuclear envelope and redistributed Nup98. Second, the interaction among these nucleoporins was altered. Third, oxidant treatment impaired Crm1 exit from the nucleus and increased its binding to Ran.

Taken together, these studies revealed that oxidative stress alters several steps of classical nuclear import and export and substantiated the hypothesis that the nuclear transport apparatus is an important target for oxidants. Some of the oxidant-sensitive components are shared by import and export pathways, which might explain why both transport routes are affected in stressed cells.

Work by other groups identified additional transport factors that are likely controlled by ROS homeostasis [72]. For instance, ceramide inhibited nuclear import through a pathway that relied on the MAPK p38 [123]. As ceramide is believed to cause oxidative stress [124, 125], these experiments provide another link between ROS imbalance and changes in nuclear trafficking. This idea is further supported by experiments in smooth muscle cells, where lysophosphatidylcholine modulated RanGAP1 activity [126]. Since lysophosphatidylcholine can induce ROS production [127], RanGAP1 and thereby the generation of RanGDP in the cytoplasm are potential candidates for ROS-dependent regulation. The role of RanGAP1 as an oxidant-sensitive target in the cytoplasm is significant, because RanGAP1 promotes the termination of protein export for all importin-β like carriers. Furthermore, RanGAP1 has emerged as target for several MAP kinases [128], emphasizing its potential to serve as a redox-sensitive transport regulator at the NPC.

The idea of redox-dependent control at the nuclear pore is consistent with a recent publication that detected the MAP kinases ERK, p38, and JNK at the NPC [129]. Importantly, all of these kinases are activated and/or redistributed by ROS (Table 1). Moreover Nup50, Nup153, and Nup214 are established ERK targets [130], and their phosphorylation changed several interactions that are important for nuclear transport. Specifically, ERK-dependent modification of Nup50 interfered with its binding to importin-β and transportin, which are both carriers of the importin-β family. Similarly, when Nup153 and Nup214 were phosphorylated by ERK, their association with importin-β was reduced.

In summary, multiple signaling pathways are activated by oxidants, MAP kinases reside at the NPC or relocate upon stress (see below), and several transport factors are targeted by these kinases. Hence, it is reasonable to propose a simplified chain of events: oxidative stress → signaling → transport factor modification and/or relocation → changes in nuclear trafficking → altered distribution of cargos. This is by no means a one-way street, as nuclear transport factors also play a critical role in modifying signaling events.

An example for the interdependence of signaling and nuclear transport is provided by RanBP3. This transport factor is not only regulated by multiple kinase modules, it also controls signaling [131, 132]. RanBP3 is predominantly located in the nucleus and a binding partner for Ran, RCC1, and Crm1. Aside from participating in Ran translocation to the cytoplasm, RanBP3 may also sequester Ran in the nucleus [131]. Phosphorylation by RSK and Akt can modulate RanBP3 function. In particular, RanBP3 modification is believed to stimulate nuclear import by regulating its interaction with RCC1. In support of this model, nonphosphorylatable mutants of RanBP3 displayed a reduced ability to stimulate RCC1 *in vitro* and caused a partial dissipation of the Ran gradient in growing cells [131]. The emerging scenario is that signaling through

Ras → MEK1/2 → ERK1/2 → RSK and PI3 kinase → Akt leads to RanBP3 phosphorylation, thereby maintaining the Ran gradient. Since both signaling pathways are modulated by ROS, it is tempting to speculate that their activation by oxidants will help to preserve or re-establish the Ran gradient in stressed cells.

Besides being a downstream target of several signaling pathways, RanBP3 has a critical role in controlling TGF-β signaling [132]. Signaling through TGF-β and its receptors have multiple links to oxidative stress [133–136], and many effects of TGF-β-like ligands are exerted by the downstream transcriptional regulators Smad2/3. Smad2/3 are shuttling proteins, and their transport to the nucleus relies on direct binding to importin-β, without involvement of the adaptor importin-α [137]. Following activation of TGF-β, Smad2/3 are phosphorylated and accumulate in nuclei, where they regulate the expression of target genes. The termination of TGF-β signaling involves the dephosphorylation of Smad2/3 and their export to the cytoplasm. Notably, Smad2/3 nuclear export is not sensitive to leptomycin B, suggesting that Crm1 is not required for exit from the nucleus. Indeed, RanBP3 was identified as a possible carrier that helps to move Smad2/3 to the cytoplasm [132]. Several lines of evidence support this idea; RanBP3 bound nonphosphorylated Smad2/3, interacted with Smad2/3 in the nucleus and promoted Smad2/3 nuclear export in a Ran-dependent fashion. Together, these studies established an essential role for RanBP3 as a negative regulator of Smad2/3 signaling, which relies on its ability to transport Smad2/3 to the cytoplasm.

The impact of ROS on nuclear transport is not limited to signaling-dependent effects, since ROS can directly induce the modification of nuclear transport components. Protein carbonylation is one of the consequences of oxidative stress, and it occurs in an age-dependent fashion for nucleoporins Nup153 and Nup93. Nucleoporin carbonylation correlated with the "leakiness" of NPCs [138], and could be particularly harmful to postmitotic cells, in which some nucleoporins are replaced only slowly. In the context of signaling, it will be interesting to determine whether the age-dependent nucleoporin carbonylation alters the NPC association of MAP kinases or nucleoporin phosphorylation.

In summary, experiments described above suggest that the stress-induced modulation of nuclear trafficking is caused by changes in the concentration, distribution, and posttranslational modification of transport factors [72, 82]. This process is further complicated by the fact that oxidant-dependent relocation of transport factors can be compartmentalized even within the nucleus or cytoplasm, as shown by the formation of cytoplasmic stress granules.

2.5. Oxidative Stress, Stress Granule Assembly, and Nuclear Transport. One of the possible consequences of oxidative stress is the formation of cytoplasmic stress granules (SGs). SGs are generated in response to stress that leads to the accumulation of stalled translation initiation complexes [139, 140]. SG assembly is part of a stress defense mechanism that helps to retain and protect mRNAs from degradation. One of the signaling events crucial for the formation of most SGs

TABLE 1: Redox-sensitive cellular targets in eukaryotic cells. Components that alter their activity and/or nucleocytoplasmic distribution when ROS concentrations increase are listed. See text for details.

Component or process	Effect of ROS
Signaling proteins, transcriptional regulators	
JNK, MAPK	Activation
p38, MAPK	Activation, nuclear translocation
ERK1/2, MAPK	Activation, nuclear accumulation
PI3 kinase (some isoforms)	Activation, changes in nucleocytoplasmic distribution
5'-AMP activated kinase	Inhibition, nuclear accumulation; possibly by reduced nuclear export *via* Crm1
Human insulin receptor kinase activity	Activation
Src family kinases	Activation
EGFR	Nuclear translocation; DNA repair
Protein tyrosine phosphatases	Inactivation
PTEN	Nuclear accumulation; association with p53
STAT3	Nuclear translocation
NF-κB, transcription factor	Nuclear accumulation; transcription
FoxO transcription factors	Nuclear translocation (i.e., FOXO1, FOXO3a, and FOXO4)
yAP-1, yeast transcription factor	Nuclear translocation
Msn2p, Msn4p, yeast transcription factors	Nuclear translocation, transcription
CREB	Phosphorylation, nuclear translocation
Nrf2	Nuclear accumulation
HMGB1	Cytoplasmic translocation
HuR, RNA-binding protein	Relocation to cytoplasm, accumulation in stress granules
Nuclear transport apparatus	
Classical nuclear import	Inhibition
Crm1-dependent nuclear export	Inhibition
Ran, small GTPase; Gsp1 in *S. cerevisiae*	Relocation to cytoplasm upon severe oxidative stress
Importin-α1, adaptor for classical nuclear import	Accumulation in nuclei, accumulation in cytoplasmic stress granules
Crm1, nuclear exporter	Accumulation at nuclear envelope
CAS, exporter for importin-α	Nuclear accumulation
Multiple nucleoporins located at different positions within the nuclear pore complex: Nup358, Nup214, Nup88, Nup62, Nup153, Nup50, Nup98, and others	Changes in the association with nuclear envelope; altered nucleocytoplasmic distribution; degradation upon severe stress, in some cases mediated by caspases.

is Ser51 phosphorylation on eIF2α (eukaryotic translation initiation factor 2) [139–141]. Ser51 can be modified by four different upstream kinases, PKR, PERK, GCN2, and HRI (heme-regulated initiation factor 2 kinase), which are activated by various stressors, including the oxidant arsenite. Other signaling events are relevant to SG biogenesis and disassembly; for instance, arsenite promotes the sequestration of Rho and ROCK1 in SGs, possibly to limit the activation of the downstream target JNK [142]. Moreover, focal adhesion kinase (FAK) controls the disassembly of SGs and can be stimulated with H_2O_2 [143, 144].

In addition to components of the small ribosomal subunit and RNA-binding proteins, arsenite-induced SGs contain importin-α1 [145]. Notably, importin-α1 knockdown delays SG formation, suggesting a role in the dynamics of SG assembly. These are important data which further substantiate the contribution of nuclear protein transport factors to the stress response. At present, we do not fully

understand these events; however, it is conceivable that SGs are one of the "hubs", where ROS-mediated signaling and nuclear transport components come together in the cytoplasm. Results for the mRNA-binding protein HuR support this idea. HuR shuttles between the nucleus and cytoplasm and relies on importin-α1 for nuclear import. Under normal growth conditions, HuR is predominantly in the nucleus, but a 4-hour DEM treatment concentrated HuR in SGs (Figures 3 and 4). At the same time, importin-α1 accumulated in nuclei, but it was still detectable in the cytoplasm [69, 117]. It should be emphasized that the association of macromolecules with SGs is dynamic. Proteins as well as RNA can shuttle between SGs and the surrounding cytoplasm [141, 146], and this may also apply to importin-α1.

What are the possible mechanisms that promote the ROS-dependent changes in importin-α1 and HuR distribution and how are these events linked to SG assembly?

The DEM-induced relocation of HuR is likely driven by the combination of importin-α1 nuclear accumulation and HuR association with SGs. In particular, concentrating importin-α1 in nuclei of stressed cells could diminish nuclear import of HuR. At the same time, importin-α1 has a role in SG biogenesis. Although details of this process have yet to be defined, importin-α1 may recruit components to cytoplasmic foci that are destined to form SGs. Given that importin-α1 binds and transports a variety of cargos, importin-α1 shuttling between SG foci and the cytoplasm could accomplish this task. If our model is correct, it could help explain the lack of SG formation in cells incubated with H_2O_2 [147, 148]. As shown in Figure 4, H_2O_2 did not induce SGs, and importin-α1 became highly concentrated in the nucleus, with little of the protein remaining in the cytoplasm. Moreover, stress can also increase nuclear retention and import of importin-α1 [113]. As a result of these events, the concentration of importin-α1 in the cytoplasm will be low when cells are treated with H_2O_2, which in turn could limit the formation of SGs.

The potential contribution of nuclear transport factors to SG assembly or function is not restricted to importin-α1. Support for this notion comes from importin-β family members importin 8 and transportin which localize to SGs upon arsenite treatment [149, 150]. At this point, we have only few examples that connect nuclear transport components with SGs, and future studies will have to unravel how nuclear trafficking, SG assembly, and ROS-dependent signaling are integrated.

2.6. Oxidative Stress and the Subcellular Distribution of Key Signaling Molecules. Elevated levels of ROS modify the activity of redox sensitive components that participate in signaling or other essential biological processes [1, 6, 9, 39, 69, 79, 87, 88, 114, 116, 151–153]. Notably, such ROS-dependent changes in activity are frequently accompanied by the intracellular relocation of the redox-sensitive factors. This scenario applies to a growing list of protein kinases, phosphatases, transcription factors, and components of the nuclear transport apparatus (Table 1). Several of the kinases and phosphatases that redistribute under oxidative stress conditions are key players in signaling circuits, where they control cell survival, growth, proliferation, or death. The interdependence of the activation status and intracellular distribution is crucial for these enzymes, as it determines the specificity and duration of signaling events [152, 154–156]. In the following, we discuss some of the kinases and phosphatases for which oxidant-dependent relocation has been established.

The activity and location of several members of the MAPK and PI3 kinase families are modulated by ROS. Such spatiotemporal control is particularly important for the response to stress, where the repair of stress-induced damage and cell survival relies on the outcome of compartment-specific signaling events. Multiple signaling modules that respond to ROS, both by activation and relocation, have been analyzed in our group [114, 116]. We focused on Akt and ERK1/2, kinases that are essential for signal transduction through PI3 $\rightarrow$ Akt and MEK $\rightarrow$ ERK1/2 modules. The stressor DEM elevated the phosphorylation of Akt on Thr308 and Ser473, which leads to Akt activation. At the same time, DEM induced the dual phosphorylation of ERK1/2, thereby activating the MAP kinases. Importantly, DEM not only activates Akt and ERK1/2, but also increased significantly the nuclear/cytoplasmic ratio of phospho-Akt(Ser473) and dually phosphorylated-ERK1/2 [114]. A possible outcome of this shift is a change in the phosphorylation profiles of nuclear and cytoplasmic targets. Notably, the compartmentalization of Akt and ERK1/2-dependent signaling events is even more complex [114], as we demonstrated in the nucleus a direct correlation between the levels of phospho-Akt(Ser473) and phospho-ERK1/2. Our studies suggested that the nuclear concentration of phospho-Akt(Ser473) is dependent on nuclear phospho-ERK1/2 and *vice versa.* Accordingly, crosstalk occurs between phospho-Akt(Ser473) and ERK1/2 in response to oxidative stress; this crosstalk is specific for the nuclear compartment.

More recent work on PI3 kinase by others further emphasizes the importance of the localized action of signaling molecules. The PI3 kinase catalytic subunit p110β carries a nuclear localization signal in its C-terminal domain, while the regulatory subunit p85β harbors a nuclear export signal. The analysis of a p110β transport mutant showed that the ability of the p85β/p110β complex to regulate cell survival was strictly dependent on its nuclear localization [157]. Although the effect of oxidative stress on the distribution of this kinase has yet to be determined, these findings provide compelling evidence for the control of cell signaling by nuclear transport.

Another example that illustrates the ROS-dependent activation and distribution of protein kinases is the heterotrimeric enzyme 5′-AMP activated kinase (AMPK). AMPK is an energy sensor which plays a pivotal role in the regulation of metabolic homeostasis by phosphorylating targets that are involved in glucose, carbohydrate, lipid, and protein metabolism [158–161]. In unstressed cells, AMPK shuttles between the nucleus and cytoplasm and this shuttling relies on the nuclear exporter Crm1 [116, 162]. However, in response to oxidative stress, AMPK α- and β-subunits concentrated in the nucleus. This could be accomplished—at least in part—by ROS-induced changes to the nuclear export apparatus, as Crm1 is one of the transport components that are affected by ROS (see above). Interestingly, the link between AMPK activity, subcellular distribution, and nuclear trafficking is even more intricate, as importin-α1, a component of the nuclear transport apparatus, is also modified by AMPK [163].

Epidermal growth factor receptor (EGFR) is a receptor tyrosine kinase that is especially important to human health, because signaling through EGFR is linked to tumorigenesis, metastasis and radioresistance. EGFR is located in the plasma membrane, but it also entered the nucleus in response to oxidative stress, heat, or radiation [164]. Moreover, incubation of cultured cells with hydroxy-nonenal, a compound generated by lipid peroxidation, promoted the nuclear accumulation of EGFR [19]. When in the nucleus, EGFR stimulated DNA repair, a process that contributes to radioresistance and potentially limits the success of radiotherapy. Since EGFR is membrane bound, details of its nuclear transport are likely to differ from soluble cargos. Nevertheless, importin-β1 and Crm1 (Figure 1) were identified as nuclear carriers that participate in EGFR trafficking [165, 166].

The link between oxidative stress and the localization of key signaling components is not limited to protein kinases. For instance, the lipid and protein phosphatase PTEN has functions in the nucleus and cytoplasm, and oxidative stress promotes PTEN nuclear accumulation [167]. In cells treated with H_2O_2, PTEN concentrated in nuclei, where it stabilizes the tumor suppressor p53. Under normal conditions, PTEN is exported from the nucleus by the carrier Crm1 in a cell-cycle dependent fashion, and this export relied on signaling through PI3 kinase [168]. However, incubation with H_2O_2 induced PTEN phosphorylation on Ser380, which inhibited its nuclear export [167]. The control of PTEN shuttling upon oxidative stress probably goes beyond the oxidant-induced phosphorylation of the enzyme. As such, the exporter Crm1 is one of the cellular targets that are sensitive to ROS, and signaling through the PI3 kinase $\rightarrow$ Akt module regulates several components of the nuclear transport apparatus [79, 117]. This interdependence of nuclear transport and signaling is further complicated by the fact that the enzymatic activity of PTEN is regulated by oxidants (see below).

For the examples discussed here, ROS-mediated changes in the nucleocytoplasmic distribution of kinases and phosphatases could reflect the requirement to modify selected substrates in specific subcellular compartments. To this end, the ROS-induced nuclear accumulation of ERK1/2, PI3 kinase, AMPK, EGFR, or PTEN will alter the phosphorylation and activity of nuclear substrates such as transcription factors and other regulators of gene expression. However, such redistribution will also impact other compartments, because the sequestration of kinases or phosphatases in the nucleus can change the phosphoproteome in the cytoplasm as well.

2.7. What Is the Interface between the Initial Oxidant Exposure and Changes in the Nuclear Transport Apparatus? As discussed in previous sections, oxidative stress targets components of the nuclear transport machinery. Moreover, different signaling cascades are implicated in the control of trafficking across the NPC, in part by regulating the posttranslational modification of nuclear transport factors. A complete mechanistic understanding of these events requires that the initial impact of the oxidant can be connected to functional changes of the nuclear transport apparatus. For many of the processes described here, the interface between the primary oxidant-induced event and changes in the posttranslational modification or function of transport factors is not fully defined. In the following, we will, therefore, speculate on some of the possible links.

In principle, two distinct mechanisms can underlie the effect of ROS on nuclear transport factors. First, ROS might react directly with the nuclear transport apparatus, leading to the covalent modification of individual components. Second, oxidative stress could activate signaling cascades that ultimately trigger the phosphorylation and/or O-GlcNAc glycosylation of the transport machinery. In the second scenario, signaling begins with a redox-sensitive target that induces a chain of events which conclude with the posttranslational modification of one or more nuclear transport factors.

Direct Modification of the Nuclear Transport Apparatus by ROS. In line with what is known about redox-sensitive residues in proteins, we expect that for nuclear transport components cysteine, methionine, lysine, arginine, and histidine residues are among the side chains that are particularly prone to direct oxidation or other ROS-dependent modifications [169]. This idea is supported by a study describing the S-nitrosylation of Crm1 on two cysteine residues and the concomitant inhibition of Crm1-mediated nuclear export [170]. Besides Crm1, nucleoporins are other candidates for a direct modification by ROS or compounds generated upon oxidative stress. Our hypothesis is supported by the increase in nucleoporin carbonylation when cells encounter oxidative stress [138].

Signaling as Possible Interface between Oxidant Exposure and Nuclear Transport Modification. Although many of the enzymes that mediate the posttranslational modification of transport factors are known, upstream events regulating these enzymes are less well understood. This applies in particular to the first step of the process, that is, the impact of ROS on its primary target. We propose that protein kinases, phosphatases, or small GTPases that are redox-sensitive [171–174] could fill this gap, as they activate signaling pathways that culminate in transport factor modification. A particularly interesting candidate in this respect is the protein kinase Src, which contains a cysteine switch that is oxidized in order to achieve full kinase activation. Moreover, the redox-dependent stimulation of Src promotes the ligand-independent transphosphorylation of EGFR and subsequent activation of PI3 and ERK kinases [175]. In line with this order of events, it is possible that the ROS-induced formation of disulfide bonds in Src will stimulate the PI3 and ERK-dependent effects on nuclear transport factors as they are discussed here.

The same reasoning applies to several phosphatases [174], including PTEN and low molecular weight protein tyrosine phosphatase (LMW-PTP). PTEN is crucial for the downregulation of PI3 kinase signaling. However, oxidant-induced thiol modification of PTEN inactivates the phosphatase, and thereby promotes signaling through the PI3 kinase $\rightarrow$ Akt module [174]. With respect to nuclear transport, ROS-induced PTEN inactivation would increase the impact of PI3 kinase on trafficking. In a similar fashion, the redox-dependent inactivation of LMW-PTP leads to sustained ERK activation [176]. This could elevate the ERK-dependent phosphorylation of soluble transport factors and nucleoporins, thus altering their function.

Aside from phosphorylation, *O*-GlcNAc glycosylation of nucleoporins is induced by oxidative stress. The oxidant-dependent increase in *O*-GlcNAc modification is possibly achieved by the complex regulation of *O*-GlcNAc transferase and *β-N*-acetylglucosaminidase. At present, these events are not fully understood [177].

Taken together, we propose that changes in the cellular redox homeostasis impact nucleocytoplasmic trafficking by two general mechanisms that are likely to operate in parallel. First, ROS or ROS-generated compounds directly modify redox-sensitive transport factors, this can alter their function. Second, the impact of ROS on redox-sensitive signaling proteins will ultimately modulate the posttranslational modification and activity of nuclear transport components.

2.8. Antioxidant Defenses Occur in a Compartmentalized Fashion. In addition to the compartmentalized activation and action of kinases and phosphatases, components of the antioxidant defense apparatus are also unequally distributed within the cell [63, 178]. This is illustrated by catalase, an enzyme concentrated in peroxisomes, and the different forms of superoxide dismutase (SOD) [64, 65, 179, 180]. While manganese-containing SOD (MnSOD) is in the mitochondrial matrix, copper- and zinc-containing SOD (Cu,ZnSOD) can be found preferentially in the cytoplasm and extracellular SOD (EC-SOD) on the cell surface. Moreover, the unequal distribution of GSH and enzymes involved in GSH metabolism will also contribute to subcellular differences in the response to ROS [59, 181–183]. Aside from these enzymes and antioxidants, the localized action of chaperones, critical factors for the repair of stress-induced damage, is well established [115, 184–186]. Since chaperone function is essential for proper signaling and also required for nuclear transport, the nucleocytoplasmic localization and function of heat shock proteins and other chaperones will have significant impact when cells experience ROS imbalances.

We propose that the unequal distribution of antioxidant defense and repair components will impact both cargos and transport factors in a compartment-specific fashion. Accordingly, the prevention and repair of oxidant-induced damage will be different in the nucleus and cytoplasm. Depending on its subcellular location, this could have differential effects on the movement and function of a shuttling protein. For example, nuclear cargos that encounter higher levels of ROS in the cytoplasm could be immobilized in this compartment. The same model can be applied to nuclear transport factors. Thus, nucleoporins on the nuclear and cytoplasmic side of the NPC could be exposed to different levels of ROS and repair. Since nuclear and cytoplasmic nucleoporins participate in different steps of trafficking, damage on either side of the nuclear pore could have unique consequences for nuclear transport.

3. Conclusions

The impact of ROS on human health is well established, and links between oxidative stress, nuclear transport, and

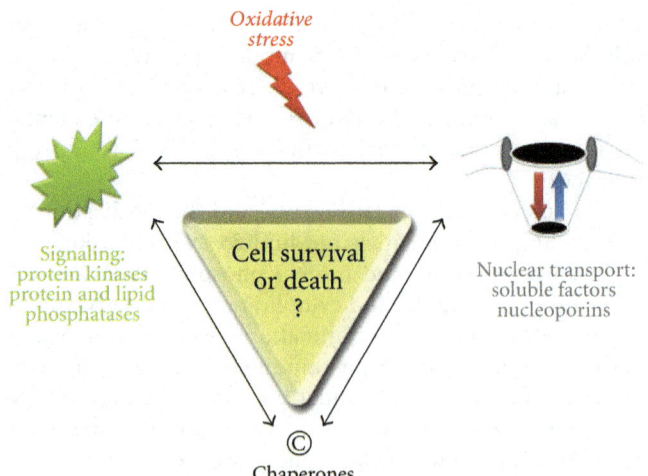

FIGURE 5: Simplified model for the crosstalk between signaling and nuclear transport in response to oxidative stress. Oxidative stress impinges on signaling molecules and the nuclear transport apparatus, with chaperones modulating both processes. Different scenarios can explain the communication between nuclear transport and signaling pathways in oxidant-treated cells. In one case, oxidative stress alters the localization and activity of transport factors. This will change the subcellular distribution of key signaling molecules, which in turn affects the modification of downstream targets. Alternatively, the signaling pathways activated by oxidative stress cause the modification and redistribution of transport factors. Both scenarios are likely to take place side-by-side, and the balance of these events will ultimately determine cell fate.

disease have been defined. For instance, oxidative stress plays a pivotal role in the hyperglycemia-induced damage of multiple tissues and organs [47, 49, 51–53, 55, 187]. GAPDH nucleocytoplasmic shuttling not only participates in these processes, but has also been connected to cancer and neurodegenerative disorders, such as ALS, Alzheimer, or Parkinson disease [88]. Hence, it is conceivable that the oxidant-induced relocation of GAPDH is common to diabetes, cancer, and some forms of neurodegeneration. This shared feature can be extended to the stress-induced nuclear trafficking of the transcriptional regulators NF-κB and Nrf2 and may include other diseases, such as Friedreich ataxia [56, 188, 189].

The examples highlight how the compartment-specific action of signaling molecules, defense and repair reactions provide sophisticated tools to regulate cell physiology. Thus, confining these processes to specific locations will limit the access to downstream targets and clients. In the context of this review, the nucleocytoplasmic distribution of kinases, phosphatases, and other factors involved in posttranslational modification or folding can be expected to directly affect the communication between cytoplasmic and nuclear compartments. This is emphasized by the fact that many of the nuclear transport components and their cargos are modified in an ROS-dependent fashion by phosphorylation, *O*-GlcNAc glycosylation, acetylation, or sumoylation.

Our current understanding of ROS, signaling, and nucleocytoplasmic transport supports the notion that these processes are intricately connected. Although many of the details are still to be discovered, the findings from different fields can be merged into a simplified model. Here, we propose that crosstalk and feedback between different components of this signaling circuit will determine how cells respond to oxidative stress (Figure 5). In one scenario, the activation of signaling pathways promotes the posttranslational modification of nuclear transport factors. This triggers the redistribution of transport factors and alters the movement of cargo across the nuclear envelope. Alternatively, oxidant-induced damage to the transport apparatus could modulate the nucleocytoplasmic localization of kinases or phosphatases, thereby changing the spatiotemporal pattern of signaling. We believe that the two scenarios will take place side by side, affecting different signaling modules and targets in the nucleus and cytoplasm. Both scenarios are further shaped by the localized action of chaperones, which impact both signaling and nuclear transport. The input from signaling, trafficking, and repair will culminate in the decision on cell survival or death.

As outlined in this review, the dynamic organization of signaling cascades and the nuclear transport apparatus are ideal to respond to internal and external cues. In this context, nucleocytoplasmic trafficking provides the switch to direct events to the nucleus or cytoplasm. The interdependence of signaling and transport pathways provides the flexibility to adjust to a wide variety of changes in cell physiology.

Acknowledgments

This research was supported by grants from FQRNT, NSERC, and HSFQ to U. Stochaj. M. Kodiha was a recipient of a postdoctoral fellowship from McGill University.

References

[1] D. P. Jones, "Radical-free biology of oxidative stress," *The American Journal of Physiology—Cell Physiology*, vol. 295, no. 4, pp. C849–C868, 2008.

[2] B. Halliwell, "Role of free radicals in the neurodegenerative diseases: therapeutic implications for antioxidant treatment," *Drugs & Aging*, vol. 18, no. 9, pp. 685–716, 2001.

[3] D.-F. Dai and P. S. Rabinovitch, "Cardiac aging in mice and humans: the role of mitochondrial oxidative stress," *Trends in Cardiovascular Medicine*, vol. 19, no. 7, pp. 213–220, 2009.

[4] J. Li and N. J. Holbrook, "Common mechanisms for declines in oxidative stress tolerance and proliferation with aging," *Free Radical Biology and Medicine*, vol. 35, no. 3, pp. 292–299, 2003.

[5] T. Finkel and N. J. Holbrook, "Oxidants, oxidative stress and the biology of ageing," *Nature*, vol. 408, no. 6809, pp. 239–247, 2000.

[6] N. J. Holbrook and S. Ikeyama, "Age-related decline in cellular response to oxidative stress: links to growth factor signaling pathways with common defects," *Biochemical Pharmacology*, vol. 64, no. 5-6, pp. 999–1005, 2002.

[7] M. C. Haigis and B. A. Yankner, "The aging stress response," *Molecular Cell*, vol. 40, no. 2, pp. 333–344, 2010.

[8] A. Y. Seo, A.-M. Joseph, D. Dutta, J. C. Y. Hwang, J. P. Aris, and C. Leeuwenburgh, "New insights into the role of mitochondria in aging: mitochondrial dynamics and more," *Journal of Cell Science*, vol. 123, no. 15, pp. 2533–2542, 2010.

[9] K. C. Kregel and H. J. Zhang, "An integrated view of oxidative stress in aging: basic mechanisms, functional effects, and pathological considerations," *The American Journal of Physiology—Regulatory Integrative and Comparative Physiology*, vol. 292, no. 1, pp. R18–R36, 2007.

[10] P. Storz, "Forkhead homeobox type O transcription factors in the responses to oxidative stress," *Antioxidants & Redox Signaling*, vol. 14, no. 4, pp. 593–605, 2011.

[11] W. Dröge, "Free radicals in the physiological control of cell function," *Physiological Reviews*, vol. 82, no. 1, pp. 47–95, 2002.

[12] W. Dröge and H. M. Schipper, "Oxidative stress and aberrant signaling in aging and cognitive decline," *Aging Cell*, vol. 6, no. 3, pp. 361–370, 2007.

[13] H.-C. Yang, M.-L. Cheng, H.-Y. Ho, and D. Tsun-Yee Chiu, "The microbicidal and cytoregulatory roles of NADPH oxidases," *Microbes and Infection*, vol. 13, no. 2, pp. 109–120, 2010.

[14] B. M. Babior, "NADPH oxidase: an update," *Blood*, vol. 93, no. 5, pp. 1464–1476, 1999.

[15] M. Reth, "Hydrogen peroxide as second messenger in lymphocyte activation," *Nature Immunology*, vol. 3, no. 12, pp. 1129–1134, 2002.

[16] M. Valko, D. Leibfritz, J. Moncol, M. T. D. Cronin, M. Mazur, and J. Telser, "Free radicals and antioxidants in normal physiological functions and human disease," *The International Journal of Biochemistry & Cell Biology*, vol. 39, no. 1, pp. 44–84, 2007.

[17] R. Pallela, Y. Na-Young, and S.-K. Kim, "Anti-photoaging and photoprotective compounds derived from marine organisms," *Marine Drugs*, vol. 8, no. 4, pp. 1189–1202, 2010.

[18] A. J. Ridley, J. R. Whiteside, T. J. McMillan, and S. L. Allinson, "Cellular and sub-cellular responses to UVA in relation to carcinogenesis," *International Journal of Radiation Biology*, vol. 85, no. 3, pp. 177–195, 2009.

[19] K. Dittmann, C. Mayer, R. Kehlbach, M. C. Rothmund, and H. P. Rodemann, "Radiation-induced lipid peroxidation activates src kinase and triggers nuclear EGFR transport," *Radiotherapy & Oncology*, vol. 92, no. 3, pp. 379–382, 2009.

[20] M. Rigoulet, E. D. Yoboue, and A. Devin, "Mitochondrial ROS generation and its regulation: mechanisms involved in H_2O_2 signaling," *Antioxidants & Redox Signaling*, vol. 14, no. 3, pp. 459–468, 2011.

[21] K.-J. Cho, J.-M. Seo, and J.-H. Kim, "Bioactive lipoxygenase metabolites stimulation of NADPH oxidases and reactive oxygen species," *Molecules and Cells*, vol. 32, no. 1, pp. 1–5, 2011.

[22] R. P. Brandes, N. Weissmann, and K. Schröder, "NADPH oxidases in cardiovascular disease," *Free Radical Biology & Medicine*, vol. 49, no. 5, pp. 687–706, 2010.

[23] T. M. Paravicini and R. M. Touyz, "NADPH oxidases, reactive oxygen species, and hypertension," *Diabetes Care*, vol. 31, supplement 2, pp. S170–S180, 2008.

[24] F. Jiang, Y. Zhang, and G. J. Dusting, "NADPH oxidase-mediated redox signaling: roles in cellular stress response, stress tolerance, and tissue repair," *Pharmacological Reviews*, vol. 63, no. 1, pp. 218–242, 2011.

[25] A. A. Fatokun, T. W. Stone, and R. A. Smith, "Oxidative stress in neurodegeneration and available means of protection," *Frontiers in Bioscience*, vol. 13, no. 9, pp. 3288–3311, 2008.

[26] V. Calabrese, C. Cornelius, A. T. Dinkova-Kostova, E. J. Calabrese, and M. P. Mattson, "Cellular stress responses, the hormesis paradigm, and vitagenes: novel targets for therapeutic intervention in neurodegenerative disorders," *Antioxidants & Redox Signaling*, vol. 13, no. 11, pp. 1763–1811, 2010.

[27] J. D. Acharya and S. S. Ghaskadbi, "Islets and their antioxidant defense," *Islets*, vol. 2, no. 4, pp. 225–235, 2010.

[28] S. V. Avery, "Molecular targets of oxidative stress," *Biochemical Journal*, vol. 434, no. 2, pp. 201–210, 2011.

[29] I. Dalle-Donne, A. Scaloni, D. Giustarini et al., "Proteins as biomarkers of oxidative/nitrosative stress in diseases: the contribution of redox proteomics," *Mass Spectrometry Reviews*, vol. 24, no. 1, pp. 55–99, 2005.

[30] B. Halliwell, "Oxidative stress and neurodegeneration: where are we now?" *Journal of Neurochemistry*, vol. 97, no. 6, pp. 1634–1658, 2006.

[31] G. I. Giles and C. Jacob, "Reactive sulfur species: an emerging concept in oxidative stress," *Biological Chemistry*, vol. 383, no. 3-4, pp. 375–388, 2002.

[32] R. P. Guttmann, "Redox regulation of cysteine-dependent enzymes," *Journal of Animal Science*, vol. 88, no. 4, pp. 1297–1306, 2010.

[33] A. Colquhoun, "Lipids, mitochondria and cell death: implications in neuro-oncology," *Molecular Neurobiology*, vol. 42, no. 1, pp. 76–88, 2010.

[34] L. M. Sayre, G. Perry, and M. A. Smith, "Oxidative stress and neurotoxicity," *Chemical Research in Toxicology*, vol. 21, no. 1, pp. 172–188, 2008.

[35] M. P. Czubryt, J. A. Austria, and G. N. Pierce, "Hydrogen peroxide inhibition of nuclear protein import is mediated by the mitogen-activated protein kinase, ERK2," *The Journal of Cell Biology*, vol. 148, no. 1, pp. 7–16, 2000.

[36] B. Halliwell, M. V. Clement, and L. H. Long, "Hydrogen peroxide in the human body," *FEBS Letters*, vol. 486, no. 1, pp. 10–13, 2000.

[37] J. A. Imlay, "Cellular defenses against superoxide and hydrogen peroxide," *Annual Review of Biochemistry*, vol. 77, no. 1, pp. 755–776, 2008.

[38] U. Stochaj, R. Rassadi, and J. Chiu, "Stress-mediated inhibition of the classical nuclear protein import pathway and nuclear accumulation of the small GTPase Gsp1p," *The FASEB Journal*, vol. 14, no. 14, pp. 2130–2132, 2000.

[39] M. Kodiha, A. Chu, N. Matusiewicz, and U. Stochaj, "Multiple mechanisms promote the inhibition of classical nuclear import upon exposure to severe oxidative stress," *Cell Death & Differentiation*, vol. 11, no. 8, pp. 862–874, 2004.

[40] Y. Miyamoto, T. Saiwaki, J. Yamashita et al., "Cellular stresses induce the nuclear accumulation of importin α and cause a conventional nuclear import block," *The Journal of Cell Biology*, vol. 165, no. 5, pp. 617–623, 2004.

[41] S. Boisnard, G. Lagniel, C. Garmendia-Torres et al., "H_2O_2 activates the nuclear localization of Msn2 and Maf1 through thioredoxins in Saccharomyces cerevisiae," *Eukaryotic Cell*, vol. 8, no. 9, pp. 1429–1438, 2009.

[42] J. Song, J. Li, J. Qiao, S. Jain, B. M. Evers, and D. H. Chung, "PKD prevents H_2O_2-induced apoptosis via NF-κB and p38 MAPK in RIE-1 cells," *Biochemical and Biophysical Research Communications*, vol. 378, no. 3, pp. 610–614, 2009.

[43] M. L. Circu and T. Y. Aw, "Reactive oxygen species, cellular redox systems, and apoptosis," *Free Radical Biology and Medicine*, vol. 48, no. 6, pp. 749–762, 2010.

[44] S. Lenzen, "Oxidative stress: the vulnerable β-cell," *Biochemical Society Transactions*, vol. 36, no. 3, pp. 343–347, 2008.

[45] B. van Loon, E. Markkanen, and U. Hübscher, "Oxygen as a friend and enemy: how to combat the mutational potential of 8-oxo-guanine," *DNA Repair*, vol. 9, no. 6, pp. 604–616, 2010.

[46] B. Halliwell, "Free radicals and antioxidants—quo vadis?" *Trends in Pharmacological Sciences*, vol. 32, no. 3, pp. 125–130, 2011.

[47] J. L. Evans, I. D. Goldfine, B. A. Maddux, and G. M. Grodsky, "Oxidative stress and stress-activated signaling pathways: a unifying hypothesis of type 2 diabetes," *Endocrine Reviews*, vol. 23, no. 5, pp. 599–622, 2002.

[48] K. Jomova, D. Vondrakova, M. Lawson, and M. Valko, "Metals, oxidative stress and neurodegenerative disorders," *Molecular and Cellular Biochemistry*, vol. 345, no. 1-2, pp. 91–104, 2010.

[49] F. Giacco and M. Brownlee, "Oxidative stress and diabetic complications," *Circulation Research*, vol. 107, no. 9, pp. 1058–1070, 2010.

[50] J. Ren, L. Pulakat, A. Whaley-Connell, and J. R. Sowers, "Mitochondrial biogenesis in the metabolic syndrome and cardiovascular disease," *Journal of Molecular Medicine*, vol. 88, no. 10, pp. 993–1001, 2010.

[51] R. Stanton, "Oxidative stress and diabetic kidney disease," *Current Diabetes Reports*, vol. 11, no. 4, pp. 330–336, 2011.

[52] C. K. Roberts and K. K. Sindhu, "Oxidative stress and metabolic syndrome," *Life Sciences*, vol. 84, no. 21-22, pp. 705–712, 2009.

[53] S. Chrissobolis, A. A. Miller, G. R. Drummond, B. K. Kemp-Harper, and C. G. Sobey, "Oxidative stress and endothelial dysfunction in cerebrovascular disease," *Frontiers in Bioscience*, vol. 16, no. 5, pp. 1733–1745, 2011.

[54] J. C. Jonas, M. Bensellam, J. Duprez, H. Elouil, Y. Guiot, and S. M. A. Pascal, "Glucose regulation of islet stress responses and β-cell failure in type 2 diabetes," *Diabetes, Obesity & Metabolism*, vol. 11, supplement 4, pp. 65–81, 2009.

[55] J. L. Rains and S. K. Jain, "Oxidative stress, insulin signaling, and diabetes," *Free Radical Biology and Medicine*, vol. 50, no. 5, pp. 567–575, 2011.

[56] S. Reuter, S. C. Gupta, M. M. Chaturvedi, and B. B. Aggarwal, "Oxidative stress, inflammation, and cancer: how are they linked?" *Free Radical Biology and Medicine*, vol. 49, no. 11, pp. 1603–1616, 2010.

[57] Y. S. Kanwar, J. Wada, L. Sun et al., "Diabetic nephropathy: mechanisms of renal disease progression," *Experimental Biology and Medicine*, vol. 233, no. 1, pp. 4–11, 2008.

[58] A. Tojo, K. Asaba, and M. L. Onozato, "Suppressing renal NADPH oxidase to treat diabetic nephropathy," *Expert Opinion on Therapeutic Targets*, vol. 11, no. 8, pp. 1011–1018, 2007.

[59] P. Diaz Vivancos, T. Wolff, J. Markovic, F. V. Pallardó, and C. H. Foyer, "A nuclear glutathione cycle within the cell cycle," *Biochemical Journal*, vol. 431, no. 2, pp. 169–178, 2010.

[60] H. R. López-Mirabal and J. R. Winther, "Redox characteristics of the eukaryotic cytosol," *Biochimica et Biophysica Acta—Molecular Cell Research*, vol. 1783, no. 4, pp. 629–640, 2008.

[61] D. P. Jones and Y. M. Go, "Redox compartmentalization and cellular stress," *Diabetes, Obesity and Metabolism*, vol. 12, no. 2, pp. 116–125, 2010.

[62] É. Margittai and R. Sitia, "Oxidative protein folding in the secretory pathway and redox signaling across compartments and cells," *Traffic*, vol. 12, no. 1, pp. 1–8, 2011.

[63] O. Blokhina, E. Virolainen, and K. V. Fagerstedt, "Antioxidants, oxidative damage and oxygen deprivation stress: a review," *Annals of Botany*, vol. 91, pp. 179–194, 2003.

[64] T. Fukai and M. Ushio-Fukai, "Superoxide dismutases: role in redox signaling, vascular function and diseases," *Antioxidants & Redox Signaling*, vol. 15, no. 6, pp. 1583–1606, 2011.

[65] A. Valdivia, S. Pérez-Álvarez, J. D. Aroca-Aguilar, I. Ikuta, and J. Jordán, "Superoxide dismutases: a physiopharmacological update," *Journal of Physiology & Biochemistry*, vol. 65, no. 2, pp. 195–208, 2009.

[66] H. Jefferies, J. Coster, A. Khalil, J. Bot, R. D. McCauley, and J. C. Hall, "Glutathione," *ANZ Journal of Surgery*, vol. 73, no. 7, pp. 517–522, 2003.

[67] N. S. Dhalla, A. B. Elmoselhi, T. Hata, and N. Makino, "Status of myocardial antioxidants in ischemia-reperfusion injury," *Cardiovascular Research*, vol. 47, no. 3, pp. 446–456, 2000.

[68] D. M. Townsend, K. D. Tew, and H. Tapiero, "The importance of glutathione in human disease," *Biomedicine & Pharmacotherapy*, vol. 57, no. 3-4, pp. 145–155, 2003.

[69] M. Kodiha, D. Tran, C. Qian et al., "Oxidative stress mislocalizes and retains transport factor importin-α and nucleoporins Nup153 and Nup88 in nuclei where they generate high molecular mass complexes," *Biochimica et Biophysica Acta—Molecular Cell Research*, vol. 1783, no. 3, pp. 405–418, 2008.

[70] K. Weis, "Regulating access to the genome: nucleocytoplasmic transport throughout the cell cycle," *Cell*, vol. 112, no. 4, pp. 441–451, 2003.

[71] S. R. Wente and M. P. Rout, "The nuclear pore complex and nuclear transport," *Cold Spring Harbor Perspectives in Biology*, vol. 2, no. 10, pp. 1–19, 2010.

[72] M. Kodiha, N. Crampton, S. Shrivastava, R. Umar, and U. Stochaj, "Traffic control at the nuclear pore," *Nucleus*, vol. 1, no. 3, pp. 237–244, 2010.

[73] I. K. H. Poon and D. A. Jans, "Regulation of nuclear transport: central role in development and transformation?" *Traffic*, vol. 6, no. 3, pp. 173–186, 2005.

[74] S. A. Adam, "The nuclear transport machinery in Caenorhabditis elegans: a central role in morphogenesis," *Seminars in Cell & Developmental Biology*, vol. 20, no. 5, pp. 576–581, 2009.

[75] D. Adam Mason and D. S. Goldfarb, "The nuclear transport machinery as a regulator of Drosophila development," *Seminars in Cell & Developmental Biology*, vol. 20, no. 5, pp. 582–589, 2009.

[76] S. Hutten and R. H. Kehlenbach, "CRM1-mediated nuclear export: to the pore and beyond," *Trends in Cell Biology*, vol. 17, no. 4, pp. 193–201, 2007.

[77] N. Kudo, N. Matsumori, H. Taoka et al., "Leptomycin B inactivates CRM1/exportin 1 by covalent modification at a cysteine residue in the central conserved region," *Proceedings of the National Academy of Sciences of the United States of America*, vol. 96, no. 16, pp. 9112–9117, 1999.

[78] D. A. Jans, C.-Y. Xiao, and M. H. C. Lam, "Nuclear targeting signal recognition: a key control point in nuclear transport?" *BioEssays*, vol. 22, no. 6, pp. 532–544, 2000.

[79] N. Crampton, M. Kodiha, S. Shrivastava, R. Umar, and U. Stochaj, "Oxidative stress inhibits nuclear protein export by multiple mechanisms that target FG nucleoporins and Crm1," *Molecular Biology of the Cell*, vol. 20, no. 24, pp. 5106–5116, 2009.

[80] M. J. Morgan and Z. G. Liu, "Crosstalk of reactive oxygen species and NF-κB signaling," *Cell Research*, vol. 21, no. 1, pp. 103–115, 2011.

[81] P. Ak and A. J. Levine, "p53 and NF-κB: different strategies for responding to stress lead to a functional antagonism," *The FASEB Journal*, vol. 24, no. 10, pp. 3643–3652, 2010.

[82] V. P. Patel and C. T. Chu, "Nuclear transport, oxidative stress, and neurodegeneration," *International Journal of Clinical and Experimental Pathology*, vol. 4, no. 3, pp. 215–229, 2011.

[83] A. Giudice, C. Arra, and M. C. Turco, "Review of molecular mechanisms involved in the activation of the Nrf2-ARE signaling pathway by chemopreventive agents," *Methods in Molecular Biology*, vol. 647, pp. 37–74, 2010.

[84] A. Martín-Montalvo, J. M. Villalba, P. Navas, and R. de Cabo, "NRF2, cancer and calorie restriction," *Oncogene*, vol. 30, no. 5, pp. 505–520, 2010.

[85] M. Theodore, Y. Kawai, J. Yang et al., "Multiple nuclear localization signals function in the nuclear import of the transcription factor Nrf2," *Journal of Biological Chemistry*, vol. 283, no. 14, pp. 8984–8994, 2008.

[86] A. K. Jain, D. A. Bloom, and A. K. Jaiswal, "Nuclear import and export signals in control of Nrf2," *Journal of Biological Chemistry*, vol. 280, no. 32, pp. 29158–29168, 2005.

[87] D. Tang, R. Kang, H. J. Zeh, and M. T. Lotze, "High-mobility group box 1, oxidative stress, and disease," *Antioxidants & Redox Signaling*, vol. 14, no. 7, pp. 1315–1335, 2011.

[88] C. Tristan, N. Shahani, T. W. Sedlak, and A. Sawa, "The diverse functions of GAPDH: views from different subcellular compartments," *Cellular Signalling*, vol. 23, no. 2, pp. 317–323, 2011.

[89] T. Bonaldi, F. Talamo, P. Scaffidi et al., "Monocytic cells hyperacetylate chromatin protein HMGB1 to redirect it towards secretion," *The EMBO Journal*, vol. 22, no. 20, pp. 5551–5560, 2003.

[90] H. Y. Ju and J.-S. Shin, "Nucleocytoplasmic shuttling of HMGB1 is regulated by phosphorylation that redirects it toward secretion," *The Journal of Immunology*, vol. 177, no. 11, pp. 7889–7897, 2006.

[91] D. Tang, Y. Shi, R. Kang et al., "Hydrogen peroxide stimulates macrophages and monocytes to actively release HMGB1," *Journal of Leukocyte Biology*, vol. 81, no. 3, pp. 741–747, 2007.

[92] K. Hayakawa, K. Arai, and E. H. Lo, "Role of ERK MAP kinase and CRM1 in IL-1β-stimulated release of HMGB1 from cortical astrocytes," *Glia*, vol. 58, no. 8, pp. 1007–1015, 2010.

[93] D. A. Butterfield, S. S. Hardas, and M. L. B. Lange, "Oxidatively modified glyceraldehyde-3-phosphate dehydrogenase (GAPDH) and Alzheimer's disease: many pathways to neurodegeneration," *Journal of Alzheimer's Disease*, vol. 20, no. 2, pp. 369–393, 2010.

[94] S. Azam, N. Jouvet, A. Jilani et al., "Human glyceraldehyde-3-phosphate dehydrogenase plays a direct role in reactivating oxidized forms of the DNA repair enzyme APE1," *Journal of Biological Chemistry*, vol. 283, no. 45, pp. 30632–30641, 2008.

[95] M. R. Hara, M. B. Cascio, and A. Sawa, "GAPDH as a sensor of NO stress," *Biochimica et Biophysica Acta*, vol. 1762, no. 5, pp. 502–509, 2006.

[96] H. J. Kwon, J. H. Rhim, I. S. Jang, G. E. Kim, S. C. Park, and E. J. Yeo, "Activation of AMP-activated protein kinase stimulates the nuclear localization of glyceraldehyde 3-phosphate dehydrogenase in human diploid fibroblasts," *Experimental & Molecular Medicine*, vol. 42, no. 4, pp. 254–269, 2010.

[97] S. Madsen-Bouterse, G. Mohammad, and R. A. Kowluru, "Glyceraldehyde-3-phosphate dehydrogenase in retinal microvasculature: implications for the development and

progression of diabetic retinopathy," *Investigative Ophthalmology & Visual Science*, vol. 51, no. 3, pp. 1765–1772, 2010.

[98] H. Nakajima, W. Amano, T. Kubo et al., "Glyceraldehyde-3-phosphate dehydrogenase aggregate formation participates in oxidative stress-induced cell death," *Journal of Biological Chemistry*, vol. 284, no. 49, pp. 34331–34341, 2009.

[99] M. A. Ortiz-Ortiz, J. M. Morán, L. M. Ruiz-Mesa, J. M. B. Pedro, and J. M. Fuentes, "Paraquat exposure induces nuclear translocation of glyceraldehyde-3-phosphate dehydrogenase (GAPDH) and the activation of the nitric oxide-GAPDH-Siah cell death cascade," *Toxicological Sciences*, vol. 116, no. 2, pp. 614–622, 2010.

[100] J. Park, D. Han, K. Kim, Y. Kang, and Y. Kim, "O-Glc-NAcylation disrupts glyceraldehyde-3-phosphate dehydrogenase homo-tetramer formation and mediates its nuclear translocation," *Biochimica et Biophysica Acta*, vol. 1794, no. 2, pp. 254–262, 2009.

[101] M. Ventura, F. Mateo, J. Serratosa et al., "Nuclear translocation of glyceraldehyde-3-phosphate dehydrogenase is regulated by acetylation," *The International Journal of Biochemistry & Cell Biology*, vol. 42, no. 10, pp. 1672–1680, 2010.

[102] N. E. Zachara, N. O'Donnell, W. D. Cheung, J. J. Mercer, J. D. Marth, and G. W. Hart, "Dynamic O-GlcNAc modification of nucleocytoplasmic proteins in response to stress," *Journal of Biological Chemistry*, vol. 279, no. 29, pp. 30133–30142, 2004.

[103] A. Martínez, M. Portero-Otin, R. Pamplona, and I. Ferrer, "Protein targets of oxidative damage in human neurodegenerative diseases with abnormal protein aggregates," *Brain Pathology*, vol. 20, no. 2, pp. 281–297, 2010.

[104] M. T. Lin and M. F. Beal, "Mitochondrial dysfunction and oxidative stress in neurodegenerative diseases," *Nature*, vol. 443, no. 7113, pp. 787–795, 2006.

[105] J. P. Morrison, M. C. Coleman, E. S. Aunan, S. A. Walsh, D. R. Spitz, and K. C. Kregel, "Aging reduces responsiveness to BSO- and heat stress-induced perturbations of glutathione and antioxidant enzymes," *The American Journal of Physiology—Regulatory Integrative & Comparative Physiology*, vol. 289, no. 4, pp. R1035–R1041, 2005.

[106] D. K. Singh, P. Winocour, and K. Farrington, "Oxidative stress in early diabetic nephropathy: fueling the fire," *Nature Reviews Endocrinology*, vol. 7, no. 3, pp. 176–184, 2010.

[107] P. M. P. Balakumar, M. K. M. Arora, J. M. Reddy, and M. B. P. Anand-Srivastava, "Pathophysiology of diabetic nephropathy: involvement of multifaceted signalling mechanism," *Journal of Cardiovascular Pharmacology*, vol. 54, no. 2, pp. 129–138, 2009.

[108] M. Brownlee, "The pathobiology of diabetic complications," *Diabetes*, vol. 54, no. 6, pp. 1615–1625, 2005.

[109] T. Nishikawa, D. Edelstein, X. L. Du et al., "Normalizing mitochondrial superoxide production blocks three pathways of hyperglycaemic damage," *Nature*, vol. 404, no. 6779, pp. 787–790, 2000.

[110] X. Cheng, R. C. M. Siow, and G. E. Mann, "Impaired redox signaling and antioxidant gene expression in endothelial cells in diabetes: a role for mitochondria and the nuclear factor-E2-related factor 2-Kelch-like ECH-associated protein 1 defense pathway," *Antioxidants & Redox Signaling*, vol. 14, no. 3, pp. 469–487, 2011.

[111] M. Brownlee, "Biochemistry and molecular cell biology of diabetic complications," *Nature*, vol. 414, no. 6865, pp. 813–820, 2001.

[112] R. G. Baker, M. S. Hayden, and S. Ghosh, "NF-κB, inflammation, and metabolic disease," *Cell Metabolism*, vol. 13, no. 1, pp. 11–22, 2011.

[113] M. Kodiha, P. Bański, D. Ho-Wo-Cheong, and U. Stochaj, "Dissection of the molecular mechanisms that control the nuclear accumulation of transport factors importin-α and CAS in stressed cells," *Cellular & Molecular Life Sciences*, vol. 65, no. 11, pp. 1756–1767, 2008.

[114] M. Kodiha, P. Bański, and U. Stochaj, "Interplay between MEK and PI3 kinase signaling regulates the subcellular localization of protein kinases ERK1/2 and Akt upon oxidative stress," *FEBS Letters*, vol. 583, no. 12, pp. 1987–1993, 2009.

[115] M. Kodiha, A. Chu, O. Lazrak, and U. Stochaj, "Stress inhibits nucleocytoplasmic shuttling of heat shock protein hsc70," *The American Journal of Physiology—Cell Physiology*, vol. 289, no. 4, pp. C1034–C1041, 2005.

[116] M. Kodiha, J. G. Rassi, C. M. Brown, and U. Stochaj, "Localization of AMP kinase is regulated by stress, cell density, and signaling through the MEK → ERK1/2 pathway," *The American Journal of Physiology—Cell Physiology*, vol. 293, no. 5, pp. C1427–C1436, 2007.

[117] M. Kodiha, D. Tran, A. Morogan, C. Qian, and U. Stochaj, "Dissecting the signaling events that impact classical nuclear import and target nuclear transport factors," *PLoS One*, vol. 4, no. 12, article e8420, 2009.

[118] Z. S. Chughtai, R. Rassadi, N. Matusiewicz, and U. Stochaj, "Starvation promotes nuclear accumulation of the hsp70 Ssa4p in yeast cells," *Journal of Biological Chemistry*, vol. 276, no. 23, pp. 20261–20266, 2001.

[119] X. Quan, P. Tsoulos, A. Kuritzky, R. Zhang, and U. Stochaj, "The carrier Msn5p/Kap142p promotes nuclear export of the hsp70 Ssa4p and relocates in response to stress," *Molecular Microbiology*, vol. 62, no. 2, pp. 592–609, 2006.

[120] X. Quan, R. Rassadi, B. Rabie, N. Matusiewicz, and U. Stochaj, "Regulated nuclear accumulation of the yeast hsp70 Ssa4p in ethanol-stressed cells is mediated by the N-terminal domain, requires the nuclear carrier Nmd5p and protein kinase C," *The FASEB Journal*, vol. 18, no. 7, pp. 899–901, 2004.

[121] A. Chu, N. Matusiewicz, and U. Stochaj, "Heat-induced nuclear accumulation of hsc70s is regulated by phosphorylation and inhibited in confluent cells," *The FASEB Journal*, vol. 15, no. 8, pp. 1478–1480, 2001.

[122] L. Sánchez, M. Kodiha, and U. Stochaj, "Monitoring the disruption of nuclear envelopes in interphase cells with GFP-beta-galactosidase," *Journal of Biomolecular Techniques*, vol. 16, no. 3, pp. 235–238, 2005.

[123] R. S. Faustino, P. Cheung, M. N. Richard et al., "Ceramide regulation of nuclear protein import," *Journal of Lipid Research*, vol. 49, no. 3, pp. 654–662, 2008.

[124] X. Li, K. A. Becker, and Y. Zhang, "Ceramide in redox signaling and cardiovascular diseases," *Cellular Physiology & Biochemistry*, vol. 26, no. 1, pp. 41–48, 2010.

[125] J.-S. Won and I. Singh, "Sphingolipid signaling and redox regulation," *Free Radical Biology & Medicine*, vol. 40, no. 11, pp. 1875–1888, 2006.

[126] R. S. Faustino, L. N. W. Stronger, M. N. Richard et al., "RanGAP-mediated nuclear protein import in vascular smooth muscle cells is augmented by lysophosphatidylcholine," *Molecular Pharmacology*, vol. 71, no. 2, pp. 438–445, 2007.

[127] J. W. Zmijewski, A. Landar, N. Watanabe, D. A. Dickinson, N. Noguchi, and V. M. Darley-Usmar, "Cell signalling by oxidized lipids and the role of reactive oxygen species in the endothelium," *Biochemical Society Transactions*, vol. 33, no. 6, pp. 1385–1389, 2005.

[128] R. S. Faustino, D. C. Rousseau, M. N. Landry, A. L. Kostenuk, and G. N. Pierce, "Effects of mitogen-activated protein kinases on nuclear protein import," *Canadian Journal of Physiology & Pharmacology*, vol. 84, no. 3-4, pp. 469–475, 2006.

[129] R. S. Faustino, T. G. Maddaford, and G. N. Pierce, "Mitogen activated protein kinase at the nuclear pore complex," *Journal of Cellular and Molecular Medicine*, vol. 15, no. 4, pp. 928–937, 2011.

[130] H. Kosako, N. Yamaguchi, C. Aranami et al., "Phospho-proteomics reveals new ERK MAP kinase targets and links ERK to nucleoporin-mediated nuclear transport," *Nature Structural and Molecular Biology*, vol. 16, no. 10, pp. 1026–1035, 2009.

[131] S.-O. Yoon, S. Shin, Y. Liu et al., "Ran-binding protein 3 phosphorylation links the Ras and PI3-kinase pathways to nucleocytoplasmic transport," *Molecular Cell*, vol. 29, no. 3, pp. 362–375, 2008.

[132] F. Dai, X. Lin, C. Chang, and X.-H. Feng, "Nuclear export of Smad2 and Smad3 by RanBP3 facilitates termination of TGF-beta signaling," *Developmental Cell*, vol. 16, no. 3, pp. 345–357, 2009.

[133] K. Koli, M. Myllärniemi, J. Keski-Oja, and V. L. Kinnula, "Transforming growth factor-β activation in the lung: focus on fibrosis and reactive oxygen species," *Antioxidants & Redox Signaling*, vol. 10, no. 2, pp. 333–342, 2008.

[134] X. Z. Shi, J. H. Winston, and S. K. Sarna, "Differential immune and genetic responses in rat models of Crohn's colitis and ulcerative colitis," *The American Journal of Physiology—Gastrointestinal & Liver Physiology*, vol. 300, no. 1, pp. G41–G51, 2011.

[135] H. Sone, H. Akanuma, and T. Fukuda, "Oxygenomics in environmental stress," *Redox Report*, vol. 15, no. 3, pp. 98–114, 2010.

[136] G. H. Tesch and A. K. Lim, "Recent insights into diabetic renal injury from the db/db mouse model of type 2 diabetic nephropathy," *The American Journal of Physiology—Renal Physiology*, vol. 300, no. 2, pp. F301–F310, 2011.

[137] C. S. Hill, "Nucleocytoplasmic shuttling of Smad proteins," *Cell Research*, vol. 19, no. 1, pp. 36–46, 2009.

[138] M. A. D'Angelo, M. Raices, S. H. Panowski, and M. W. Hetzer, "Age-dependent deterioration of nuclear pore complexes causes a loss of nuclear integrity in postmitotic cells," *Cell*, vol. 136, no. 2, pp. 284–295, 2009.

[139] P. Anderson and N. Kedersha, "Stress granules: the Tao of RNA triage," *Trends in Biochemical Sciences*, vol. 33, no. 3, pp. 141–150, 2008.

[140] M. G. Thomas, M. Loschi, M. A. Desbats, and G. L. Boccaccio, "RNA granules: the good, the bad and the ugly," *Cellular Signalling*, vol. 23, no. 2, pp. 324–334, 2011.

[141] J. R. Buchan and R. Parker, "Eukaryotic stress granules: the ins and outs of translation," *Molecular Cell*, vol. 36, no. 6, pp. 932–941, 2009.

[142] N.-P. Tsai and L.-N. Wei, "RhoA/ROCK1 signaling regulates stress granule formation and apoptosis," *Cellular Signalling*, vol. 22, no. 4, pp. 668–675, 2010.

[143] N.-P. Tsai, P.-C. Ho, and L.-N. Wei, "Regulation of stress granule dynamics by Grb7 and FAK signalling pathway," *The EMBO Journal*, vol. 27, no. 5, pp. 715–726, 2008.

[144] S. Basuroy, M. Dunagan, P. Sheth, A. Seth, and R. K. Rao, "Hydrogen peroxide activates focal adhesion kinase and c-Src by a phosphatidylinositol 3 kinase-dependent mechanism and promotes cell migration in Caco-2 cell monolayers," *The American Journal of Physiology—Gastrointestinal & Liver Physiology*, vol. 299, no. 1, pp. G186–G195, 2010.

[145] K. Fujimura, T. Suzuki, Y. Yasuda, M. Murata, J. Katahira, and Y. Yoneda, "Identification of importin α1 as a novel constituent of RNA stress granules," *Biochimica et Biophysica Acta—Molecular Cell Research*, vol. 1803, no. 7, pp. 865–871, 2010.

[146] S. Mollet, N. Cougot, A. Wilczynska et al., "Translationally repressed mRNA transiently cycles through stress granules during stress," *Molecular Biology of the Cell*, vol. 19, no. 10, pp. 4469–4479, 2008.

[147] W. J. Kim, S. H. Back, V. Kim, I. Ryu, and S. K. Jang, "Sequestration of TRAF2 into stress granules interrupts tumor necrosis factor signaling under stress conditions," *Molecular and Cellular Biology*, vol. 25, no. 6, pp. 2450–2462, 2005.

[148] N. Kedersha and P. Anderson, "Mammalian stress granules and processing bodies," *Methods in Enzymology*, vol. 431, pp. 61–81, 2007.

[149] L. Weinmann, J. Höck, T. Ivacevic et al., "Importin 8 is a gene silencing factor that targets argonaute proteins to distinct mRNAs," *Cell*, vol. 136, no. 3, pp. 496–507, 2009.

[150] W.-L. Chang and W.-Y. Tarn, "A role for transportin in deposition of TTP to cytoplasmic RNA granules and mRNA decay," *Nucleic Acids Research*, vol. 37, no. 19, pp. 6600–6612, 2009.

[151] M. Ito, K. Miyado, K. Nakagawa et al., "Age-associated changes in the subcellular localization of phosphorylated p38 MAPK in human granulosa cells," *Molecular Human Reproduction*, vol. 16, no. 12, pp. 928–937, 2010.

[152] N. R. Leslie, "The redox regulation of PI 3-kinase-dependent signaling," *Antioxidants & Redox Signaling*, vol. 8, no. 9-10, pp. 1765–1774, 2006.

[153] P. Storz, "Reactive oxygen species-mediated mitochondria-to-nucleus signaling: a key to aging and radical-caused diseases," *Science's STKE*, vol. 2006, no. 332, p. re3, 2006.

[154] J.-F. L. Bodart, "Extracellular-regulated kinase—mitogen-activated protein kinase cascade: unsolved issues," *Journal of Cellular Biochemistry*, vol. 109, no. 5, pp. 850–857, 2010.

[155] L. T. May and S. J. Hill, "ERK phosphorylation: spatial and temporal regulation by G protein-coupled receptors," *The International Journal of Biochemistry & Cell Biology*, vol. 40, no. 10, pp. 2013–2017, 2008.

[156] B. Ananthanarayanan, Q. Ni, and J. Zhang, "Signal propagation from membrane messengers to nuclear effectors revealed by reporters of phosphoinositide dynamics and Akt activity," *Proceedings of the National Academy of Sciences of the United States of America*, vol. 102, no. 42, pp. 15081–15086, 2005.

[157] A. Kumar, J. Redondo-Muñoz, V. Perez-García, I. Cortes, M. Chagoyen, and A. C. Carrera, "Nuclear but not cytosolic phosphoinositide 3-kinase beta has an essential function in cell survival," *Molecular and Cellular Biology*, vol. 31, no. 10, pp. 2122–2133, 2011.

[158] M. Kodiha and U. Stochaj, "Targeting AMPK for therapeutic intervention in type 2 diabetes," in *Medical Complications of Type 2 Diabetes*, C. Croniger, Ed., InTech, 2011, http://www.intechopen.com/articles/show/title/targeting-ampk-for-therapeutic-intervention-in-type-2-diabetes.

[159] D. G. Hardie, "AMPK: a key regulator of energy balance in the single cell and the whole organism," *International Journal of Obesity*, vol. 32, supplement 4, pp. S7–S12, 2008.

[160] G. R. Steinberg and B. E. Kemp, "AMPK in health and disease," *Physiological Reviews*, vol. 89, no. 3, pp. 1025–1078, 2009.

[161] B. Viollet, S. Horman, J. Leclerc et al., "AMPK inhibition in health and disease," *Critical Reviews in Biochemistry & Molecular Biology*, vol. 45, no. 4, pp. 276–295, 2010.

[162] N. Kazgan, T. Williams, L. J. Forsberg, and J. E. Brenman, "Identification of a nuclear export signal in the catalytic subunit of AMP-activated protein kinase," *Molecular Biology of the Cell*, vol. 21, no. 19, pp. 3433–3442, 2010.

[163] W. Wang, X. Yang, T. Kawai et al., "AMP-activated protein kinase-regulated phosphorylation and acetylation of importin α1: involvement in the nuclear import of RNA-binding protein HuR," *Journal of Biological Chemistry*, vol. 279, no. 46, pp. 48376–48388, 2004.

[164] H. W. Lo and M. C. Hung, "Nuclear EGFR signalling network in cancers: linking EGFR pathway to cell cycle progression, nitric oxide pathway and patient survival," *The British Journal of Cancer*, vol. 94, no. 2, pp. 184–188, 2006.

[165] Y.-N. Wang, H. Yamaguchi, L. Huo et al., "The translocon Sec61β localized in the inner nuclear membrane transports membrane-embedded EGF receptor to the nucleus," *Journal of Biological Chemistry*, vol. 285, no. 49, pp. 38720–38729, 2010.

[166] H.-W. Lo, M. Ali-Seyed, Y. Wu, G. Bartholomeusz, S. C. Hsu, and M. C. Hung, "Nuclear-cytoplasmic transport of EGFR involves receptor endocytosis, importin β1 and CRM1," *Journal of Cellular Biochemistry*, vol. 98, no. 6, pp. 1570–1583, 2006.

[167] C.-J. Chang, D. J. Mulholland, B. Valamehr, S. Mosessian, W. R. Sellers, and H. Wu, "PTEN nuclear localization is regulated by oxidative stress and mediates p53-dependent tumor suppression," *Molecular and Cellular Biology*, vol. 28, no. 10, pp. 3281–3289, 2008.

[168] J.-L. Liu, Z. Mao, T. A. LaFortune et al., "Cell cycle-dependent nuclear export of phosphatase and tensin homologue tumor suppressor is regulated by the phosphoinositide-3-kinase signaling cascade," *Cancer Research*, vol. 67, no. 22, pp. 11054–11063, 2007.

[169] I. Dalle-Donne, G. Aldini, M. Carini, R. Colombo, R. Rossi, and A. Milzani, "Protein carbonylation, cellular dysfunction, and disease progression," *Journal of Cellular and Molecular Medicine*, vol. 10, no. 2, pp. 389–406, 2006.

[170] P. Wang, G.-H. Liu, K. Wu et al., "Repression of classical nuclear export by S-nitrosylation of CRM1," *Journal of Cell Science*, vol. 122, no. 20, pp. 3772–3779, 2009.

[171] E. Giannoni, M. L. Taddei, and P. Chiarugi, "Src redox regulation: again in the front line," *Free Radical Biology and Medicine*, vol. 49, no. 4, pp. 516–527, 2010.

[172] T. Adachi, D. R. Pimentel, T. Heibeck et al., "S-glutathiolation of Ras mediates redox-sensitive signaling by angiotensin II in vascular smooth muscle cells," *Journal of Biological Chemistry*, vol. 279, no. 28, pp. 29857–29862, 2004.

[173] A. Aghajanian, E. S. Wittchen, S. L. Campbell, and K. Burridge, "Direct activation of RhoA by reactive oxygen species requires a redox-sensitive motif," *PloS One*, vol. 4, no. 11, article e8045, 2009.

[174] N. Brandes, S. Schmitt, and U. Jakob, "Thiol-based redox switches in eukaryotic proteins," *Antioxidants & Redox Signaling*, vol. 11, no. 5, pp. 997–1014, 2009.

[175] E. Giannoni, F. Buricchi, G. Grimaldi et al., "Redox regulation of anoikis: reactive oxygen species as essential mediators of cell survival," *Cell Death & Differentiation*, vol. 15, no. 5, pp. 867–878, 2008.

[176] E. Giannoni, G. Raugei, P. Chiarugi, and G. Ramponi, "A novel redox-based switch: LMW-PTP oxidation enhances Grb2 binding and leads to ERK activation," *Biochemical &*

[177] C. Butkinaree, K. Park, and G. W. Hart, "O-linked β-N-acetylglucosamine (O-GlcNAc): extensive crosstalk with phosphorylation to regulate signaling and transcription in response to nutrients and stress," *Biochimica et Biophysica Acta—General Subjects*, vol. 1800, no. 2, pp. 96–106, 2010.

[178] R. M. Green, M. Graham, M. R. O'Donovan, J. K. Chipman, and N. J. Hodges, "Subcellular compartmentalization of glutathione: correlations with parameters of oxidative stress related to genotoxicity," *Mutagenesis*, vol. 21, no. 6, pp. 383–390, 2006.

[179] F. Johnson and C. Giulivi, "Superoxide dismutases and their impact upon human health," *Molecular Aspects of Medicine*, vol. 26, no. 4-5, pp. 340–352, 2005.

[180] M. Schrader and H. D. Fahimi, "Peroxisomes and oxidative stress," *Biochimica et Biophysica Acta—Molecular Cell Research*, vol. 1763, no. 12, pp. 1755–1766, 2006.

[181] P. D. Vivancos, Y. Dong, K. Ziegler et al., "Recruitment of glutathione into the nucleus during cell proliferation adjusts whole-cell redox homeostasis in Arabidopsis thaliana and lowers the oxidative defence shield," *The Plant Journal*, vol. 64, no. 5, pp. 825–838, 2010.

[182] J. Markovic, N. J. Mora, A. M. Broseta et al., "The depletion of nuclear glutathione impairs cell proliferation in 3t3 fibroblasts," *PLoS One*, vol. 4, no. 7, article e6413, 2009.

[183] K. Kamada, S. Goto, T. Okunaga et al., "Nuclear glutathione S-transferase π prevents apoptosis by reducing the oxidative stress-induced formation of exocyclic DNA products," *Free Radical Biology & Medicine*, vol. 37, no. 11, pp. 1875–1884, 2004.

[184] J. C. Young, J. M. Barral, and F. U. Hartl, "More than folding: localized functions of cytosolic chaperones," *Trends in Biochemical Sciences*, vol. 28, no. 10, pp. 541–547, 2003.

[185] P. Bański, M. Kodiha, and U. Stochaj, "Chaperones and multitasking proteins in the nucleolus: networking together for survival?" *Trends in Biochemical Sciences*, vol. 35, no. 7, pp. 361–367, 2010.

[186] P. Bański, M. Kodiha, and U. Stochaj, "Exploring the nuclear proteome: novel concepts for chaperone trafficking and function," *Current Proteomics*, vol. 8, no. 1, pp. 59–82, 2011.

[187] O. Huet, L. Dupic, A. Harrois, and J. Duranteau, "Oxidative stress and endothelial dysfunction during sepsis," *Frontiers in Bioscience*, vol. 16, no. 5, pp. 1986–1995, 2011.

[188] J. Pi, Q. Zhang, J. Fu et al., "ROS signaling, oxidative stress and Nrf2 in pancreatic beta-cell function," *Toxicology and Applied Pharmacology*, vol. 244, no. 1, pp. 77–83, 2010.

[189] V. Paupe, E. P. Dassa, S. Goncalves et al., "Impaired nuclear Nrf2 translocation undermines the oxidative stress response in Friedreich ataxia," *PLoS One*, vol. 4, no. 1, article e4253, 2009.

10

Dopamine D_2 Receptor-Mediated Heterologous Sensitization of AC5 Requires Signalosome Assembly

Karin F. K. Ejendal,[1] Carmen W. Dessauer,[2] Terence E. Hébert,[3] and Val J. Watts[1]

[1] Department of Medicinal Chemistry and Molecular Pharmacology, College of Pharmacy, Purdue University,
575 Stadium Mall Drive, West Lafayette, IN 47907-2051, USA

[2] Department of Integrative Biology and Pharmacology, University of Texas Health Science Center at Houston,
Houston, TX 77030, USA

[3] Department of Pharmacology Therapeutics, McGill University, McIntyre Medical Sciences Building, Montréal, QC, Canada H3G 1Y6

Correspondence should be addressed to Val J. Watts, wattsv@purdue.edu

Academic Editor: J. Adolfo García-Sáinz

Chronic dopamine receptor activation is implicated in several central nervous system disorders. Although acute activation of $G\alpha_i$-coupled D_2 dopamine receptors inhibits adenylyl cyclase, persistent activation enhances adenylyl cyclase activity, a phenomenon called heterologous sensitization. Previous work revealed a requirement for $G\alpha_s$ in D_2-induced heterologous sensitization of AC5. To elucidate the mechanism of $G\alpha_s$ dependency, we expressed $G\alpha_s$ mutants in $G\alpha_s$-deficient $Gnas^{E2-/E2-}$ cells. Neither $G\alpha_s$-palmitoylation nor $G\alpha_s$-$G\beta\gamma$ interactions were required for sensitization of AC5. Moreover, we found that coexpressing βARKct-CD8 or Sar1(H79G) blocked heterologous sensitization. These studies are consistent with a role for $G\alpha_s$-AC5 interactions in sensitization however, $G\beta\gamma$ appears to have an indirect role in heterologous sensitization of AC5, possibly by promoting proper signalosome assembly.

1. Introduction

Dopamine receptors and dopamine signaling have been implicated in various neurological and psychiatric disorders including Parkinson's disease, schizophrenia, and drug abuse [1–3]. Dopamine receptors are divided into two subfamilies, the $G\alpha_s$-coupled D_1 and D_5 receptors and the $G\alpha_{i/o}$-coupled D_2, D_3, and D_4 dopamine receptors that have stimulatory and inhibitory effects on adenylyl cyclase (AC), respectively (see [3] for a recent review). Acute stimulation of D_2 dopamine receptors leads to inhibition of AC activity, however, persistent activation of this $G\alpha_{i/o}$-coupled receptor paradoxically results in its enhancement [4]. This phenomenon, called heterologous sensitization of AC, is also known as cAMP overshoot, supersensitization, or superactivation of AC. D_2 dopamine receptor-induced heterologous sensitization of cyclic AMP signaling has been demonstrated in several cellular systems as well as in animal models and has also been suggested to occur in humans [4–6]. For

example, it was observed that repeated administration of the D_2 receptor agonist quinpirole enhances AC activity in the caudate putamen, increases CREB phosphorylation, and also alters behavior in rodents [5, 6]. Although this mode of AC regulation has been recognized for over three decades [7], the molecular signaling mechanism causing heterologous sensitization of AC is only partially understood, attributed to some extent to differences in AC isoform-specific regulation [4].

There are nine differentially regulated membrane-bound AC isoforms in mammalian cells [4, 8]. Whereas all AC isoforms are stimulated by stimulatory $G\alpha_s$, only a subset is inhibited by inhibitory $G\alpha_i$, and some AC isoforms are differentially regulated by $G\beta\gamma$ [4, 8]. Here, we studied human adenylyl cyclase type 5 (AC5) that is potently stimulated by $G\alpha_s$, inhibited by acute activation of $G\alpha_i$, and conditionally activated by $G\beta\gamma$ [8]. AC5 is expressed at high levels in the central nervous system and has been identified as a primary effector of D_2 dopamine receptors in the striatum [9, 10].

The aim of the current study was to investigate the role(s) of heterotrimeric G proteins in D_2 receptor-mediated heterologous sensitization of AC5. By exploring sensitization in cells devoid of endogenous $G\alpha_s$ [11], we were able to examine the ability of $G\alpha_s$ mutants to support sensitization without interference from endogenous $G\alpha_s$. Additionally, this $G\alpha_s$-deficient cellular model expresses very low levels of AC5 making them a reasonable model for studies of recombinant AC5 [12]. Heterologous sensitization of AC5 was readily rescued by wild-type $G\alpha_s$ and by mutants deficient in palmitoylation [13] or $G\beta\gamma$ interaction [14]. We also assessed the role of $G\beta\gamma$ and the signalosome in D_2 receptor-induced heterologous sensitization of AC5 by sequestering $G\beta\gamma$ subunits with βARKct-CD8 [15, 16] and coexpressing a dominant-negative mutant of the Sar1 GTPase [17]. These experiments revealed that both βARKct-CD8 and Sar1(H79G) attenuated sensitization, suggesting that the components of the signaling complex utilized in heterologous sensitization, presumably AC5 and $G\alpha_s$, assemble postsynthesis in the endoplasmic reticulum (ER). Together with previous findings, the present data support a model in which $G\alpha_s$ directly interacts with AC5. In contrast, $G\beta\gamma$ appears to have an indirect role in heterologous sensitization of AC5.

2. Materials and Methods

2.1. Constructs. The human D_{2L} receptor and AC5 or ΔAC5 [18] were cloned into the dual expression vector pBUDCE4 (Invitrogen, Carlsbad, CA) creating pBUD/hAC5, D_2R and pBUD/ΔAC5, D_2R. pcDNA3/βARKct-CD8 [15, 16] and pcDNA/vsvg-Sar1 (wild type and H79G) [19] were used. pcDNA1/$G\alpha_s$-CFP [20] was a gift from Dr. Catherine Berlot. The pcDNA3.1/$G\alpha_s$-IEK+ mutant [21] was a gift from Dr. Philip Wedegaertner. The C3S mutation was created by site-directed mutagenesis, and the fragment containing the IEK+ mutations was amplified by PCR. The resulting constructs, pcDNA1/$G\alpha_s$-CFP(C3S) and pcDNA1/$G\alpha_s$-CFP(IEK+) were sequenced.

2.2. Cell Culture and Transient Transfection. All reagents were purchased from Sigma-Aldrich (St. Louis, MO) unless otherwise noted. $G\alpha_s$-deficient murine embryonic fibroblast cells, $Gnas^{E2-/E2-}$ cells [11, 12], were a gift from Dr. Murat Bastepe. Cells were cultured in 50 : 50 mix of F12 : DMEM media supplemented with 5% FBS (HyClone, Logan, UT), 1% Ant-Anti (Invitrogen, Carlsbad, CA) in a humidified incubator at 33°C with 5% CO_2. Approximately 80,000 cells/well were seeded in 24-well plates the day before transient transfection. DNA (400 ng pBUD/hAC5 or ΔAC5, D_2R alone or in combination with 10 ng pcDNA/$G\alpha_s$-CFP, 300 ng pcDNA3/βARKct-CD8, or 300 ng pcDNA/vsvg-Sar1) was mixed with Opti-MEM and 1 μL/well Lipofectamine 2000 (Invitrogen, Carlsbad, CA). The medium was replaced with 200 μL/well prewarmed Opti-MEM, and the DNA/Lipofectamine mixture was added to the cells. After 4 hr, culture medium (500 μL/well) was added, and the cells were analyzed after 48 hr. For microscopy, the amount of pcDNA/$G\alpha_s$-CFP was increased to 100 ng/well.

2.3. Acute cAMP Accumulation. The assays were carried out in assay buffer (EBSS supplemented with 0.2% ascorbic acid, 15 mM HEPES, and 2% BCS (HyClone, Logan, UT), and 500 μM IBMX) with 100 nM forskolin (Tocris Bioscience, Ellisville, MO) as noted for 37°C for 15 min. The media was decanted, ice-cold trichloroacetic acid was added, and the lysates were stored at 4°C. Cyclic AMP was quantified using a competitive binding assay as described previously [22]. Data were collected from a minimum of three independent experiments carried out in duplicate and were normalized to either basal or vehicle conditions. The GraphPad Prism 5 software (GraphPad Software Inc., LaJolla, CA) was used for data and statistical analyses. A P value of $\leq$0.05 was considered statistically significant.

2.4. Heterologous Sensitization. The cells were pretreated with 1 μM quinpirole or vehicle in assay buffer (without IBMX) for 2 hr followed by three washes. cAMP was measured as described above for acute cAMP accumulation, with the addition of 1 μM spiperone to block the action of any residual quinpirole.

2.5. Microscopy. Cells were seeded in cover glass slides (Nunc, Rochester, NY). A 12 bit photometric CoolSNAP (Roper Scientific) CCD camera mounted on a TE-2000 inverted epifluorescence microscope (Nikon Instruments Inc., Melville, NY) with filters (ex. 500/20, em. 535/30) from Chroma (Rockingham, VT) was used. Images were acquired with the MetaMorph software (Molecular Devices, Sunnyvale, CA) and analyzed using Image J (http://rsbweb.nih.gov/ij/).

3. Results and Discussion

3.1. $G\alpha_s$ Mutants Rescue Heterologous Sensitization of AC5. Our laboratory has previously shown that mutants of canine AC5 that do not interact with $G\alpha_s$ are deficient in sensitization [23, 24] and that D_2-mediated heterologous sensitization of AC5 has an absolute requirement for $G\alpha_s$ [12]. Our present objective was to elucidate the mechanism of $G\alpha_s$-dependent heterologous sensitization of human AC5 by utilizing two different $G\alpha_s$-CFP [20] mutants (Figure 1(a)). The C3S substitution eliminates the N-terminal palmitoylation site, which causes $G\alpha_s$ to mislocalize to the cytosolic fraction [13]. The IEK+ mutant contains a series of substitutions, yielding a $G\beta\gamma$-binding deficient $G\alpha_s$ that also displays a reduction in palmitoylation [21].

The $G\alpha_s$-CFP constructs were coexpressed with AC5 and D_2. Since both C3S and IEK+ are deficient in responses to receptor stimulation [13, 21], we used direct stimulation of AC5 with forskolin throughout this study. Basal cAMP accumulation without any $G\alpha_s$ was 0.73 $\pm$ 0.09 pmol/ well, whereas co-expression of $G\alpha_s$-CFP increased cAMP accumulation to 3.12 $\pm$ 0.22 pmol/well (wild-type, wt), 4.22 $\pm$ 0.06 pmol/well (C3S), and 5.88$\pm$ 0.05 pmol/well (IEK+). Forskolin further stimulated cAMP with values 2.5–3-fold over basal levels (Figure 1(b)), indicating that wild-type and both $G\alpha_s$ mutants functionally couple to AC5.

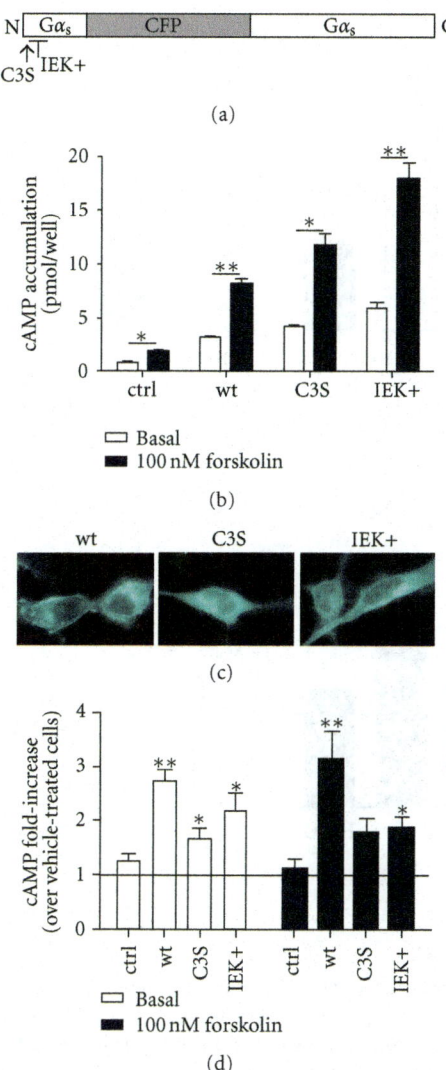

FIGURE 1: Gα_s-CFP mutants are functional and rescue heterologous sensitization of AC5. (a) Schematic of Gα_s-CFP constructs. (b) Acute cAMP accumulation in cells expressing AC5 and D$_2$ alone (ctrl) or in combination with 10 ng Gα_s-CFP (wild type, C3S, or IEK+) was measured under basal (open bars) or forskolin-stimulated conditions (black bars). $**= P < 0.01$, $*= P < 0.05$, using a paired, one-tailed t-test comparing basal and forskolin-stimulated values. (c) Expression and localization of Gα_s-CFP mutants. (d) Heterologous sensitization of AC5 in cells expressing AC5 and D$_2$ in the absence or presence of Gα_s-CFP. Data shown represent fold-increase of cAMP accumulation observed in quinpirole-treated cells. $**= P < 0.01$, $*= P < 0.05$, using a one-sample, two-tailed t-test comparing ctrl to each Gα_s-CFP construct.

Next, expression and subcellular localization of the Gα_s-CFP constructs (in the presence of AC5 and D$_2$) were evaluated by fluorescence microscopy (Figure 1(c)). Wild-type Gα_s-CFP showed both plasma membrane and intracellular localization, whereas the C3S and IEK+ mutants were predominantly localized intracellularly (Figure 1(c)), consistent with previous reports [14, 21].

To assess whether the Gα_s-CFP mutants could rescue heterologous sensitization, cells were pretreated with vehicle or quinpirole followed by cAMP accumulation. Consistent with our previous report [12], no sensitization of AC5 was observed in the absence of Gα_s (Figure 1(d), ctrl). In contrast, coexpression of wild-type Gα_s-CFP resulted in robust sensitization of AC5 under both basal and forskolin-stimulated conditions (Figure 1(d)). Surprisingly, expression of the Gα_s mutants also significantly rescued heterologous sensitization under basal conditions (white bars) and to a lesser degree forskolin-stimulated conditions (black bars). As both mutants are deficient in palmitoylation and membrane localization, neither palmitoylation *per se*, nor membrane localization of Gα_s appears to be essential for heterologous sensitization of AC5.

3.2. Role of G$\beta\gamma$ Subunits in Heterologous Sensitization of AC5. Although we have established that Gα_s is required for heterologous sensitization, our findings above for the IEK+ mutant suggest that direct interactions between Gα_s and G$\beta\gamma$ are not critical. This prompted us to further investigate the role of G$\beta\gamma$ in D$_2$ receptor-mediated heterologous sensitization of AC5. The C-terminus of β-adrenergic kinase or GRK2 (βARKct) has been used to sequester G$\beta\gamma$ subunits and inhibit G$\beta\gamma$-mediated signaling events, including heterologous sensitization [15, 25, 26]. In the absence of βARKct-CD8 (membrane bound βARKct), AC5 displayed robust heterologous sensitization (open bars, Figure 2(a)). Sequestering G$\beta\gamma$ blocked sensitization of AC5, under both basal and forskolin-stimulated conditions, revealing the necessity of G$\beta\gamma$ for heterologous sensitization of AC5 (black bars, Figure 2(a)). In contrast, βARKct-CD8 had no substantial effects on acute D$_2$ receptor activation; quinpirole produced significant inhibition of cAMP accumulation in the presence of βARKct-CD8 ($77 \pm 10\%$ inhibition; $n = 2$, data not shown). In an effort to explore the site of action for G$\beta\gamma$-dependent sensitization, we used an N-terminal deletion mutant of AC5, ΔAC5. This mutant is functional and responds to Gα_s stimulation but is deficient in binding G$\beta\gamma$ [18]. The ΔAC5 mutant displayed significant sensitization that was also blocked by βARKct-CD8 (Figure 2(b)), suggesting that N-terminal G$\beta\gamma$ binding is not intimately involved in heterologous sensitization of AC5. Instead, there are clearly additional, unidentified G$\beta\gamma$ interaction sites in AC5 that are necessary for heterologous sensitization. Such an assumption is supported by FRET and *in vitro* activation studies of the AC5 deletion mutant [18] as well as studies of AC2, which possesses multiple motifs for G$\beta\gamma$ interaction and regulation that are located in the C1b and C2b domains of AC2 [27]. Other possibilities are that ΔAC5 interacts with endogenous AC isoforms in an AC dimer (see [28]) that binds G$\beta\gamma$ or that specific Gβ and Gγ subunits or G$\beta\gamma$ pairs are involved. However, it is also possible that the G$\beta\gamma$ mechanisms involving sensitization of AC may be indirect [4].

3.3. Disruption of Signalosome Assembly Affects Heterologous Sensitization of AC5. Because sequestering G$\beta\gamma$ subunits alters signalosome assembly [15], we hypothesized that a specific signaling complex could be required for heterologous sensitization of AC5. Several small GTPases, including Sar1,

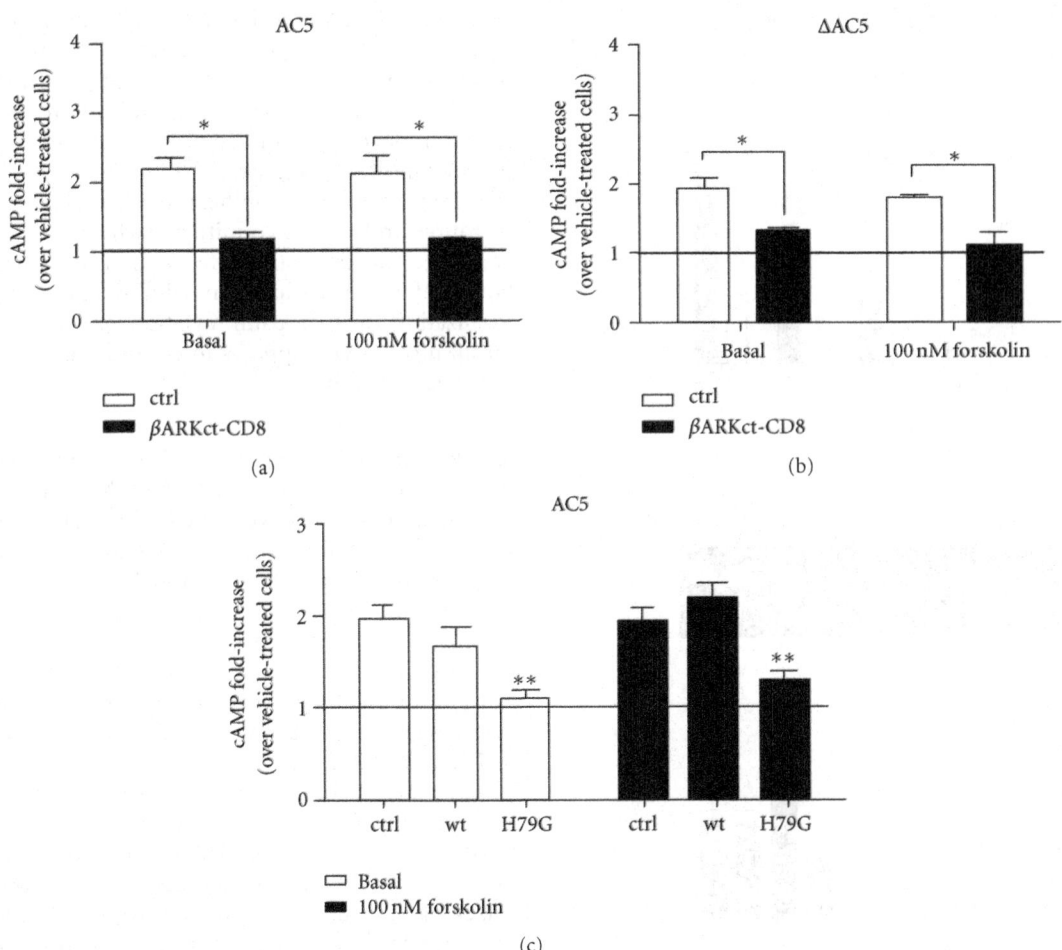

FIGURE 2: Sequestration of $G\beta\gamma$ with βARKct-CD8 or coexpression of dominant negative Sar1(H79G) attenuate heterologous sensitization of AC5. Cells expressing $G\alpha_s$-CFP, D_2R and (a and c) AC5 or (b) ΔAC5 in combination with either empty vector (ctrl), (a-b) βARKct-CD8, or (c) indicated Sar1 construct. Data shown represent the fold-increase of cAMP accumulation observed in quinpirole-treated cells. (a-b) *=$P < 0.05$, using a paired, one-tailed t-test. (c) **=$P < 0.01$, using a one-way ANOVA and Dunnett's *post hoc* test, comparing ctrl to Sar1(wt) or Sar1(H79G).

are involved in signal complex assembly and anterograde protein trafficking [29]. A series of studies using dominant negative mutants of these GTPases shows that $G\alpha_s$ and $G\beta\gamma$ interact with AC2 during trafficking to the plasma membrane [30, 31] and that the $G\alpha_s$-AC2 interaction is disrupted by Sar1(H79G) [30].

To study the possibility that interactions between AC5 and its specific signaling partners play a role, we utilized Sar1 and Sar1(H79G) and noted that coexpression with the dominant negative mutant prevented heterologous sensitization of AC5 (Figure 2(c)). In contrast, acute D_2 receptor-mediated inhibition of AC5 was not significantly blocked in the presence of Sar1(H79G) (data not shown). Our data are consistent with the findings that Sar1(H79G) disrupts AC-$G\alpha_s$ interactions (as measured by BRET or coimmuno-precipitation) to a larger degree than AC-$G\alpha_i$ interactions [30]. In contrast, Sar1(H79G) did not affect the interactions between AC and $G\beta\gamma$ [30], suggesting that the AC interacts with $G\beta\gamma$ at an early step in the endoplasmic reticulum (ER), but that the interaction with $G\alpha_s$ occurs after ER export. The observation that signaling mechanisms of acute activity and

heterologous sensitization are differentially affected further supports the hypothesis that heterologous sensitization and acute stimulation are dependent on separate mechanisms and possibly separate signalosome components.

4. Conclusion

The present data support a complex model of D_2 dopamine receptor-induced heterologous sensitization of AC5 where $G\alpha_s$ appears to directly interact with AC5. A role for $G\beta\gamma$ was confirmed; however, our observations suggest an indirect role for $G\beta\gamma$ that may be involved during the formation of the sensitization signaling complex. A critical role for AC5 in mediating dopamine responses has been previously demonstrated in AC5 deficient mice, which show impaired responses to D_2 receptor activation [9]. Therefore, these results have implications in brain regions where D_2 dopamine receptors and AC5 are coexpressed, such as the striatum [32], which is implicated in drug addiction, motivation, mood, and voluntary movement. Persistent D_2 dopamine receptor activation has also been linked to psychiatric disorders (e.g., schizophrenia and drug abuse) and to the adaptive responses associated with drug therapy in Parkinson's disease. Enhancing our understanding of the underlying components and mechanisms of heterologous sensitization and regulation of specific AC activity (in the striatum) may aid in the development of improved and future therapies for these disorders. For example, recent studies have identified small molecule inhibitors of G$\beta\gamma$-mediated signaling [33] and AC isoform-specific inhibitors [34] that may offer novel therapeutic strategies for modulating complex CNS behaviors involving dopamine receptor signaling.

Abbreviations

AC: Adenylyl cyclase
cAMP: Cyclic adenosine monophosphate
CFP: Cyan fluorescent protein
D$_2$R: Dopamine D$_{2L}$ receptor
GPCR: G protein-coupled receptor
βARKct: β-adrenergic kinase c-terminus
ER: Endoplasmic reticulum

Acknowledgments

This work was supported by Purdue University and by NIH grants MH060397 (V. J. Watts) and GM60419 (C. W. Dessauer). T. E. Hebért is a Chercheur National of the Fonds de la Recherche en Santé du Québec (FRSQ). The authors would like to thank Dr. Pierre-Alexandre Vidi for help with cloning of constructs. They would also like to thank Jason Conley and Elisabeth Garland-Kuntz for proofreading and making suggestions to improve the present paper.

References

[1] S. D. Iversen and L. L. Iversen, "Dopamine: 50 years in perspective," *Trends in Neurosciences*, vol. 30, no. 5, pp. 188–193, 2007.

[2] B. Le Foll, A. Gallo, Y. L. Strat, L. Lu, and P. Gorwood, "Genetics of dopamine receptors and drug addiction: a comprehensive review," *Behavioural Pharmacology*, vol. 20, no. 1, pp. 1–17, 2009.

[3] J.-M. Beaulieu and R. R. Gainetdinov, "The physiology, signaling, and pharmacology of dopamine receptors," *Pharmacological Reviews*, vol. 63, no. 1, pp. 182–217, 2011.

[4] V. J. Watts and K. A. Neve, "Sensitization of adenylate cyclase by Gαi/o-coupled receptors," *Pharmacology and Therapeutics*, vol. 106, no. 3, pp. 405–421, 2005.

[5] J. A. Chester, A. J. Mullins, C. H. Nguyen, V. J. Watts, and R. L. Meisel, "Repeated quinpirole treatments produce neurochemical sensitization and associated behavioral changes in female hamsters," *Psychopharmacology*, vol. 188, no. 1, pp. 53–62, 2006.

[6] K. E. Culm, A. M. Lim, J. A. Onton, and R. P. Hammer, "Reduced Gi and Go protein function in the rat nucleus accumbens attenuates sensorimotor gating deficits," *Brain Research*, vol. 982, no. 1, pp. 12–18, 2003.

[7] S. K. Sharma, W. A. Klee, and M. Nirenberg, "Dual regulation of adenylate cyclase accounts for narcotic dependence and tolerance," *Proceedings of the National Academy of Sciences of the United States of America*, vol. 72, no. 8, pp. 3092–3096, 1975.

[8] X. Gao, R. Sadana, C. W. Dessauer, and T. B. Patel, "Conditional stimulation of type V and VI adenylyl cyclases by G protein $\beta\gamma$ subunits," *Journal of Biological Chemistry*, vol. 282, no. 1, pp. 294–302, 2007.

[9] K. W. Lee, J. H. Hong, I. Y. Choi et al., "Impaired D$_2$ dopamine receptor function in mice lacking type 5 adenylyl cyclase," *Journal of Neuroscience*, vol. 22, no. 18, pp. 7931–7940, 2002.

[10] T. Iwamoto, S. Okumura, K. Iwatsubo et al., "Motor dysfunction in type 5 adenylyl cyclase-null mice," *Journal of Biological Chemistry*, vol. 278, no. 19, pp. 16936–16940, 2003.

[11] M. Bastepe, Y. Gunes, B. Perez-Villamil, J. Hunzelman, L. S. Weinstein, and H. Jüppner, "Receptor-mediated adenylyl cyclase activation through XLαs, the extra-large variant of the stimulatory G protein α-subunit," *Molecular Endocrinology*, vol. 16, no. 8, pp. 1912–1919, 2002.

[12] T. A. Vortherms, C. H. Nguyen, M. Bastepe, H. Jüppner, and V. J. Watts, "D$_2$ dopamine receptor-induced sensitization of adenylyl cyclase type 1 is Gαs independent," *Neuropharmacology*, vol. 50, no. 5, pp. 576–584, 2006.

[13] P. B. Wedegaertner, D. H. Chu, P. T. Wilson, M. J. Levis, and H. R. Bourne, "Palmitoylation is required for signaling functions and membrane attachment of G(q)α and G(s)α," *Journal of Biological Chemistry*, vol. 268, no. 33, pp. 25001–25008, 1993.

[14] D. S. Evanko, M. M. Thiyagarajan, D. P. Siderovski, and P. B. Wedegaertner, "G$\beta\gamma$ isoforms selectively rescue plasma membrane localization and palmitoylation of mutant Gα_s and Gα_q," *Journal of Biological Chemistry*, vol. 276, no. 26, pp. 23945–23953, 2001.

[15] D. J. Dupré, M. Robitaille, R. V. Rebois, and T. E. Hébert, "The role of G$\beta\gamma$ subunits in the organization, assembly, and function of GPCR signaling complexes," *Annual Review of Pharmacology and Toxicology*, vol. 49, pp. 31–56, 2009.

[16] P. Crespo, T. G. Cachero, N. Xu, and J. S. Gutkind, "Dual effect of β-adrenergic receptors on mitogen-activated protein kinase. Evidence for a $\beta\gamma$-dependent activation and a Gα(s)-cAMP-mediated inhibition," *Journal of Biological Chemistry*, vol. 270, no. 42, pp. 25259–25265, 1995.

[17] D. J. Dupré, M. Robitaille, N. Éthier, L. R. Villeneuve, A. M. Mamarbachi, and T. E. Hébert, "Seven transmembrane receptor core signaling complexes are assembled prior to plasma membrane trafficking," *Journal of Biological Chemistry*, vol. 281, no. 45, pp. 34561–34573, 2006.

[18] R. Sadana, N. Dascal, and C. W. Dessauer, "N terminus of type 5 adenylyl cyclase scaffolds Gs heterotrimer," *Molecular Pharmacology*, vol. 76, no. 6, pp. 1256–1264, 2009.

[19] M. Robitaille, N. Ramakrishnan, A. Baragli, and T. E. Hébert, "Intracellular trafficking and assembly of specific Kir3 channel/G protein complexes," *Cellular Signalling*, vol. 21, no. 4, pp. 488–501, 2009.

[20] T. R. Hynes, S. M. Mervine, E. A. Yost, J. L. Sabo, and C. H. Berlot, "Live cell imaging of Gs and the β2-adrenergic receptor demonstrates that both αs and β 1γ7 internalize upon stimulation and exhibit similar trafficking patterns that differ from that of the β2-adrenergic receptor," *Journal of Biological Chemistry*, vol. 279, no. 42, pp. 44101–44112, 2004.

[21] D. S. Evanko, M. M. Thiyagarajan, and P. B. Wedegaertner, "Interaction with G$\beta\gamma$ is required for membrane targeting and palmitoylation of Gα(s) and Gα(q)," *Journal of Biological Chemistry*, vol. 275, no. 2, pp. 1327–1336, 2000.

[22] J. A. Przybyla and V. J. Watts, "Ligand-induced regulation and localization of cannabinoid CB1 and dopamine D$_2$L recep-

tor heterodimers," *Journal of Pharmacology and Experimental Therapeutics*, vol. 332, no. 3, pp. 710–719, 2009.

[23] V. J. Watts, R. Taussig, R. L. Neve, and K. A. Neve, "Dopamine D_2 receptor-induced heterologous sensitization of adenylyl cyclase requires Gαs: characterization of Gαs-insensitive mutants of adenylyl cyclase V," *Molecular Pharmacology*, vol. 60, no. 6, pp. 1168–1172, 2001.

[24] G. Zimmermann, D. Zhou, and R. Taussig, "Genetic selection of mammalian adenylyl cyclases insensitive to stimulation by G(sα)," *Journal of Biological Chemistry*, vol. 273, no. 12, pp. 6968–6975, 1998.

[25] C. H. Nguyen and V. J. Watts, "Dexras1 blocks receptor-mediated heterologous sensitization of adenylyl cyclase 1," *Biochemical and Biophysical Research Communications*, vol. 332, no. 3, pp. 913–920, 2005.

[26] T. Avidor-Reiss, I. Nevo, R. Levy, T. Pfeuffer, and Z. Vogel, "Chronic opioid treatment induces adenylyl cyclase V superactivation. Involvement of G($\beta\gamma$)," *Journal of Biological Chemistry*, vol. 271, no. 35, pp. 21309–21315, 1996.

[27] S. Weitmann, G. Schultz, and C. Kleuss, "Adenylyl cyclase type II domains involved in G$\beta\gamma$ stimulation," *Biochemistry*, vol. 40, no. 36, pp. 10853–10858, 2001.

[28] A. Baragli, M. L. Grieco, P. Trieu, L. R. Villeneuve, and T. E. Hébert, "Heterodimers of adenylyl cyclases 2 and 5 show enhanced functional responses in the presence of Gαs," *Cellular Signalling*, vol. 20, no. 3, pp. 480–492, 2008.

[29] D. J. Dupré and T. E. Hébert, "Biosynthesis and trafficking of seven transmembrane receptor signalling complexes," *Cellular Signalling*, vol. 18, no. 10, pp. 1549–1559, 2006.

[30] D. J. Dupré, A. Baragli, R. V. Rebois, N. Éthier, and T. E. Hébert, "Signalling complexes associated with adenylyl cyclase II are assembled during their biosynthesis," *Cellular Signalling*, vol. 19, no. 3, pp. 481–489, 2007.

[31] R. V. Rebois, M. Robitaille, C. Galés et al., "Heterotrimeric G proteins form stable complexes with adenylyl cyclase and Kir3.1 channels in living cells," *Journal of Cell Science*, vol. 119, no. 13, pp. 2807–2818, 2006.

[32] P. D. Gortari and G. Mengod, "Dopamine D_1, D_2 and mu-opioid receptors are co-expressed with adenylyl cyclase 5 and phosphodiesterase 7B mRNAs in striatal rat cells," *Brain Research*, vol. 1310, pp. 37–45, 2010.

[33] A. L. Dessal, R. Prades, E. Giralt, and A. V. Smrcka, "Rational design of a selective covalent modifier of G protein $\beta\gamma$ subunits," *Molecular Pharmacology*, vol. 79, no. 1, pp. 24–33, 2011.

[34] H. Wang, H. Xu, L. J. Wu et al., "Identification of an adenylyl cyclase inhibitor for treating neuropathic and inflammatory pain," *Science Translational Medicine*, vol. 3, no. 65, article 65ra3, 2011.

11

An Fc Gamma Receptor-Mediated Upregulation of the Production of Interleukin 10 by Intravenous Immunoglobulin in Bone-Marrow-Derived Mouse Dendritic Cells Stimulated with Lipopolysaccharide *In Vitro*

Akihiro Fujii, Yuko Kase, Chiaki Suzuki, Akihito Kamizono, and Teruaki Imada

Japan Blood Products Organization, Central Research Laboratory, Protein Pharmacology Research Section,
1-5-2 Minatojima Minami-machi, Chuo-ku, Kobe, Hyogo 650-0047, Japan

Correspondence should be addressed to Akihiro Fujii; fujii-akihiro@jbpo.or.jp

Academic Editor: Rudi Beyaert

Intravenous immunoglobulin (IVIG), a highly purified immunoglobulin fraction prepared from pooled plasma of several thousand donors, increased anti-inflammatory cytokine IL-10 production, while decreased proinflammatory cytokine IL-12p70 production in bone-marrow-derived mouse dendritic cells (BMDCs) stimulated with lipopolysaccharide (LPS). The changes of cytokine production were confirmed with the transcription levels of these cytokines. To study the mechanisms of this bidirectional effect, we investigated changes of intracellular molecules in the LPS-induced signaling pathway and observed that IVIG upregulated ERK1/2 phosphorylation while downregulated p38 MAPK phosphorylation. Using chemical inhibitors specific to protein kinases involved in activation of Fc gamma receptors (FcγRs), which mediate IgG signals, we found that hyperphosphorylation of ERK1/2 and Syk phosphorylation occurred after stimulation of BMDC with LPS and IVIG, and the increasing effect on IL-10 production was abolished by these inhibitors. Furthermore, an antibody specific to FcγRI, one of FcγRs involved in immune activation, inhibited IVIG-induced increases in IL-10 production, but not IL-12p70 decreases, whereas the anti-IL-10 antibody restored the decrease in IL-12p70 induced by IVIG. These findings suggest that IVIG induced the upregulation of IL-10 production through FcγRI activation, and IL-10 was indispensable to the suppressing effect of IVIG on the production of IL-12p70 in LPS-stimulated BMDC.

1. Introduction

Dendritic cells (DCs) are potent and specialized antigen presenting cells and important regulators of innate and adaptive immunity with the ability to induce T cell activation or its suppression. After the migration from peripheral tissues to the lymphoid organs, DCs trigger immune responses by secreting proinflammatory and anti-inflammatory cytokines to regulate T cell polarization [1, 2]. Bone-marrow-derived mouse dendritic cells (BMDCs) produce proinflammatory cytokine IL-12p70 and anti-inflammatory cytokine IL-10 when stimulated with LPS [3]. Development and proliferation of type 1 effector helper T cells (Th1) is known to be under the influence of IL-12p70. IL-12p70 activates NK and T cells and its production is inhibited by IL-10 [4, 5].

DC maturation is impaired by IL-10, and Th1-mediated immune responses are attenuated by immature DC [6, 7]. It is thought to be an important role of DC to control the balance between the development of effector and regulatory helper T cells in determination of the direction toward efficient immunosuppression and immune activation.

Intravenous immunoglobulin (IVIG) is a highly purified immunoglobulin (IgG) fraction prepared from pooled plasma of several thousand donors and, based on its immunoregulatory role, is widely applied for the therapy of inflammatory and autoimmune diseases [8]. IgG consists of two major functional regions, Fab and Fc. The Fab region is mainly responsible for antigen binding including the blockade of certain receptors and neutralization of bacterial toxins, autoantibodies, or cytokines. The Fc region couples the antibody to IgG receptors, named Fc gamma receptors (FcγRs), of the innate immune effector cells, such as neutrophils, mast cells, macrophages, and dendritic cells [8]. Although the precise mechanisms of the regulatory functions of IVIG in the immune system have not been cleared yet, several mechanisms of action have been proposed, such as the interaction of an anti-idiotypic antibody, modulation of cytokine production, inhibition of T-cell proliferation, and modulation of serum complement action on target cells [9–11].

Bayry et al. reported an interesting bidirectional effect of IVIG [12]. They showed that IVIG inhibited the production of IL-12p70 and stimulated the secretion of IL-10 in LPS-activated human monocyte-derived dendritic cells (mo-DC). As a consequence, in the presence of IVIG during mo-DC maturation or developmental stages, the T-cell stimulatory activity of mo-DC is impaired and its T-cell suppressive function appears [12]. The mechanisms of this bidirectional effect of IVIG on cytokine production are not clear. To understand the immunoregulatory function of IVIG more clearly, we focused on the relationship between this modulatory effect of IVIG on cytokine production and its actions on the signaling pathway in mouse BMDC stimulated with LPS.

LPS signal is mediated by the transmembrane receptor, Toll-like receptor 4 (TLR4), for the induction of cytokine production in immune cells [13]. The LPS-triggered TLR4 activation induces the phosphorylation of intracellular signaling proteins including transcription factor NFκ-B and members of the extracellular signal-regulated kinases (ERKs) family, ERK1/2, p38 MAPK, and c-Jun N-terminal kinase (JNK). Activation of TLR4 is necessary for the maturation and functional responses of BMDC including cytokine production, phagocytosis, antigen presentation, and T-cell activation/suppression [14, 15]. Because IVIG contains a wide range of antibodies that harbor a broad repertoire of antigen binding variable regions present in normal serum, an LPS-binding fraction in IVIG is a possible factor that blocks TLR4 signaling and reduces cytokine production in DC stimulated with LPS [16]. However, it is difficult to explain that only an inhibition of TLR4 signaling results in the upregulation of cytokine production in these LPS-stimulated cells.

BMDCs express two general classes of FcγRs [17]. One is activation receptors, the high affinity receptor FcγRI (CD64) and the low affinity receptor FcγRIII (CD16), which mediate activating functions in immune responses. The α-chain of these two activation receptors associates with the cell-signaling common γ-chain (FcRγ) subunit containing the immunoreceptor tyrosine-based activation motif (ITAM), and ITAM is indispensable in the immune responses after receptor activation. The other is the inhibitory receptor FcγRIIB (CD32B) containing the immunoreceptor tyrosine-based inhibitory motif (ITIM) within the sequence and it has been shown to be critical for its inhibitory function [17]. In the case of signal transduction by FcγR after its engagement with immune complexes, the activation of several molecules in the signaling cascade of ITAM including ERK family kinases occurs and this is an important step for immune responses mediated by FcγR activation [18, 19]. The molecular targets of IVIG in immune modulation are not

clear; however, activation and inhibitory FcγRs are promising candidates through which IVIG triggers receptor functions and modulates immune responses.

To investigate the mechanisms of modulatory effect of IVIG on the cytokine production, we hypothesized that IVIG could affect the signaling pathway of FcγR as well as TLR-4 signal transduction in LPS-stimulated BMDC, which may affect cytokine production in these cells. In this study, we investigated changes in FcγR-mediated signaling molecules and cytokine production when cells were activated by LPS in the presence of IVIG and found that FcγRI activation was necessary to enhance IL-10 production in LPS-stimulated BMDC by IVIG.

2. Materials and Methods

2.1. Reagents and Antibodies. Venoglobulin-IH (Japan Blood Products Organization, Tokyo, Japan), which is used as an intravenous immunoglobulin (IVIG), was dialyzed against phosphate-buffered saline (PBS) at 4°C for one day and filtered through a $0.22\,\mu$m membrane (Millipore, Temecula, CA). Lipopolysaccharide (LPS) from *Escherichia coli* serotype O55:B5 and penicillin/streptomycin were purchased from Sigma (St. Louis, MO). LPS was used at a concentration of 500 ng/mL or $1\,\mu$g/mL. Fetal calf serum (FCS) was obtained from Gibco (Rockville, MD). Recombinant murine granulocyte-macrophage colony-stimulating factor (rmGM-CSF) was purchased from PeproTech (Rocky Hill, NJ). The culture medium was RPMI1640 supplemented with penicillin (100 u/mL), streptomycin (100 μg/mL), and 10% heat-inactivated FCS. Human pooled plasma was prepared by Japan Blood Products Organization and used after heat inactivation. Protein tyrosine kinase inhibitors, piceatannol for Syk and PP2 for Hck/Lyn, were purchased from Wako (Osaka, Japan) and Enzo (Plymouth Meeting, PA), respectively [20–22].

For immunoblotting, monoclonal rabbit antinuclear factor kappa (NFκ-B) p65 (C22B4), monoclonal rabbit anti-phospho-NFκ-B p65 (Ser536, 93H1), polyclonal rabbit anti-p38, monoclonal mouse anti-phospho-p38 (Thr180/Tyr182, 28B10), monoclonal rabbit antiextracellular signal-regulated kinase 1/2 (ERK1/2, 137F5), monoclonal rabbit anti-phospho-ERK1/2 (Thr202/Tyr204, D13.14.4E), monoclonal rabbit anti-c-Jun N-terminal kinase (JNK, 56G8), monoclonal mouse anti-phospho-JNK (Thr183/Tyr185, G9), and polyclonal rabbit anti-phospho-Syk (Tyr525/526) were purchased from Cell Signaling Technology (Danvers, MA) and were used for 1,000 times in dilution. Monoclonal mouse anti-Syk (SYK-01, 1:1,000) was from EXBIO (Vestec u Prahy, Czech). Horseradish-peroxidase- (HRP-) conjugated, monoclonal mouse anti-phosphotyrosine antibody (4G10 Platinum, 1:1,000) was from Millipore. HRP-conjugated goat anti-mouse IgG and HRP-conjugated goat anti-rabbit IgG (number 7074, 1:1,000) were purchased from DAKO (Glostrup, Denmark) and Cell Signaling Technology, respectively. All other materials used in this study were of reagent grade.

2.2. Mice. C57BL/6 female mice were purchased from Charles River Laboratories (Kanagawa, Japan) and were maintained under specific pathogen-free conditions in accordance with the ethics and safety guidelines for animal experiments of Japan Blood Products Organization.

2.3. Preparation and Culture of BMDC.

2.3. Preparation and Culture of BMDC. Methods for the preparation of BMDC were performed according to Lutz et al. with some modifications [23]. Briefly, on day 0, bone marrow cells prepared from the femurs and tibiae of 7–9-week-old female mice were adjusted to 2×10^5/mL in 10 mL culture medium containing rmGM-CSF (20 ng/mL) and were maintained in 100 mm dishes (Asahi Glass, Tokyo, Japan) at 37°C in a humidified incubator with 5% CO_2. On day 2, another 10 mL of culture medium supplemented with rmGM-CSF was added to these plates. On day 4 or 5, half of the medium was centrifuged and cells were suspended in 10 mL fresh culture medium containing rmGM-CSF and were returned to the original plates. On day 7 or 8, cells were collected and used as BMDC. At this point, over 90% of CD11c expression was confirmed by cell surface maker analysis using an FC500 flow cytometer (Beckman-Coulter, Miami, FL).

2.4. Cytokine Production and Treatment with the Anti-FcγRI Antibody or Anti-IL-10 Antibody. Cells (5×10^5/mL) were cultured in 48 well plates (0.5 mL/well, Asahi Glass) with or without LPS (500 ng/mL) for 6 h and 18 h. IVIG was added simultaneously at concentrations of 2.5, 5, and 10 mg/mL according to our previous study with some modifications [24]. Cell culture supernatants were assayed for IL-10 and IL-12p70 concentrations by an enzyme-linked immunosorbent assay (ELISA) using the Quantikine mouse IL-10 immunoassay and mouse IL-12p70 immunoassay (R&D Systems, Minneapolis, MN, USA), respectively, according to manufacturer's procedures. In our study, without LPS stimulation, IL-10 and IL-12p70 concentrations in the culture medium of cells were under the lower limits of the standard ELISA curves (lower limit values of standard curves of ELISA were 15.6 pg/mL for IL-10 and 7.8 pg/mL for IL-12p70). IVIG (2.5–10 mg/mL) showed no production of either cytokine in cells without LPS stimulation. IVIG did not inhibit the cell growth *in vitro*.

To test whether FcγRI was involved in the increase in IL-10 by IVIG, the rat monoclonal anti-mouse FcγRI/CD64 antibody (290322, R&D systems, Minneapolis, MN) and a matched control antibody (rat IgG$_{2A}$, R&D systems) at a concentration of 1 μg/mL were added to the culture medium of cells in the presence or absence of IVIG (10 mg/mL) and were stimulated with LPS (500 ng/mL) for 18 h. To study the effects of the anti-IL-10 antibody on the production of IL-12p70, cells were stimulated with LPS (1 μg/mL) in the presence or absence of IVIG (5 mg/mL) and the rat monoclonal ant-mouse IL-10 (1 μg/mL, JES5-25A, Southern Biotech, Birmingham, AL) or a matched control antibody (rat IgG$_1$, Southern Biotech) for 18 h. Supernatants were collected and cytokine production was assayed in the same manner as that described earlier.

2.5. Effects of Protein Tyrosine Kinase Inhibitors on IL-10 Production. Cells (5×10^5/mL) were stimulated with LPS

(500 ng/mL) in the presence or absence of IVIG (10 mg/mL) and protein tyrosine kinase inhibitors for 18 h. Cytokine production in the culture supernatant was measured as described earlier. The concentrations of the inhibitors used were 5 μM for piceatannol and 0.05 μM for PP2, respectively. These concentrations effectively inhibited the phosphorylation of the respective kinase [20–22].

2.6. Quantitative-PCR of IL-10, IL-12a, and IL-12b mRNAs. Cells (5×10^5/mL) were stimulated with or without LPS (500 ng/mL) in the presence or absence of IVIG in 48 well plates for 6 h and 18 h. The expressions of IL-10 mRNA and IL-12a and IL-12b mRNA, which codes the IL-12p35 and IL-12p40 subunit of IL-12p70, respectively, were measured by a quantitative reverse transcription-polymerase chain reaction (RT-PCR) using a 7500 Real-Time PCR System (Applied Biosystems, Foster City, CA). Briefly, total RNA was extracted from cells using the PureLink RNA Mini kit and Turbo DNA-free kit (Life Technologies, Carlsbad, CA) and cDNA was constructed by the High Capacity RNA-to-cDNA kit (Applied Biosystems). Real-time PCR was subsequently performed using TaqMan Gene Expression Assays (Applied Biosystems), sequence specific primers, and probes according to the manufacturer's protocol. The expression of each mRNA was standardized to GAPDH mRNA, and they were expressed as ratios to the mean value for cells without stimulation. Each mRNA expression was analyzed by the ∆∆Ct method as per the manufacturer's instructions [25]. The following sequence specific primers and probes were used for real-time PCR: IL-10, Mm01288386_m1; IL-12a, Mm00434169_m1; IL-12b, Mm01288993_m1; GAPDH, TaqMan Rodent GAPDH control reagents (Applied Biosystems).

2.7. Immunoblot and Immunoprecipitation. Immunoblot assays were performed as described next.

Cells ($0.5–1 \times 10^6$/mL) were treated with LPS (500 ng/mL) with or without IVIG (10 mg/mL) at 37°C for 15 min. When protein tyrosine kinase inhibitors were used in the assay, they were added to the culture medium at concentrations of 0.05 or 0.1 μM for PP2 and 5 or 10 μM for piceatannol. Reactions were stopped by rapid cooling on ice and cells were washed with ice-cold PBS once. Cells were lysed with lysis buffer containing 50 mM Tris-HCl, 1% NP40, protease inhibitors cocktail, Complete (Roche Diagnostic, Basel, Switzerland), 1 mM β-glycerophosphoric acid, 1 mM Na_3VO_4, and 5 mM NaF and were centrifuged at 12,000 ×g at 4°C for 15 min. Supernatants were collected and used as cell lysates. The protein concentrations of supernatants were measured by the BCA protein assay kit (Pierce, Rockford, IL).

Cell lysates (25 or 50 μg protein) were separated on 10% Nu-PAGE gels (Life Technologies) and electrotransferred onto nitrocellulose membranes using the iBlot transfer system (Life Technologies). After the transfer, membranes were blocked with 5% skim milk in PBS containing 0.1% Tween 20 (PBS-T) for 1 h at room temperature. After blocking, membranes were reacted with the primary antibodies described earlier at 4°C overnight. After washing with PBS-T, membranes were treated with HRP-conjugated secondary antibodies for 1-2 h at room temperature. Blots were developed with enhanced chemiluminescence reagents (Immobilon Western Chemiluminescent HRP Substrate kit, Millipore). Chemiluminescence signals were imaged using a Molecular Imager Pharos FX (Bio-Rad, Hercules, CA).

To detect Syk phosphorylation after stimulation with LPS for 15 min with or without IVIG, cell lysates (100 μg protein) were incubated with the anti-Syk antibody (1 μg) and precipitated by Protein A/G (Santa Cruz, Santa Cruz, CA) at 4°C for one day. Immunoprecipitates were analyzed by immunoblotting with the HRP-conjugated, anti-phosphotyrosine antibody (4G10), anti-Phospho-Syk antibody, or anti-Syk antibody, in the same manner as that described earlier.

2.8. Statistical Analysis. Results were expressed as mean values and standard error of the mean (SEM, $n = 3$). Data were analyzed by Student's t-test (for comparison between two group) or Dunnett's multiple comparison test (for multiple group) using the SAS system (ver. 9.1.3, SAS Institute, Cary, NC). Differences with P values less than 0.05 were considered to be significant. Results were representative of two or three independent experiments.

3. Results

3.1. IVIG Increased IL-10 Production Whereas Decreased IL-12p70 Production in BMDC Stimulated with LPS. First, we evaluated IL-10 and IL-12p70 production from BMDC stimulated with LPS and the effects of IVIG on the production of these two cytokines. After the stimulation of cells with LPS for 18 h, both IL-10 and IL-12p70 productions were clearly detected in the culture medium (Figure 1). The addition of IVIG concentration dependently increased IL-10 production which was statistically significant at concentrations of 5 and 10 mg/mL (Figure 1(a)). On the other hand, a clear decrease in IL-12p70 production was observed in the culture medium 18 h after stimulation in the presence of 2.5, 5, and 10 mg/mL IVIG (Figure 1(b)). The similar effects of IVIG were observed in cells 6 h after stimulation with LPS (Supplement data, Figure S1 available online at http://dx.doi.org/10.1155/2013/239320). These observed effects of IVIG in mouse BMDC stimulated with LPS were similar to those reported using human blood DC (12). To confirm whether another human protein had the same effect, we tested the effects of human pooled plasma on IL-10 production in BMDC stimulated with LPS. When human pooled plasma (2.5 to 10 mg/mL) was added to the culture medium of BMDC stimulated with LPS, a clear decrease in IL-10 production was observed in a concentration-dependent manner (Figure 1(c)). This indicated that human pooled plasma contained unknown factors that inhibited IL-10 production in LPS-stimulated BMDC and a xenobiotic protein exerted various influences on cytokine production in these cells.

3.2. IVIG Increased IL-10 mRNA Transcription Whereas Decreased IL-12 mRNA Transcription in BMDC Stimulated

with LPS. To investigate the effects of IVIG on the transcription levels of these cytokines, we next measured the mRNA expression of IL-10 as well as IL-12a and IL-12b, which codes the IL-12p35 and IL-12p40 subunits of IL-12p70, respectively, in cells stimulated with LPS. The expression of all three mRNAs was seen 6 h after the LPS treatment (Figure 2). IVIG at concentrations of 2.5, 5, and 10 mg/mL significantly increased the IL-10 mRNA expression 6 h after LPS treatment in a concentration-dependent manner (Figure 2(a)). On the other hand, 5 and 10 mg/mL IVIG clearly decreased IL-12a mRNA and 2.5, 5, and 10 mg/mL IVIG suppressed IL-12b expression in cells 6 h after stimulation (Figures 2(b) and 2(c)). The similar effects of IVIG on the expression of these three mRNA were observed 18 h after stimulation with LPS (Supplement data, Figure S2). These results suggest that IVIG affects the production and expression of both IL-10 and IL-12p70 in BMDC stimulated with LPS.

3.3. IVIG Affected Signaling Molecules in TLR4 Signaling Cascade of LPS-Stimulated BMDC. IL-10 and IL-12p70 production in cells stimulated with LPS is mediated by activation of Toll-like receptor 4 (TLR4) on the cell membrane [13–15]. TLR4 signal induces the phosphorylation of NFκ-B and the ERK family members, ERK1/2, p38 MAPK, and JNK. To investigate effects of IVIG on the LPS-TLR4 signal transduction, the phosphorylation of these proteins after the stimulation of cells with LPS was evaluated using specific antibodies by immunoblotting. The clear phosphorylation of NFκ-B, ERK1/2, and p38 MAPK and a very weak JNK phosphorylation signal were observed in the cell lysates 15 min after stimulation with LPS (Figure 3). IVIG decreased phosphorylation of p38 MAPK in cells stimulated with LPS. IVIG (10 mg/mL) showed no clear influence on NFκ-B phosphorylation. We could not detect any significant change in JNK phosphorylation by IVIG. On the other hand, an increase in ERK1/2 phosphorylation was detected in the same cell lysates (Figure 3). Although ERK1/2 hyperphosphorylation occurred by the treatment, these results suggest that IVIG at least inhibited activation of one signaling protein in TLR4 signaling cascade in BMDC stimulated with LPS.

3.4. IVIG Induced Syk Phosphorylation in BMDC Stimulated with LPS. As p38 MAPK and JNK activations are reported to be required for IL-12p70 production in DC [26, 27], the fact that IVIG inhibits p38 MAPK phosphorylation could explain the decrease in IL-12p70 production in BMDC stimulated with LPS and IVIG. In contrast, ERK1/2 phosphorylation is reported to be necessary for the induction of IL-10 [28–30]. As IVIG treatment induced an increase in ERK1/2 phosphorylation, we thought that hyperphosphorylation of ERK1/2 could contribute to an increase in IL-10 production by IVIG. IgG exerts its effects through FcγRs on the cell membrane [8, 10]. We then hypothesized that when BMDCs are stimulated with LPS in the presence of IVIG, activating signals from FcγR are initiated and these result in ERK1/2 hyperphosphorylation. Therefore, we examined the effects of IVIG on phosphorylation of the Syk protein, which is required for the activation of high affinity FcγRI and low

An Fc Gamma Receptor-Mediated Upregulation of the Production of Interleukin 10 by Intravenous Immunoglobulin in
Bone-Marrow-Derived Mouse Dendritic Cells Stimulated with Lipopolysaccharide In Vitro

131

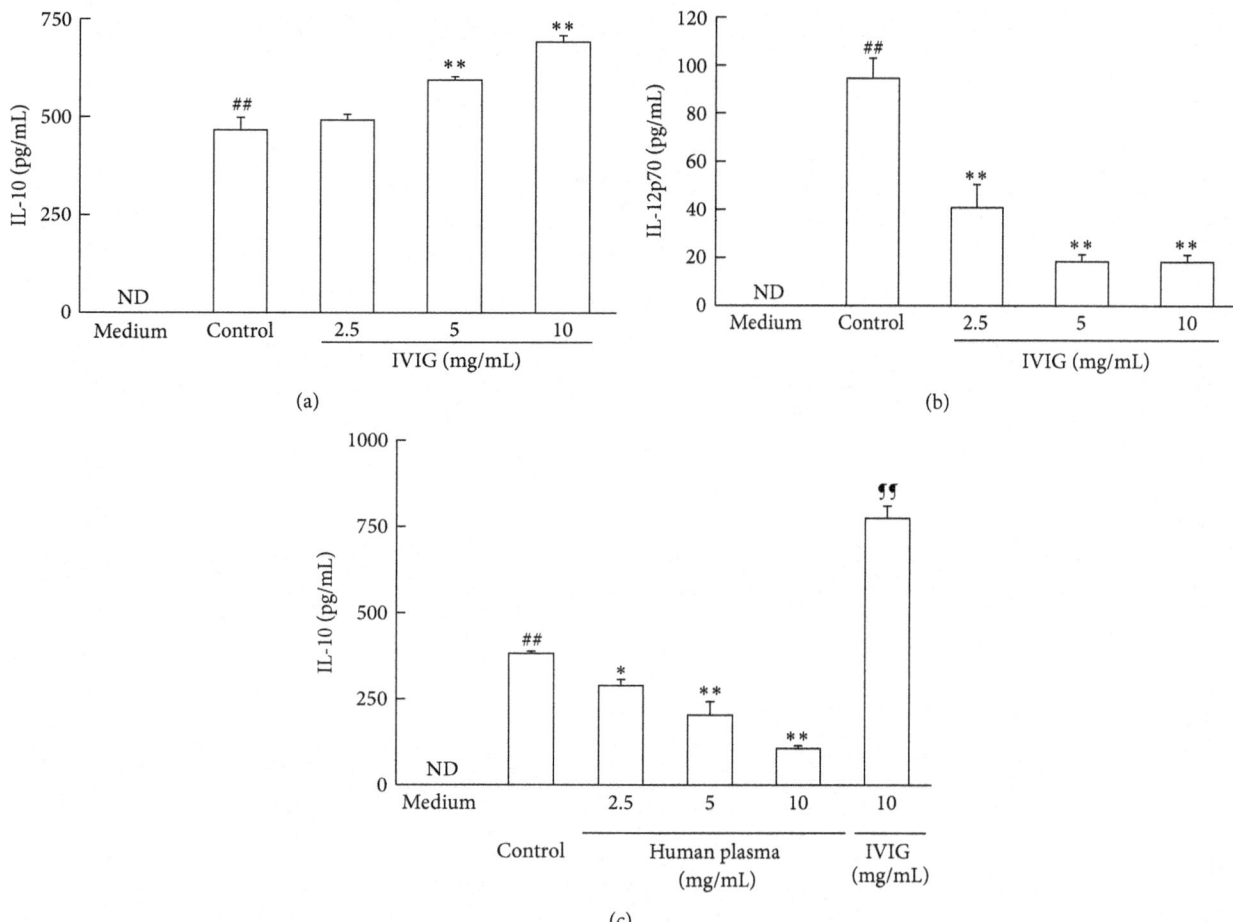

FIGURE 1: IVIG increased IL-10 production whereas decreased IL-12p70 production in BMDC stimulated with LPS. Cells were stimulated with LPS ($1 \mu g/mL$) in the presence of IVIG or human pooled plasma for 18 h. Cytokine concentrations in the culture medium were determined using respective ELISA kits. (a) Production of IL-10; (b) production of IL-12p70; (c) production of IL-10 in the presence of human pooled plasma. Results were expressed as mean ± SEM ($n = 3$). $^{##}P < 0.01$, significantly different from the medium alone (without LPS stimulation, Student's t-test); $^{*}P < 0.05$, $^{**}P < 0.01$, significantly different from the Control (LPS stimulation without IVIG, Dunnett's multiple comparison test); $^{¶¶}P < 0.01$, significantly different from the Control, Student's t-test; ND, IL-10 and IL-12p70 concentrations were under the lower limit values of the standard ELISA curves. At least three independent experiments were conducted and representative results were shown.

affinity FcγRIII, after the stimulation of cells with LPS [31, 32]. Analysis by the immunoprecipitation of cell lysates with the anti-Syk antibody and HRP-conjugated phosphotyrosine specific 4G10 antibody revealed that a clear increase in Syk phosphorylation was detected upon stimulation in DC stimulated with LPS and IVIG (Figure 4). In contrast, no increase in Syk phosphorylation was observed in cells stimulated with LPS alone (Figure 4). This suggests that IVIG triggers FcγR activation of BMDC when these cells are stimulated with LPS.

3.5. PP2 and Piceatannol Inhibited the Enhancement of IL-10 Production Induced by IVIG. The activation of FcγR is mediated by several protein tyrosine kinases. Of these kinases, the Src family kinases, Hck/Lyn, are essential for tyrosine phosphorylation in an ITAM motif of FcRγ subunit of FcγRI and FcγRIII, and ITAM-phosphorylated FcRγ activation is

required for Syk activation [31–34]. Therefore, to confirm that IVIG-induced FcγR activation is involved in the enhancing effect on IL-10 production in BMDC stimulated with LPS, we tested whether the inhibition of these protein tyrosine kinases could affect the upregulation of IL-10 production by IVIG. First, the Hck/Lyn inhibitor, PP2, was added to the culture and the production of IL-10 was assessed. Treatment with PP2 at $0.05 \mu M$ reduced the increase in IL-10 production by IVIG (Figure 5(a)). Next, to investigate the effects of the Syk inhibitor, piceatannol, cells were cultured with IVIG and stimulated with LPS in the presence of piceatannol ($5 \mu M$) and IL-10 production was measured. The addition of piceatannol diminished the enhancing effect of IVIG on IL-10 increase (Figure 5(b)). Analysis by immunoblotting and immunoprecipitation confirmed that PP2 and piceatannol inhibited the phosphorylation of ERK1/2 and Syk induced by IVIG in cells treated with LPS (Figures 5(c) and 5(d)).

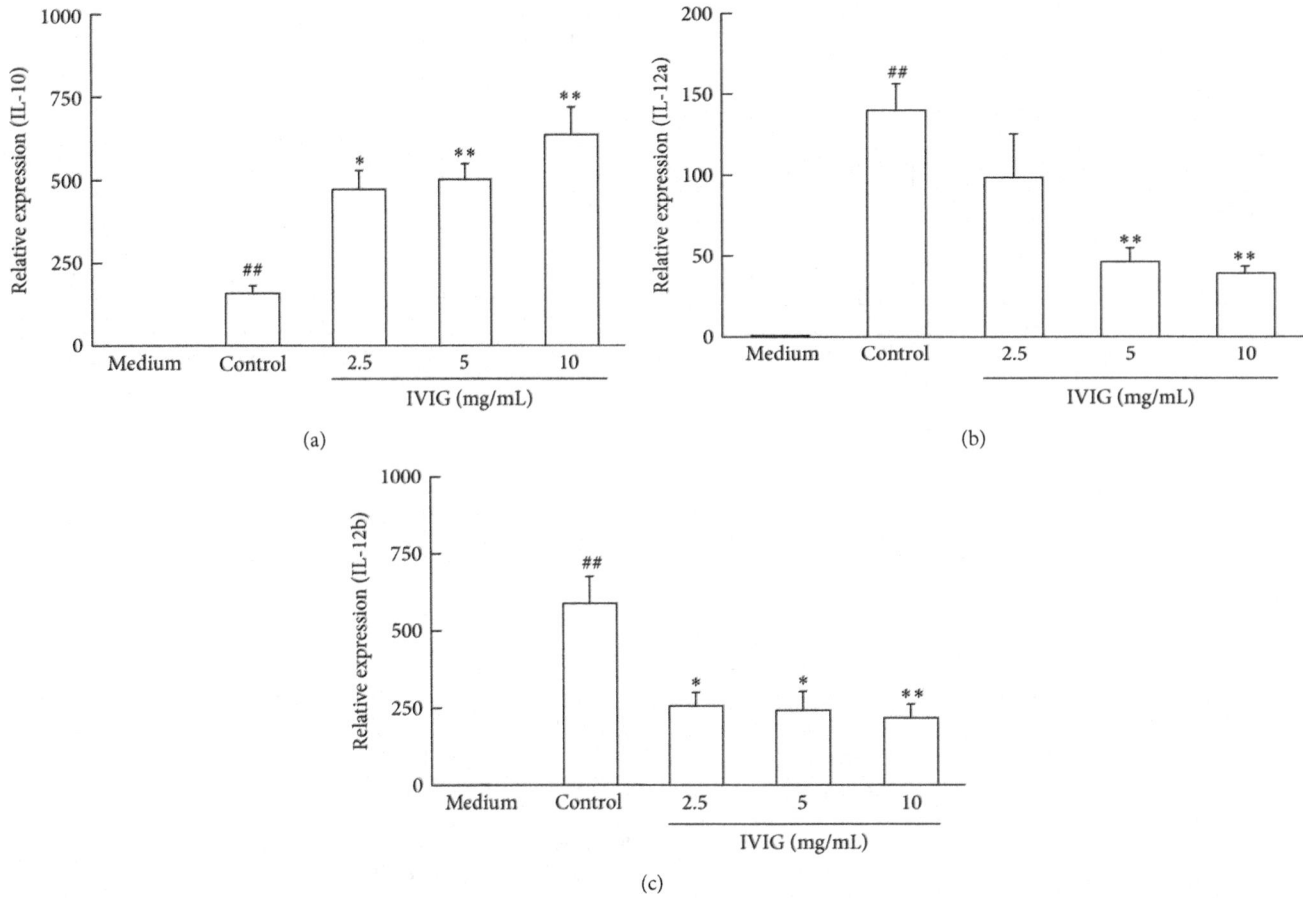

FIGURE 2: IVIG increased IL-10 mRNA transcription whereas decreased IL-12 mRNA transcription in BMDC stimulated with LPS. Cells were stimulated with LPS ($1\,\mu g/mL$) in the presence of IVIG for 6 h. The expressions of mRNA for IL-10, IL-12a, and IL-12b were determined by real-time quantitative RT-PCR. Results were expressed as mean ± SEM ($n = 3$). $^{\#\#}P < 0.01$, significantly different from the medium alone (without LPS stimulation, Student's t-test); $^{*}P < 0.05$, $^{**}P < 0.01$, significantly different from the Control (LPS stimulation without IVIG, Dunnett's multiple comparison test). At least three independent experiments were conducted and representative results were shown. (a) Expression of IL-10; (b) expression of IL-12a; (c) expression of IL-12b.

These results suggest that FcγR activation induced by IVIG is necessary to increase IL-10 production in BMDC stimulated with LPS.

3.6. FcγRI Was Required for the IL-10 Production Induced by IVIG.

To study the role of FcγR activation in the modulatory effects of IVIG described earlier more clearly, we evaluated the effect of anti-FcγRI antibody on IL-10 and IL-12p70 production in BMDC treated with LPS and IVIG. In the presence of anti-FcγRI antibody, increment of IVIG-induced IL-10 production was clearly negated. Control antibody had no effect. Both antibodies had no influence on IL-10 production in cells stimulated with LPS and the control antibody also had not affect the IL-10 production induced by IVIG (Figure 6(a)). On the other hand, the suppressing effect of IVIG on IL-12p70 production did not change in the presence of the anti-FcγRI antibody in the assay (Figure 6(b)). These findings suggest that activation of FcγRI is necessary for IVIG to enhance the production of IL-10 but is not required for the suppression of IL-12p70 production induced by IVIG in LPS-stimulated BMDC.

3.7. Suppressive Effect of IVIG on the IL-12p70 Production Was Inhibited by Anti-IL-10 Antibody.

It has been reported that IL-12p70 production in BMDC stimulated with LPS is regulated by IL-10 [5]. We thought that IL-10 in the culture medium could affect and decrease IL-12p70 production. Thus, we cultured the cells with LPS in the presence of IVIG and an anti-IL-10 antibody and measured IL-12p70 production in the medium. The addition of the anti-IL-10 antibody, but not its control antibody, clearly negated the effect of IVIG on IL-12p70 production. Both antibodies did not show clear effect on IL-12p70 production from the cells stimulated with LPS alone, and the control antibody also had no influence on the suppressing effect of IVIG on the production of IL-12p70 (Figure 7). These results indicate that IL-10 in the culture medium is required for the suppressing effect of IVIG on the production of IL-12p70 in BMDC stimulated with LPS.

An Fc Gamma Receptor-Mediated Upregulation of the Production of Interleukin 10 by Intravenous Immunoglobulin in
Bone-Marrow-Derived Mouse Dendritic Cells Stimulated with Lipopolysaccharide In Vitro

133

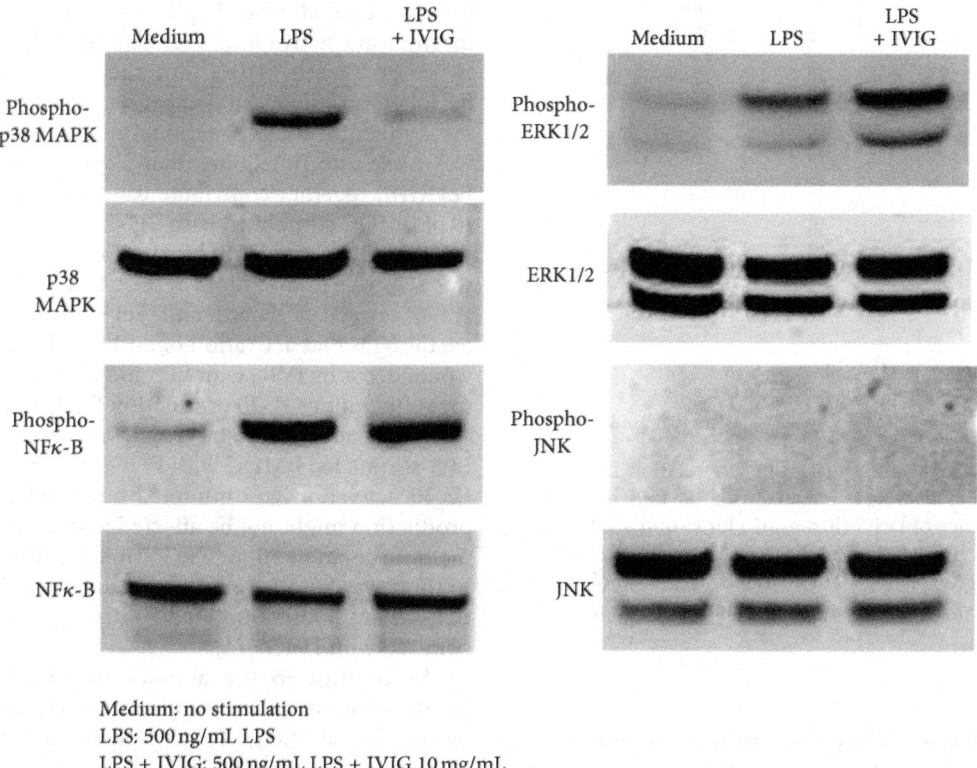

Medium: no stimulation
LPS: 500 ng/mL LPS
LPS + IVIG: 500 ng/mL LPS + IVIG 10 mg/mL

FIGURE 3: IVIG induced hyperphosphorylation of ERK1/2 and downregulated p38 MAPK phosphorylation in BMDC stimulated with
LPS. Cells were stimulated with LPS (500 ng/mL) in the presence or absence of IVIG (10 mg/mL) for 15 min. Cell lysates were incubated
with specific antibodies against NFκ-B, ERK1/2, p38 MAPK, and JNK and their phosphorylated forms and were analyzed by respective
immunoblottings.

4. Discussion

IVIG shows immunomodulatory effects in inflammatory and
autoimmune diseases [8, 9].

Although the direct effects of IVIG such as on the
cytokine production in peripheral blood mononuclear cells
(PBMCs) induced by bacterial components, the proliferation
of and cytokine production in T-cells, and TLR-mediated B-
cell responses have been reported previously [24, 35–37], the
molecular mechanisms of immunomodulation by IVIG are
still under extensive research. To investigate the molecular
targets of IVIG in the modulation of cytokine productions,
we used mouse BMDC stimulated with LPS and observed
that IVIG had an enhancing effect on the production of
the anti-inflammatory cytokine IL-10 and, at a same time, a
suppressing effect on the proinflammatory cytokine IL-12p70
production, similar to human mo-DC as reported by Bayry et
al. [12]. We also confirmed that these modulations of cytokine
production by IVIG occurred at the transcription level of
each cytokine gene. In addition, we found the upregulation
of ERK1/2 phosphorylation as well as the downregulation
of p38 MAPK phosphorylation after LPS stimulation in the
presence of the drug. The results of immune blotting were out
of our expectation, as we hypothesized that neutralization by
IVIG would inhibit LPS-induced TLR4 signaling. The exact
reasons of the unexpected results were not clear, but we could

not deny the possibility of neutralization by IVIG because
we thought that our experimental conditions might not be
suitable to detect the clear changes in NF-κB phosphorylation
and the phosphorylation signal of JNK was very faint and
hard to detect the reduction of phosphorylation by IVIG. It
was also reasonable to think that ERK1/2 phosphorylation
was reduced by neutralization, but we thought that the effect
of activated FcγRs would exceed that of neutralization as
discussed later.

Several studies have reported that ERK1/2 phosphorylation is necessary for the production of IL-10 by DC after some
ligand stimulations [28–30]. The fact that the upregulation of
ERK1/2 phosphorylation of BMDC stimulated with LPS in
the presence of IVIG correlates well with the increase in IL-10
production under the same culture conditions. It seems that
IVIG exerts its action through a different pathway including
ERK1/2 phosphorylation other than LPS-TLR4 signaling.
FcγRI and FcγRIII are members of IgG receptor, named FcγR,
which mediate activating functions in immune responses.
FcγR activation is mediated by tyrosine phosphorylation of
the ITAM motif in the FcRγ subunit, which associates with
the ligand binding subunit of each receptor [30–32, 38].
Members of the Src family kinase, such as Hck and Lyn, are
necessary for tyrosine phosphorylation of the ITAM motif
in FcRγ [33, 39]. Tyrosine phosphorylated ITAM serves as
a docking site for Syk, a member of the Syk protein kinase

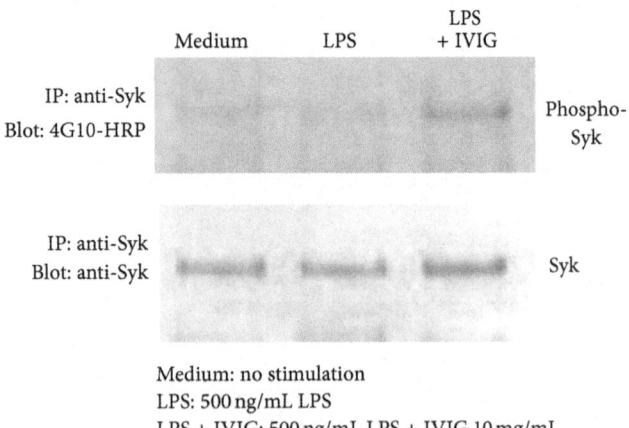

Medium: no stimulation
LPS: 500 ng/mL LPS
LPS + IVIG: 500 ng/mL LPS + IVIG 10 mg/mL

FIGURE 4: IVIG induced Syk tyrosine phosphorylation in BMDC stimulated with LPS. Cells were stimulated with LPS (500 ng/mL) in the presence or absence of IVIG (10 mg/mL) for 15 min. Cell lysates were incubated with the anti-Syk antibody and precipitated by Protein A/G. Immunoprecipitates were analyzed by immunoblotting with HRP-conjugated, anti-phosphotyrosine antibody (4G10) or the anti-Syk antibody.

family, and the phosphorylation of tyrosine residues within Syk occurred by Hck/Lyn as well as by autophosphorylation [34, 39–43]. Tyrosine-phosphorylated Syk is an important molecule in downstream signal transduction from FcγR activation after ligand binding and receptor aggregation [19, 39, 43].

We thought that when BMDC was stimulated with LPS in the presence of IVIG, FcγRI and/or FcγRIII signaling pathways were activated and both Syk and ERK1/2 were phosphorylated to increase IL-10 production. Hence, we first examined whether IVIG could induce Syk phosphorylation in BMDC stimulated with LPS. As we expected, Syk phosphorylation was observed when cells were treated with IVIG and LPS, but not with LPS alone. Next, to confirm that IVIG induced FcγR activation, we added two novel protein tyrosine kinase inhibitors, the Hck/Lyn inhibitor PP2 and Syk inhibitor piceatannol, to the culture of LPS-stimulated BMDC together with IVIG and evaluated both IL-10 production and the phosphorylation of ERK1/2 and Syk. We found that the enhancing effect of IVIG on IL-10 production diminished when cells were stimulated with LPS in the presence of PP2 and piceatannol. Furthermore, the increase in the phosphorylation of ERK1/2 and Syk by IVIG after stimulation with LPS was reduced by the treatment with PP2 and piceatannol. These results suggest that FcγR activation is an important factor in the enhancing effect of IVIG on the production of IL-10, and Src family kinases, such as Hck/Lyn, and the Syk family kinase, Syk, are together involved in the regulation of cytokine production in LPS-stimulated BMDC in the presence of IVIG.

It is interesting that the increase in IL-10 production by IVIG disappeared when LPS-stimulated BMDCs were cultured with IVIG and the anti-FcγRI antibody, whereas a decreasing effect on IL-12p70 production was not affected by the antibody in the same culture conditions. These findings indicate that at least FcγRI, one of two FcγRs involved in immune activation, mediates the upregulation of IL-10 production by IVIG, but the same receptor seems to have had no suppressing effect on IL-12p70 production. The mechanism of these functional differences is not clear, but we think one possibility that FcγRI and FcγRIII (if any, FcγRIIB) together contribute to the hyperproduction of IL-10 of BMDC stimulated with LPS in the presence of IVIG. As this production of IL-10 by IVIG in LPS-stimulated BMDC was sensitive to inhibitors of Hck/Lyn and Syk (both kinases are necessary to FcγRI and FcγRIII signal transduction), we thought that activation of an FcγRIII-mediated signaling would occur by IVIG with LPS and the signal from this receptor could induce IL-10 production likely in the case of FcγRI. When we added the anti-FcγRI antibody in the culture of LPS-stimulated BMDC with IVIG, IL-10 production through FcγRI activation was inhibited but FcγRIII-mediated IL-10 production might not be affected and IL-10 remaining in the medium could be enough to inhibit the IL-12 p70 production. In this regard, Lories et al. reported that anti-FcγRI and anti-FcγRIII antibodies inhibited IL-10 production in human DC cultured with IVIG [44].

In contrast to the absence of an effect by the anti-FcγRI antibody on the suppressing activity of IVIG on the production of IL-12p70, the anti-IL-10 antibody treatment clearly restored the IL-12p70 decrease by IVIG. All isotype antibodies used in these experiments had no influence on the cytokine production in BMDC stimulated with LPS. These findings suggest that the IL-10 hyperproduced by IVIG through FcγRI activation is important for the suppression of IL-12p70 production. However, the possibility of FcγRIII-mediated signal transduction and the contribution of inhibitory FcγRIIB should be also considered to understand the effects of IVIG on the production of IL-10 and IL-12p70 more clearly. As our preliminary study using an antibody that binds FcγRIIB and FcγRIII showed an inhibitory effect on IL-10 production by IVIG in cells stimulated with LPS (data not shown), we thought that receptors other than FcγRI, FcγRIII, and FcγRIIB may play important roles in the modulatory functions of IVIG. Furthermore, whether FcγRIIB could exert its inhibitory effects on signal transduction of TLR4 and cytokine production in BMDC induced by FcγR activation needs to be investigated.

The functionally important structures of IVIG in its immunomodulatory function were not determined in this study. Without LPS stimulation, IVIG showed no influence on cytokine production in BMDC in our study. As IVIG contains an LPS-binding fraction, it seems that IVIG could exert immunomodulatory effects on cells through an immune complex with LPS. LPS is a possible partner in the formation of an immune complex with IVIG, although further studies are required to confirm this [16]. In our preliminary experiments, neither Fab nor F(ab$'$)$_2$ fragments increased IL-10 production in LPS-stimulated BMDC (data not shown). We suppose that the binding activities of Fab and F(ab$'$)$_2$ fragments against antigens in LPS were not enough for IVIG to express its modulatory effects on the production of the cytokine and a help of Fc region might be required for the immunoregulatory function of IVIG.

An Fc Gamma Receptor-Mediated Upregulation of the Production of Interleukin 10 by Intravenous Immunoglobulin in
Bone-Marrow-Derived Mouse Dendritic Cells Stimulated with Lipopolysaccharide In Vitro

135

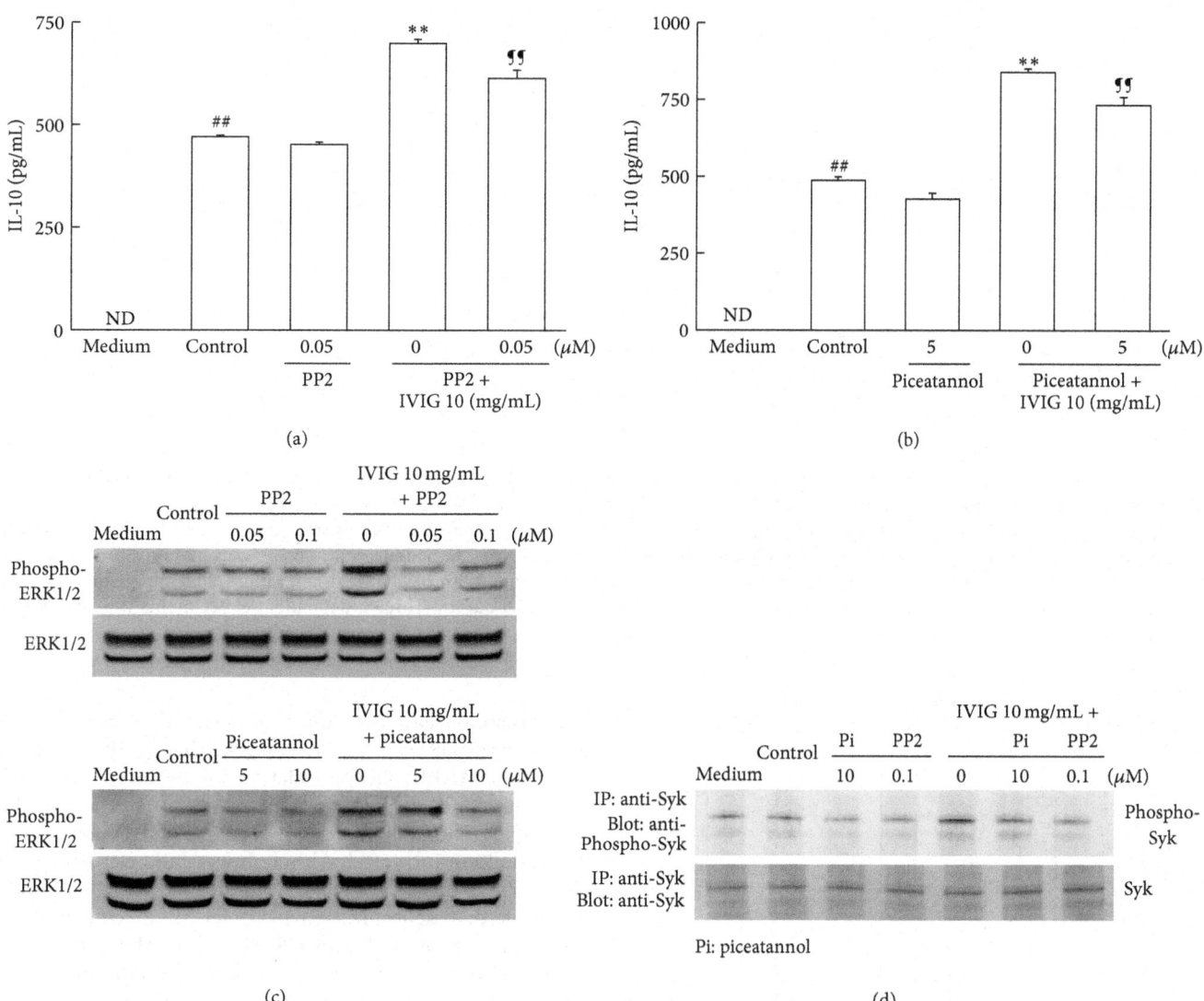

FIGURE 5: Protein tyrosine kinase inhibitors PP2 and piceatannol affected the enhancing effect of IVIG on IL-10 production in BMDC stimulated with LPS. Cells (5×10^5/mL) were stimulated with LPS (500 ng/mL) in the presence or absence of IVIG (10 mg/mL) and/or protein tyrosine kinase inhibitors for 18 h. IL-10 production in the culture supernatant was measured using an ELISA kit and results were expressed as mean ± SEM ($n = 3$). $^{\#\#}P < 0.01$, significantly different from the medium alone (without LPS stimulation, Student's t-test); $^{**}P < 0.01$, significantly different from the Control (LPS stimulation without IVIG, Dunnett's multiple comparison test); $^{\P\P}P < 0.01$, significantly different from LPS stimulation with IVIG, Student's t-test. ND, IL-10 concentrations were under the lower limit values of the standard ELISA curves. The enhancing effect of IVIG on IL-10 production was abolished by (a) the Hck/Lyn inhibitor PP2 and (b) Syk inhibitor piceatannol. Three independent experiments were conducted and representative results were shown. The tyrosine phosphorylation of ERK1/2 and Syk in cells was detected by immunoblotting as described in the Materials and Methods. PP2 and piceatannol inhibited ERK1/2 and Syk phosphorylation by IVIG in mouse BMDC stimulated with LPS. (c) ERK1/2; (d) Syk.

In contrast to the mechanisms of the enhancing effect of IVIG on the production of IL-10 in BMDC stimulated with LPS, those of the suppressing effect on IL-12p70 production by IVIG are thought to be more controversial. There may be at least two possibilities for the mechanisms of the suppressing effect of IVIG on the production of IL-12p70 in the cells stimulated with LPS. One is LPS-binding neutralizing antibodies in IVIG [16]. Signals required for IL-12p70 production may be inhibited by blocking LPS-induced activation in target cells. We observed that p38 MAPK phosphorylation was reduced

in LPS-stimulated BMDC in the presence of IVIG. p38 MAPK and JNK activation has been reported to be necessary for the production of IL-12p70 by DC after stimulation with LPS [26, 27]. We first thought that IL-10 had a possibility to reduce the phosphorylation of p38 MAPK. But if IL-10 could affect p38 MAPK phosphorylation, the production of this cytokine was seemed too early (within 15 min after stimulation) and considerably small amount in quantity (seems about several pg/mL) to show its reducing effect. Furthermore, Donnelly and coworkers reported that IL-10

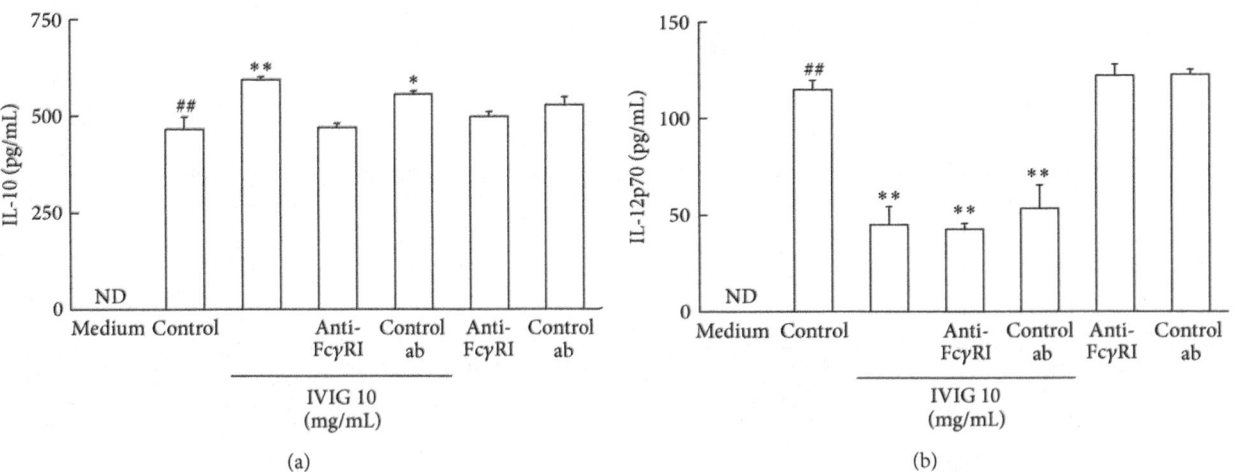

(a)   (b)

FIGURE 6: Anti-FcγRI antibody affects the cytokine productions in the presence of IVIG in BMDC stimulated with LPS. The anti-mouse FcγRI antibody and a matched control antibody were added to the cells in the presence or absence of IVIG (10 mg/mL) and cells were stimulated with LPS (500 ng/mL) for 18 h. Productions of cytokines in the culture supernatant were measured using respective ELISA kits and results were expressed as mean ± SEM ($n = 3$). $^{\#\#}P < 0.01$, significantly different from the medium alone (without LPS stimulation, Student's t-test); $^{*}P < 0.05$, $^{**}P < 0.01$, significantly different from the Control (LPS stimulation without IVIG, Dunnett's multiple comparison test). ND, Cytokine concentrations were under the lower limit values of the standard ELISA curves. Three independent experiments were conducted and representative results were shown. (a) IL-10; (b) IL-12p70.

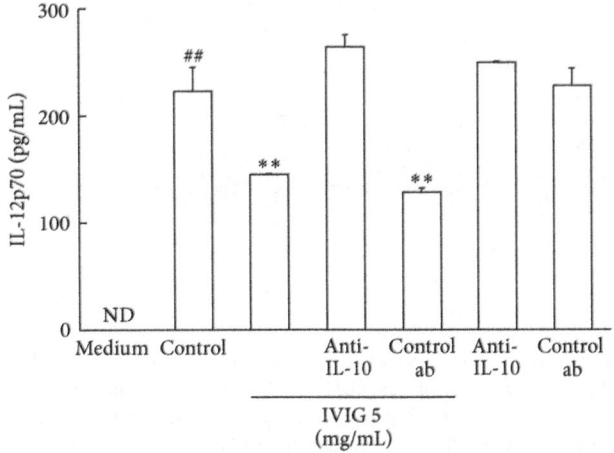

FIGURE 7: Anti-IL-10 antibody abolished the effect of IVIG on the suppression of IL-12p70 production in BMDC stimulated with LPS. Cells were stimulated with LPS (1 μg/mL) in the presence or absence of IVIG (5 mg/mL) and the anti-IL-10 or its control antibody for 18 h. IL-12p70 production in the culture supernatant was measured using the ELISA kit. Results were expressed as mean ± SEM ($n = 3$). $^{\#\#}P < 0.01$, significantly different from the medium alone (without LPS stimulation, Student's t-test); $^{**}P < 0.01$, significantly different from the Control (LPS stimulation without IVIG, Dunnett's multiple comparison test). ND, cytokine concentrations were under the lower limit values of the standard ELISA curves. Three independent experiments were conducted and representative results were shown.

showed no clear inhibitory effect on the phosphorylation of p38 MAPK of human monocyte stimulated with LPS *in vitro* [45]. In their report, purified human monocytes were pretreated with IL-10 (10 ng/mL) for 1 hour and were incubated with LPS (100 ng/mL) for 0 to 60 min and they

found that pretreatment with IL-10 did not decrease the levels of phospho-p38 MAPK. We thought that IL-10 might not affect p38 MAPK phosphorylation in the immediate early phase after LPS stimulation and an inhibitory effect of this anti-inflammatory cytokine would appear at later phase when its production increased. Although we could not detect any clear change of JNK phosphorylation by IVIG in our study, we think that neutralization by IVIG might contribute to the reduction of phospho-p38 MAPK in the early phase (within 15 min after stimulation) after LPS stimulation and result in the suppression of IL-12p70 production. Another possibility was the unidirectional negative regulation of IL-12p70 by IL-10 in LPS-activated DC as reported by Kao [5]. They demonstrated the reverse relationship between the production of IL-10 and IL-12p70 in activated DC. In their study, it was found that exogenous IL-10 suppressed the production of IL-12p70, while the addition of IL-12p70 did not suppress IL-10 production in LPS-activated DC [5]. They also reported that an ERK inhibitor significantly suppressed IL-10 and increased IL-12p70 production. It is likely that IL-10 and the IL-10 receptor-mediated signaling pathway suppresses the production of IL-12p70 in DC. In our study, when cells were stimulated with LPS, IVIG induced the upregulation of ERK1/2 phosphorylation by activation of FcγR-mediated mechanism and this led to an increase in IL-10 production. Increased IL-10 could suppress IL-12p70 production by its negative regulation on cytokine production and may maintain DC in an immature state to exert immunosuppressive functions. These putative mechanisms of modulatory effect of IVIG on cytokine production were illustrated in in Supplement data Figure S3.

Signal transduction through FcγRI activation by the immune complex of IVIG and LPS is one possible mechanism to explain this enhancing effect of IVIG on the production of IL-10 in BMDC stimulated with LPS. However, a clear mechanism including FcγRIIB and FcγRIII for the effects of IVIG on IL-10 and L-12p70 production remains to be determined, and further studies are necessary to demonstrate that the same mechanism works in human DC stimulated with LPS.

In conclusion, the results of this study clearly showed that IVIG had an enhancing effect on IL-10 production in mouse BMDC stimulated with LPS through FcγR activation. The suppression of IL-12p70 production by IVIG depends on IL-10 secreted, and inhibition of the LPS-TLR4 signaling pathway may also contribute to the suppressive effect of IVIG. In conjunction with inhibitory FcγRIIB in mouse DC, signals from activated FcγR may be a novel mechanism through which IVIG expresses its immunosuppressing functions.

Abbreviations

BMDC: Bone-marrow-derived dendritic cells
FcγR: Fc gamma receptor
FCS: Fetal calf serum
rmGM-CSF: Recombinant murine granulocyte-macrophage colony-stimulating factor
IL-10: Interleukin 10
IL-12p70: Interleukin 12p70
IVIG: Intravenous immunoglobulin
LPS: Lipopolysaccharide
TLR4: Toll-like receptor 4.

Conflict of Interests

Akihiro Fujii, Yuko Kase, Chiaki Suzuki, Akihito Kamizono, and Teruaki Imada are all employees of Japan Blood Products Organization and do not have any direct financial relation with the commercial identities mentioned in this study.

References

[1] J. W. Young and R. M. Steinman, "The hematopoietic development of dendritic cellsa distinct pathway for myeloid differentiation," *Stem Cells*, vol. 14, no. 4, pp. 376–387, 1996.

[2] J. Bancherau and R. M. Steinman, "Dendritic cells and the control of immunity," *Nature*, vol. 392, no. 6673, pp. 245–252, 1998.

[3] H.-R. Jiang, E. Muckersie, M. Robertson, H. Xu, J. Liversidge, and J. V. Forrester, "Secretion of interleukin-10 or interleukin-12 by LPS-activated dendritic cells is critically dependent on time of stimulus relative to initiation of purified DC culture," *Journal of Leukocyte Biology*, vol. 72, no. 5, pp. 978–985, 2002.

[4] G. Trinchieri, "Interleukin-12: a proinflammatory cytokine with immunoregulatory functions that bridge innate resistance and antigen-specific adaptive immunity," *Annual Review of Immunology*, vol. 13, pp. 251–276, 1995.

[5] C.-Q. Xia and K. J. Kao, "Suppression of interleukin-12 production through endogenously secreted interleukin-10 in activated dendritic cells: involvement of activation of extracellular signal-regulated protein kinase," *Scandinavian Journal of Immunology*, vol. 58, no. 1, pp. 23–32, 2003.

[6] R. de Waal Malefyt, J. Haanen, H. Spits et al., "Interleukin 10 (IL-10) and viral IL-10 strongly reduce antigen-specific human T cell proliferation by diminishing the antigen-presenting capacity of monocytes via downregulation of class II major histocompatibility complex expression," *Journal of Experimental Medicine*, vol. 174, no. 4, pp. 915–924, 1991.

[7] K. Steinbrink, M. Wölfl, H. Jonuleit, J. Knop, and A. H. Enk, "Induction of tolerance by IL-10-treated dendritic cells," *Journal of Immunology*, vol. 159, no. 10, pp. 4772–4780, 1997.

[8] M. D. Kazatchkine and S. V. Kaveri, "Immunomodulation of autoimmune and inflammatory diseases with intravenous immune globulin," *The New England Journal of Medicine*, vol. 345, no. 10, pp. 747–755, 2001.

[9] V. S. Negi, S. Elluru, S. Sibéril et al., "Intravenous immunoglobulin: an update on the clinical use and mechanisms of action," *Journal of Clinical Immunology*, vol. 27, no. 3, pp. 233–245, 2007.

[10] M. Ballow and C. Allen, "Intravenous immunoglobulin modulates the maturation of TLR 4-primed peripheral blood monocytes," *Clinical Immunology*, vol. 139, no. 2, pp. 208–214, 2011.

[11] J. Kwekkeboom, "Modulation of dendritic cells and regulatory T cells by naturally occurring antibodies," *Advances in Experimental Medicine and Biology*, vol. 750, chapter 10, pp. 133–144, 2012.

[12] J. Bayry, S. Lacroix-Desmazes, C. Carbonneil et al., "Inhibition of maturation and function of dendritic cells by intravenous immunoglobulin," *Blood*, vol. 101, no. 2, pp. 758–765, 2003.

[13] M. Guha and N. Mackman, "LPS induction of gene expression in human monocytes," *Cellular Signalling*, vol. 13, no. 2, pp. 85–94, 2001.

[14] B. M. Neves, M. T. Cruz, V. Francisco et al., "Differential roles of PI3-Kinase, MAPKs and NF-κB on the manipulation of dendritic cell T_h1/T_h2 cytokine/chemokine polarizing profile," *Molecular Immunology*, vol. 46, no. 13, pp. 2481–2492, 2009.

[15] J.-F. Arrighi, M. Rebsamen, F. Rousset, V. Kindler, and C. Hauser, "A critical role for p38 mitogen-activated protein kinase in the maturation of human blood-derived dendritic cells induced by lipopolysaccharide, TNF-α, and contact sensitizers," *Journal of Immunology*, vol. 166, no. 6, pp. 3837–3845, 2001.

[16] S. von Gunten, D. F. Smith, R. D. Cummings et al., "Intravenous immunoglobulin contains a broad repertoire of anticarbohydrate antibodies that is not restricted to the IgG2 subclass," *Journal of Allergy and Clinical Immunology*, vol. 123, no. 6, pp. 1268–1276, 2009.

[17] A. Yada, S. Ebihara, K. Matsumura et al., "Accelerated antigen presentation and elicitation of humoral response in vivo by FcγRIIB- and FcγRI/RIII-mediated immune complex uptake," *Cellular Immunology*, vol. 225, no. 1, pp. 21–32, 2003.

[18] J. V. Ravetch and S. Bolland, "IgG Fc receptors," *Annual Review of Immunology*, vol. 19, pp. 275–290, 2001.

[19] C. Sedlik, D. Orbach, P. Veron et al., "A critical role for Syk protein tyrosine kinase in Fc receptor-mediated antigen presentation and induction of dendritic cell maturation," *Journal of Immunology*, vol. 170, no. 2, pp. 846–852, 2003.

[20] J. M. Oliver, D. L. Burg, B. S. Wilson, J. L. McLaughlin, and R. L. Geahlen, "Inhibition of mast cell FcεRI-mediated signaling and effector function by the Syk-selective inhibitor, piceatannol," *Journal of Biological Chemistry*, vol. 269, no. 47, pp. 29697–29703, 1994.

[21] J. H. Hanke, J. P. Gardner, R. L. Dow et al., "Discovery of a novel, potent, and Src family-selective tyrosine kinase inhibitor," *Journal of Biological Chemistry*, vol. 271, no. 2, pp. 695–701, 1996.

[22] A. Sobota, A. Strzelecka-Kiliszek, E. Gladkowska, K. Yoshida, K. Mrozińska, and K. Kwiatkowska, "Binding of IgG-opsonized particles to FcγR is an active stage of phagocytosis that involves receptor clustering and phosphorylation," *Journal of Immunology*, vol. 175, no. 7, pp. 4450–4457, 2005.

[23] M. B. Lutz, N. Kukutsch, A. L. J. Ogilvie et al., "An advanced culture method for generating large quantities of highly pure dendritic cells from mouse bone marrow," *Journal of Immunological Methods*, vol. 223, no. 1, pp. 77–92, 1999.

[24] K. Murakami, C. Suzuki, F. Kobayashi et al., "Intravenous immunoglobulin preparation attenuates LPS-induced production of pro-inflammatory cytokines in human monocytic cells by modulating TLR4-mediated signaling pathways," *Naunyn-Schmiedeberg's Archives of Pharmacology*, vol. 385, no. 9, pp. 891–898, 2012.

[25] T. D. Schmittgen and K. J. Livak, "Analyzing real-time PCR data by the comparative CT method," *Nature Protocols*, vol. 3, no. 6, pp. 1101–1108, 2008.

[26] S. M. Mäkelä, M. Strengell, T. E. Pietilä, P. Österlund, and I. Julkunen, "Multiple signaling pathways contribute to synergistic TLR ligand-dependent cytokine gene expression in human monocyte-derived macrophages and dendritic cells," *Journal of Leukocyte Biology*, vol. 85, no. 4, pp. 664–672, 2009.

[27] T. Nakahara, H. Uchi, K. Urabe, Q. Chen, M. Furue, and Y. Moroi, "Role of c-Jun N-terminal kinase on lipopolysaccharide induced maturation of human monocyte-derived dendritic cells," *International Immunology*, vol. 16, no. 12, pp. 1701–1709, 2004.

[28] A.-K. Yi, J.-G. Yoon, S.-J. Yeo, S.-C. Hong, B. K. English, and A. M. Krieg, "Role of mitogen-activated protein kinases in CpG DNA-mediated IL-10 and IL-12 production: central role of extracellular signal-regulated kinase in the negative feedback loop of the CpG DNA-mediated Th1 response," *Journal of Immunology*, vol. 168, no. 9, pp. 4711–4720, 2002.

[29] C. Qian, X. Jiang, H. An et al., "TLR agonists promote ERK-mediated preferential IL-10 production of regulatory dendritic cells (diffDCs), leading to NK-cell activation," *Blood*, vol. 108, no. 7, pp. 2307–2315, 2006.

[30] Y. Yanagawa and K. Onoé, "Enhanced IL-10 production by TLR4- and TLR2-primed dendritic cells upon TLR restimulation," *Journal of Immunology*, vol. 178, no. 10, pp. 6173–6180, 2007.

[31] O. Letourneur, I. C. S. Kennedy, A. T. Brini, J. R. Ortaldo, J. J. O'Shea, and J.-P. Kinet, "Characterization of the family of dimers associated with Fc receptors (FcεRI and FcγRIII)," *Journal of Immunology*, vol. 147, no. 8, pp. 2652–2656, 1991.

[32] P. R. Scholl and R. S. Geha, "Physical association between the high-affinity IgG receptor (FcγRI) and the γ subunit of the high-affinity IgE receptor (FcεRIγ)," *Proceedings of the National Academy of Sciences of the United States of America*, vol. 90, no. 19, pp. 8847–8850, 1993.

[33] A. V. T. Wang, P. R. Scholl, and R. S. Geha, "Physical and functional association of the high affinity immunoglobulin G receptor (FcγRI) with the kinases Hck and Lyn," *Journal of Experimental Medicine*, vol. 180, no. 3, pp. 1165–1170, 1994.

[34] D. L. Durden and Y. B. L. Yen bou Liu, "Protein-tyrosine kinase p72(syk) in FcγRI receptor signaling," *Blood*, vol. 84, no. 7, pp. 2102–2108, 1994.

[35] H. F. MacMillan, T. Lee, and A. C. Issekutz, "Intravenous immunoglobulin G-mediated inhibition of T-cell proliferation reflects an endogenous mechanism by which IgG modulates T-cell activation," *Clinical Immunology*, vol. 132, no. 2, pp. 222–233, 2009.

[36] M. S. Maddur, M. Sharma, P. Hegde, S. Lacroix-Desmazes, S. V. Kaveri, and J. Bayry, "Inhibitory effects of IVIG on IL-17 production by Th17 cells is independent of anti-IL-17 antibodies in the immunoglobulin preparations," *Journal of Clinical Immunology*, vol. 33, supplement 1, pp. S62–S66, 2013.

[37] J.-F. Séité, T. Guerrier, D. Cornec, C. Jamin, P. Youinou, and S. Hillion, "TLR9 responses of B cells are repressed by intravenous immunoglobulin through the recruitment of phosphatase," *Journal of Autoimmunity*, vol. 37, no. 3, pp. 190–197, 2011.

[38] L. K. Ernst, A.-M. Duchemin, and C. L. Anderson, "Association of the high-affinity receptor for IgG (FcγRI) with the γ subunit of the IgE receptor," *Proceedings of the National Academy of Sciences of the United States of America*, vol. 90, no. 13, pp. 6023–6027, 1993.

[39] R. O. de Castro, "Regulation and function of Syk tyrosine kinase in mast cell signaling and beyond," *Journal of Signal Transduction*, vol. 2011, Article ID 507291, 9 pages, 2011.

[40] C. Darby, R. L. Geahlen, and A. D. Schreiber, "Stimulation of macrophage FcγRIIIA activates the receptor-associated protein tyrosine kinase Syk and induces phosphorylation of multiple proteins including p95Vav and p62/GAP-associated protein," *Journal of Immunology*, vol. 152, no. 11, pp. 5429–5437, 1994.

[41] Z. K. Indik, J.-G. Park, S. Hunter, and A. D. Schreiber, "The molecular dissection of Fcγ receptor mediated phagocytosis," *Blood*, vol. 86, no. 12, pp. 4389–4399, 1995.

[42] A. Strzelecka, K. Kwiatkowska, and A. Sobota, "Tyrosine phosphorylation and Fcγ receptor-mediated phagocytosis," *FEBS Letters*, vol. 400, no. 1, pp. 11–14, 1997.

[43] D. Cox and S. Greenberg, "Phagocytic signaling strategies: Fcγ receptor-mediated phagocytosis as a model system," *Seminars in Immunology*, vol. 13, no. 6, pp. 339–345, 2001.

[44] R. J. Lories, M. Casteels-Van Daele, J. L. Ceuppens, and S. W. Van Gool, "Polyclonal immunoglobulins for intravenous use induce interleukin 10 release in vivo and in vitro," *Annals of the Rheumatic Diseases*, vol. 63, no. 6, pp. 747–748, 2004.

[45] R. P. Donnelly, H. Dickensheets, and D. S. Finbloom, "The interleukin-10 signal transduction pathway and regulation of gene expression in mononuclear phagocytes," *Journal of Interferon and Cytokine Research*, vol. 19, no. 6, pp. 563–573, 1999.

12

RGD-Dependent Epithelial Cell-Matrix Interactions in the Human Intestinal Crypt

Yannick D. Benoit,[1,2] **Jean-François Groulx,**[1] **David Gagné,**[1] **and Jean-François Beaulieu**[1]

[1] *Département d'Anatomie et Biologie Cellulaire, Faculté de Médecine et des Sciences de la Santé, Université de Sherbrooke, Sherbrooke, QC, Canada J1H 5N4*
[2] *Pharmacology Department, Weill Cornell Medical College, New York, NY 10065, USA*

Correspondence should be addressed to Jean-François Beaulieu, jean-francois.beaulieu@usherbrooke.ca

Academic Editor: Claire Brown

Interactions between the extracellular matrix (ECM) and integrin receptors trigger structural and functional bonds between the cell microenvironment and the cytoskeleton. Such connections are essential for adhesion structure integrity and are key players in regulating transduction of specific intracellular signals, which in turn regulate the organization of the cell microenvironment and, consequently, cell function. The RGD peptide-dependent integrins represent a key subgroup of ECM receptors involved in the maintenance of epithelial homeostasis. Here we review recent findings on RGD-dependent ECM-integrin interactions and their roles in human intestinal epithelial crypt cells.

1. Introduction

Cell contacts with the extracellular matrix (ECM) provide both cohesive and functional properties in a variety of tissues, such as epithelia, nerves, muscle, and stroma, through specific interactions with cell membrane receptors [1, 2]. All ECMs are made up of collagen fibrils and/or networks, proteoglycans as well as specialized glycoproteins such as fibronectin and laminins that are archetypal of interstitial ECM and basement membrane (BM), respectively [3, 4]. Cells from multiple origins interact with ECM molecules using a variety of receptors, most of them being members of the integrin superfamily [2]. Integrins are noncovalent transmembrane α/β heterodimers. In mammals, over 24 distinct integrin heterodimers have been characterized to date, describing the association between 18α and 8β subunits [5–7]. The fact that integrin-mediated connections between the ECM and the cytoplasm regulate key cell functions such as adhesion, migration, proliferation, apoptosis, and differentiation is well recognized [8–11].

Epithelia express a wide variety of typical integrin receptors such as the $\alpha1\beta1$, $\alpha2\beta1$, $\alpha3\beta1$, and $\alpha6\beta4$ integrins that serve as collagen and/or laminin receptors [12–15].

Although less well documented in epithelia, the RGD-dependent integrins are another group of receptors that appears to be involved in epithelial cell homeostasis [15–17]. RGD-dependent integrins include $\alpha5\beta1$-, $\alpha8\beta1$-, and αV-containing integrins and are named as such because they specifically recognize the RGD motif, a sequence of three amino acids (Arg-Gly-Asp) found in many ECM molecules such as fibronectin and osteopontin [5, 12, 14, 15]. Collectively, these interactions are termed the "RGD-dependent adhesion system" (Figure 1). Interestingly, RGD-dependent cell interactions represent a key role in hierarchical assembly and maturation of adhesion structures including focal complexes (FXs), focal adhesions (FAs), and fibrillar adhesions (FBs) [1, 2, 18].

Therefore, RGD adhesion can by divided into three distinct components, the extracellular component (e.g., fibronectin), the membrane receptor (e.g., the $\alpha5\beta1$ integrin), and the intracellular molecule (e.g., vinculin). Moreover, each component acts in concert with the others to organize and regulate RGD adhesion dynamics. In this paper, we will focus on the importance of the RGD-dependent adhesion system for human intestinal crypt cell homeostasis (Section 2). We chose to elaborate on recent findings from

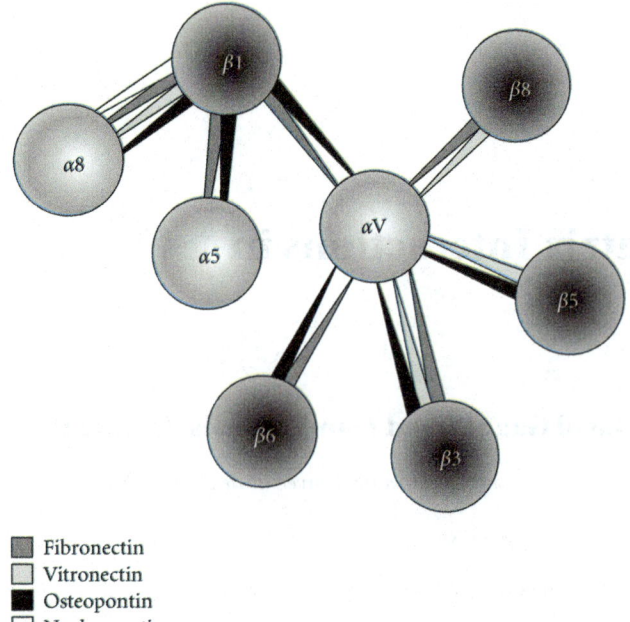

Fibronectin
Vitronectin
Osteopontin
Nephronectin

FIGURE 1: The RGD-dependent integrins. The RGD peptide (Arg-Gly-Asp) binding integrins represent a subclass of integrin receptors that specifically interact with the RGD motif found in several ECM elements. RGD integrins are formed by $\alpha 8/\alpha 5$ subunits coupled with the $\beta 1$ subunit and the αV subunit coupled with $\beta 3/\beta 5/\beta 6/\beta 8$ subunits. RGD-dependent α and β heterodimers are connected to each other with respect to their specific RGD containing ligands. The major RGD ligands are fibronectin (dark gray), vitronectin (light gray), osteopontin (black), and nephronectin (white).

our laboratory related to each of the RGD adhesion components, the $\alpha 8\beta 1$ integrin (receptor, Section 3), integrin-linked kinase (ILK) (intracellular molecule, Section 4), and type VI collagen (ECM, Section 5).

2. Cell-Matrix Interactions in the Human Intestinal Crypt

The small intestinal epithelium is a useful model to investigate the relationship between cell state and interaction with the ECM because of the well-defined architecture of its renewing unit, the crypt-villus axis. Indeed, proliferative cells, differentiating cells, and mature functional cells are topologically restricted to distinct compartments: the lower two-thirds of the crypt, upper third of the crypt, and villus, respectively. Gene expression in intestinal crypt cells must therefore be tightly regulated to efficiently control stemness, proliferation, migration, and differentiation in order to ensure the right equilibrium for the production of functional cells destined to renew the villus epithelium [19, 20]. There is strong evidence that cell-matrix interactions are involved in the regulation of these cell functions in the crypt [12, 21, 22]. For instance, differential spatial expression of laminins in the epithelial BM and their epithelial integrin receptors were observed along the crypt axis while in vitro studies have revealed functional relationships between laminin-binding

integrins and specific intestinal cell functions such as proliferation, migration, and differentiation [23–30]. A schematic illustration of the human crypt-villus axis and the spatial expression of laminins, laminin receptors of the integrin family, and the two classic RGD components fibronectin and the $\alpha 5\beta 1$ integrin (as depicted by dark areas) is shown in Figure 2. Moreover, another example is the transient expression of the tenascin and osteopontin receptor $\alpha 9\beta 1$ integrin in the lower third of the crypt of the immature small intestine as well as in proliferative epithelial crypt cells [31] and its reexpression in colon adenocarcinoma cells [32].

The RGD archetype fibronectin is another ECM component that was found strongly expressed in the epithelial BM of the crypts in both human and small laboratory animals [33–36]. Synthesis and deposition of fibronectin by proliferating intestinal epithelial cells was confirmed in vitro [26, 34]. Furthermore, expression of the fibronectin receptors, $\alpha 5\beta 1$ and αV-containing integrins, was found to be associated with intestinal cell proliferation [21, 29, 37]. Taken together, these observations suggest that fibronectin may significantly contribute to the RGD system regulating intestinal crypt cell functions.

To investigate this hypothesis, we used a strategy combining expression studies in the intact human intestine and functional studies using HIEC cells, a human intestinal epithelial crypt cell model well-characterized for the expression of typical features of intestinal crypt cells [38–41]. As summarized in the next sections, this experimental approach has led to the identification and characterization of new components of the RGD-dependent adhesion system that emphasize the importance of this adhesion system in human intestinal crypt homeostasis.

3. Integrin $\alpha 8\beta 1$ as a Crucial Mediator of Crypt Cell-Matrix Interaction

3.1. Integrin $\alpha 8\beta 1$ Is a Novel Regulator of Epithelial Cell Adhesion. Initially characterized in the chicken nervous system [42, 43], integrin $\alpha 8\beta 1$ represents an important RGD-dependent receptor [44]. Ligand binding to integrin $\alpha 8\beta 1$ was shown to be important for RhoA GTPase activation and subsequent actin stress fiber assembly in vascular smooth muscle cells [45–47]. Integrin $\alpha 8\beta 1$ was also recently found to play an important role in microfilament organization which was central to RGD-dependent intestinal epithelial crypt cell adhesion [48]. $\alpha 8$ subunit knockdown experiments, carried out in HIEC cells, showed that this integrin is important for proper vinculin recruitment to adhesion structures [48] (Figure 3). Intestinal epithelial crypt cells in which $\alpha 8$ was knocked down exhibited lower numbers of vinculin-positive FAs compared to controls, while paxillin localization was not affected [48]. It is well known that RhoA/ROCK signalling enhances actin stress fiber assembly and increases cell adhesion [49–51]. RhoA activity was shown to promote scaffolding protein recruitment, including vinculin, to the developing adhesion structures [51, 52]. Thus, the increased RhoA activity displayed by $\alpha 8$ knockdown cells leads to the absence or reduced levels of vinculin observed within these cells [48, 53].

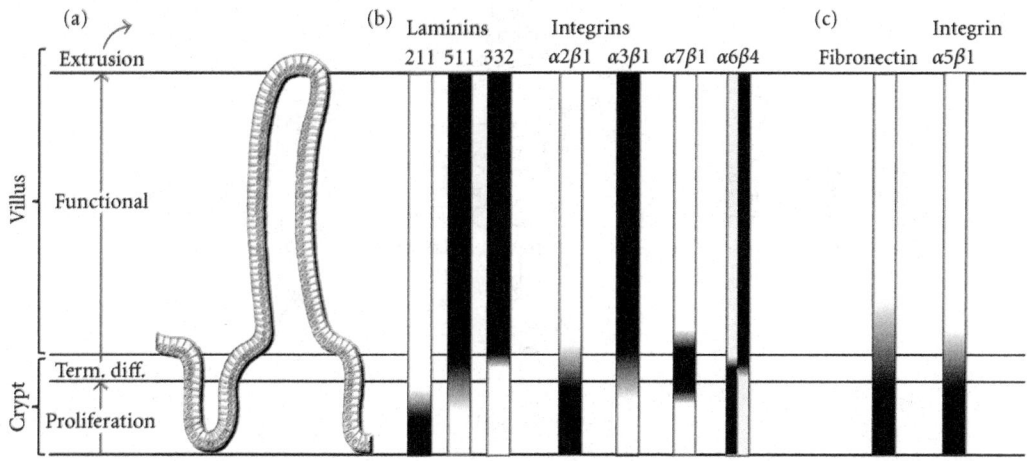

FIGURE 2: Distribution of laminins and laminin receptors of the integrin family as well as the RGD components fibronectin and the $\alpha 5\beta 1$ integrin receptor along the crypt-villus axis in the human small intestine. (a) Organization of the crypt-villus epithelial renewing unit. Villi are lined by functional epithelial cells responsible for digestion and absorption of nutrients. Stem cells located at the bottom of the gland generate transit amplifying cells that expand in the middle of the gland until they reach the upper gland region where they stop proliferating and undertake their terminal differentiation program before reaching the base of the villus. (b) Patterns of distribution of laminins at the epithelial BM as well as laminin receptors of the integrin family revealed differential expression of these molecules along the crypt-villus axis according to the cell state as shown by dark areas. (c) The RGD components fibronectin and its specific integrin receptor $\alpha 5\beta 1$ were found mostly confined to the crypt region (dark areas).

Based on the scheme of adhesion structures hierarchical assembly, vinculin recruitment occurs at later stages of FX formation, while paxillin is recruited at early stages [54]. Thus, observations made in intestinal epithelial crypt cells suggest that integrin $\alpha 8\beta 1$ is essential, at this particular stage of FX maturation into FA, via its role in RhoA activation [48] (Figure 3(a)). A similar function could also be predicted for the collagen-binding integrin $\alpha 2\beta 1$, considering the expression of this receptor in undifferentiated intestinal epithelium cells and its participation in RhoA activation [44, 55, 56].

Interestingly, ectopic expression of the enterocytic differentiation associated factor GATA-4 in intestinal epithelial crypt cells caused a depletion of $\alpha 8$ subunit expression [39, 48]. In these same cells, reduced levels of $\alpha 8\beta 1$ were associated with a decrease in cell growth, marked by Cyclin D1 inhibition and accumulation of cells in the G1 phase [48]. Similarly, decreased RhoA activity was observed in differentiated and nonproliferative HT29 cells compared to their undifferentiated and proliferative counterparts [55]. Together with the role of integrin $\alpha 8\beta 1$ in RGD-dependent adhesion, these findings support the concept that cell-ECM interactions are crucial to maintaining a proliferative state in epithelial cells, which is anchorage and cell position dependent, reflecting its exclusive localization in the lower crypt of the intact intestine.

3.2. Integrin $\alpha 8\beta 1$ Regulates Crypt Cell Migration.

Due to the role of integrin $\alpha 8\beta 1$ in RGD-dependent cell adhesion and RhoA GTPase activity, this receptor was shown to exert a critical influence on intestinal epithelial crypt cell motility [48]. Alteration of RhoA activity was found to modulate migration in different systems [49, 57]. We recently reported that loss of RGD-$\alpha 8\beta 1$ interactions in intestinal

epithelial cells caused increased cell migration [48]. From a physiological perspective, proliferating intestinal epithelial cells must be restricted to the lower two-thirds of the crypt to avoid premature terminal differentiation and loss of proliferative capacity [38, 40]. Therefore, without necessarily affecting the expression of differentiation master regulator genes, RGD-dependent adhesion plays a major role in regulating cell migration, which in turn is crucial for wound healing, cell differentiation, and tissue integrity [24, 58, 59].

3.3. Integrin $\alpha 8\beta 1$ RGD-Dependent Interactions Act as a Check Point in the Intestinal Crypt Epithelium.

Cell survival is tightly regulated by RGD-dependent ECM-integrin interactions [11]. Indeed, integrin receptors, such as $\alpha 5\beta 1$ and αV integrins, play a central role in controlling anoikis or apoptosis by loss of attachment [10, 11, 60]. Specifically, engagement of $\beta 1$ integrins was found to be essential to intestinal epithelial cell survival through FAK signalling [60, 61].

As mentioned above, integrin $\alpha 8\beta 1$ is involved in efficient vinculin recruitment to developing adhesion structures [48, 53]. The presence of vinculin in cell-ECM adhesion structures affects cell survival signal transduction. As previously described, HIEC cells share a number of features with intestinal epithelial stem cells, including a proliferative and undifferentiated state as well as the expression of several putative stem cell markers [39]. Interestingly, silencing of vinculin expression in F9 embryonic teratocarcinoma cells, another cell model closely related to stem cells [62], has shown increased resistance to anoikis, while ectopic reexpression of vinculin restored sensitivity to anchorage-dependent survival [63]. A similar phenomenon was observed in nonadherent $\alpha 8$ knockdown intestinal epithelial crypt cells [53]. In both studies, elevated levels of FAK phosphorylation

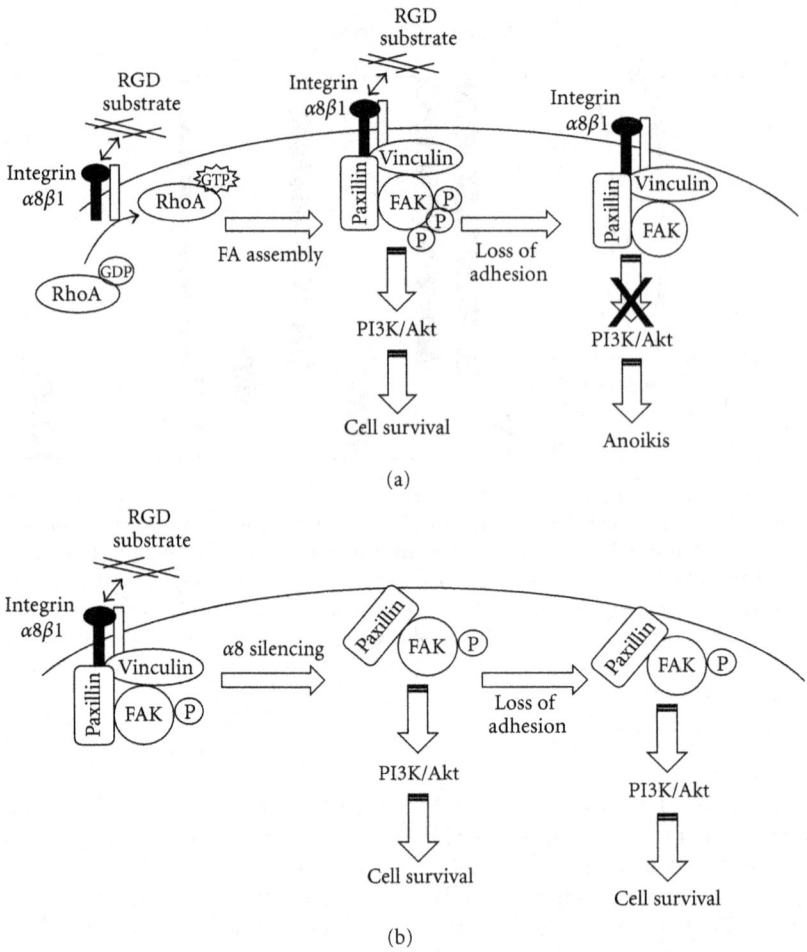

(a)

(b)

FIGURE 3: RGD-dependent adhesion influences anoikis sensitivity in undifferentiated epithelial cells. (a) Schematic representation of the proposed mechanism by which integrin $\alpha 8\beta 1$ and RGD-dependent adhesion regulates anoikis sensitivity, through differential interactions between vinculin, paxillin, and FAK in intestinal epithelial crypt cells. As described in Section 3, $\alpha 8\beta 1$ is essential to vinculin recruitment within maturing adhesion structures, while paxillin localization is not affected by $\alpha 8$ subunit silencing. (b) Following $\alpha 8$ subunit silencing, the absence of vinculin, combined with the presence of paxillin in the adhesion complexes, leads to an anchorage-independent activation of FAK and, consequently, anoikis resistance.

on tyrosine 397 were noted in nonadherent cell cultures. The absence of vinculin combined with the presence of paxillin in primitive adhesion structures prior to loss of adhesion could explain such a phenomenon (Figure 3). At the molecular level, it has been shown that paxillin exhibits partially overlapping binding sites for FAK and vinculin [64]. Thus, the vinculin tail domain appears to compete with FAK for paxillin binding. In the presence of vinculin, FAK activation would depend on ECM-integrin binding. However, absence of vinculin leads to a conformational change in adhesion structures which results in constitutive activation of FAK when bound to paxillin [63] where FAK activity no longer relies on ECM-integrin interactions [53, 63]. Additionally, nonadherent $\alpha 8\beta 1$-depleted intestinal epithelial cells showed increased activity of the PI3 K/Akt signalling pathway compared to nonadherent controls [53]. A summary of integrin $\alpha 8\beta 1$ contribution to anoikis regulation in epithelial intestinal crypt cells is presented in Figure 3.

Considering the proliferative and highly adaptive capacities of crypt cells, such as stem and transit amplifying cells, RGD-dependent $\alpha 8\beta 1$ interactions with ECM are suggested to act as a security switch that keeps the detachment of undifferentiated epithelial cells in check. It is worth noting that none of the five human colorectal cancer cell lines tested were found to express the integrin $\alpha 8$ subunit and that ectopic expression of this RGD-dependent receptor restored sensitivity of malignant cells to anoikis [53]. The mechanism by which colon cancer cells repress $\alpha 8$ expression to bypass this checkpoint remains unknown. However, in normal cells, this security step mediated by $\alpha 8\beta 1$ occupancy is potentially important to support homeostasis in the human intestinal crypt. New evidence from the literature has shown that colon cancer may originate from defective crypt stem cells [65]. Therefore, in light of the expression of $\alpha 8\beta 1$ in the region associated with intestinal stem cells, combined with its role in sensitizing epithelial cells to anoikis [53], it could

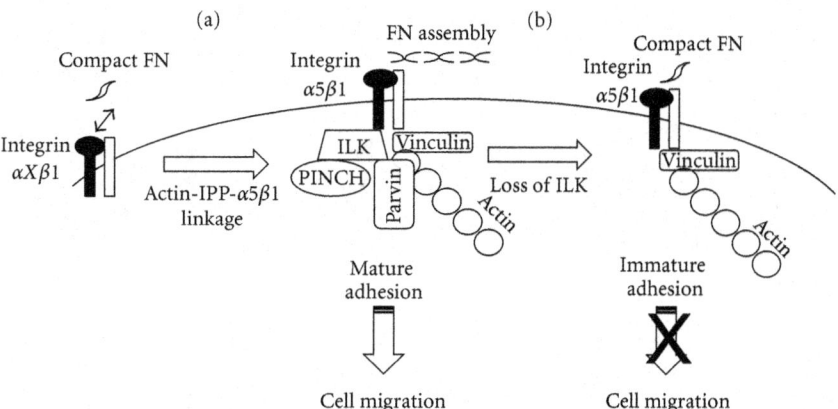

FIGURE 4: Regulation of the dynamic assembly of fibronectin by ILK. Schematic representation of the proposed mechanism by which ILK regulates FN assembly in HIEC. (a) Following cellular adhesion, the ILK/IPP complex is recruited to focal adhesions providing the link between the actin cytoskeleton and integrin α5β1. IPP recruitment mediates the formation of mature focal adhesions that allow fibronectin deposition into the BM of HIEC. (b) Depletion of ILK in HIEC results in the disruption of the IPP complex which prevents actin cytoskeleton-α5β1 linkage and focal adhesions cannot mature. Consequently, loss of the IPP complex reduces FN deposition and decreases migration of HIEC.

be speculated that α8 integrin silencing represents a key step in cancer initiation, in order to escape apoptosis upon modification of the malignant stem cell niche or location. In this context, α8β1 could promote defective progenitor cell elimination, and consequently prevent the onset of ecto-cryptal proliferative structures. Such specific involvement of RGD-dependent integrins is not without precedent since altered expression of other heterodimers has been reported in colon cancer. For instance, integrin αVβ3 expression has been found to be specifically decreased in anoikis-resistant Caco-2 cells [66].

4. Integrin-Linked Kinase (ILK) as an Integrator of Cell-Fibronectin Interaction

The intestinal epithelial cell mediates RGD interactions through expression of specific integrin receptors, as observed with α8β1, as well as through the production and deposition of RGD ligands, such as fibronectin. The efficient deposition of fibronectin into the BM relies upon its recognition by RGD-dependent integrins, which mediate its unfolding to expose specific fibronectin structural domains, which in turn mediates the formation of insoluble fibronectin fibrils [67]. Fibronectin deposition is characterized by the formation of specialized cell-matrix contact structures containing integrins, cytosolic proteins, and actin referred to as fibrillar adhesion (FB) points [67].

The integrin-linked kinase (ILK) is a constituent of integrin containing adhesion sites where it mediates multiple cellular processes. ILK is a pseudokinase and scaffolding protein ubiquitously expressed in mammalian cells forming a trimeric complex with PINCH and parvins named the IPP complex [68–70]. ILK interacts with the cytoplasmic domain of integrin β1 and β3 subunits to create a physical link between integrins and the actin cytoskeleton [68, 71]. Interestingly, it has been suggested that ILK regulates fibronectin expression/deposition [72–74] and other studies

have placed IPP complex members within FA points [75, 76]. In vivo, fibronectin expression is restricted to the BM underlying epithelial crypt cells and HIEC cells produce copious amount of fibronectin and generate numerous well-defined adhesion structures. The expression and roles of ILK were therefore investigated in human intestinal crypt cells.

We first focused on the localization of ILK-related components in the small intestine. As previously observed for fibronectin and integrin α5β1 in the intact intestine [21, 29, 33], ILK, PINCH-1 α-parvin, and β-parvin were found to be predominantly expressed by the proliferative epithelial cells of the crypts [58]. In HIEC cells, ILK, PINCH-1, α-parvin, and β-parvin were all closely associated with FA points (Figure 4(a)). A siRNA strategy was used to knock down ILK expression in HIEC cells in order to further investigate the role of ILK in intestinal crypt cells [58]. Interestingly, ILK knockdown in HIEC was accompanied by severe disruption of the IPP complex including the loss of PINCH-1 and parvins as well as major alterations in fibronectin synthesis and functional matrix deposition (Figure 4(b)). Overexpression of ILK was previously shown to increase fibronectin deposition in rat intestinal cells [76] while ILK knockdown decreases fibronectin expression in mice and human colon cancer cells. Indeed, the fibronectin gene promoter contains response elements that have been shown to be potentially regulated by ILK-mediated signalling [68, 77]. However, in HIEC cells, although a reduction of fibronectin was observed at the transcript level, ILK knockdown had no net effect on fibronectin protein amounts found in the culture medium suggesting that it was mainly the ability to process and deposit soluble fibronectin that was altered by the loss of the IPP complex [58]. The exact mechanism by which ILK knockdown impairs fibronectin deposition remains to be elucidated. Expression levels of the fibronectin integrin receptors were not altered in HIEC ILK knockdown cells suggesting that the required receptors for fibrillogenesis [67] remain available for binding. However,

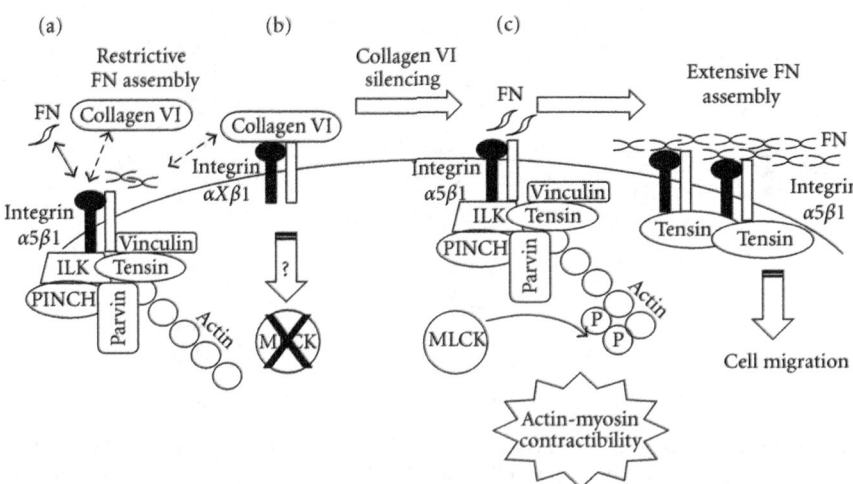

FIGURE 5: Regulation of dynamic assembly of fibronectin by type VI collagen. Schematic representation of the proposed mechanism by which collagen VI regulates FN fibrillogenesis. In HIEC, collagen VI is deposited into the ECM and interferes with fibronectin assembly by three distinct mechanisms. (a) First, in HIEC collagen VI competes with fibronectin for β1 integrin binding in focal adhesions. (b) Second, collagen VI limits cellular accessibility of fibronectin through a direct interaction with FN preventing fibronectin association with other fibronectin molecules, a step required for the extensive formation of the fibronectin matrix. (c) The third mechanism involves the regulation of MLCK by collagen VI. When collagen VI is depleted from the ECM, the MLCK/MLC pathway is activated by an unknown mechanism and mediates fibrillar actin contractility that allows the recruitment of tensin to FBs generating extensive fibrillogenesis. The increase in fibronectin deposition followed the depletion of collagen VI is accompanied by an increase in migration.

because of the important scaffolding role of ILK and IPP complexes, the decrease of fibronectin deposition in these ILK-deficient cells may reflect a reduction in the cytoskeletal tension necessary for fibrillogenesis [78, 79]. Alternatively, alteration in signalization pathways may also be involved. Indeed, key signalling molecules such as Src, PI3 K, and ERK have been shown to modulate fibronectin deposition in various cell models [80–82] and ILK and the IPP complexes can regulate these signalling molecules [83–85].

In addition to an alteration in fibronectin deposition, ILK knockdown severely affected basic intestinal crypt cell functions such as cell spreading, migration restitution abilities as well as cell proliferation [58]. Alterations in these functions in ILK-knockdown HIEC cells were not surprising since these functions can be stimulated by fibronectin in intestinal epithelial cells [86–89]. Interestingly, exogenously deposited fibronectin was found to fully rescue the ILK-knockdown HIEC phenotype with regard to cell proliferation, spreading and migration [58].

Taken together, as summarized in Figure 4, these data reveal that ILK and, by extension, the IPP complexes, perform crucial roles in the control of human intestinal crypt cell homeostasis, especially as key mediator of fibronectin deposition in the BM, which in turn regulates cell proliferation, migration, and restitution.

5. BM Collagen VI as a Regulator of Crypt-Cell-Fibronectin Interaction

Type VI collagen is a ubiquitously expressed ECM component [90]. In interstitial ECM, collagen VI acts as an anchoring meshwork bridging collagen fibers to the surrounding matrix [91, 92]. Collagen VI has also been shown to directly

interact with the BM-specific type IV collagen [93] supporting a key role for this collagen in connecting BM to ECM [94, 95]. However, we recently identified collagen VI as a *bona fide* component of the basal lamina in the intestinal BM and found that it is synthesized in significant amounts by crypt epithelial cells [59].

To investigate the function of type VI collagen in the intestinal epithelial crypt cell, we used a similar knockdown strategy with HIEC cells as described in the previous sections for integrin the α8 subunit and ILK. Surprisingly, abolition of collagen VI expression resulted in a striking increase in cell size and spreading accompanied by a significant increase in the number of stress fibers and tensin recruitment at the FB points [59]. The observations that removal of collagen VI emphasized features normally associated with fibronectin suggested that collagen VI regulates fibronectin assembly in epithelial cells. Interactions between collagen VI and fibronectin have been previously reported [93, 96]. Further investigation in collagen-VI-depleted HIEC cells revealed that fibronectin was increased at both protein and transcript levels and was subjected to extracellular rearrangement into long, parallel fibrils. Importantly, exogenous collagen VI, but not collagen I or IV, was able to fully rescue the knockdown phenotype indicating that the effect is specific for type VI collagen [59]. Considering that exposure of fibronectin-binding sites is critical for both cell binding and fibrillogenesis [67, 97], one may hypothesize that, under normal conditions, collagen VI acts by limiting cellular accessibility to fibronectin through competition for integrin receptors (Figure 5(a)) or by a direct interaction with fibronectin in the ECM (Figure 5(b)). Consistent with this possibility, collagen VI has been reported to be recognized by the RGD-binding α5β1 and αV integrins [98–100]. Furthermore,

HIEC binding to collagen VI is integrin $\beta1$ dependent and it was the FB complexes, specifically enriched in tensin and $\alpha5\beta1$ integrin [6, 54, 67], that were enhanced in collagen-VI-depleted HIEC [59].

To further investigate the mechanism underlying the generation of FB complexes in collagen-VI-depleted intestinal crypt cells, the regulation of actomyosin forces was analyzed. Actin contractility depends on the phosphorylation of the myosin light chain (MLC), which is mainly mediated by the kinases MLC (MLCK) and Rho (ROCK) acting on MLC and myosin phosphatase, respectively [101–104]. Interestingly, MLCK-dependent activation of MLC phosphorylation was observed in poor collagen VI/rich fibronectin ECM environments consistent with the observed generation of higher numbers of tensin-enriched FB complexes and extensive fibronectin fibrillar deposition [59] (Figure 5(c)).

As summarized in Figure 5, these data identified collagen VI as a major regulator of fibronectin synthesis and fibrillogenesis and suggest that collagen VI influences intestinal epithelial crypt cell behaviour by restraining cell-fibronectin interactions and their downstream events.

6. Conclusions

Described as a predominant epithelial BM component in the intestinal crypt more than 3 decades ago [33–36], fibronectin has been confirmed to play an important role in the RGD system regulating crypt epithelial cell functions. The recent findings summarized herein further emphasize the crucial importance of this RGD-adhesion system and its regulatory mechanisms. Indeed, intestinal epithelial cells can regulate RGD interactions through expression of specific integrin receptors, as exemplified by $\alpha8\beta1$, which exerts major regulatory influences on key cell functions such as cell proliferation, migration, and survival [48, 53]. Regulation of RGD interactions can also be accomplished by regulating production and deposition of their ligands, such as fibronectin, as illustrated by the finding that ILK/IPP complexes are key mediators of fibronectin deposition into the BM, which in turn regulates cell proliferation, migration, and restitution [58]. Finally, regulation of RGD-dependent cell interactions can also be achieved by interaction with other ECM molecules as shown with type VI collagen, a basement membrane component that regulates epithelial cell-fibronectin interactions. Taken together, these studies define new molecular elements and shed new light on the relative complexity of specific cell-matrix interactions in a well-defined environment such as the intestinal crypt and the critical impact these interactions have on cell function.

Authors' Contribution

Y. D. Benoit and J.-F. Groulx contributed equally to this work.

Acknowledgments

The authors thank Nuria Basora, Tamara Weissman, and Naira C. Rezende for comments and advice on the paper and Elizabeth Herring for reviewing the paper. The work was supported by grants from the Canadian Institutes for Health Research. J.-F. Beaulieu holds the Canada Research Chair in Intestinal Physiopathology and is a member of the FRSQ-funded Centre de Recherche Clinique Etienne-Le Bel of the CHUS.

References

[1] R. O. Hynes and A. Naba, "Overview of the matrisome—an inventory of extracellular matrix constituents and functions," *Cold Spring Harbor Perspectives in Biology*, vol. 4, no. 1, Article ID a004903, 2012.

[2] B. Geiger and K. M. Yamada, "Molecular architecture and function of matrix adhesions," *Cold Spring Harbor Perspectives in Biology*, vol. 3, no. 5, Article ID a005033, 2011.

[3] S. Ricard-Blum, "The collagen family," *Cold Spring Harbor Perspectives in Biology*, vol. 3, no. 1, Article ID a004978, 2011.

[4] P. D. Yurchenco, "Basement membranes: cell scaffoldings and signaling platforms," *Cold Spring Harbor Perspectives in Biology*, vol. 3, no. 2, Article ID a004911, 2011.

[5] M. Barczyk, S. Carracedo, and D. Gullberg, "Integrins," *Cell and Tissue Research*, vol. 339, no. 1, pp. 269–280, 2010.

[6] A. L. Berrier and K. M. Yamada, "Cell-matrix adhesion," *Journal of Cellular Physiology*, vol. 213, no. 3, pp. 565–573, 2007.

[7] Y. Takada, X. Ye, and S. Simon, "The integrins," *Genome Biology*, vol. 8, no. 5, article no. 215, 2007.

[8] F. G. Giancotti, "Integrin signaling: specificity and control of cell survival and cell cycle progression," *Current Opinion in Cell Biology*, vol. 9, no. 5, pp. 691–700, 1997.

[9] J. G. Lock, B. Wehrle-Haller, and S. Strömblad, "Cell-matrix adhesion complexes: master control machinery of cell migration," *Seminars in Cancer Biology*, vol. 18, no. 1, pp. 65–76, 2008.

[10] P. J. Reddig and R. L. Juliano, "Clinging to life: cell to matrix adhesion and cell survival," *Cancer and Metastasis Reviews*, vol. 24, no. 3, pp. 425–439, 2005.

[11] P. H. Vachon, "Integrin signaling, cell survival, and anoikis: distinctions, differences, and differentiation," *Journal of Signal Transduction*, vol. 2011, Article ID 738137, 18 pages, 2011.

[12] J. F. Beaulieu, "Extracellular matrix components and integrins in relationship to human intestinal epithelial cell differentiation," *Progress in Histochemistry and Cytochemistry*, vol. 31, no. 4, pp. 1–78, 1997.

[13] A. M. Mercurio, "Laminin receptors: achieving specificity through cooperation," *Trends in Cell Biology*, vol. 5, no. 11, pp. 419–423, 1995.

[14] A. Pozzi and R. Zent, "Extracellular matrix receptors in branched organs," *Current Opinion in Cell Biology*, vol. 23, no. 5, pp. 547–553, 2011.

[15] D. Sheppard, "Epithelial integrins," *BioEssays*, vol. 18, no. 8, pp. 655–660, 1996.

[16] J. F. Beaulieu, "Integrins and human intestinal cell functions," *Frontiers in Bioscience*, vol. 4, pp. D310–D321, 1999.

[17] E. Fong, S. Tzlil, and D. A. Tirrell, "Boundary crossing in epithelial wound healing," *Proceedings of the National Academy of Sciences of the United States of America*, vol. 107, no. 45, pp. 19302–19307, 2010.

[18] J. E. Schwarzbauer and D. W. DeSimone, "Fibronectins, their fibrillogenesis, and in vivo functions," *Cold Spring Harbor Perspectives in Biology*, vol. 3, no. 7, Article ID a005041, 2011.

[19] D. K. Podolsky and M. W. Babyatsky, "Growth and development of the gastrointestinal tract," in *Textbook of Gastroenterology*, T. Yamada, Ed., pp. 547–584, J.B. Lippincott, Philadelphia, Pa, USA, 1999.

[20] D. Ménard, J. -F. Beaulieu, F. Boudreau, N. Perreault, N. Rivard, and P. H. Vachon, "Gastrointestinal tract," in *Cell Signaling and Growth Factors in Development: from Molecules to Organogenesis*, K. Unsicker and K. Krieglstein, Eds., vol. 2, chapter 20, pp. 755–790, Wiley-Vch, Weinheim, Germany, 2006.

[21] C. Lussier, N. Basora, Y. Bouatrouss, and J.-F. Beaulieu, "Integrins as mediators of epithelial cell-matrix interactions in the human small intestinal mucosa," *Microscopy Research and Technique*, vol. 51, no. 2, pp. 169–178, 2000.

[22] I. C. Teller and J. F. Beaulieu, "Interactions between laminin and epithelial cells in intestinal health and disease," *Expert Reviews in Molecular Medicine*, vol. 3, no. 24, pp. 1–18, 2001.

[23] A. B. Dydensborg et al., "Differential expression of the integrins $\alpha 6A\beta 4$ and $\alpha 6B\beta 4$ along the crypt–villus axis in the human small intestine," *Histochemistry and Cell Biology*, vol. 131, no. 4, pp. 531–536, 2009.

[24] A. Seltana, N. Basora, and J. F. Beaulieu, "Intestinal epithelial wound healing assay in an epithelial-mesenchymal co-culture system," *Wound Repair and Regeneration*, vol. 18, no. 1, pp. 114–122, 2010.

[25] I. C. Teller, J. Auclair, E. Herring, R. Gauthier, D. Ménard, and J. F. Beaulieu, "Laminins in the developing and adult human small intestine: relation with the functional absorptive unit," *Developmental Dynamics*, vol. 236, no. 7, pp. 1980–1990, 2007.

[26] P. H. Vachon, A. Simoneau, F. E. Herring-Gillam, and J. F. Beaulieu, "Cellular fibronectin expression is down-regulated at the mRNA level in differentiating human intestinal epithelial cells," *Experimental Cell Research*, vol. 216, no. 1, pp. 30–34, 1995.

[27] J. F. Beaulieu and P. H. Vachon, "Reciprocal expression of laminin A-chain isoforms along the crypt-villus axis in the human small intestine," *Gastroenterology*, vol. 106, no. 4, pp. 829–839, 1994.

[28] P. Simon-Assmann, B. Duclos, V. Orian-Rousseau et al., "Differential expression of laminin isoforms and $\alpha 6$-$\beta 4$ integrin subunits in the developing human and mouse intestine," *Developmental Dynamics*, vol. 201, no. 1, pp. 71–85, 1994.

[29] J. F. Beaulieu, "Differential expression of the VLA family of integrins along the crypt-villus axis in the human small intestine," *Journal of Cell Science*, vol. 102, no. 3, pp. 427–436, 1992.

[30] N. Basora, F. E. Herring-Gillam, F. Boudreau et al., "Expression of functionally distinct variants of the $\beta 4A$ integrin subunit in relation to the differentiation state in human intestinal cells," *Journal of Biological Chemistry*, vol. 274, no. 42, pp. 29819–29825, 1999.

[31] N. Desloges, N. Basora, N. Perreault, Y. Bouatrouss, D. Sheppard, and J.-F. Beaulieu, "Regulated expression of the integrin $\alpha 9\beta 1$ in the epithelium of the developing human gut and in intestinal cell lines: relation with cell proliferation," *Journal of Cellular Biochemistry*, vol. 71, no. 4, pp. 536–545, 1998.

[32] N. Basora, N. Desloges, Q. Chang et al., "Expression of the $\alpha 9\beta 1$ integrin in human colonic epithelial cells: resurgence of the fetal phenotype in a subset of colon cancers and adenocarcinoma cell lines," *International Journal of Cancer*, vol. 75, no. 5, pp. 738–743, 1998.

[33] J. F. Beaulieu, P. H. Vachon, and S. Chartrand, "Immunolocalization of extracellular matrix components during organogenesis in the human small intestine," *Anatomy and Embryology*, vol. 183, no. 4, pp. 363–369, 1991.

[34] A. Quaroni, K. J. Isselbacher, and E. Ruoslahti, "Fibronectin synthesis by epithelial crypt cells of rat small intestine," *Proceedings of the National Academy of Sciences of the United States of America*, vol. 75, no. 11, pp. 5548–5552, 1978.

[35] P. Simon-Assmann, M. Kedinger, and K. Haffen, "Immunocytochemical localization of extracellular-matrix proteins in relation to rat intestinal morphogenesis," *Differentiation*, vol. 32, no. 1, pp. 59–66, 1986.

[36] G. W. Laurie, C. P. Leblond, and G. R. Martin, "Localization of type IV collagen, laminin, heparan sulfate proteoglycan, and fibronectin to the basal lamina of basement membranes," *Journal of Cell Biology*, vol. 95, no. 1, pp. 340–344, 1982.

[37] J. Zhang, W. Li, M. A. Sanders, B. E. Sumpio, A. Panja, and M. D. Basson, "Regulation of the intestinal epithelial response to cyclic strain by extracellular matrix proteins," *The FASEB Journal*, vol. 17, no. 8, pp. 926–928, 2003.

[38] Y. D. Benoit et al., "Polycomb repressive complex 2 impedes intestinal cell terminal differentiation," *Journal of Cell Science*. In press.

[39] Y. D. Benoit, F. Paré, C. Francoeur et al., "Cooperation between HNF-1α, Cdx2, and GATA-4 in initiating an differentiation program in a normal human intestinal epithelial progenitor cell line," *American Journal of Physiology. Gastrointestinal and Liver Physiology*, vol. 298, no. 4, pp. G504–G517, 2010.

[40] L. P. Pageot, N. Perreault, N. Basora, C. Francoeur, P. Magny, and J. F. Beaulieu, "Human cell models to study small intestinal functions: recapitulation of the crypt-villus axis," *Microscopy Research and Technique*, vol. 49, no. 4, pp. 394–406, 2000.

[41] C. Francoeur, F. Escaffit, P. H. Vachon, and J. F. Beaulieu, "Proinflammatory cytokines TNF-alpha; and IFN-γ alter laminin expression under an apoptosis-independent mechanism in human intestinal epithelial cells," *American Journal of Physiology. Gastrointestinal and Liver Physiology*, vol. 287, no. 3, pp. G592–G598, 2004.

[42] L. M. Schnapp, J. M. Breuss, D. M. Ramos, D. Sheppard, and R. Pytela, "Sequence and tissue distribution of the human integrin $\alpha 8$ subunit: a $\beta 1$-associated α subunit expressed in smooth muscle cells," *Journal of Cell Science*, vol. 108, no. 2, pp. 537–544, 1995.

[43] B. Bossy, E. Bossy-Wetzel, and L. F. Reichardt, "Characterization of the integrin $\alpha 8$ subunit: a new integrin $\beta 1$-associated subunit, which is prominently expressed on axons and on cells in contact with basal laminae in chick embryos," *EMBO Journal*, vol. 10, no. 9, pp. 2375–2385, 1991.

[44] B. Bieritz, P. Spessotto, A. Colombatti, A. Jahn, F. Prols, and A. Hartner, "Role of $\alpha 8$ integrin in mesangial cell adhesion, migration, and proliferation," *Kidney International*, vol. 64, no. 1, pp. 119–127, 2003.

[45] R. Zargham and G. Thibault, "$\alpha 8$ Integrin expression is required for maintenance of the smooth muscle cell differentiated phenotype," *Cardiovascular Research*, vol. 71, no. 1, pp. 170–178, 2006.

[46] R. Zargham, R. M. Touyz, and G. Thibault, "$\alpha 8$ Integrin overexpression in de-differentiated vascular smooth muscle cells attenuates migratory activity and restores the characteristics of the differentiated phenotype," *Atherosclerosis*, vol. 195, no. 2, pp. 303–312, 2007.

[47] R. Zargham, B. R. Wamhoff, and G. Thibault, "RNA interference targeting α8 integrin attenuates smooth muscle cell growth," *FEBS Letters*, vol. 581, no. 5, pp. 939–943, 2007.

[48] Y. D. Benoit, C. Lussier, P. A. Ducharme et al., "Integrin α8β1 regulates adhesion, migration and proliferation of human intestinal crypt cells via a predominant RhoA/ROCK dependent mechanism," *Biology of the Cell*, vol. 101, no. 12, pp. 695–708, 2009.

[49] S. Cetin, H. R. Ford, L. R. Sysko et al., "Endotoxin inhibits intestinal epithelial restitution through activation of Rho-GTPase and increased focal adhesions," *Journal of Biological Chemistry*, vol. 279, no. 23, pp. 24592–24600, 2004.

[50] J. M. Russo, P. Florian, L. Shen et al., "Distinct temporal-spatial roles for rho kinase and myosin light chain kinase in epithelial purse-string wound closure," *Gastroenterology*, vol. 128, no. 4, pp. 987–1001, 2005.

[51] R. Zaidel-Bar, C. Ballestrem, Z. Kam, and B. Geiger, "Early molecular events in the assembly of matrix adhesions at the leading edge of migrating cells," *Journal of Cell Science*, vol. 116, no. 22, pp. 4605–4613, 2003.

[52] S. T. Barry and D. R. Critchley, "The RhoA-dependent assembly of focal adhesions in Swiss 3T3 cells is associated with increased tyrosine phosphorylation and the recruitment of both pp125FAK and protein kinase C-δ to focal adhesions," *Journal of Cell Science*, vol. 107, no. 7, pp. 2033–2045, 1994.

[53] Y. D. Benoit, J. F. Larrivée, J. F. Groulx, J. Stankova, P. H. Vachon, and J. F. Beaulieu, "Integrin α8β1 confers anoikis susceptibility to human intestinal epithelial crypt cells," *Biochemical and Biophysical Research Communications*, vol. 399, no. 3, pp. 434–439, 2010.

[54] R. Zaidel-Bar, M. Cohen, L. Addadi, and B. Geiger, "Hierarchical assembly of cell-matrix adhesion complexes," *Biochemical Society Transactions*, vol. 32, no. 3, pp. 416–420, 2004.

[55] S. P. Gout, M. R. Jacquier-Sarlin, L. Rouard-Talbot, P. Rousselle, and M. R. Block, "RhoA-dependent switch between α2β1 and α3β1 integrins is induced by laminin-5 during early stage of HT-29 cell differentiation," *Molecular Biology of the Cell*, vol. 12, no. 10, pp. 3268–3281, 2001.

[56] C. S. Haas, K. Amann, J. Schittny, B. Blaser, U. Müller, and A. Hartner, "Glomerular and renal vascular structural changes in α8 integrin-deficient mice," *Journal of the American Society of Nephrology*, vol. 14, no. 9, pp. 2288–2296, 2003.

[57] S. Cetin, C. L. Leaphart, J. Li et al., "Nitric oxide inhibits enterocyte migration through activation of RhoA-GTPase in a SHP-2-dependent manner," *American Journal of Physiology. Gastrointestinal and Liver Physiology*, vol. 292, no. 5, pp. G1347–G1358, 2007.

[58] D. Gagné, J. F. Groulx, Y. D. Benoit et al., "Integrin-linked kinase regulates migration and proliferation of human intestinal cells under a fibronectin-dependent mechanism," *Journal of Cellular Physiology*, vol. 222, no. 2, pp. 387–400, 2010.

[59] J. F. Groulx, D. Gagné, Y. D. Benoit, D. Martel, N. Basora, and J. F. Beaulieu, "Collagen VI is a basement membrane component that regulates epithelial cell-fibronectin interactions," *Matrix Biology*, vol. 30, no. 3, pp. 195–206, 2011.

[60] V. Bouchard, C. Harnois, M. J. Demers et al., "β1 integrin/Fak/Src signaling in intestinal epithelial crypt cell survival: integration of complex regulatory mechanisms," *Apoptosis*, vol. 13, no. 4, pp. 531–542, 2008.

[61] V. Bouchard, M. J. Demers, S. Thibodeau et al., "Fak/Src signaling in human intestinal epithelial cell survival and anoikis:

[62] differentiation state-specific uncoupling with the PI3-K/Akt-1 and MEK/Erk pathways," *Journal of Cellular Physiology*, vol. 212, no. 3, pp. 717–728, 2007.

[62] R. F. Gillespie and L. J. Gudas, "Retinoic acid receptor isotype specificity in F9 teratocarcinoma stem cells results from the differential recruitment of coregulators to retinoic acid response elements," *Journal of Biological Chemistry*, vol. 282, no. 46, pp. 33421–33434, 2007.

[63] M. C. Subauste, O. Pertz, E. D. Adamson, C. E. Turner, S. Junger, and K. M. Hahn, "Vinculin modulation of paxillin-FAK interactions regulates ERK to control survival and motility," *Journal of Cell Biology*, vol. 165, no. 3, pp. 371–381, 2004.

[64] C. E. Turner, "Paxillin interactions," *Journal of Cell Science*, vol. 113, no. 23, pp. 4139–4140, 2000.

[65] N. Barker, R. A. Ridgway, J. H. Van Es et al., "Crypt stem cells as the cells-of-origin of intestinal cancer," *Nature*, vol. 457, no. 7229, pp. 608–611, 2009.

[66] G. E. Morozevich, N. I. Kozlova, A. N. Chubukina, and A. E. Berman, "Role of integrin alphavbeta3 in substrate-dependent apoptosis of human intestinal carcinoma cells," *Biochemistry*, vol. 68, no. 4, pp. 416–423, 2003.

[67] Y. Mao and J. E. Schwarzbauer, "Fibronectin fibrillogenesis, a cell-mediated matrix assembly process," *Matrix Biology*, vol. 24, no. 6, pp. 389–399, 2005.

[68] K. R. Legate, E. Montañez, O. Kudlacek, and R. Fässler, "ILK, PINCH and parvin: the tIPP of integrin signalling," *Nature Reviews Molecular Cell Biology*, vol. 7, no. 1, pp. 20–31, 2006.

[69] J. L. Sepulveda and C. Wu, "The parvins," *Cellular and Molecular Life Sciences*, vol. 63, no. 1, pp. 25–35, 2006.

[70] S. A. Wickström, A. Lange, E. Montanez, and R. Fässler, "The ILK/PINCH/parvin complex: the kinase is dead, long live the pseudokinase!," *EMBO Journal*, vol. 29, no. 2, pp. 281–291, 2010.

[71] Y. Zhang, L. Guo, K. Chen, and C. Wu, "A critical role of the PINCH-integrin-linked kinase interaction in the regulation of cell shape change and migration," *Journal of Biological Chemistry*, vol. 277, no. 1, pp. 318–326, 2002.

[72] K. Assi, J. Mills, D. Owen et al., "Integrin-linked kinase regulates cell proliferation and tumour growth in murine colitis-associated carcinogenesis," *Gut*, vol. 57, no. 7, pp. 931–940, 2008.

[73] V. Vouret-Craviari, E. Boulter, D. Grall, C. Matthews, and E. Van Obberghen-Schilling, "ILK is required for the assembly of matrix-forming adhesions and capillary morphogenesis in endothelial cells," *Journal of Cell Science*, vol. 117, no. 19, pp. 4559–4569, 2004.

[74] C. Wu, S. Y. Keightley, C. Leung-Hagesteijn et al., "Integrin-linked protein kinase regulates fibronectin matrix assembly, E-cadherin expression, and tumorigenicity," *Journal of Biological Chemistry*, vol. 273, no. 1, pp. 528–536, 1998.

[75] L. Guo and C. Wu, "Regulation of fibronectin matrix deposition and cell proliferation by the PINCH-ILK-CH-ILKBP complex," *The FASEB Journal*, vol. 16, no. 10, pp. 1298–1300, 2002.

[76] C. Wu, "The PINCH-ILK-parvin complexes: assembly, functions and regulation," *Biochimica et Biophysica Acta*, vol. 1692, no. 2-3, pp. 55–62, 2004.

[77] P. C. McDonald, A. B. Fielding, and S. Dedhar, "Integrin-linked kinase—essential roles in physiology and cancer biology," *Journal of Cell Science*, vol. 121, no. 19, pp. 3121–3132, 2008.

[78] G. Baneyx, L. Baugh, and V. Vogel, "Fibronectin extension and unfolding within cell matrix fibrils controlled by

cytoskeletal tension," *Proceedings of the National Academy of Sciences of the United States of America*, vol. 99, no. 8, pp. 5139–5143, 2002.

[79] A. Yoneda, D. Ushakov, H. A. B. Multhaupt, and J. R. Couchman, "Fibronectin matrix assembly requires distinct contributions from Rho kinases I and -II," *Molecular Biology of the Cell*, vol. 18, no. 1, pp. 66–75, 2007.

[80] K. A. Brenner, S. A. Corbett, and J. E. Schwarzbauer, "Regulation of fibronectin matrix assembly by activated Ras in transformed cells," *Oncogene*, vol. 19, no. 28, pp. 3156–3163, 2000.

[81] P. E. Hughes, M. W. Renshaw, M. Pfaff et al., "Suppression of integrin activation: a novel function of a Ras/Raf- initiated MAP kinase pathway," *Cell*, vol. 88, no. 4, pp. 521–530, 1997.

[82] I. Wierzbicka-Patynowski and J. E. Schwarzbauer, "Regulatory role for Src and phosphatidylinositol 3-kinase in initiation of fibronectin matrix assembly," *Journal of Biological Chemistry*, vol. 277, no. 22, pp. 19703–19708, 2002.

[83] M. Delcommenne, C. Tan, V. Gray, L. Rue, J. Woodgett, and S. Dedhar, "Phosphoinositide-3-OH kinase-dependent regulation of glycogen synthase kinase 3 and protein kinase B/AKT by the integrin-linked kinase," *Proceedings of the National Academy of Sciences of the United States of America*, vol. 95, no. 19, pp. 11211–11216, 1998.

[84] Y. B. Kim, S. Choi, M. C. Choi et al., "Cell adhesion-dependent cofilin serine 3 phosphorylation by the integrin-linked kinase·c-Src complex," *Journal of Biological Chemistry*, vol. 283, no. 15, pp. 10089–10096, 2008.

[85] T. Fukuda, K. Chen, X. Shi, and C. Wu, "PINCH-1 Is an obligate partner of Integrin-linked Kinase (ILK) functioning in cell shape modulation, motility, and survival," *Journal of Biological Chemistry*, vol. 278, no. 51, pp. 51324–51333, 2003.

[86] M. Göke, A. Zuk, and D. K. Podolsky, "Regulation and function of extracellular matrix in intestinal epithelial restitution in vitro," *American Journal of Physiology. Gastrointestinal and Liver Physiology*, vol. 271, no. 5, pp. G729–G740, 1996.

[87] S. K. Kuwada and X. Li, "Integrin $\alpha5/\beta1$ mediates fibronectin-dependent epithelial cell proliferation through epidermal growth factor receptor activation," *Molecular Biology of the Cell*, vol. 11, no. 7, pp. 2485–2496, 2000.

[88] E. M. Hagerman, S. H. H. Chao, J. C. Y. Dunn, and B. M. Wu, "Surface modification and initial adhesion events for intestinal epithelial cells," *Journal of Biomedical Materials Research A*, vol. 76, no. 2, pp. 272–278, 2006.

[89] J. Zhang, C. R. Owen, M. A. Sanders, J. R. Turner, and M. D. Basson, "The motogenic effects of cyclic mechanical strain on intestinal epithelial monolayer wound closure are matrix dependent," *Gastroenterology*, vol. 131, no. 4, pp. 1179–1189, 2006.

[90] R. R. Bruns, W. Press, and E. Engvall, "Type VI collagen in extracellular, 100-nm periodic filaments and fibrils: identification by immunoelectron microscopy," *Journal of Cell Biology*, vol. 103, no. 2, pp. 393–404, 1986.

[91] P. Bonaldo, V. Russo, F. Bucciotti, R. Doliana, and A. Colombatti, "Structural and functional features of the $\alpha3$ chain indicate a bridging role for chicken collagen VI in connective tissues," *Biochemistry*, vol. 29, no. 5, pp. 1245–1254, 1990.

[92] D. R. Keene, E. Engvall, and R. W. Glanville, "Ultrastructu4re of type VI collagen in human skin and cartilage suggests an anchoring function for this filamentous network," *Journal of Cell Biology*, vol. 107, no. 5, pp. 1995–2006, 1988.

[93] H. J. Kuo, C. L. Maslen, D. R. Keene, and R. W. Glanville, "Type VI collagen anchors endothelial basement membranes by interacting with type IV collagen," *Journal of Biological Chemistry*, vol. 272, no. 42, pp. 26522–26529, 1997.

[94] P. Bonaldo, P. Braghetta, M. Zanetti, S. Piccolo, D. Volpin, and G. M. Bressan, "Collagen VI deficiency induces early onset myopathy in the mouse: an animal model for Bethlem myopathy," *Human Molecular Genetics*, vol. 7, no. 13, pp. 2135–2140, 1998.

[95] A. K. Lampe and K. M. D. Bushby, "Collagen VI related muscle disorders," *Journal of Medical Genetics*, vol. 42, no. 9, pp. 673–685, 2005.

[96] E. Tillet et al., "Recombinant expression and structural and binding properties of alpha 1(VI) and alpha 2(VI) chains of human collagen type VI," *European Journal of Biochemistry*, vol. 221, no. 1, pp. 177–185, 1994.

[97] R. Pankov, E. Cukierman, B. Z. Katz et al., "Integrin dynamics and matrix assembly: tensin-dependent translocation of $\alpha5\beta1$ integrins promotes early fibronectin fibrillogenesis," *Journal of Cell Biology*, vol. 148, no. 5, pp. 1075–1090, 2000.

[98] M. Aumailley, K. Mann, H. Von Der Mark, and R. Timpl, "Cell attachment properties of collagen type VI and Arg-Gly-Asp dependent binding to its $\alpha2(VI)$ and $\alpha3(VI)$ chains," *Experimental Cell Research*, vol. 181, no. 2, pp. 463–474, 1989.

[99] S. L. Du, H. Pan, W. Y. Lu, J. Wang, J. Wu, and J. Y. Wang, "Cyclic Arg-Gly-Asp peptide-labeled liposomes for targeting drug therapy of hepatic fibrosis in rats," *Journal of Pharmacology and Experimental Therapeutics*, vol. 322, no. 2, pp. 560–568, 2007.

[100] M. Pfaff, M. Aumailley, U. Specks, J. Knolle, H. G. Zerwes, and R. Timpl, "Integrin and Arg-Gly-Asp dependence of cell adhesion to the native and unfolded triple helix of collagen type VI," *Experimental Cell Research*, vol. 206, no. 1, pp. 167–176, 1993.

[101] Y. Fukata, K. Kaibuchi, M. Amano, and K. Kaibuchi, "Rho-Rho-kinase pathway in smooth muscle contraction and cytoskeletal reorganization of non-muscle cells," *Trends in Pharmacological Sciences*, vol. 22, no. 1, pp. 32–39, 2001.

[102] K. Kimura, M. Ito, M. Amano et al., "Regulation of myosin phosphatase by Rho and Rho-associated kinase (Rho-kinase)," *Science*, vol. 273, no. 5272, pp. 245–248, 1996.

[103] K. Iizuka, A. Yoshii, K. Samizo et al., "A major role for the Rho-associated coiled coil forming protein kinase in G-protein-mediated Ca2+ sensitization through inhibition of myosin phosphatase in rabbit trachea," *British Journal of Pharmacology*, vol. 128, no. 4, pp. 925–933, 1999.

[104] G. Totsukawa, Y. Wu, Y. Sasaki et al., "Distinct roles of MLCK and ROCK in the regulation of membrane protrusions and focal adhesion dynamics during cell migration of fibroblasts," *Journal of Cell Biology*, vol. 164, no. 3, pp. 427–439, 2004.

13

The Concept of Divergent Targeting through the Activation and Inhibition of Receptors as a Novel Chemotherapeutic Strategy: Signaling Responses to Strong DNA-Reactive Combinatorial Mimicries

Heather L. Watt, Zakaria Rachid, and Bertrand J. Jean-Claude

Cancer Drug Research Laboratory, Division of Oncology, Department of Medicine, McGill University Health Centre, Royal Victoria Hospital, Montreal, QC, Canada H3A 1A1

Correspondence should be addressed to Bertrand J. Jean-Claude, bertrandj.jean-claude@mcgill.ca

Academic Editor: Laura Cerchia

Recently, we reported the combination of multitargeted ErbB1 inhibitor–DNA damage combi-molecules with OCT in order to downregulate ErbB1 and activate SSTRs. Absence of translation to cell kill was believed to be partially due to insufficient ErbB1 blockage and DNA damage. In this study, we evaluated cell response to molecules that damage DNA more aggressively and induce stronger attenuation of ErbB1 phosphorylation. We used three cell lines expressing low levels (U87MG) or transfected to overexpress wildtype (U87/EGFR) or a variant (U87/EGFRvIII) of ErbB1. The results showed that Iressa ± HN2 and the combi-molecules, ZRBA4 and ZR2003, significantly blocked ErbB1 phosphorylation in U87MG cells. Addition of OCT significantly altered cell cycle distribution. Analysis of the DNA damage response pathway revealed strong upregulation of p53 by HN2 and the combi-molecules. Apoptosis was only induced by a 48 h exposure to HN2. All other treatments resulted in cell necrosis. This is in agreement with Akt-Bad pathway activation and survivin upregulation. Despite strong DNA damaging properties and downregulation of ErbB1 phosphorylation by these molecules, the strongest effect of SSTR activation was on cell cycle distribution. Therefore, any enhanced antiproliferative effects of combining ErbB1 inhibition with SSTR activation must be addressed in the context of cell cycle arrest.

1. Background

The genetic heterogeneity of solid tumours presents a challenge to cancer therapy such that single-targeted approaches, whether with nonselective cytotoxic drugs or highly specific kinase inhibitors, often fail due to the development of drug resistance. Invariably, as one receptor or pathway is blocked, alternate pathways substitute for the drug target. Moreover, if the target is not completely blocked, downstream components may be able to compensate. Therefore, modern chemotherapeutic strategies must adopt a more divergent targeting approach. Chemogenomic strategies seek to identify molecules which can target, upon minor modification, multiple members of the same family of proteins (e.g., protein kinases, GPCRs, or nuclear hormone receptors) [1, 2]. However, this remains a strategy whereby similar receptors with potentially similar functions within a tumour are targeted. The optimal strategy for an efficient multitargeting approach should be divergent to avoid the adverse effects of target redundancy at the advanced states of tumour progression. Over the past few years, we have designed molecules capable of targeting structurally unrelated cellular components (i.e., receptors and DNA). The fact that our unimolecular drugs that target both ErbB1 and DNA can be 10–20 times more potent than the combination of their single-target counterparts confirms the efficiency of divergent targeting [3–7]. Within the same context, we and others recently reported interactions between SSTRs (GPCRs) and ErbBs (RTKs) suggesting that these two receptor families might be ideal targets for our divergent strategy (Scheme 1) [8–10]. Therefore,

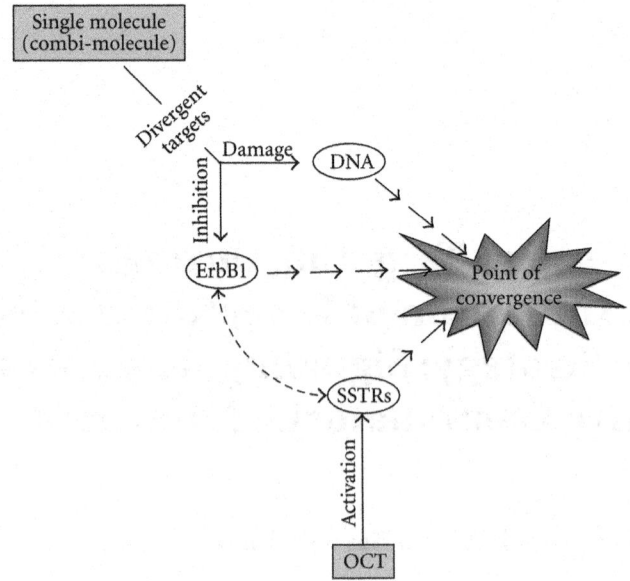

SCHEME 1: Principle of divergent targeting.

we recently designed a divergent targeting strategy whereby we activated somatotstatin (SST) receptors (SSTRs) with octreotide (OCT), blocked epidermal growth factor (EGF) receptor (ErbB1/EGFR) with kinase inhibitors, and ErbB1-DNA targeting combi-molecules and induced DNA damage.

SST functions as a potent inhibitor of hormone and growth factor secretion as well as a modulator of cell proliferation through its cognate receptors SSTR1–5 and regulates a variety of signal transduction pathways including the mitogen-activated protein kinase (MAPK) pathway [11–16]. In contrast to SSTRs, ErbBs play fundamental roles in development, proliferation, differentiation, survival, and transformation [17–19]. Major ErbB1 downstream signalling pathways include Ras/Raf/MEK/MAPK, PI3K/Akt, STAT, and PLCγ [18, 20, 21]. While both SSTRs and ErbBs activate the MAPK pathway, SST-induced MAPK activation results in delayed cell cycle progression and EGF activation promotes proliferation. Therefore, SSTR and ErbB1 are true divergent targets.

In a recent study, we showed exacerbation of cell cycle perturbations following the combination of multitargeted ErbB1-DNA combi-molecules with OCT, a SSTR agonist [22]. The lack of translation into cell kill was believed to be in part due to insufficient ErbB1 inhibition and DNA damage. Here, we report the analysis of cell response following exposure to concurrent treatment of OCT with combinations of single-target molecules and unimolecular multitargeted combi-molecules that damage DNA more aggressively and induce stronger attenuation of ErbB1 phosphorylation.

In this study, we combined strong ErbB1 TKIs with more potent chloroethylating DNA damaging drugs and investigated the cell signalling response to divergent targeting that induced concomitant ErbB1 inhibition, DNA damage, and SSTR activation. To this end, we analyzed the modulation of key proteins in the SSTR, MAPK, ErbB1-related signalling, and DNA damage response pathway (Scheme 2) as well as

cell cycle distributions with the purpose of identifying a pharmacological effect (see point of convergence, Scheme 1) that is significantly enhanced by the divergent targeting process.

2. Methods

2.1. Materials. EGF was obtained from Roche Diagnostics (Indianapolis, IN). Mouse monoclonal antibodies against p21 (sc-817) and rabbit polyclonal antibodies against ErbB1 (sc-03), GADD45 (sc-797) and phosphotyrosine (sc-7020), were from Santa Cruz (Santa Cruz, CA). Rabbit polyclonal antibodies against phospho- and total Erk 1/2 (9101, 9102), phospho- and total p38 (9211, 9212), phospho- and total JNK (9251, 9252), phospho- and total p53 (9284, 2527), phospho- and total Akt (4060, 9272), and phospho- and total Bad (9291, 9295, 9292) were purchased from Cell Signalling Technology (Mississauga, ON). Rabbit polyclonal antibodies against survivin (AF886) were obtained from R&D Systems (Minneapolis, MN). Mouse monoclonal antibodies against XRCC1 (MS-434) and ERCC1 (MS-647) were purchased from LabVision (Fremont, CA). Ciprofloxacin and mouse monoclonal antibodies against α-actinin (A-5044) were from Sigma. Horseradish peroxidase-conjugated goat anti-rabbit and goat anti-mouse secondary antibodies (IgG) were from Jackson ImmunoResearch Laboratories (West Grove, PA). Cell culture media, Amphotericin B, HEPES, L-glutamine, and gentamycin sulfate were purchased from Wisent (St. Bruno, QC), while G418 was obtained from EMD Chemicals (Gibbstown, NJ). All other reagents were of analytical grade and purchased from various local suppliers.

2.2. Drug Treatment. ZRBA4 and ZR2003 were synthesized in our laboratory according to previously published procedures [23, 24]. Iressa (gefitinib) was provided by

The Concept of Divergent Targeting through the Activation and Inhibition of Receptors as a Novel Chemotherapeutic Strategy: Signaling Responses to Strong DNA-Reactive Combinatorial Mimicries

151

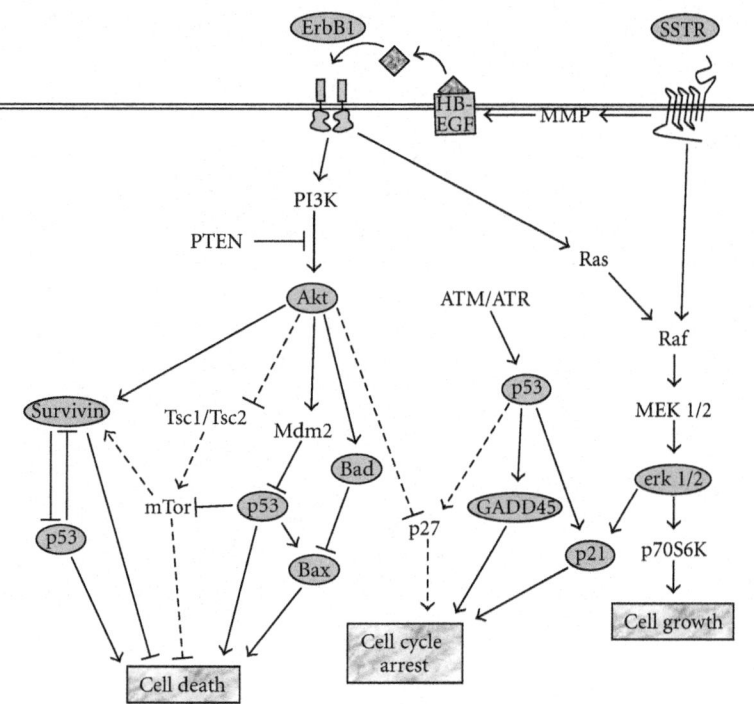

SCHEME 2: Key signalling pathways targeted with our divergent targeting strategy. The multitargeted approach includes activating SSTRs, inhibiting ErbB1, and inducing DNA damage. Key proteins analysed in this study are circled, while pathways not investigated are represented by dotted lines.

AstraZeneca, while mechlorethamine (HN2) was from Sigma and OCT was purchased from Bachem (Torrance, CA). The structures of these five drugs are presented in Figure 1. In all assays, drugs were resuspended in dimethyl sulfoxide (DMSO) and subsequently diluted in serum-supplemented medium immediately prior to use, unless otherwise specified. DMSO concentration never exceeded 0.2% (v/v).

We combined Iressa and HN2 at equimolar concentrations to maintain the same ratio of ErbB1 TKI : DNA damage molecules as the combi-molecules.

2.3. Cell Lines and Culture. U87MG glioma cells (American Type Culture Collection, Manassas, VA) and isogenic U87/EGFR and U87/EGFRvIII glioma cells (generous gifts from Dr. Frank Furnari, University of California, La Jolla, CA) were maintained in DMEM medium supplemented with 10% FBS, L-glutamine (1.76 μM), HEPES (5.25 mg/mL), and antibiotics (26.8 μM ciprofloxacin, 0.04 mg/mL gentamycin sulfate, 0.11 μg/mL Amphotericin B) at 37°C in an atmosphere of 5% CO_2/95% air. Selection pressure on the two transfected cell lines was maintained by supplementing the culture media with 400 μg/mL G418. All experiments were performed on cells between passage 2 and 4. In all assays, cells were plated in DMEM without G418 24 h prior to treatment of subconfluent monolayers.

2.4. Alamar Blue Assay. Inhibition of cell proliferation was monitored with CellTiter Blue (Promega) as per the manufacturer's instructions. Briefly, cells were plated in 96-well

plates and allowed to attach overnight. Cells were exposed to individual or combination treatments for six days. Treatments were terminated by the addition of 60 μL CellTiter Blue (1:4 dilution in PBS). Plates were incubated at 37°C for an additional 2.5 h, while viable cells metabolized resazurin (maximum absorbance of 605 nm) into resorufin, a fluorescent metabolite (maximum absorbance of 573 nm). This translated into a fluorometric colour change that was captured using SOFTmax Pro 4.3LS (Molecular Devices, Sunnyvale, CA) connected to a SpectraMAX Gemini plate reader (Molecular Devices, Sunnyvale, CA). The following filters were used: 580 nm for excitation and 600 nm for fluorescence emission. Data were analysed using GraphPad Prism 4 (GraphPad Software Inc, San Diego, CA). IC$_{50}$ values were calculated from three independent experiments run in triplicate. Statistical analysis was carried out using a one-way ANOVA, followed by a post hoc Tukey's test. P values < 0.05 were considered statistically significant.

2.5. Cell Cycle Analysis. Flow cytometric analysis of cell cycle profiles was performed on nonsynchronized cell populations as previously described with minor adjustments [25, 26]. Briefly, cells were plated in 6-well plates, allowed to grow until 65–75% confluency in serum-supplemented medium, and subsequently exposed to serial dilutions of drugs, alone or in combination, for 24 or 48 h at 37°C. Treatments were terminated by aspirating the media and rinsing the wells with PBS. Cells were subsequently collected by trypsinization, centrifuged (3500 rpm for 5 min) and washed twice with

Iressa	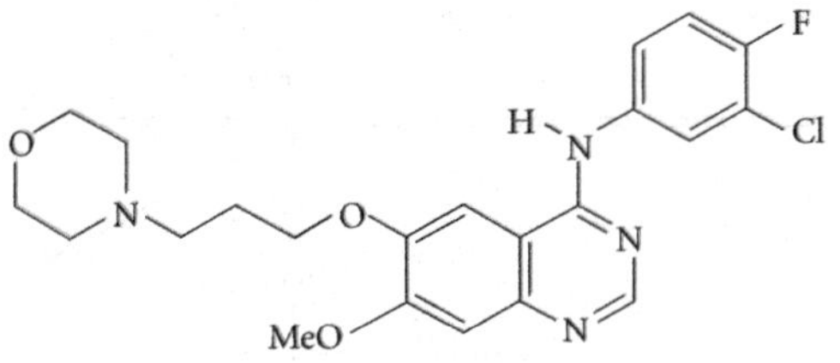
HN2	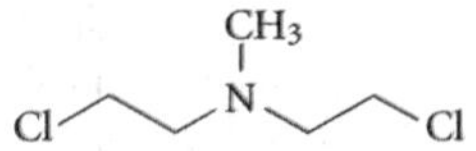
ZRBA4	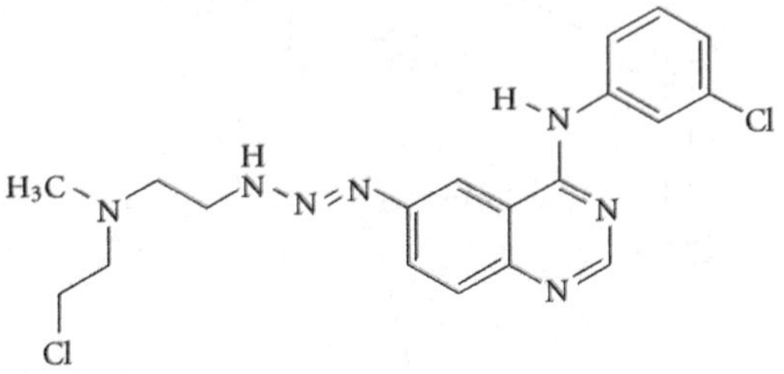
ZR2003	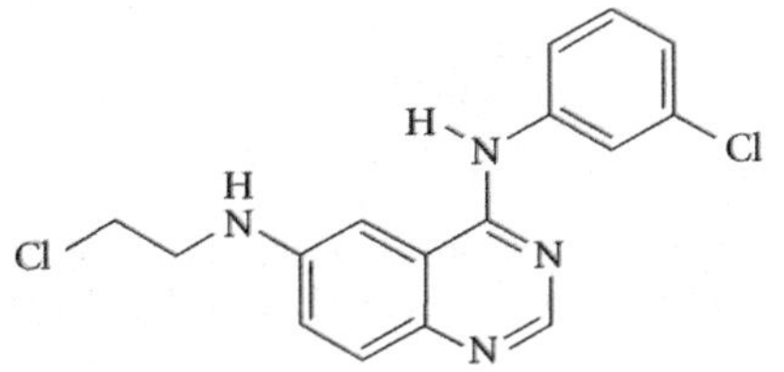
Octreotide (OCT)	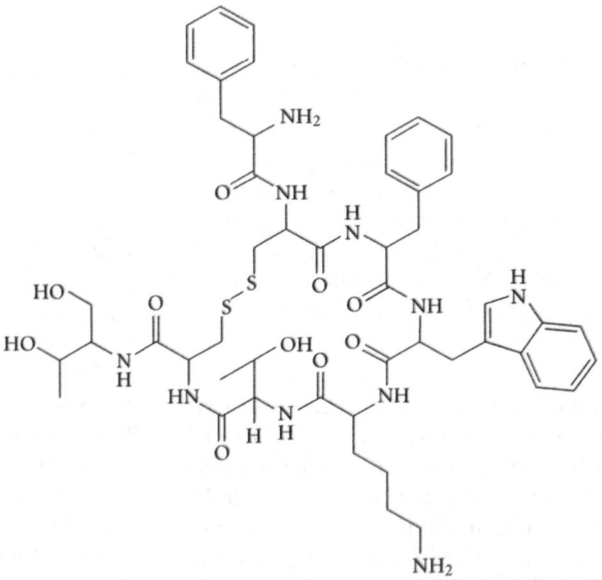

FIGURE 1: Chemical structures of Iressa, mechlorethamine (HN2), binary ErbB1-DNA damage combi-molecules (ZRBA4 and ZR2003), and octreotide (OCT).

PBS. Cells were fixed by slowly adding 1 mL ethanol (70%) with continuous vortexing and then stored at 4°C for up to eight days. The day of analysis, cells were pelleted by centrifugation (3500 rpm for 5 min), rinsed twice with PBS and incubated with 200 μL freshly prepared propidium iodide (PI)/RNAse solution (50 μg/mL, 100 μg/mL, resp.) in the dark for 30 min at 37°C. Data were collected using a BD FACSCalibur (BD Biosciences, Mississauga, ON) and the percentage of cells in each phase was calculated using FlowJo 8.4.6 (Tree Star, Ashland, OR). Data represent two independent experiments run in duplicate. Unpaired two-tailed t-test were used to identify significant changes in cell cycle distributions upon the addition of OCT. P values < 0.05 were considered statistically significant.

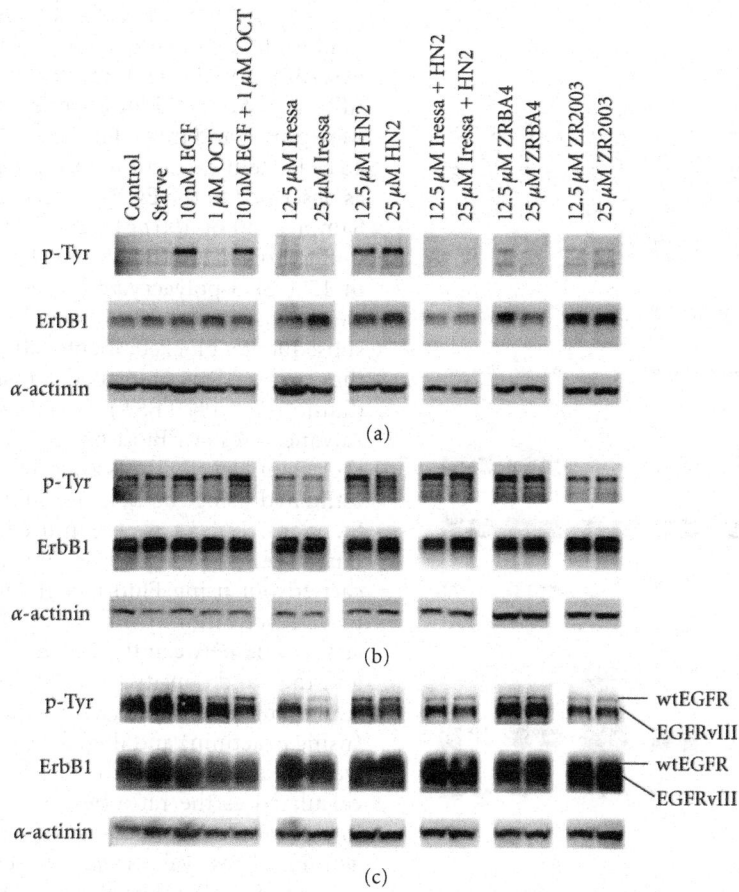

FIGURE 2: Dose-dependent inhibition of EGF-induced ErbB1 activation in U87MG, (a) U87/EGFR (b), and U87/EGFRvIII (c) glioma cells. Serum-starved cells were treated with the indicated concentrations of Iressa ± mechlorethamine (HN2), ZRBA4, or ZR2003 for 2 h followed by a 20 min EGF (50 ng/mL) stimulation. Cell lysates (40 μg) were fractionated by SDS-PAGE and probed with antiphosphotyrosine (1:1000) antibodies (see Materials and Methods for details). Blots were subsequently stripped and reprobed for total ErbB1 (1:1000) followed by α-actinin (1:1500). Major protein bands of 170 (ErbB1) and 100 kDa (α-actinin) were obtained.

2.6. Apoptosis. Cell kill was determined by Annexin V-FITC binding as previously described with minor modifications [27]. Briefly, cells were plated in 6-well plates and allowed to attach overnight. Cells (65–75% confluent) were treated with a range of drug dilutions prepared in serum-supplemented medium for 24 or 48 h at 37°C. Treatments were terminated by rinsing the wells with PBS, and cells were collected by trypsinization followed by centrifugation (3500 rpm for 5 min). Cell pellets were washed twice with PBS and then resuspended in 1X binding buffer for a final concentration of 1×10^6 cells/mL. Cells were treated with Annexin V-FITC and PI using the Apoptosis Detection Kit (BD Bioscience Pharmingen, San Jose, CA) according to the manufacturer's protocol. The reactions were subsequently quenched by the addition of 150 μL 1X binding buffer. Data were collected using a BD FACSCalibur, and quadrant analysis of co-ordinate dot blots was performed using FlowJo 8.4.6. Data represent two independent experiments run in duplicate.

2.7. EGF-Induced Autophosphorylation Assay. U87MG cells were plated in 6-well plates using serum-supplemented medium and allowed to attach overnight. At 85–90%

confluency, the wells were rinsed with PBS and the cells were starved for 24 h. Treatments consisted of 2 h exposures to the drugs followed by a quick rinse with PBS and a further 20 min treatment with 50 ng/mL EGF. Treatments were terminated by rinsing the wells with ice cold PBS and placing the plates on ice. Cells were scraped using a rubber policeman, and cell suspensions were transferred to labelled eppendorf tubes. Samples were centrifuged for two minutes at 10 000 rpm at 4°C, and the supernatant was removed. Cell pellets were homogenized in ice-cold lysis buffer (50 mM Tris-HCl pH 7.5, 150 nM NaCl, 1% NP-40, 1 mM EDTA, 5 mM NaF, 1 mM Na_3VO_4, 1 complete protease inhibitor tablet Roche Biochemicals, Laval, QC) and incubated for 30 min on ice. Samples were centrifuged at 10 000 rpm for 20 min at 4°C to remove cellular debris. Protein concentrations of the supernatants were determined by Bradford assay using known dilutions of BSA as standards. Samples (40 μg) were solubilized in Laemmli sample buffer, placed in boiling water for 5 min and fractionated by electrophoresis on a 10% SDS-polyacrylamide gel. The fractionated proteins were transferred by electrophoresis to 0.2 μm polyvinyli-dene difluoride (PVDF) membranes (Millipore, Bedford,

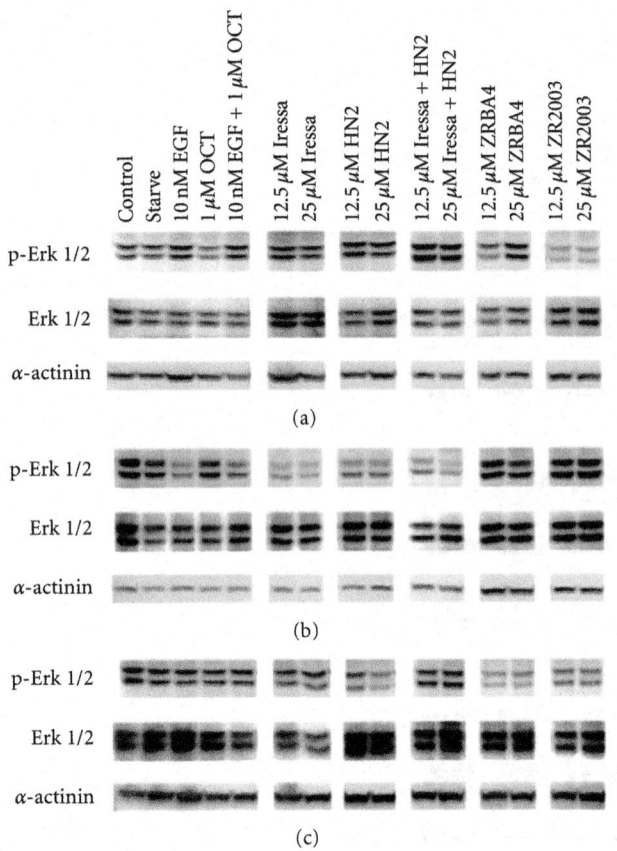

(a)

(b)

(c)

FIGURE 3: Dose-dependent inhibition of EGF-induced Erk 1/2 activation in U87MG (a), U87/EGFR (b) and U87/EGFRvIII (c) glioma cells. Serum-starved cells were treated with the indicated concentrations of Iressa ± mechlorethamine (HN2), ZRBA4 or ZR2003 for 2 h followed by a 20 min EGF (50 ng/mL) stimulation. Cell lysates (40 μg) were fractionated by SDS-PAGE and probed with anti-phospho-Erk 1/2 (1:1000) antibodies (see Materials and Methods for details). Blots were subsequently stripped and reprobed for total Erk 1/2 (1:1000) followed by α-actinin (1:1500). Major protein bands of 44, 42 (Erk 1/2) and 100 kDa (α-actinin) were obtained.

MA). Membranes were blocked, incubated with primary antibodies and then HRP-conjugated secondary antibodies (1:25 000 in 0.1% TBST) followed by chemiluminescence detection with the ECL Advance Western Blotting Detection kit (Amersham Biosciences) in accordance with the manufacturer's instructions. Molecular weights were estimated using the BenchMark prestained Western Protein Standard (Invitrogen). Images were captured using an Alpha Innotech FluorChem 8800 gel box imager, and densitometry was carried out using FluorChem software (Alpha Innotech Co.). Percent changes in ErbB1 tyrosine phosphorylation expression were calculated as the ratio between the density of the phosphorylated tyrosine band (185 kDa) and the band density for EGFR. These values were subsequently corrected for loading (using α-actinin) and then for basal expression (control level was set at 1).

2.8. Western Blot Analysis. To investigate Erk 1/2 and Akt inhibition, U87 glioma cells were cultured and treated as described for the EGF-induced autophosphorylation assay. All other Western Blot analyses were executed on cells that were grown and treated in serum-supplemented medium for 48 h. Protein extraction and quantification were performed as described in the EGF-induced autophosphorylation assay. Samples (40 or 100 μg) were solubilized in Laemmli sample buffer, boiled, and fractionated by electrophoresis on 10, 12, or 15% SDS-polyacrylamide gels. The fractionated proteins were transferred to PVDF membranes. The membranes were subsequently blocked, incubated with primary antibody and then with HRP-conjugated secondary antibody (1:25 000 dilution in 0.1% TBST). Signals were detected with the ECL Advance Western Blotting Detection kit in accordance with the manufacturer's instructions. Molecular weights were estimated using the BenchMark prestained Western Protein Standard. Images were captured using an Alpha Innotech FluorChem 8800 gel box imager, and densitometry was carried out using FluorChem software. Percent changes in protein activation (p-Erk 1/2, p-Akt, p-Bad) were calculated as the ratio between the density of the phosphorylated band and the band density for total Erk 1/2, Akt, or Bad, respectively. These values were subsequently corrected for loading (using α-actinin) and then for basal expression (control level was set at 1). Expression levels of all other proteins were calculated as the ratio between the density of the band of interest and the band density for the loading control (i.e., α-actinin). These values were subsequently corrected for basal expression (control level was set as 1).

3. Results

3.1. Inhibition of ErbB1-Mediated Signalling. Recent studies have reported strong ErbB1 TK inhibitory activity for ZRBA4 (4.4 nM) and ZR2003 (26 nM) [23, 24]. Therefore, we first investigated their ability to inhibit ErbB1 activation in our isogenic panel of brain tumour cells. All ErbB1 TKIs (Iressa, ZRBA4 and ZR2003) attenuated EGF-induced ErbB1 tyrosine phosphorylation in U87MG as well as U87/EGFRvIII cells (Figure 2). Moreover, Iressa and ZR2003 slightly decreased EGFRvIII phosphorylation. Similarly, at the concentrations tested, only Iressa and ZR2003 blocked ErbB1 phosphorylation in U87/EGFR cells.

We next determined whether inhibition of ErbB1 phosphorylation translated into attenuation of the downstream MAPK pathway, through which EGF induces proliferation (Figure 3). Iressa and ZR2003 inhibited Erk 1/2 phosphorylation in U87MG cells, while only Iressa attenuated Erk 1/2 activation in U87/EGFR cells. While ErbB1 phosphorylation in the U87/EGFRvIII cell line was inhibited by all TKIs or combi-molecules, they only induced moderate inhibition of EGFRvIII phosphorylation. Therefore, we had in hand all the levels of effects needed to examine cell response to the divergent targeting approach. When the combi-molecules or combination of Iressa + HN2 were coadministered with the SSTR agonist octreotide (OCT), no significant change in Erk1/2 phosphorylation status of the cells was observed

The Concept of Divergent Targeting through the Activation and Inhibition of Receptors as a Novel Chemotherapeutic Strategy: Signaling Responses to Strong DNA-Reactive Combinatorial Mimicries

155

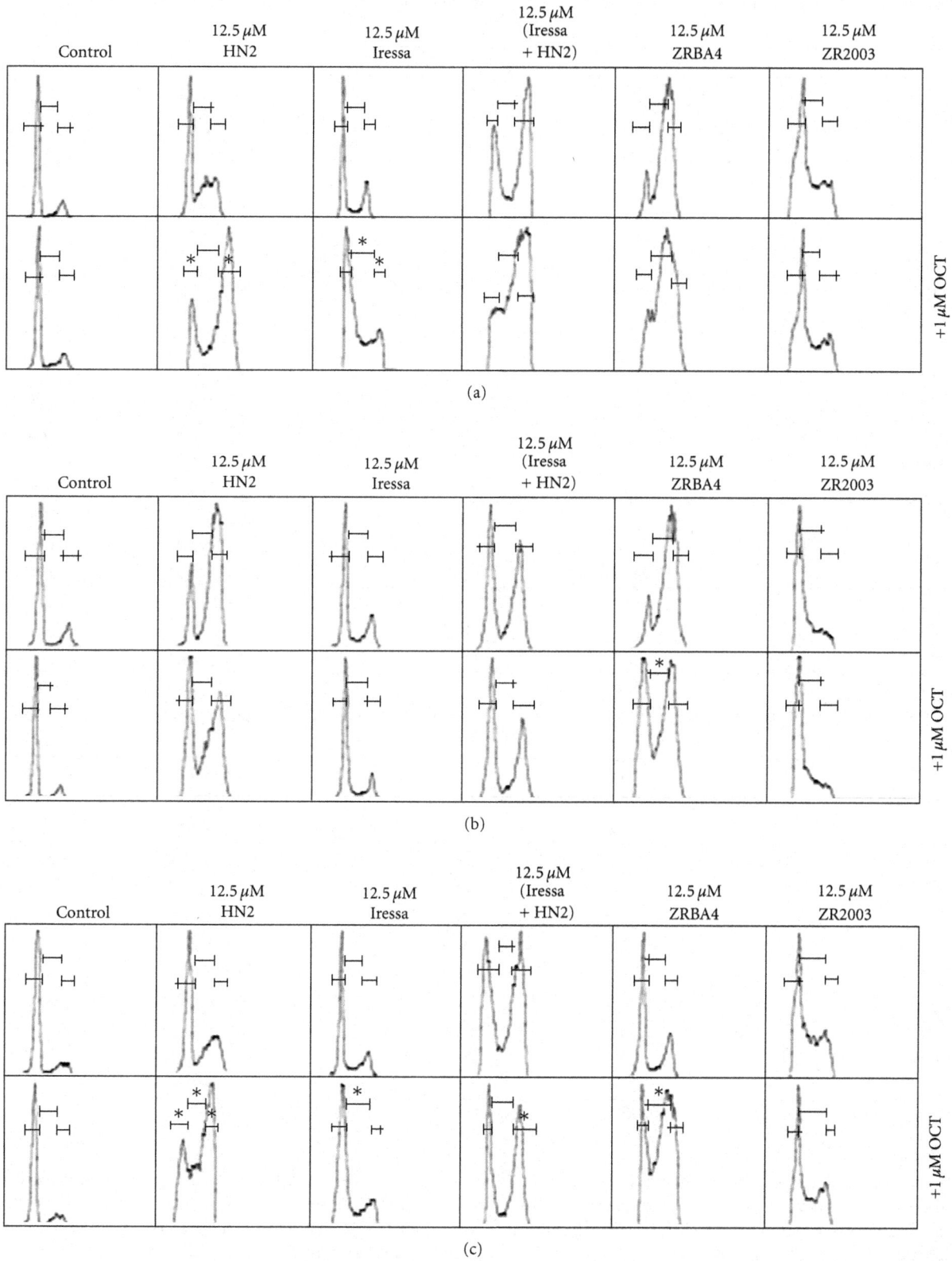

FIGURE 4: Representative histograms illustrating Iressa, mechlorethamine (HN2), Iressa + HN2, ZRBA4, and ZR2003-induced cell cycle arrest in U87MG (a), U87/EGFR (b), and U87/EGFRvIII (c) glioma cells following a 48 h treatment. Cell cycle perturbations following concomitant treatment with 1 μM octreotide (OCT) are shown in the lower panels. *Shows statistical differences, within the same phase of the cell cycle, between drug alone and drug + OCT (P < 0.05).

TABLE 1: Relative distribution of U87MG, U87/EGFR, and U87/EGFRvIII glioma cells across the G1, S, and G2 phases of the cell cycle. Cells were treated for 48 h with Iressa, mechlorethamine (HN2), Iressa + HN2, ZRBA4, and ZR2003 in the absence or presence of 1 μM octreotide (OCT).

		U87MG	U87/EGFR	U87/EGFRvIII
Control	G1	73.0 ± 3.4	80.0 ± 2.2	83.3 ± 0.2
	S	10.2 ± 1.5	4.2 ± 2.1	7.6 ± 0.6
	G2	17.3 ± 1.6	15.7 ± 0.1	9.1 ± 0.3
1 μM OCT	G1	77.2 ± 0.8	82.7 ± 2.9	82.7 ± 1.2
	S	9.3 ± 0.3	5.9 ± 3.0	7.0 ± 1.1
	G2	18.0 ± 2.6	11.5 ± 0.1	10.3 ± 0.7
12.5 μM HN2	G1	51.5 ± 7.8	20.7 ± 2.7	55.0 ± 0.2
	S	36.1 ± 1.7	49.1 ± 8.6	24.8 ± 1.8
	G2	20.1 ± 0.7	45.5 ± 0.9	20.1 ± 1.7
12.5 μM HN2 + 1 μM OCT	G1	18.7 ± 2.2*	30.6 ± 3.8	19.6 ± 4.7*
	S	48.7 ± 7.5	28.9 ± 2.7	71.7 ± 2.2*
	G2	59.5 ± 2.3*	35.0 ± 2.4	41.8 ± 1.8*
12.5 μM Iressa	G1	49.6 ± 5.7	63.6 ± 0.4	58.2 ± 2.3
	S	18.6 ± 1.2	15.3 ± 2.3	15.7 ± 0.5
	G2	21.9 ± 1.0	22.1 ± 2.9	22.5 ± 1.2
12.5 μM Iressa + 1 μM OCT	G1	53.1 ± 4.7	58.3 ± 2.5	66.3 ± 2.8
	S	40.5 ± 2.6*	22.7 ± 2.1	24.7 ± 2.3*
	G2	16.6 ± 1.7*	16.0 ± 1.7	13.6 ± 1.4
12.5 μM (Iressa + HN2)	G1	25.7 ± 6.4	32.0 ± 3.4	32.5 ± 9.3
	S	19.7 ± 1.8	32.0 ± 5.9	23.5 ± 9.5
	G2	39.6 ± 17.4	33.6 ± 1.8	44.7 ± 0.3
12.5 μM (Iressa + HN2) + 1 μM OCT	G1	23.5 ± 3.9	39.5 ± 3.8	34.9 ± 3.9
	S	51.9 ± 10.1	18.9 ± 2.4	17.2 ± 5.3
	G2	19.0 ± 2.9	22.3 ± 2.2	52.1 ± 1.2*
12.5 μM ZRBA4	G1	12.2 ± 0.3	15.6 ± 0.2	60.5 ± 0.3
	S	56.1 ± 1.3	71.4 ± 1.8	12.9 ± 0.3
	G2	31.1 ± 0.8	33.5 ± 2.5	26.5 ± 0.1
12.5 μM ZRBA4 + 1 μM OCT	G1	20.3 ± 6.9	31.4 ± 2.3	22.9 ± 4.7
	S	59.3 ± 4.0	39.0 ± 4.1*	50.6 ± 3.2*
	G2	23.7 ± 3.4	28.8 ± 2.1	28.3 ± 0.8
12.5 μM ZR2003	G1	52.1 ± 4.6	28.3 ± 1.9	35.3 ± 1.5
	S	26.3 ± 2.3	54.3 ± 2.7	53.5 ± 0.9
	G2	15.7 ± 2.0	12.7 ± 0.2	13.9 ± 1.7
12.5 μM ZR2003 + 1 μM OCT	G1	49.5 ± 4.6	32.6 ± 3.6	28.7 ± 1.9
	S	25.7 ± 1.6	57.8 ± 0.9	57.1 ± 0.5
	G2	19.3 ± 1.5	12.5 ± 1.3	12.1 ± 2.6

*Shows statistical differences, within the same phase of the cell cycle, between drug alone and drug + OCT ($P < 0.05$).

(data not shown). Total Erk 1/2 was relatively even across all treatments in U87 and U87/EGFR cell lines, while a dose-dependent increase was observed in U87/EGFRvIII calls, an effect that may be specific to the latter cell type.

3.2. Cell Cycle Analysis

3.2.1. HN2 + Iressa ± OCT-Induced Cell Cycle Perturbations. HN2 is a bifunctional alkylating agent that induces high levels of DNA cross-links. It is known to induce cell cycle arrest at all phases of the cell cycle. At high concentrations, it blocks cells in G1 and at low concentrations, it induces cell cycle arrest in S and G2/M. On the other hand, Iressa is known to arrest cells in G1. As demonstrated in Figure 4 and Table 1, treatment with 12.5 μM of HN2 induced cell cycle arrest in S in U87MG and U87/EGFRvIII transfectant cells but strong S (late) and G2/M arrest in the U87/EGFR cells. Surprisingly, Iressa induced some cell cycle arrest in

The Concept of Divergent Targeting through the Activation and Inhibition of Receptors as a Novel Chemotherapeutic Strategy: Signaling Responses to Strong DNA-Reactive Combinatorial Mimicries

157

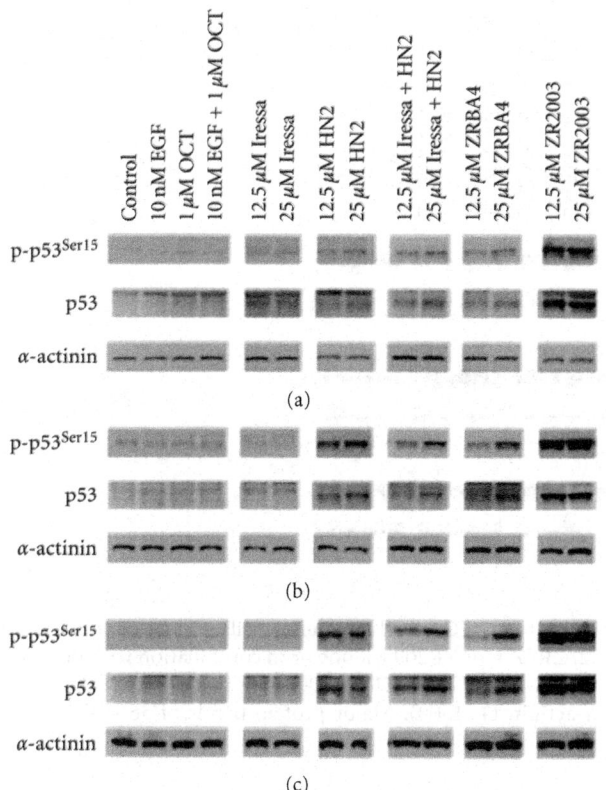

FIGURE 5: Dose-dependent changes in p53 phosphorylation (Ser15) and expression in U87MG (a), U87/EGFR (b), and U87/EGFRvIII (c) glioma cells treated for 48 h. Cell lysates (40 μg) were fractionated by SDS-PAGE and probed with antiphospho-p53 (1 : 1000) antibodies (see Materials and Methods for details). Blots were subsequently stripped and reprobed for total p53 (1 : 1000) followed by α-actinin (1 : 1500). Major protein bands of 53 (p53) and 100 kDa (α-actinin) were obtained.

the S phase. When the two drugs (HN2 and Iressa) were combined, a dramatic change in cell cycle distribution was induced leading to increased S (late) and G2/M arrest in all three cell types. More importantly, addition of OCT shifted the cell cycle arrests to S.

3.2.2. ZRBA4 ± OCT-Induced Cell Cycle Perturbations.
ZRBA4 is designed to be a prodrug of a DNA cross-linking alkylating species similar to HN2 and an ErbB1 TKI. It is therefore a unimolecular mimic of the HN2 + Iressa combination. ZRBA4 induced cell cycle arrest in S and G2M in U87MG and U87/EGFR cells (Figure 4, Table 1). Addition of OCT further perturbed cell cycle distribution profiles in a cell-dependent manner. U87MG cells shifted from S and G2/M arrest to the S phase. In contrast, OCT enhanced the accumulation of U87/EGFR cells in G1 at the expense of the S phase while leaving the G2/M population unchanged. Meanwhile, U87/EGFRvIII cells accumulated in the G2/M phase of the cell cycle in the absence of OCT. However, addition of OCT dramatically changed the cell cycle profile, leading to strong cell cycle arrest in late S and G2M.

3.2.3. ZR2003 ± OCT-Induced Cell Cycle Perturbations.
ZR2003 is a combi-molecule that does not require metabolic activation to generate its DNA damaging species: it can either block ErbB1 tyrosine kinase activity or damage DNA, and, unlike ZRBA4 and HN2, it cannot generate DNA cross-links. Therefore, its mechanism of action is different from that of ZRBA4. Interestingly, while ZR2003 induced S phase arrest in all three isogenic cell lines (Figure 4, Table 1), its effect was not altered by OCT, indicating the effects of OCT may be dependent on the type of DNA lesions induced by these drugs.

3.3. p53 Expression and Ser15 Phosphorylation.
Upon DNA damage, Ataxia-telangiectasia (ATM), ATM and Rad3-related (ATR), and DNA-dependent protein kinase (DNA-PK) activate p53 through phosphorylation at Ser15 [28, 29]. We detected a dose-dependent phosphorylation of p53 at Ser15 in all samples treated with HN2, alone or in combination with Iressa, and ZRBA4 (Figure 5). Moreover, treatment with HN2, HN2 + Iressa, and ZRBA4 enhanced p53 accumulation. Meanwhile, ZR2003, a type II combi-molecule, elicited the greatest activation as well as accumulation of p53 in all three cell lines. Finally, combination of OCT with these treatments did not enhance p53 activation nor expression.

3.4. Alterations of Key Players in the Cell Cycle.
To elucidate the pathway through which SSTR activation could enhance HN2 ± Iressa and ZRBA4-induced cell cycle arrest, we investigated changes in p21, a signalling intermediate for SSTRs as well as other pathways that play a role in cell cycle arrest. Since OCT enhanced HN2- and ZRBA4-induced S and G2/M arrest, we investigated whether this effect was mediated by p21. Unfortunately, p21 was not detectable in these cells, potentially due to downregulation by Akt. Based on these results, we decided to verify the expression of GADD45, another signalling intermediate in p53-induced G2/M arrest. The results showed that GADD45 was activated wherever p53 was phosphorylated (data not shown).

3.5. Effect of ErbB1 Inhibition on DNA Repair Proteins.
Eukaryotes have developed multiple types of DNA repair systems to ensure genomic fidelity before replication. ATM, ATR, and DNA-PK kinases check genomic integrity at the G1/S and G2/M checkpoints. Moreover, stimulation of ErbB1 has been reported to induce DNA repair proteins such as ERCC1 and XRCC1 [30]. The former plays a role in nucleotide excision repair (NER) and recombination repair, while the latter is involved in base excision repair (BER) and nonhomologous end-joining (NHEJ). HN2, as a bifunctional alkylator, damages DNA by alkylating its bases mainly at the N7 position of guanine [31–33]. This can result in DNA base pair mismatches as well as intra- and interstrand crosslinks. The N7-alkyl guanine can be repaired by BER, while the crosslinks are generally repaired by homologous recombination repair (HRR) and NHEJ. ERCC1 was upregulated in all three cell lines following a 48 h exposure to Iressa + HN2, ZRBA4, or ZR2003 (Figure 6). ZR2003

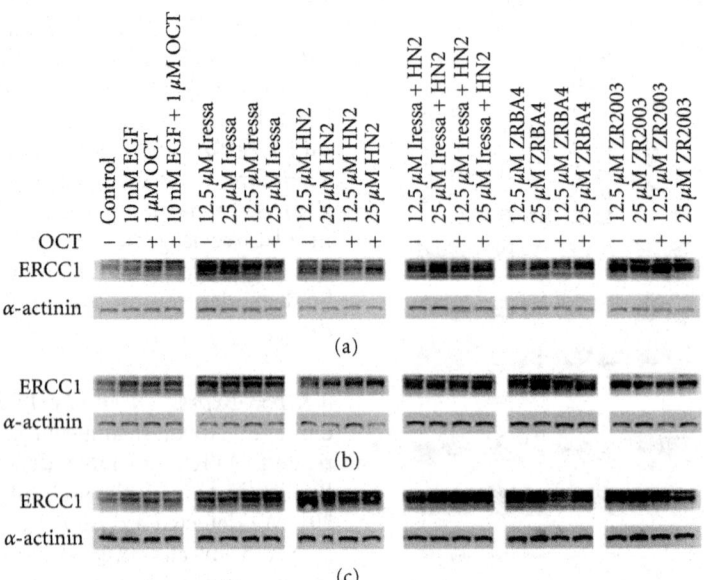

FIGURE 6: Upregulation of ERCC1 expression in U87MG (a), U87/EGFR (b), and U87/EGFRvIII (c) glioma cells. Cells were treated with the indicated concentrations of Iressa, mechlorethamine (HN2), Iressa + HN2, ZRBA4, or ZR2003, alone or in combination with octreotide (OCT) for 48 h. Cell lysates (40 μg) were fractionated by SDS-PAGE and probed with anti-ERCC1 (1 : 1000) antibodies (see Materials and Methods for details). Blots were subsequently stripped and reprobed for α-actinin (1 : 1500). Major protein bands of 36 (ERCC1) and 100 kDa (α-actinin) were obtained.

TABLE 2: Inhibition of U87MG, U87/EGFR, and U87/EGFRvIII cell growth by Iressa ± mechlorethamine (HN2), ZRBA4, and ZR2003, alone or in combination with 1 μM octreotide (OCT), as assessed by the alamar blue assay.

	U87 IC$_{50}$ (μM)	U87/EGFR IC$_{50}$ (μM)	U87/EGFRvIII IC$_{50}$ (μM)
OCT	n/a	n/a	n/a
Iressa	11.89 ± 8.40	2.96 ± 0.05	34.14 ± 3.53
Iressa + OCT	13.01 ± 9.70	3.27 ± 0.28	32.23 ± 3.80
HN2	9.58 ± 1.20	1.52 ± 0.59	19.74 ± 2.85
HN2 + OCT	n/a	1.81 ± 0.68	13.33 ± 3.78
Iressa + HN2	14.51 ± 0.20	0.77 ± 0.27	15.82 ± 1.97
Iressa + HN2 + OCT	12.24 ± 1.53	0.66 ± 0.13	n/a
ZRBA4	8.27 ± 0.57	3.91 ± 0.62	7.50 ± 0.82
ZRBA4 + OCT	8.20 ± 0.59	3.58 ± 0.52	7.45 ± 0.62
ZR2003	0.82 ± 0.24	0.87 ± 0.14	0.54 ± 0.18
ZR2003 + OCT	0.77 ± 0.19	0.73 ± 0.08	0.43 ± 0.14

Values are presented as mean ± SEM and are representative of 3 experiments run in triplicate.

elicited the strongest response in U87MG cells, while ERCC1 expression in U87/EGFR cells was most strongly upregulated in response to ZRBA4. Moreover, U87/EGFRvIII cells showed the strongest upregulation of ERCC1 with Iressa + HN2, ZRBA4, and ZR2003 eliciting similar degrees of upregulation. In contrast, XRCC1 was not detected over the course of the 48 h treatments (data not shown).

3.6. Antiproliferative Activity of ZRBA4, ZR2003, Iressa, HN2, and OCT. We next investigated the anti-proliferative effects of ZRBA4, ZR2003, Iressa, and HN2, alone as well as in combination with OCT, using a 6-day alamar blue assay (Table 2).

ZRBA4, a type I combi-molecule, demonstrated 1.4-and-4.5 fold superior antiproliferative activity ($P < 0.05$) over Iressa in U87MG and U87/EGFRvIII cells, respectively. ZRBA4 also slightly enhanced growth inhibition over HN2 in U87MG cells, while it induced a 2.6-fold increase in cell kill compared with HN2 in U87/EGFRvIII cells. Consistent with the combi-targeting concept, a 6-day treatment with ZRBA4 resulted in a 1.8-to 2.1-fold superior inhibition of proliferation ($P < 0.05$) compared with the two-drug Iressa + HN2 combination in U87MG and U87/EGFRvIII cells (Figure 7, Table 2). In addition, ZRBA4 showed 2.1-fold selectivity for ErbB1-overexpressing cells ($P < 0.05$); however, in U87/EGFR cells,

The Concept of Divergent Targeting through the Activation and Inhibition of Receptors as a Novel Chemotherapeutic Strategy: Signaling Responses to Strong DNA-Reactive Combinatorial Mimicries

159

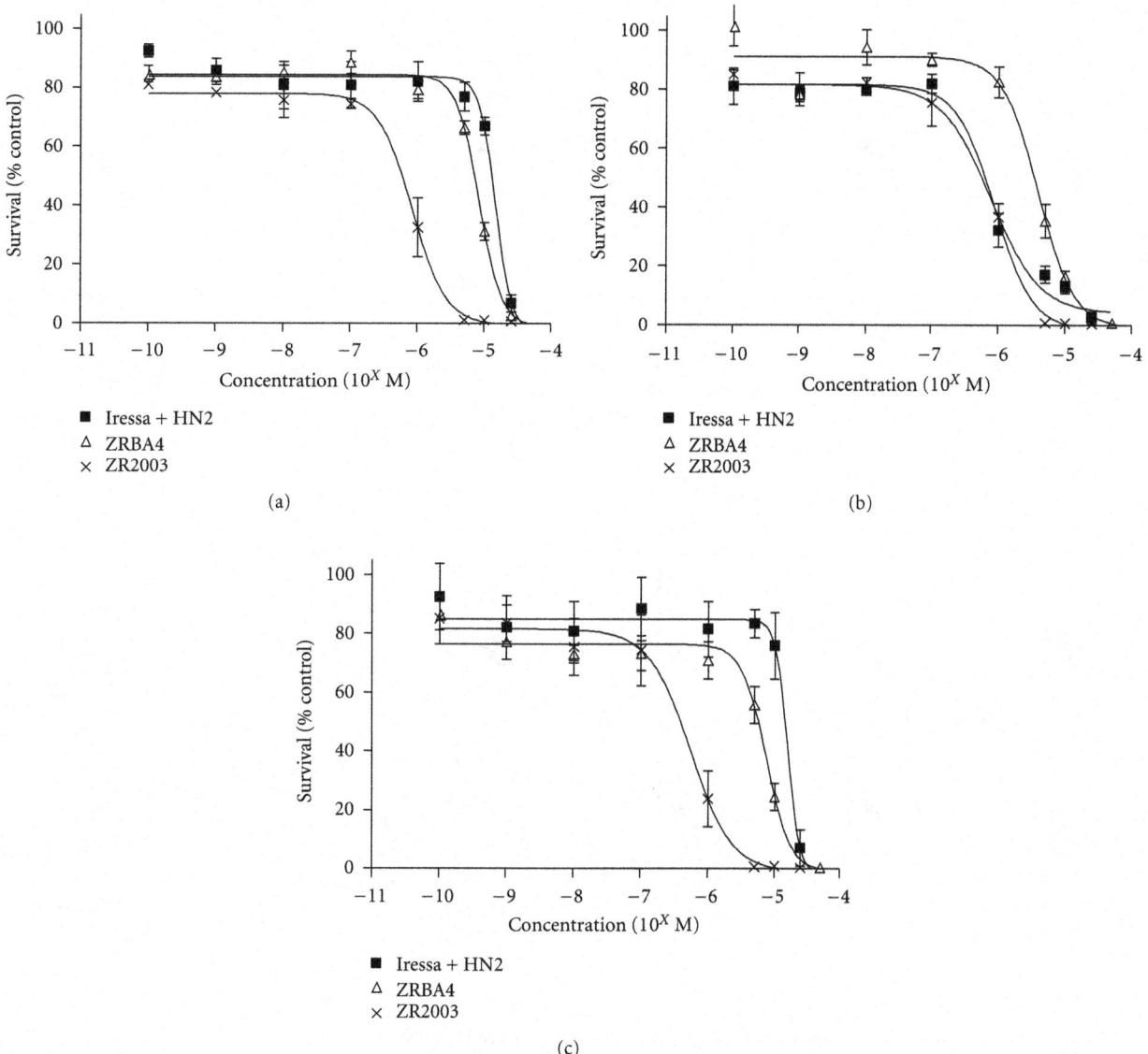

FIGURE 7: Relative growth inhibition of ZRBA4, ZR2003, and equimolar combination of Iressa + mechlorethamine (HN2) in U87MG (a), U87/EGFR (b), and U87/EGFRvIII (c) isogenic glioma cells. Cells were exposed to each drug for 6 days, and growth inhibition was measured by alamar blue assay (see Materials and Methods for details). Each point represents three independent experiments run in triplicate.

it was less effective at inhibiting proliferation than Iressa, HN2, and Iressa + HN2. In contrast, ZR2003, a type II combi-molecule, demonstrated a slight selectivity (1.5-fold) for the EGFRvIII mutation. It showed 14.5-, 3.4-, and 63-fold superior antiproliferative activity ($P < 0.05$) over Iressa in U87MG, U87/EGFR, and U87/EGFRvIII cells, respectively. Moreover, in U87/EGFRvIII cells, ZR2003 demonstrated a statistically significant ($P < 0.05$) 29.3-fold enhancement of cell kill over Iressa + HN2 (Figure 7). A more moderate 11.7-and 17.7-fold increase in growth inhibition ($P < 0.05$) was detected in U87MG cells treated with HN2 or Iressa + HN2, respectively. We also investigated whether simultaneous activation of SSTRs with OCT would enhance the antiproliferative activity of the binary-targeted combi-molecules but did not detect any significant interactions.

3.7. Apoptosis. We subsequently determined how the observed cell cycle perturbations would translate into apoptosis (Figures 8 and 9). Cell death was induced in the three cell lines by HN2 as well as Iressa + HN2. Interestingly, a shorter (24 h) treatment with HN2 mainly induced a nonapoptotic cell death pathway, while we detected some cells undergoing apoptosis following a longer (48 h) exposure (Figure 8). Meanwhile, ZRBA4 induced minimal cell death in U87/EGFRvIII (data not shown) and U87MG cells and nonapoptotic cell death in U87/EGFR cells (Figure 8). Moreover, ZR2003 showed dose-dependent induction of cell death with relatively strong early (within 24 h) induction of nonapoptotic cell death (Figure 8). Finally, when we combined 1 μM OCT with the above treatments, we did not detect any potentiation of cell death.

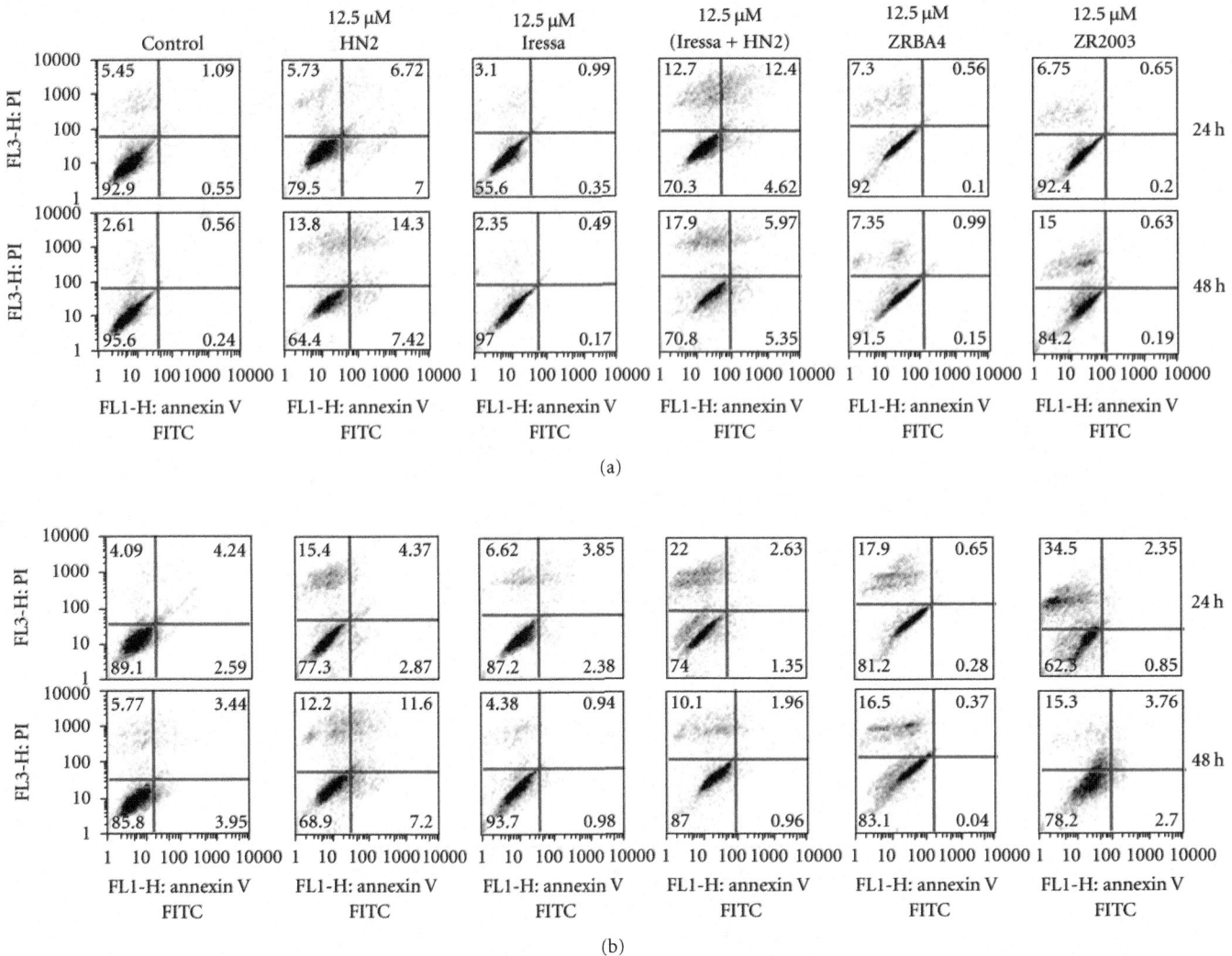

FIGURE 8: Representative Annexin V/propidium iodide (PI) intensity dot blots of U87MG (a) and U87/EGFR (b) cells treated for 24 (upper panels) or 48 h (lower panels) with Iressa, mechlorethamine (HN2), Iressa + HN2, ZRBA4, or ZR2003. Cell death was determined by Annexin V and propidium iodide (PI) staining (see Materials and Methods for details). Data are the mean of two independent experiments run in duplicate.

3.8. Modulation of Apoptotic as well as Antiapoptotic Signalling. To rationalize the lack of apoptosis, we extended our investigation to the analysis of key components of the DNA damage response pathway and the intrinsic apoptotic pathway. Based upon reports that DNA alkylators, including HN2, induce apoptosis partially through JNK activation, we investigated JNK and p38 activation by Western Blot analysis [34, 35]. Neither JNK nor p38 activation were detected (data not shown). This is consistent with the lack of induced apoptosis.

The PI3K/Akt pathway, another major downstream effector pathway of ErbB1, promotes cell survival by inhibiting apoptosis as well as modulating cell cycle arrest. We, therefore, verified whether the combi-molecules could alter Akt phosphorylation. However, due to a PTEN mutation in these cells, Akt was constitutively phosphorylated at Ser473 and unresponsive to ErbB1 inhibition (data not shown).

Since these cells responded to DNA damage with p53 activation as well as upregulation, we further extended our investigation and verified Bad phosphorylation at both Ser112 and Ser136. Phosphorylation of these two sites (by MEK1 and Akt, respectively) plays a critical role in cell survival through sequestration of Bad with 14-3-3 proteins thereby preventing Bad from binding Bcl-2 or Bcl-xL and subsequently releasing proapoptotic Bax. Therefore, we determined the extent to which our drugs modulated Bad phosphorylation. We also investigated whether combining OCT with the above treatments would further alter Bad phosphorylation. Bad was constitutively phosphorylated at Ser112 and Ser136 in U87 and U87/EGFRvIII cells (data not shown). In contrast, total Bad was barely detectable in U87/EGFR cells (data not shown). No treatment reduced Bad phosphorylation at either site. Moreover, OCT had no effect on Bad phosphorylation (data not shown).

The Concept of Divergent Targeting through the Activation and Inhibition of Receptors as a Novel Chemotherapeutic Strategy: Signaling Responses to Strong DNA-Reactive Combinatorial Mimicries

161

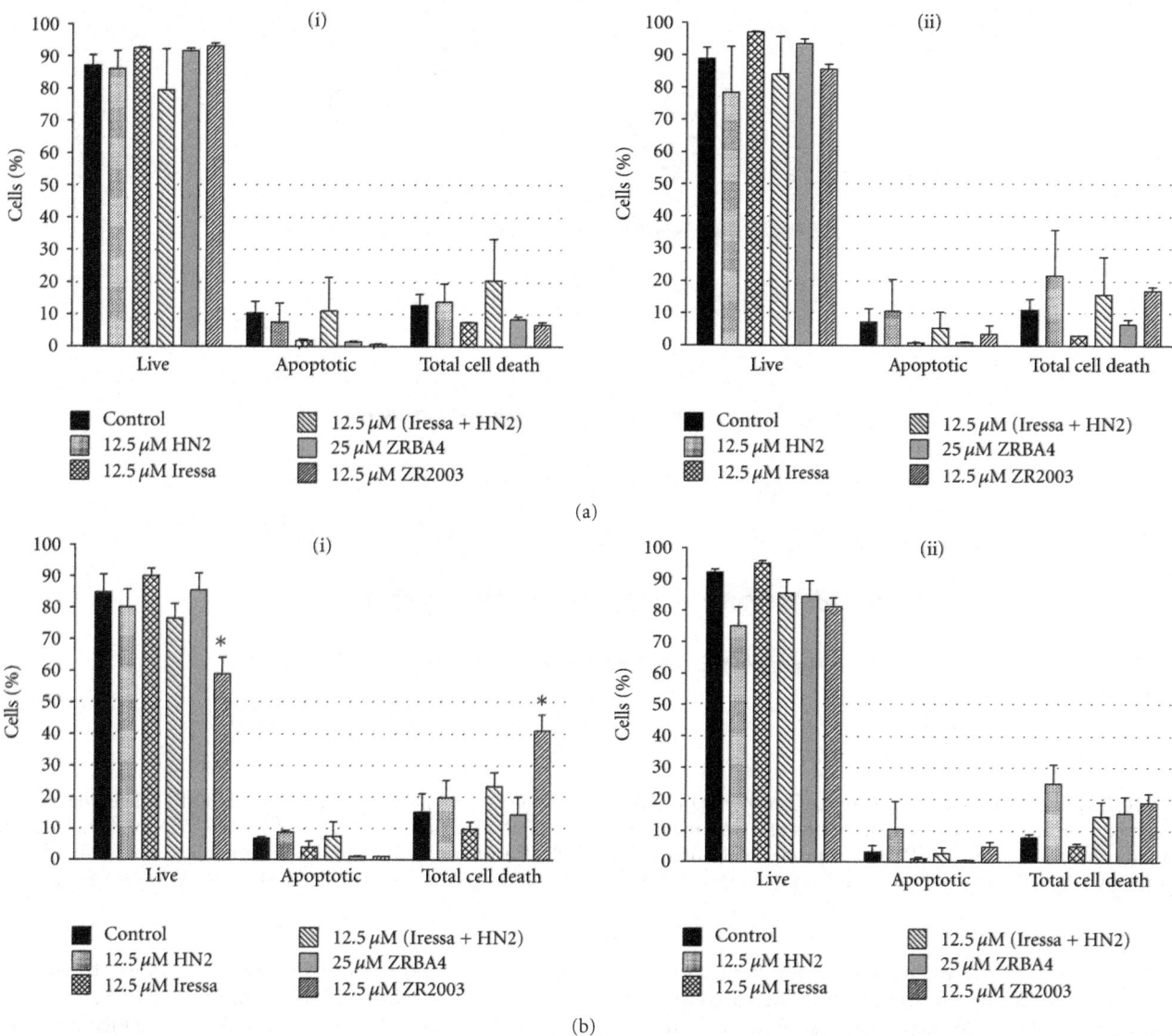

FIGURE 9: Assessment of apoptotic effects induced by Iressa ± mechlorethamine (HN2), ZRBA4, and ZR2003. U87MG (a) and U87/EGFR (b) cells were treated for 24 (i) or 48 h (ii). Levels of cell death were determined by Annexin V and propidium iodide (PI) staining. Bars for apoptotic cell death represent the mean percentage of Annexin-V-positive cells. Total cell death encompasses early and late apoptotic as well as necrotic cell death. Data are the mean of two independent experiments run in duplicate. *Statistically different from control ($P < 0.05$).

SSTR3 has been shown to play a role in p53-mediated apoptosis, while the other four SSTRs induce cell cycle arrest via p21 or p27. With no clear enhancement of p53, Bad, p21, or GADD45 by OCT, we extended our study to include another key protein in apoptosis, survivin. Survivin, an inhibitor of apoptosis protein (IAP), is most recognized for its role in chromosome segregation and cytokinesis [36, 37]. In addition to its role in cell division, survivin overexpression is associated with inhibition of apoptosis via both the extrinsic as well as intrinsic pathways although it is more efficient at blocking the latter pathway [38, 39]. In general, survivin and p53 negatively regulate each other's expression. However, as illustrated in Figure 10, ZRBA4 enhanced survivin as well as p53 (Figure 5) expression confirming blockage of apoptosis. In contrast, in HN2-

and ZR2003-treated gliomas cells, p53 and survivin were inversely related (Figures 5 and 10) while Iressa attenuated the HN2-mediated inhibition of survivin. We did not detect any OCT-induced regulation of survivin expression (data not shown).

4. Discussion

The effectiveness of single-targeted cancer therapies is mitigated by the inevitable onset of drug resistance. This may arise due to alternate pathways compensating for the drug target or to the accumulation of mutations within the target or components of downstream signalling pathways. Therefore, classical cancer therapies generally combine multiple drugs with different mechanisms of action to prevent drug

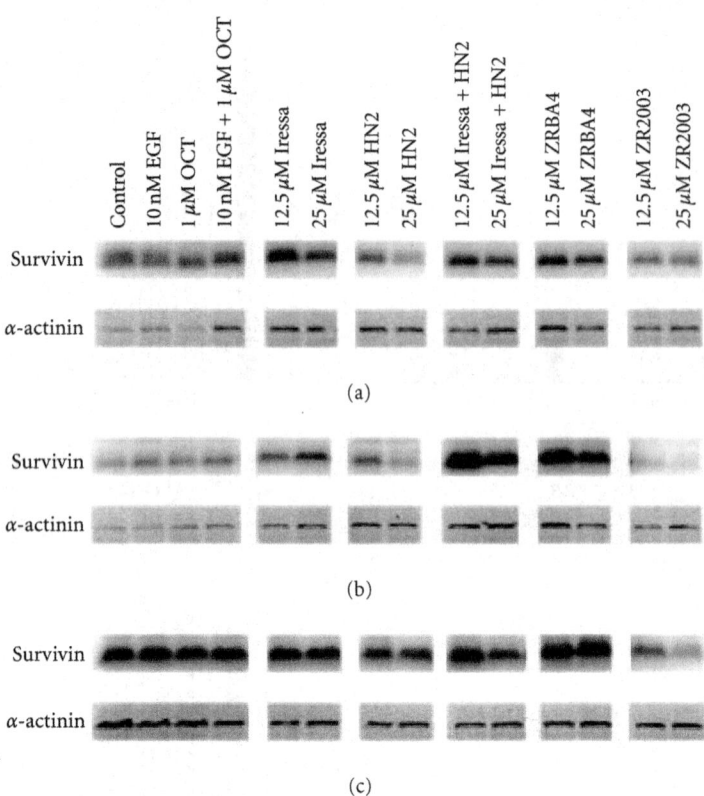

FIGURE 10: Treatment-dependent regulation of survivin expression in U87MG (a), U87/EGFR (b), and U87/EGFRvIII (c) glioma cells. Cells were treated with the indicated concentrations of Iressa, mechlorethamine (HN2), Iressa + HN2, ZRBA4 or ZR2003 for 48 h. Cell lysates (40 μg) were fractionated by SDS-PAGE and probed with antisurvivin (1 : 2000) antibodies (see Materials and methods for details). Blots were subsequently stripped and reprobed for α-actinin (1 : 1500). Major protein bands of 16 (survivin) and 100 kDa (α-actinin) were obtained.

resistance. However, due to the nonspecific nature of their binding, some combinations can result in increased toxicity. Moreover, the potency of these drugs is often mitigated by DNA repair pathways. Therefore, novel chemotherapeutic approaches are urgently needed. In this study, we examined our divergent targeting strategy using DNA damage, ErbB1 TK inhibition, and SSTR activation. We used OCT as our SSTR agonist, while HN2 + Iressa, ZRBA4 and ZR2003, chloroethylating combi-molecules, induced concurrent DNA damage and ErbB1 inhibition.

Previous studies have demonstrated the binary ErbB1-DNA targeting properties of ZRBA4 as well as its ability to induce DNA interstrand crosslinks in a manner similar to that of HN2 [23]. Consistent with literature, ZRBA4, as a partially irreversible ErbB1 inhibitor, showed selectivity for ErbB1-overexpressing cells. Furthermore, it manifested characteristics of both components (DNA damage and ErbB1 inhibition) as outlined by the similarity of the cell cycle perturbation profile that it induced when compared with equivalent two-drug combinations of HN2 + Iressa. Likewise, cell cycle arrest induced by the two forms of combinations (i.e., individual drugs or unimolecular combi-molecules) was significantly enhanced by OCT activation of SSTRs in these cells. Notably, OCT altered the cell cycle distribution profile of cells exposed to the DNA damaging

agent HN2 more dramatically than those treated with the ErbB1 inhibitor Iressa. However, its effect was more dramatic when HN2 was combined with the ErbB1 inhibitor, suggesting that ErbB1 inhibition plays a role in the overall cell cycle perturbation. As outlined in Scheme 2, SSTR activation induces cell cycle inhibitors, while ErbB1 phosphorylation downregulates them. Thus, inhibition of ErbB1 that leads to downregulation of downstream signalling (e.g., Erk1/2 activation) may relieve any antagonistic effect to SSTR-mediated cell cycle arrest.

In general, SSTR1, 2, 4, and 5 induce G1 arrest in a p53-independent manner while SSTR3 induces apoptosis through a p53/Bax-dependent mechanism [40–43]. Previous studies have shown that SSTR3-mediated p53 activation occurs independently of cell cycle arrest and p21 induction [44]. Moreover, p53-mediated activation of p21 promotes G1 arrest while loss of G1/S checkpoint control generally sensitizes cells to DNA damage. We did not detect p21 in our samples nor did the nitrogen mustard-containing compounds (HN2, ZRBA4, and ZR2003) induce significant G1 arrest, suggesting that the p53 activation and upregulation observed in the Western Blot analyses may not be related to cell cycle arrest. Thus the increased effect conferred by OCT may be due to a direct effect of SSTR activation on the cell cycle through induction of cell cycle inhibitors or other

The Concept of Divergent Targeting through the Activation and Inhibition of Receptors as a Novel Chemotherapeutic Strategy: Signaling Responses to Strong DNA-Reactive Combinatorial Mimicries

163

proteins that trigger the cells to arrest earlier in the cycle in response to the DNA damage induced by HN2 and our combi-molecules.

While p53 is generally associated with the induction of apoptosis, the absence of Bax upregulation and Bad dephosphorylation demonstrates that the p53-mediated apoptotic pathway is blocked. Moreover, the increased expression of survivin, an inhibitor of apoptosis protein (IAP), provides further evidence that the drugs tested in this study cannot induce apoptosis. However, HN2 (but not Iressa + HN2) activated and upregulated p53 as well as downregulated survivin expression after a 48 h treatment which translated into cells dying by both apoptosis (ca. 50%) and a nonapoptotic form of cell death. In contrast, ZR2003 showed the strongest p53 activation of all the drugs and combinations of drugs tested in this study. Yet, the concomitant decrease in survivin levels did not translate into increased apoptosis suggesting that the observed decline was not due to drug-induced inhibition, as observed with HN2, but was perhaps due to rapid turnover ($t1/2 = 30$ min) of the protein in the G1 phase of the cell cycle [45]. *In toto*, these data suggest that the concomitant inhibition of survivin may allow these cells to undergo apoptosis.

5. Conclusions

In summary, the results presented herein demonstrate that ErbB1 TKIs inhibit ErbB1 but not EGFRvIII phosphorylation. Moreover, due to a PTEN mutation, Akt was constitutively active and Bad remained phosphorylated, preventing cells from undergoing apoptosis upon ErbB1 inhibition. This may have played a role in p21 downregulation which could explain the absence of OCT-induced cell cycle arrest on its own. However, OCT potentiated arrest in the S-phase of the cell cycle when combined with Iressa ± HN2, or ZRBA4. Moreover, both Bax unresponsiveness to p53 activation and survivin upregulation despite p53 activation may contribute to the cells dying via a nonapoptotic pathway. Thus, future studies to improve the divergent targeting strategy should be directed at bridging the strong cell cycle perturbation observed to a cell death pathway.

Conflict of Interests

The authors declare that they have no competing interests.

Authors' Contributions

Dr. H. L. Watt performed the experimental work and prepared the paper. Dr. Z. Rachid synthesized ZRBA4 and ZR2003. Dr. B. Jean-Claude revised the paper.

Abbreviations

BER: Base excision repair
DMSO: Dimethyl sulfoxide
EGF: Epidermal growth factor
ErbB: Epidermal growth factor receptor
GPCR: G protein-coupled receptor
HN2: Mechlorethamine
HRR: Homologous recombination repair
ICL: Interstrand crosslink
MAPK: Mitogen-activated protein kinase
NER: Nucleotide excision repair
NHEJ: Nonhomologous end joining
OCT: Octreotide
PI: Propidium iodide
PVDF: Polyvinylidene difluoride
RTK: Receptor tyrosine kinase
SST: Somatostatin
SSTR: Somatostatin receptor
TK: Tyrosine kinase
TKI: Tyrosine kinase inhibitor
TMZ: Temozolomide.

Acknowledgments

The authors would like to acknowledge the Canadian Institute for Health Research (CIHR) and the Brain Tumour Foundation of Canada for financial support. H. L. Watt was supported by a McGill University Health Centre Research Institute Studentship.

References

[1] M. Bredel and E. Jacoby, "Chemogenomics: an emerging strategy for rapid target and drug discovery," *Nature Reviews Genetics*, vol. 5, no. 4, pp. 262–275, 2004.

[2] C. Harris and A. Stevens, "Chemogenomics: structuring the drug discovery process to gene families," *Drug Discovery Today*, vol. 11, no. 19-20, pp. 880–888, 2006.

[3] N. Merayo, Z. Rachid, Q. Qiu, F. Brahimi, and B. Jean-Claude, "The combi-targeting concept: evidence for the formation of a novel inhibitor in vivo," *Anti-Cancer Drugs*, vol. 17, no. 2, pp. 165–171, 2006.

[4] R. Banerjee, Z. Rachid, J. McNamee, and B. Jean-Claude, "Synthesis of a prodrug designed to release multiple inhibitors of the epidermal growth factor receptor tyrosine kinase and an alkylating agent: a novel tumor targeting concept," *Journal of Medicinal Chemistry*, vol. 46, no. 25, pp. 5546–5551, 2003.

[5] Q. Qiu, F. Dudouit, S. Matheson et al., "The combi-targeting concept: a novel 3,3-disubstituted nitrosourea with EGFR tyrosine kinase inhibitory properties," *Cancer Chemotherapy and Pharmacology*, vol. 51, no. 1, pp. 1–10, 2003.

[6] F. Brahimi, S. Matheson, F. Dudouit, J. McNamee, A. Tari, and B. Jean-Claude, "Inhibition of epidermal growth factor receptor-mediated signaling by "combi-triazene" BJ2000, a new probe for combi-targeting postulates," *Journal of Pharmacology and Experimental Therapeutics*, vol. 303, no. 1, pp. 238–246, 2002.

[7] S. Matheson, J. McNamee, and B. Jean-Claude, "Design of a chimeric 3–methyl–1,2,3–triazene with mixed receptor tyrosine kinase and DNA damaging properties: a novel tumor targeting strategy," *Journal of Pharmacology and Experimental Therapeutics*, vol. 296, no. 3, pp. 832–840, 2001.

[8] Y. He, X. Yuan, P. Lei et al., "The antiproliferative effects of somatostatin receptor subtype 2 in breast cancer cells," *Acta Pharmacologica Sinica*, vol. 30, no. 7, pp. 1053–1059, 2009.

[9] H. Watt, G. Kharmate, and U. Kumar, "Somatostatin receptors 1 and 5 heterodimerize with epidermal growth factor receptor: agonist-dependent modulation of the downstream MAPK signalling pathway in breast cancer cells," *Cellular Signalling*, vol. 21, no. 3, pp. 428–439, 2009.

[10] B. Burghardt, K. Barabás, Z. Marcsek, L. Flautner, T. Gress, and G. Varga, "Inhibitory effect of a long-acting somatostatin analogue on EGF-stimulated cell proliferation in Capan-2 cells," *Journal of Physiology Paris*, vol. 94, no. 1, pp. 57–62, 2000.

[11] Y. Patel, "Basic aspects of somatostatin receptors," in *Advances in Molecular and Cellular Endocrinology*, D. LeRoith and C. T. Greenwich, Eds., JAI Press, 1998.

[12] Y. Patel, "Somatostatin and its receptor family," *Frontiers in Neuroendocrinology*, vol. 20, no. 3, pp. 157–198, 1999.

[13] Y. Patel, M. Greenwood, R. Panetta, L. Demchyshyn, H. Niznik, and C. Srikant, "Mini review: the somatostatin receptor family," *Life Sciences*, vol. 57, no. 13, pp. 1249–1265, 1995.

[14] Z. Csaba and P. Dournaud, "Cellular biology of somatostatin receptors," *Neuropeptides*, vol. 35, no. 1, pp. 1–23, 2001.

[15] T. Florio, S. Thellung, S. Arena et al., "Somatostatin and its analog lanreotide inhibit the proliferation of dispersed human non-functioning pituitary adenoma cells *in vitro*," *European Journal of Endocrinology*, vol. 141, no. 4, pp. 396–408, 1999.

[16] H. Lahlou, J. Guillermet, M. Hortala et al., "Molecular signaling of somatostatin receptors," *Annals of the New York Academy of Sciences*, vol. 1014, pp. 121–131, 2004.

[17] D. C. Lev, L. S. Kim, V. Melnikova, M. Ruiz, H. N. Ananthaswamy, and J. E. Price, "Dual blockade of EGFR and ERK1/2 phosphorylation potentiates growth inhibition of breast cancer cells," *British Journal of Cancer*, vol. 91, no. 4, pp. 795–802, 2004.

[18] S. Okubo, J. Kurebayashi, T. Otsuki, Y. Yamamoto, K. Tanaka, and H. Sonoo, "Additive antitumour effect of the epidermal growth factor receptor tyrosine kinase inhibitor gefitinib (Iressa, ZD1839) and the antioestrogen fulvestrant (Faslodex, ICI 182,780) in breast cancer cells," *British Journal of Cancer*, vol. 90, no. 1, pp. 236–244, 2004.

[19] M. A. Olayioye, R. M. Neve, H. Lane, and N. E. Hynes, "The ErbB signaling network: receptor heterodimerization in development and cancer," *The EMBO Journal*, vol. 19, no. 13, pp. 3159–3167, 2000.

[20] S. Huang, E. A. Armstrong, S. Benavente, P. Chinnaiyan, and P. M. Harari, "Dual-agent molecular targeting of the epidermal growth factor receptor (EGFR): combining anti-EGFR antibody with tyrosine kinase inhibitor," *Cancer Research*, vol. 64, no. 15, pp. 5355–5362, 2004.

[21] S. Matheson, *The Combi-Targeting Concept: A Novel Tumour Targeting Strategy*, McGill University, Montreal, Canada, 2003.

[22] H. L. Watt, Z. Rachid, and B. J. Jean-Claude, "Receptor activation and inhibition in cellular response to chemotherapeutic combinational mimicries: the concept of divergent targeting," *Journal of Neuro-Oncology*, vol. 100, no. 3, pp. 345–361, 2010.

[23] Z. Rachid, F. Brahimi, Q. Qiu et al., "Novel nitrogen mustard-armed combi-molecules for the selective targeting of epidermal growth factor receptor overexpressing solid tumors: discovery of an unusual structure-activity relationship," *Journal of Medicinal Chemistry*, vol. 50, no. 11, pp. 2605–2608, 2007.

[24] Z. Rachid, F. Brahimi, J. Domarkas, and B. Jean-Claude, "Synthesis of half-mustard combi-molecules with fluorescence properties: correlation with EGFR status," *Bioorganic and Medicinal Chemistry Letters*, vol. 15, no. 4, pp. 1135–1138, 2005.

[25] S. Matheson, J. McNamee, T. Wang, M. Alaoui-Jamali, A. Tari, and B. Jean-Claude, "The combi-targeting concept: dissection of the binary mechanism of action of the combi-triazene SMA41 in vitro and antitumor activity in vivo," *Journal of Pharmacology and Experimental Therapeutics*, vol. 311, no. 3, pp. 1163–1170, 2004.

[26] Q. Qiu, F. Dudouit, R. Banerjee, J. McNamee, and B. Jean-Claude, "Inhibition of cell signaling by the combi-nitrosourea FD137 in the androgen independent DU145 prostate cancer cell line," *Prostate*, vol. 59, no. 1, pp. 13–21, 2004.

[27] F. Brahimi, Z. Rachid, J. McNamee, M. Alaoui-Jamali, A. Tari, and B. Jean-Claude, "Mechanism of action of a novel "combi-triazene" engineered to possess a polar functional group on the alkylating moiety: evidence for enhancement of potency," *Biochemical Pharmacology*, vol. 70, no. 4, pp. 511–519, 2005.

[28] S. Caporali, S. Falcinelli, G. Starace et al., "DNA damage induced by temozolomide signals to both ATM and ATR: role of the mismatch repair system," *Molecular Pharmacology*, vol. 66, no. 3, pp. 478–491, 2004.

[29] A. Senderowicz, "Targeting cell cycle and apoptosis for the treatment of human malignancies," *Current Opinion in Cell Biology*, vol. 16, no. 6, pp. 670–678, 2004.

[30] A. Yacoub, R. McKinstry, D. Hinman, T. Chung, P. Denta, and M. Hagan, "Epidermal growth factor and ionizing radiation up-regulate the DNA repair genes XRCC1 and ERCC1 in DU145 and LNCaP prostate carcinoma through MAPK signaling," *Radiation Research*, vol. 159, no. 4, pp. 439–452, 2003.

[31] W. Mattes, C. Lee, J. Laval, and T. O'Connor, "Excision of DNA adducts of nitrogen mustards by bacterial and mammalian 3-methyladenine-DNA glycosylases," *Carcinogenesis*, vol. 17, no. 4, pp. 643–648, 1996.

[32] S. Rink and P. Hopkins, "Direct evidence for DNA intrastrand cross-linking by the nitrogen mustard mechlorethamine in synthetic oligonucleotides," *Bioorganic and Medicinal Chemistry Letters*, vol. 5, no. 23, pp. 2845–2850, 1995.

[33] I. Giuliani, E. Boivieux-Ulrich, O. Houcine, C. Guennou, and F. Marano, "Toxic effects of mechlorethamine on mammalian respiratory mucociliary epithelium in primary culture," *Cell Biology and Toxicology*, vol. 10, no. 4, pp. 231–246, 1994.

[34] G. Small, Y. Shi, L. Higgins, and R. Orlowski, "Mitogen-activated protein kinase phosphatase-1 is a mediator of breast cancer chemoresistance," *Cancer Research*, vol. 67, no. 9, pp. 4459–4466, 2007.

[35] S. Somasundaram, N. Edmund, D. Moore, G. Small, Y. Shi, and R. Orlowski, "Dietary curcumin inhibits chemotherapy-induced apoptosis in models of human breast cancer," *Cancer Research*, vol. 62, no. 13, pp. 3868–3875, 2002.

[36] A. Mita, M. Mita, S. Nawrocki, and F. Giles, "Survivin: key regulator of mitosis and apoptosis and novel target for cancer therapeutics," *Clinical Cancer Research*, vol. 14, no. 16, pp. 5000–5005, 2008.

[37] D. Altieri, "The case for survivin as a regulator of microtubule dynamics and cell-death decisions," *Current Opinion in Cell Biology*, vol. 18, no. 6, pp. 609–615, 2006.

[38] D. Altieri, "Molecular circuits of apoptosis regulation and cell division control: the survivin paradigm," *Journal of Cellular Biochemistry*, vol. 92, no. 4, pp. 656–663, 2004.

[39] D. Altieri, "Survivin, versatile modulation of cell division and apoptosis in cancer," *Oncogene*, vol. 22, no. 35, pp. 8581–8589, 2003.

[40] M. Li, X. Wang, W. Li et al., "Somatostatin receptor-1 induces cell cycle arrest and inhibits tumor growth in pancreatic cancer," *Cancer Science*, vol. 99, no. 11, pp. 2218–2223, 2008.

The Concept of Divergent Targeting through the Activation and Inhibition of Receptors as a Novel Chemotherapeutic Strategy: Signaling Responses to Strong DNA-Reactive Combinatorial Mimicries

165

[41] B. Zhao, H. Zhao, N. Zhao, and X. Zhu, "Cholangiocarcinoma cells express somatostatin receptor subtype 2 and respond to octreotide treatment," *Journal of Hepato-Biliary-Pancreatic Surgery*, vol. 9, no. 4, pp. 497–502, 2002.

[42] K. Sharma, Y. Patel, and C. B. Srikant, "C-terminal region of human somatostatin receptor 5 is required for induction of Rb and G1 cell cycle arrest," *Molecular Endocrinology*, vol. 13, no. 1, pp. 82–90, 1999.

[43] K. Sharma, Y. Patel, and C. Srikant, "Subtype-selective induction of wild-type p53 and apoptosis, but not cell cycle arrest, by human somatostatin receptor 3," *Molecular Endocrinology*, vol. 10, no. 12, pp. 1688–1696, 1996.

[44] K. Sharma and C. Srikant, "Induction of wild-type p53, Bax, and acidic endonuclease during somatostatin-signaled apoptosis in MCF-7 human breast cancer cells," *International Journal of Cancer*, vol. 76, no. 2, pp. 259–266, 1998.

[45] J. Zhao, T. Tenev, L. Martins, J. Downward, and N. Lemoine, "The ubiquitin-proteasome pathway regulates survivin degradation in a cell cycle-dependent manner," *Journal of Cell Science*, vol. 113, part 23, pp. 4363–4371, 2000.

14

The Roles of Mitogen-Activated Protein Kinase Pathways in TGF-β-Induced Epithelial-Mesenchymal Transition

Ting Gui, Yujing Sun, Aiko Shimokado, and Yasuteru Muragaki

First Department of Pathology, Wakayama Medical University School of Medicine, 811-1 Kimiidera, Wakayama 641-0012, Japan

Correspondence should be addressed to Yasuteru Muragaki, ymuragak@wakayama-med.ac.jp

Academic Editor: Karl Matter

The mitogen-activated protein kinase (MAPK) pathway allows cells to interpret external signals and respond appropriately, especially during the epithelial-mesenchymal transition (EMT). EMT is an important process during embryonic development, fibrosis, and tumor progression in which epithelial cells acquire mesenchymal, fibroblast-like properties and show reduced intercellular adhesion and increased motility. TGF-β signaling is the first pathway to be described as an inducer of EMT, and its relationship with the Smad family is already well characterized. Studies of four members of the MAPK family in different biological systems have shown that the MAPK and TGF-β signaling pathways interact with each other and have a synergistic effect on the secretion of additional growth factors and cytokines that in turn promote EMT. In this paper, we present background on the regulation and function of MAPKs and their cascades, highlight the mechanisms of MAPK crosstalk with TGF-β signaling, and discuss the roles of MAPKs in EMT.

1. Introduction

Signal transduction networks allow cells to perceive changes in the intra- and extracellular environment and respond to them appropriately. Mitogen-activated protein kinase (MAPK) cascades are one of the most thoroughly studied signal transduction systems and have been shown to participate in a diverse array of cellular programs, including cell differentiation, movement, division, and death [1]. MAPKs are serine/threonine kinases that play important roles in a vast array of pathophysiological processes. The family is divided into four main subfamilies: extracellular-regulated kinases (ERKs), Jun N-terminal kinases (JNKs), p38 MAPK, and ERK5. All of these proteins are characterized by the presence of a typical activation module and a conserved activation domain [2]. ERK1 and ERK2 are activated by mitogenic stimuli, whereas JNK and p38 MAPK, which are also called stress-activated protein kinases (SAPKs), are activated by environmental and genotoxic stresses [3–5]. The ERK5 cascade is a MAPK pathway that transmits both mitogenic and stress signals, yet its mechanism of activation is not fully understood [6]. MAPK can be regulated by TGF-β stimulation [7], which represents an important mechanism for Smad-independent TGF-β signaling. Here, we focus mainly on the cross-talk between MAPK and TGF-β signaling.

The TGF-β superfamily of signaling molecules controls a diverse set of cellular responses, including cell proliferation, differentiation, extracellular matrix remodeling, and embryonic development. Consequently, when not strictly controlled, TGF-β signaling can contribute to the pathogenesis of cancer as well as fibrotic, cardiovascular, and autoimmune diseases [8, 9]. Members of the TGF-β superfamily (e.g., TGF-βs, activins, and bone morphogenetic proteins (BMPs)) signal via heteromeric serine/threonine kinase transmembrane receptor complexes [10–13]. The effects of TGF-β are mediated by three TGF-β ligands, TGF-β1, 2, and 3 via TGF-β type I and II receptors [9, 14, 15]. The binding of the ligand to its primary (type II) receptor, a constitutively active kinase, allows the recruitment, trans-phosphorylation, and activation of the signaling (type I) receptor. The receptor, also known as activin receptor-like kinase 5 (ALK5), is then able to exert its phosphorylation-dependent serine-threonine kinase activity to phosphorylate Smad2 and Smad3 [16–18]. These receptor-activated Smads (R-Smads) interact directly with and are phosphorylated by activated TGF-β receptor type I [19, 20]. Smad1, Smad5, and Smad8 are specific substrates of the BMP receptors, whereas Smad2 and Smad3 are activated by both TGF-β and activin receptors [17, 21]. Upon phosphorylation, they form heteromeric complexes with Smad4 [22], a common mediator of all Smad pathways. The resulting Smad heterocomplexes are then translocated into the nucleus where they activate target genes by either binding DNA directly or in association with other transcription factors [10, 12, 13, 17, 18]. Members of the third group of Smads, known as inhibitory Smads (Smad6 and Smad7) [23], control Smad signaling by preventing the phosphorylation and/or nuclear translocation of receptor-associated Smads and by inducing receptor complex degradation through the recruitment of ubiquitin ligases [24–26]. More recently, Smad7 was shown to recruit the protein phosphatase complex, type 1 protein serine/threonine phosphatase (PP1), and growth arrest and DNA damage-inducible protein 34 (GADD34) to activated TGF-β receptors, stabilizing them and thereby inducing receptor dephosphorylation and deactivation [26]. Following target gene transcription, Smad complexes are released from the chromatin and may undergo ubiquitination and subsequent proteasomal degradation.

These Smad pathways are not the only means by which TGF-βs regulate cellular functions. Smad-independent pathways including the mitogen-activated protein kinase (MAPK), nuclear factor κ-light chain-enhancer of activated B cells (NF-κB), and PI3 kinase/AKT pathways also participate in TGF-β signaling, and these pathways can either be induced by TGF-β or modulate the outcome of TGF-β-induced Smad signaling [21, 27, 28]. Indeed, broad evidence suggests that Smad signaling is tightly integrated within a complex network of signaling pathways with cross-talk that modify the initial Smad signals and allow the pleiotropic activities of TGF-β. There are also instances in which Smad signaling is not required for some TGF-β responses, as exemplified by the Smad-independent activation of the cyclin kinase inhibitors p15 and p21 in HaCaT keratinocytes, and the transcriptional activation of the fibronectin promoter via MAPK-dependent mechanisms. It appears clear that Smad proteins are not only the primary substrates for the TGF-β receptor kinases but may also be phosphorylated by MAPKs in response to either TGF-β itself or to various cytokines. Such R-Smad phosphorylation by MAPKs may serve to regulate Smad by modulating either its transcriptional activity or its capacity to translocate into the cell nucleus [28, 29]. Smad proteins are also capable of physically interacting with transcription factors that are also substrates of MAPKs, adding more complexity to the already intricate relationship between the MAPK and Smad pathways.

The epithelial-mesenchymal transition (EMT) is a complex, stepwise phenomenon that occurs during embryonic development and tumor progression [30]. EMT is also associated with chronic inflammatory and fibrogenic diseases that affect the lungs, the liver, and the peritoneum of patients undergoing peritoneal dialysis [31, 32]. EMT and the reverse process, termed the mesenchymal-epithelial transition (MET), play central roles in embryogenesis, cancer invasion and metastasis, and fibrosis [33, 34]. EMT is characterized by the disruption of intercellular junctions, the replacement of apical-basolateral polarity with front-to-back polarity, and the acquisition of migratory and invasive phenotypes. Cells that have undergone EMT also acquire the capacity to produce extracellular matrix (ECM) components and a wide spectrum of inflammatory, fibrogenic, and angiogenic factors [35]. EMT is triggered by the interplay of several extracellular signals, such as ECM components, soluble growth factors, and cytokines. These signals include members of the TGF-β and fibroblast growth factor families, epidermal growth factor, and hepatocyte growth factor [30]. TGF-β was first described as an inducer of EMT in normal mammary epithelial cells, and several studies have established crucial roles for TGF-β-induced EMT [36].

A key question in studies of MAPK is how a ubiquitously active regulatory enzyme generates a specific and biologically appropriate cellular response during EMT. This paper will summarize some of the latest data from the literature regarding the interactions among MAPK, TGF-β, and other factors, with a major focus on the cellular events that contribute to EMT.

2. Four Subfamilies of MAP Kinases and Their Substrates in Each Signaling Cascade

MAP kinases are a large group of proteins that allow numerous extracellular signals to rapidly activate nuclear transcription factors [37] (Figure 1). They consist of at least four subfamilies: the extracellular signal-regulated kinases (ERK1 and ERK2), the stress-activated protein (SAP) kinases, known as c-Jun N-terminal kinases (JNK1, JNK2, and JNK3), the p38 MAPKs (α, β, γ, and δ) [2], and ERK5 [38]. ERK5, which is also known as big MAP kinase 1 (BMK1) and has been described as a mediator of Src activation [39], is twice as large as other MAPKs [40].

Signaling initiated by each MAPK pathway occurs through the sequential phosphorylation of a MAPK kinase kinase (MAPKKK), a MAPK kinase (MAPKK), and a MAPK by membrane-associated kinases, such as cytokine or growth factor receptors [41]. MAPK activation leads to the downstream phosphorylation of nuclear kinases or, most commonly, transcription factors. Figure 1 provides a simplified view of the various MAPK pathways and includes most of the MAPK members and substrates cited in the text below.

ERK1 and ERK2, isoforms of the classical MAPK, are phosphorylated by the MAPKKs MEK1 (for MAPK/ERK kinase 1) and MEK2, which are substrates of the MAPKKK Mos and Raf-1 [42]. Raf-1 is activated by the membrane-bound small G-protein Ras following induction by mitogenic stimuli, such as epidermal growth factor (EGF), upon binding and activation of their respective receptors (i.e., EFGR). ERK-mediated pathways are mainly involved in proliferation and differentiation and are generally considered antiapoptotic.

JNK family members are the substrates of MAPK kinase 4 (MKK4, also known as SEK1) and MKK7. p38 MAPK is phosphorylated by MKK3 and MKK6, which are the substrates of apoptosis signal-regulating kinase-1 (ASK1), mixed lineage kinases (MLK), and TGF-β-activated kinase-1

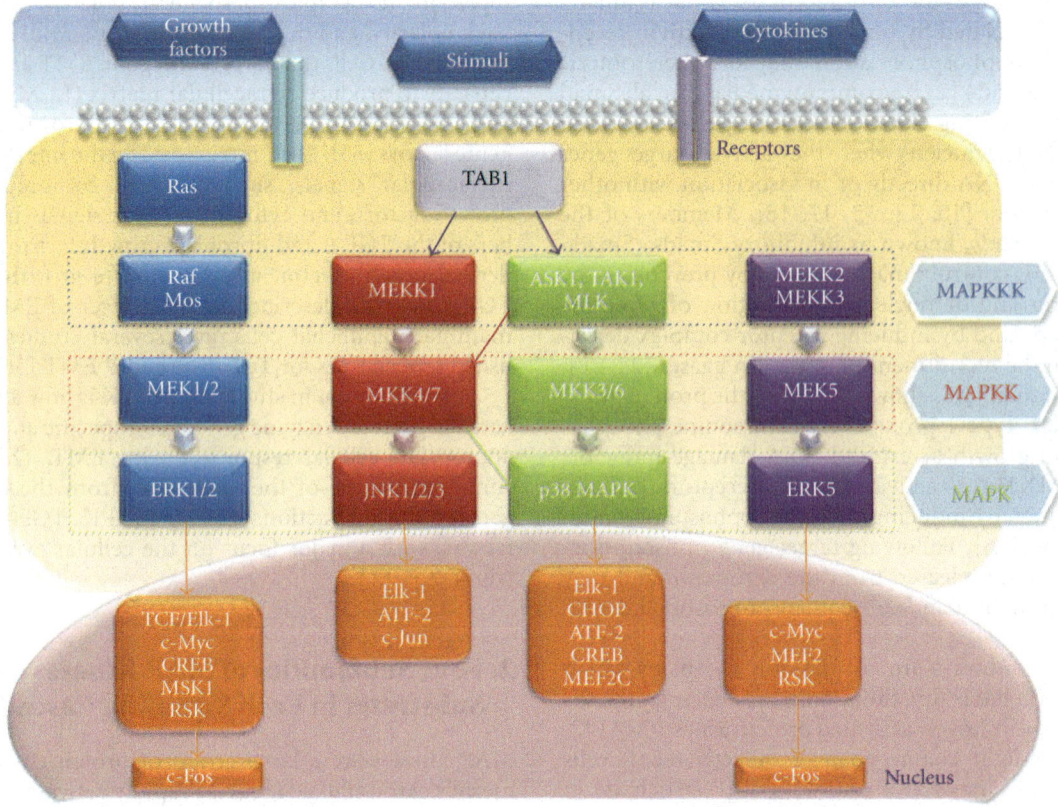

FIGURE 1: The network of the mitogen-activated protein kinase (MAPK) family. Extracellular stimuli transduce signals to the nucleus. The sequential phosphorylation of MAPKKK, MAPKK, and MAPK activates their nuclear targets, kinases, and transcription factors. For details, refer to the text.

(TAK1) [43, 44]. MEK kinase (MEKK1) and TAK1 activate JNK through MKK4 or MKK7 and activate p38 MAPK through MKK3 or MKK6. JNK and p38-signaling pathways are activated by stress stimuli, many of which induce apoptosis, but, in some cellular systems, they have also been implicated in proliferation and differentiation [45, 46].

Upon ERK5 stimulation, two members of the MAPKKK family, MEKK2 and MEKK3, activate MEK5, a MAPKK that is specific for ERK5 [47]. Unlike the first three groups of MAPKs, this pathway has not yet been clearly shown to be activated by TGF-β or to interfere with Smad signaling.

MAPK pathways control the cell response to changes in the extracellular environment through the regulation of transcription factors in the nucleus [48]. Thus, to transmit extracellular signals to the nucleus, the terminal components of the MAPK pathways, such as ERK1/2, JNK, and p38 MAPK, must translocate to the nucleus.

A variety of transcription factors and downstream kinases serve as substrates for activated MAPKs [49, 50]. These include activating protein-1 (AP-1), a family of pleiotropic transcription factors comprised of homo- and heterodimers of Fos, Jun, and activating transcription factor (ATF) family members that are involved in the control of cell proliferation, death, and survival, as well as tumorigenesis [51, 52]. Activated ERK1/2 phosphorylates many substrates, including TCF/Elk-1 and c-Myc, and activates cAMP response element

binding protein (CREB) and protein kinases, such as mitogen- and stress-activated protein kinase 1 (MSK1) and ribosomal S6 kinase (RSK), which subsequently induces the immediate early gene c-Fos [53, 54].

p38 MAPKs activate many substrates including E twenty six-like transcription factor 1 (Elk-1), CCAAT/enhancer binding protein homologous protein (CHOP), ATF-2, CREB, and myocyte-specific enhancer factor 2C (MEF2C) [55]. JNK is the only MAPK that phosphorylates c-Jun, the main component of AP-1 complexes, and also acts on ATF-2 and Elk-1 [2, 56]. Phosphorylation of c-Jun activates this key member of the AP-1 family of transcription factors, which can then bind the specific AP-1 recognition sites TGAG/CTCA to transactivate target genes [57]. Upon activation, CREB and ATF-2 bind to CRE sites (TGACGTCA) within target gene promoters [58]. Heterodimers of c-Jun and ATF-2 have also been shown to bind to CRE sites [59]. ERK5, similar to ERK1/2, phosphorylates c-Myc, MEF2, and RSK, subsequently inducing c-Fos [60, 61].

3. Smad-Dependent and -Independent MAPK Activation by TGF-β

TGF-β has been shown to activate all ERK, p38 MAPK, and JNK MAPKs in numerous cell types [62–65] through Smad-dependent and -independent transcriptional mechanisms.

Because MAPK activation is not a specific feature of TGF-β signaling and may be produced by various extracellular stimuli, including cytokines, ultraviolet irradiation, cell-cell or cell-matrix contacts [66–68], the outcome of Smad-dependent or -independent MAPK interactions should be viewed not only as the result of TGF-β signaling but also as a consequence of cytokine networks acting in concert to modulate MAPK signals.

As an example of Smad-dependent MAPK activation, in mink lung epithelial cells, TGF-β-induced activation of JNK mediates Smad3 phosphorylation, which is required for Smad3-dependent transcriptional responses [69] (Figure 2).

However, the initial evidence for Smad-independent activation of MAPK by TGF-β came from the observation that the activation of JNK in response to the TGF-β pathway was possible in Smad4-deficient cells and cells overexpressing dominant-negative Smads, despite the deficient Smad cascade. It has also been shown that a mutated TGF-β type I receptor that cannot phosphorylate R-Smad can still activate p38 MAPK signaling in response to TGF-β [70, 71].

Several other Smad-independent signaling examples have been described in the literature. TGF-β can activate ERK via rapid activation of Ras in rat intestine [72] (Figure 3). TGF-β type I receptor could phosphorylate the ShcA adaptor protein that subsequently associates with Grb2 and Sos in the cytoplasm in the absence of ligand stimulation [73, 74] (Figure 3). The ShcA/Grb/Sos complex is a well-established link between receptor tyrosine kinases and the MEK and ERK pathway via Ras and Raf activation [75].

The mechanisms of ERK, JNK, or p38 MAPK activation by TGF-β and the associated biological consequences are not fully characterized. ERK activation by TGF-β in epithelial cells may involve Ras signaling [76], while JNK and p38 MAPK signaling could be activated by various MAPKKKs in response to various stimuli. The first MAPKKK known to be activated by TGF-β family members was TGF-β-activated kinase 1 (TAK1), which was originally identified as a MAPKKK activated by TAB1 (TGF-β-activated kinase-binding protein-1) downstream of TGF-β/BMP receptors. TAK1 positively regulates the JNK and p38 kinase pathways [77] (Figure 2).

TGF-β1 may induce rapid and prolonged activation of p38 MAPK, depending on the cell type. Rapid and transient p38 MAPK activation has been described in certain cell types, including human neutrophils, HEK293, and C2C12 cells, and may be mediated by the induction of TAK1 in an R-Smad-independent manner. On the other hand, the prolonged and sustained p38 MAPK activation observed in pancreatic carcinoma cells, hepatocytes, and osteoblasts requires Smad signaling. Smad activation induces the expression of GADD45β, an upstream activator of MKK4, and thus promotes the prolonged activation of p38 MAPK [78] (Figure 2). Functional differences between rapid and prolonged activation of p38 MAPK may be dependent on cell type, but, at least in pancreatic cells, prolonged activation through the Smad-mediated induction of GADD45β may contribute to the tumor-suppressive effect of TGF-β [78].

4. The Association between MAPK and TGF-β Signaling in EMT

EMT is a complex process involving a restructuring of the cytoskeleton, cell membrane, and cell-cell junctions. Previous studies have implicated several molecules in different aspects of EMT. However, the aspects of EMT that might be mediated by MAPK signaling have not yet been defined.

ERK activation may be important for several key features of EMT that could cause the loss of epithelial characteristics and acquisition of mesenchymal properties, including the downregulation of adherens junctions and their affiliated proteins (e.g., E-cadherin), increased MMP activity, the induction of actin stress fibers, and the acquisition of motile and invasive properties [79–81]. ERK activation is one of the Smad-independent events that is necessary for TGF-β-mediated EMT [82, 83]. ERK is required for the disassembly of cell adherens junctions and the induction of cell motility by TGF-β. In a transcriptomic screen of genetic programs for TGF-β-induced EMT, TGF-β-stimulated ERK activation regulates a subset of target genes, a large proportion of which have defined roles in cell-matrix interactions, cell motility, and endocytosis [82]. These genes are known to function in the remodeling of integrin-based cell-matrix adhesion and in promoting cell motility.

The loss of E-cadherin is a critical step in EMT [84]. There is compelling evidence that ERKs repress E-cadherin expression to drive EMT in many experimental systems [85]. Previous studies have demonstrated that ERK is rapidly activated by TGF-β in culture models of EMT, and a specific inhibitor of MEK (upstream of ERK) blocks key morphologic features of EMT, such as the disassembly of E-cadherin-mediated adherens junctions, in various models [86, 87]. Several transcriptional repressors of E-cadherin have now been identified, including two members of the Snail superfamily of the zinc-finger transcription factors, Snail [88] and Slug [89]. Choi et al. found that TGF-β1-induced Slug expression was significantly inhibited by MEK- and JNK-specific inhibitors, indicating that MAPK pathways are involved in the regulation of Slug expression by TGF-β1 [90].

Recent data suggest that the aberrant activation of ERK may play an important role in diverting the TGF-β response towards EMT in kidney epithelial cells. Raf activation confers protection against TGF-β-induced apoptosis while enhancing the proinvasive effects of TGF-β [91]. Furthermore, the induction of EMT in breast tumor cells is dependent on the presence of both activated Ras and a functional TGF-β autocrine loop that is enhanced by Ras [86, 91]. Gene array data obtained from human keratinocytes induced to undergo EMT by TGF-β provided the first insights into ERK-dependent gene targets with roles in cell-matrix interactions and cell motility [92].

Perhaps the best-characterized interaction between TGF-β and MAPK signaling involves the JNK and p38 MAPK signaling cascades (Figure 2). TGF-β can rapidly activate JNK through MKK4 [69, 93] and p38 MAPK through MKK3/6 in various cell lines [70, 94]. Further upstream, MKKs are activated by the MAPKKKs; TAK1 is one of these activating MAPKKKs. Because TAK1 is rapidly induced by TGF-β1 and

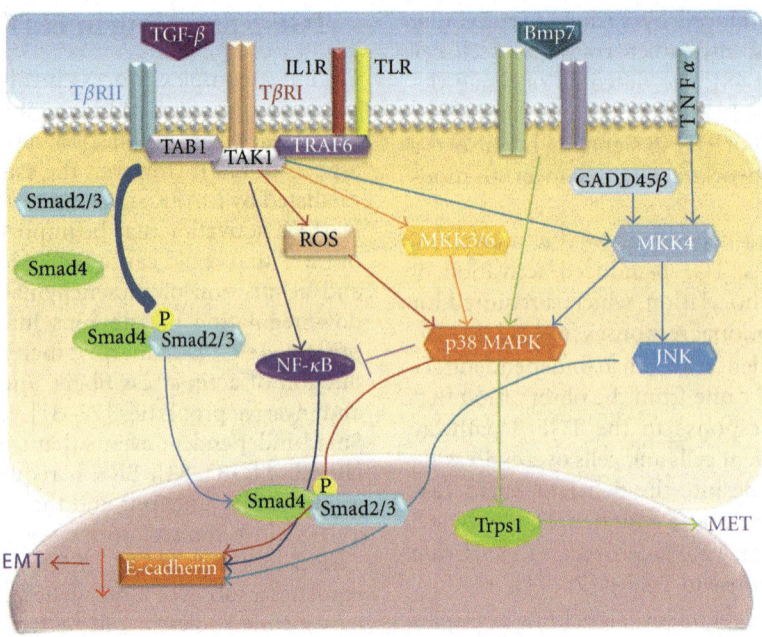

FIGURE 2: The involvement of JNK and p38 MAPK pathways in the TGF-β-induced epithelial-mesenchymal transition. Upon TGF-β ligation, the receptor phosphorylates Smad2/3 and interacts with TRAF6, which recruits TAK1 and TAB1 to activate JNK and p38 MAPK. The activated JNK and p38 MAPK can act in a Smad-dependent or -independent manner to regulate EMT by controlling the downstream transcriptional factors. This figure depicts the cross-talk between JNK, p38 MAPK, and TGF-β signaling in different cellular systems and illustrates how these networks may function in a stimuli-dependent manner to determine the EMT response.

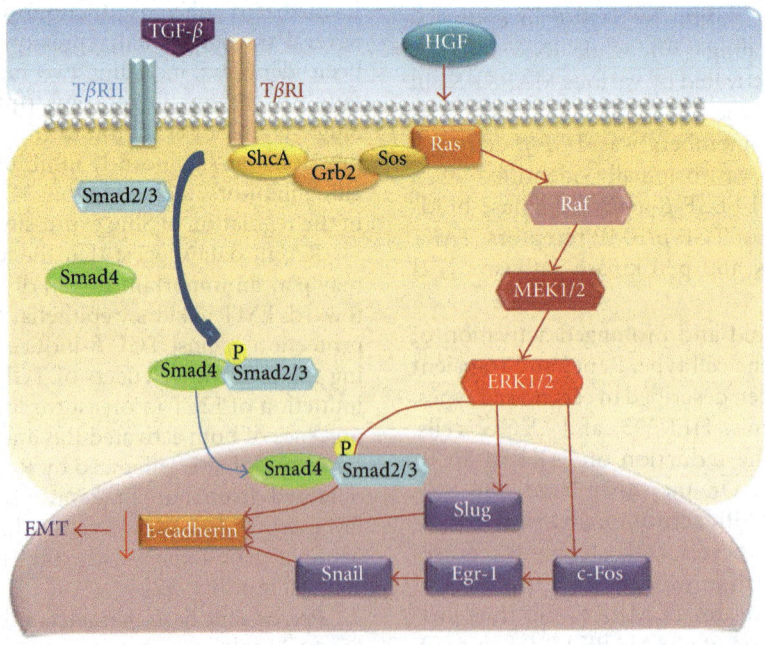

FIGURE 3: The involvement of the ERK pathway in the TGF-β-induced epithelial-mesenchymal transition. After TGF-β induces the phosphorylation of serine and/or tyrosine on TβRI and/or ShcA, ShcA is capable of recruiting Grb2 and Sos to active ERK1/2 through Ras, Raf, and MEK1/2. The activation of Ras can also be induced by HGF to control the EMT, which is regulated by Snail. This figure depicts the cross-talk between ERK, TGF-β, and other factors in different cellular systems and illustrates how these networks may function in a stimuli-dependent manner to determine the EMT response.

plays a role in p38 MAPK activation and JNK and NF-κB signaling [95], some researchers have focused on TAK1 and found that p38 MAPK maintains E-cadherin expression by suppressing TAK1/NF-κB signaling, thus impeding the induction of EMT in human primary mesothelial cells [96].

TNF receptor associated factor 6 (TRAF6), which plays an important role in the activation of TAK1 in interleukin-1 receptor (IL-1R) and Toll-like-receptor-(TLR-) mediated signaling pathways, was found to be crucial for the TGF-β-induced activation of the TAK1-JNK/p38 MAPK pathways [97, 98]. The TRAF6-TAK1-JNK/p38 MAPK pathway plays an important role in TGF-β-induced EMT (Figure 2). Inhibiting p38 activity using a p38 inhibitor or dominant-negative forms of MKK3 or p38 impairs TGF-β-mediated reorganization of the actin cytoskeleton and results in changes in cell shape [99]. Knocking down TRAF6 expression also inhibits TGF-β-mediated EMT [98]. Thus, activation of the TRAF6-TAK1-p38 MAPK pathway is another requirement for TGF-β-induced EMT.

Studies of the roles of MAPK family proteins in the genesis of EMT have produced conflicting results, likely due to the heterogeneity of the models and the different experimental approaches used. p38 MAPK appears to promote EMT during development and in tumors [100, 101]. According to an earlier study, p38 MAPK can regulate actin organization via heat shock protein 27 (HSP27) [102]. Therefore, p38 MAPK may function in the TGF-β-induced reorganization of the actin cytoskeleton parallel to or upstream of the RhoA/Rock pathway [103]. In addition, p38 MAPK may contribute to the expression of TGF-β target genes that are casually involved in EMT because p38 MAPK has been implicated in TGF-β transcriptional responses through its activation of ATF2 and Sp1 [104]. Taken together, these results suggest that the MAPK pathway contributes to TGF-β-induced changes in the actin cytoskeleton and in cell shape during EMT.

In recent years, significant evidence has indicated that the p38 MAPK pathway is an important intracellular signal transduction pathway in TGF-β1-induced EMT in renal tubular epithelial cells [105, 106]. Activated p38 MAPK can directly regulate the protein synthesis of α-smooth muscle cell actin (α-SMA) and thus indirectly activate the Smad pathway, leading to excessive matrix deposition and finally inducing fibrosis. For example, reactive oxygen species (ROS), which have been shown to mediate TGF-β-induced cellular responses in various cells [107], play an important role in EMT in rat proximal tubular epithelial cells, primarily through the activation of MAPK but also indirectly through ERK and subsequently through the phospho-Smad2 pathway [108] (Figure 2).

Semaphorin-4C (Sema4C) is essential for the activation of p38 MAPK [109]. The semaphorins are a large family of secreted or membrane-bound proteins that share a conserved Sema domain, which is known to regulate tumor progression [110], angiogenesis [111], nervous system development [112], and immune cell interactions [113]. Sema4C plays an important role in TGF-β1-induced EMT through its activation of p38 MAPK in proximal tubular epithelial cells [114]. Sema4C knockdown strongly inhibits the phosphorylation of p38 and reverses TGF-β1-induced EMT. Trps1, an

atypical member of the GATA-type family of transcription factors [115], acts downstream of bone morphogenetic protein 7 (BMP7) via p38 [116]. Knockdown of Trps1 or p38 MAPK inhibits the BMP7-induced MET.

In advanced stages of tumor development, TGF-β promotes tumor metastasis by stimulating EMT, matrix metalloproteinase (MMP) expression, and by angiogenesis and inhibiting immune surveillance [117–119]. Numerous studies have revealed that TGF-β-induced EMT can be blocked by inhibiting MAPK activation. Synergy between TNF-α and TGF-β signaling enables p38 MAPK activation to promote the rapid morphological conversion of colon carcinoma epithelia to dispersed cells with mesenchymal phenotypes [85, 120]. Hepatocyte growth factor/scatter factor (HGF) has several functions in the induction of epithelial cell scattering, motility, and tumor progression. One underlying mechanism that could explain this observation is that HGF upregulates Snail, a transcriptional repressor involved in EMT, through MAPK and early growth response factor-1 (Egr-1) (Figure 3).

5. Future Perspective and Conclusions

Within the past few years, considerable progress has been made toward understanding the signaling cascades and multiple pathways that involve MAPKs. At present, it is clear that cooperation between TGF-β-induced Smad signaling and the MAPK pathway determines the final cellular response to TGF-β, especially during EMT. It will not be surprising if more associations between the MAPK pathway and EMT are discovered in the future. The computational and mathematical modeling of biological systems has become increasingly valuable in recent years, and a wide variety of mathematical models of the MAPK pathway have led to some novel insights and predictions about how this system functions [121]. Further cross-talk research will undoubtedly rely on the development of new computational systems and will reveal novel mechanisms that contribute to TGF-β-dependent and -independent MAPK signaling, advancing our understanding of how MAPK can induce a plethora of diverse biological responses, including EMT. A major goal will be to determine how the specificity in MAPK downstream signaling is achieved in different cell lines and animal models; this information could be used to seek out clinical advantages in combination therapy.

References

[1] H. J. Schaeffer and M. J. Weber, "Mitogen-activated protein kinases: specific messages from ubiquitous messengers," *Molecular and Cellular Biology*, vol. 19, no. 4, pp. 2435–2444, 1999.

[2] L. Chang and M. Karin, "Mammalian MAP kinase signalling cascades," *Nature*, vol. 410, no. 6824, pp. 37–40, 2001.

[3] E. F. Wagner and A. R. Nebreda, "Signal integration by JNK and p38 MAPK pathways in cancer development," *Nature Reviews Cancer*, vol. 9, no. 8, pp. 537–549, 2009.

[4] L. Bardwell and K. Shah, "Analysis of mitogen-activated protein kinase activation and interactions with regulators and substrates," *Methods*, vol. 40, no. 3, pp. 213–223, 2006.

[5] S. J. Lee, T. Zhou, and E. J. Goldsmith, "Crystallization of MAP kinases," *Methods*, vol. 40, no. 3, pp. 224–233, 2006.

[6] Z. Yao, S. Yoon, E. Kalie, Z. Raviv, and R. Seger, "Calcium regulation of EGF-induced ERK5 activation: role of Lad1-MEKK2 interaction," *PLoS One*, vol. 5, no. 9, Article ID e12627, pp. 1–10, 2010.

[7] X. Guo and X. F. Wang, "Signaling cross-talk between TGF-β/BMP and other pathways," *Cell Research*, vol. 19, no. 1, pp. 71–88, 2009.

[8] K. H. Wrighton, X. Lin, and X. H. Feng, "Phospho-control of TGF-β superfamily signaling," *Cell Research*, vol. 19, no. 1, pp. 8–20, 2009.

[9] H. Ikushima and K. Miyazono, "TGFβ signalling: a complex web in cancer progression," *Nature Reviews Cancer*, vol. 10, no. 6, pp. 415–424, 2010.

[10] R. Derynck and X. H. Feng, "TGF-β receptor signaling," *Biochimica et Biophysica Acta*, vol. 1333, no. 2, pp. F105–F150, 1997.

[11] X. H. Feng and R. Derynck, "A kinase subdomain of transforming growth factor-β (TGF-β) type I receptor determines the TGF-β intracellular signaling specificity," *EMBO Journal*, vol. 16, no. 13, pp. 3912–3923, 1997.

[12] D. Javelaud and A. Mauviel, "Transforming growth factor-betas: smad signaling and roles in physiopathology," *Pathologie Biologie*, vol. 52, no. 1, pp. 50–54, 2004.

[13] P. Ten Dijke and C. S. Hill, "New insights into TGF-β-Smad signalling," *Trends in Biochemical Sciences*, vol. 29, no. 5, pp. 265–273, 2004.

[14] C. H. Heldin, K. Miyazono, and P. Ten Dijke, "TGF-β signalling from cell membrane to nucleus through SMAD proteins," *Nature*, vol. 390, no. 6659, pp. 465–471, 1997.

[15] X. H. Feng and R. Derynck, "Specificity and versatility in TGF-β signaling through smads," *Annual Review of Cell and Developmental Biology*, vol. 21, pp. 659–693, 2005.

[16] R. Derynck, Y. Zhang, and X. H. Feng, "Smads: transcriptional activators of TGF-β responses," *Cell*, vol. 95, no. 6, pp. 737–740, 1998.

[17] K. Miyazono, P. Ten Dijke, and C. H. Heldin, "TGF-β signaling by Smad proteins," *Advances in Immunology*, vol. 75, pp. 115–157, 2000.

[18] Y. Shi and J. Massagué, "Mechanisms of TGF-β signaling from cell membrane to the nucleus," *Cell*, vol. 113, no. 6, pp. 685–700, 2003.

[19] M. Schiller, D. Javelaud, and A. Mauviel, "TGF-β-induced SMAD signaling and gene regulation: consequences for extracellular matrix remodeling and wound healing," *Journal of Dermatological Science*, vol. 35, no. 2, pp. 83–92, 2004.

[20] C. M. Zimmerman and R. W. Padgett, "Transforming growth factor β signaling mediators and modulators," *Gene*, vol. 249, no. 1-2, pp. 17–30, 2000.

[21] J. Massagué, S. W. Blain, and R. S. Lo, "TGFβ signaling in growth control, cancer, and heritable disorders," *Cell*, vol. 103, no. 2, pp. 295–309, 2000.

[22] N. A. Ali, M. J. McKay, and M. P. Molloy, "Proteomics of Smad4 regulated transforming growth factor-beta signalling in colon cancer cells," *Molecular BioSystems*, vol. 6, no. 11, pp. 2332–2338, 2010.

[23] A. Nakao, M. Afrakhte, A. Morén et al., "Identification of Smad7, a TGFβ-inducible antagonist of TGF-β signalling," *Nature*, vol. 389, no. 6651, pp. 631–635, 1997.

[24] Y. Zhang, C. Chang, D. J. Gehling, A. Hemmati-Brivanlou, and R. Derynck, "Regulation of Smad degradation and activity by Smurf2, an E3 ubiquitin ligase," *Proceedings of the National Academy of Sciences of the United States of America*, vol. 98, no. 3, pp. 974–979, 2001.

[25] T. Ebisawa, M. Fukuchi, G. Murakami et al., "Smurf1 interacts with transforming growth factor-β type I receptor through Smad7 and induces receptor degradation," *Journal of Biological Chemistry*, vol. 276, no. 16, pp. 12477–12480, 2001.

[26] W. Shi, C. Sun, B. He et al., "GADD34-PP1c recruited by Smad7 dephosphorylates TGFβ type I receptor," *Journal of Cell Biology*, vol. 164, no. 2, pp. 291–300, 2004.

[27] J. Massagué, "How cells read TGF-β signals," *Nature Reviews Molecular Cell Biology*, vol. 1, no. 3, pp. 169–178, 2000.

[28] R. Derynck and Y. E. Zhang, "Smad-dependent and Smad-independent pathways in TGF-β family signalling," *Nature*, vol. 425, no. 6958, pp. 577–584, 2003.

[29] M. Lutz and P. Knaus, "Integration of the TGF-β pathway into the cellular signalling network," *Cellular Signalling*, vol. 14, no. 12, pp. 977–988, 2002.

[30] J. P. Thiery, H. Acloque, R. Y. J. Huang, and M. A. Nieto, "Epithelial-mesenchymal transitions in development and disease," *Cell*, vol. 139, no. 5, pp. 871–890, 2009.

[31] L. S. Aroeira, A. Aguilera, J. A. Sánchez-Tomero et al., "Epithelial to mesenchymal transition and peritoneal membrane failure in peritoneal dialysis patients: pathologic significance and potential therapeutic interventions," *Journal of the American Society of Nephrology*, vol. 18, no. 7, pp. 2004–2013, 2007.

[32] R. Kalluri and R. A. Weinberg, "The basics of epithelial-mesenchymal transition," *Journal of Clinical Investigation*, vol. 119, no. 6, pp. 1420–1428, 2009.

[33] J. M. Pérez-Pomares, A. Phelps, M. Sedmerova et al., "Experimental studies on the spatiotemporal expression of WT1 and RALDH2 in the embryonic avian heart: a model for the regulation of myocardial and valvuloseptal development by epicardially derived cells (EPDCs)," *Developmental Biology*, vol. 247, no. 2, pp. 307–326, 2002.

[34] J. P. Thiery and J. P. Sleeman, "Complex networks orchestrate epithelial-mesenchymal transitions," *Nature Reviews Molecular Cell Biology*, vol. 7, no. 2, pp. 131–142, 2006.

[35] S. Thomson, F. Petti, I. Sujka-Kwok et al., "A systems view of epithelial-mesenchymal transition signaling states," *Clinical and Experimental Metastasis*, vol. 28, no. 2, pp. 137–155, 2011.

[36] A. Moustakas and C. H. Heldin, "Signaling networks guiding epithelial-mesenchymal transitions during embryogenesis and cancer progression," *Cancer Science*, vol. 98, no. 10, pp. 1512–1520, 2007.

[37] A. J. Whitmarsh and R. J. Davis, "Signal transduction by MAP kinases: regulation by phosphorylation-dependent switches," *Sciences STKE*, vol. 1999, no. 1, p. PE1, 1999.

[38] X. Wang and C. Tournier, "Regulation of cellular functions by the ERK5 signalling pathway," *Cellular Signalling*, vol. 18, no. 6, pp. 753–760, 2006.

[39] G. Zhou, Z. Q. Bao, and J. E. Dixon, "Components of a new human protein kinase signal transduction pathway," *Journal of Biological Chemistry*, vol. 270, no. 21, pp. 12665–12669, 1995.

[40] P. Rafiee, J. K. Lee, C. C. Leung, and T. A. Raffin, "TNF-α induces tyrosine phosphorylation of mitogen-activated protein kinase in adherent human neutrophils," *Journal of Immunology*, vol. 154, no. 9, pp. 4785–4792, 1995.

[41] V. L. Lowes, N. Y. Ip, and Y. H. Wong, "Integration of signals from receptor tyrosine kinases and G protein-coupled receptors," *NeuroSignals*, vol. 11, no. 1, pp. 5–19, 2002.

[42] T. Joneson, J. A. Fulton, D. J. Volle, O. V. Chaika, D. Bar-Sagi, and R. E. Lewis, "Kinase suppressor of Ras inhibits the activation of extracellular ligand-regulated (ERK) mitogen-activated Protein (MAP) kinase by growth factors, activated

Ras, and Ras effectors," *Journal of Biological Chemistry*, vol. 273, no. 13, pp. 7743–7748, 1998.

[43] Y. T. Ip and R. J. Davis, "Signal transduction by the c-Jun N-terminal kinase (JNK)—from inflammation to development," *Current Opinion in Cell Biology*, vol. 10, no. 2, pp. 205–219, 1998.

[44] S. Davis, P. Vanhoutte, C. Pagès, J. Caboche, and S. Laroche, "The MAPK/ERK cascade targets both Elk-1 and cAMP response element- binding protein to control long-term potentiation-dependent gene expression in the dentate gyrus in vivo," *Journal of Neuroscience*, vol. 20, no. 12, pp. 4563–4572, 2000.

[45] R. Eferl and E. F. Wagner, "AP-1: a double-edged sword in tumorigenesis," *Nature Reviews Cancer*, vol. 3, no. 11, pp. 859–868, 2003.

[46] R. Zenz, H. Scheuch, P. Martin et al., "c-Jun regulates eyelid closure and skin tumor development through EGFR signaling," *Developmental Cell*, vol. 4, no. 6, pp. 879–889, 2003.

[47] W. Sun, K. Kesavan, B. C. Schaefer et al., "MEKK2 associates with the adapter protein Lad/RIBP and regulates the MEK5-BMK1/ERK5 pathway," *Journal of Biological Chemistry*, vol. 276, no. 7, pp. 5093–5100, 2001.

[48] S. Pelet, F. Rudolf, M. Nadal-Ribelles, E. De Nadal, F. Posas, and M. Peter, "Transient activation of the HOG MAPK pathway regulates bimodal gene expression," *Science*, vol. 332, no. 6030, pp. 732–735, 2011.

[49] R. Treisman, "Regulation of transcription by MAP kinase cascades," *Current Opinion in Cell Biology*, vol. 8, no. 2, pp. 205–215, 1996.

[50] D. Javelaud and A. Mauviel, "Crosstalk mechanisms between the mitogen-activated protein kinase pathways and Smad signaling downstream of TGF-β: implications for carcinogenesis," *Oncogene*, vol. 24, no. 37, pp. 5742–5750, 2005.

[51] M. Karin, Z. G. Liu, and E. Zandi, "AP-1 function and regulation," *Current Opinion in Cell Biology*, vol. 9, no. 2, pp. 240–246, 1997.

[52] E. Shaulian and M. Karin, "AP-1 as a regulator of cell life and death," *Nature Cell Biology*, vol. 4, no. 5, pp. E131–E136, 2002.

[53] C. Hauge and M. Frödin, "RSK aand MSK in MAP kinase signalling," *Journal of Cell Science*, vol. 119, no. 15, pp. 3021–3023, 2006.

[54] M. D. Godeny and P. P. Sayeski, "ERK1/2 regulates ANG II-dependent cell proliferation via cytoplasmic activation of RSK2 and nuclear activation of elk1," *American Journal of Physiology*, vol. 291, no. 6, pp. C1308–C1317, 2006.

[55] C. A. Hazzalin and L. C. Mahadevan, "MAPK-regulated transcription: a continuously variable gene switch?" *Nature Reviews Molecular Cell Biology*, vol. 3, no. 1, pp. 30–40, 2002.

[56] D. Hao, P. Gao, P. Liu et al., "AC3-33, a novel secretory protein, inhibits Elk1 transcriptional activity via ERK pathway," *Molecular Biology Reports*, vol. 38, no. 2, pp. 1375–1378, 2011.

[57] P. Angel and M. Karin, "The role of Jun, Fos and the AP-1 complex in cell-proliferation and transformation," *Biochimica et Biophysica Acta*, vol. 1072, no. 2-3, pp. 129–157, 1991.

[58] T. Smeal, M. Hibi, and M. Karin, "Altering the specificity of signal transduction cascades: positive regulation of c-Jun transcriptional activity by protein kinase A," *EMBO Journal*, vol. 13, no. 24, pp. 6006–6010, 1994.

[59] T. Hai and T. Curran, "Cross-family dimerization of transcription factors Fos/Jun and ATF/CREB alters DNA binding specificity," *Proceedings of the National Academy of Sciences of the United States of America*, vol. 88, no. 9, pp. 3720–3724, 1991.

[60] S. Kamakura, T. Moriguchi, and E. Nishida, "Activation of the protein kinase ERK5/BMK1 by receptor tyrosine kinases. Identification and characterization of a signaling pathway to the nucleus," *Journal of Biological Chemistry*, vol. 274, no. 37, pp. 26563–26571, 1999.

[61] S. Bailey, A. G. Hall, A. D. J. Pearson, and C. P. F. Redfern, "The role of AP-1 in glucocorticoid resistance in leukaemia," *Leukemia*, vol. 15, no. 3, pp. 391–397, 2001.

[62] L. M. Wakefield and A. B. Roberts, "TGF-β signaling: positive and negative effects on tumorigenesis," *Current Opinion in Genetics and Development*, vol. 12, no. 1, pp. 22–29, 2002.

[63] J. Li, Z. Zhao, J. Liu et al., "MEK/ERK and p38 MAPK regulate chondrogenesis of rat bone marrow mesenchymal stem cells through delicate interaction with TGF-β1/Smads pathway," *Cell Proliferation*, vol. 43, no. 4, pp. 333–343, 2010.

[64] M. L. Burch, S. N. Y. Yang, M. L. Ballinger, R. Getachew, N. Osman, and P. J. Little, "TGF-β stimulates biglycan synthesis via p38 and ERK phosphorylation of the linker region of Smad2," *Cellular and Molecular Life Sciences*, vol. 67, no. 12, pp. 2077–2090, 2010.

[65] R. Mao, Y. Fan, Y. Mou, H. Zhang, S. Fu, and J. Yang, "TAK1 lysine 158 is required for TGF-β-induced TRAF6-mediated Smad-independent IKK/NF-κB and JNK/AP-1 activation," *Cellular Signalling*, vol. 23, no. 1, pp. 222–227, 2011.

[66] M. Guma, D. Stepniak, H. Shaked et al., "Constitutive intestinal NF-κB does not trigger destructive inflammation unless accompanied by MAPK activation," *The Journal of Experimental Medicine*, vol. 208, no. 9, pp. 1889–1900, 2011.

[67] S. Holland, O. Coste, D. D. Zhang, S. C. Pierre, G. Geisslinger, and K. Scholich, "The ubiquitin ligase MYCBP2 regulates transient receptor potential vanilloid receptor 1 (TRPV1) internalization through inhibition of p38 MAPK signaling," *Journal of Biological Chemistry*, vol. 286, no. 5, pp. 3671–3680, 2011.

[68] M. C. Lawrence, B. Naziruddin, M. F. Levy, A. Jackson, and K. McGlynn, "Calcineurin/nuclear factor of activated T cells and MAPK signaling induce TNF-α gene expression in pancreatic islet endocrine cells," *Journal of Biological Chemistry*, vol. 286, no. 2, pp. 1025–1036, 2011.

[69] M. E. Engel, M. A. McDonnell, B. K. Law, and H. L. Moses, "Interdependent SMAD and JNK signaling in transforming growth factor-β- mediated transcription," *Journal of Biological Chemistry*, vol. 274, no. 52, pp. 37413–37420, 1999.

[70] L. Yu, M. C. Hébert, and Y. E. Zhang, "TGF-β receptor-activated p38 MAP kinase mediates smad-independent TGF-β responses," *EMBO Journal*, vol. 21, no. 14, pp. 3749–3759, 2002.

[71] M. M. Martin, J. A. Buckenberger, J. Jiang et al., "TGF-β1 stimulates human at1 receptor expression in lung fibroblasts by cross talk between the Smad, p38 MAPK, JNK, and PI3K signaling pathways," *American Journal of Physiology*, vol. 293, no. 3, pp. L790–L799, 2007.

[72] K. M. Mulder and S. L. Morris, "Activation of p21(ras) by transforming growth factor β in epithelial cells," *Journal of Biological Chemistry*, vol. 267, no. 8, pp. 5029–5031, 1992.

[73] A. Wong, B. Lamothe, A. Lee, J. Schlessinger, and I. Lax, "FRS2α attenuates FGF receptor signaling by Grb2-mediated recruitment of the ubiquitin ligase Cbl," *Proceedings of the National Academy of Sciences of the United States of America*, vol. 99, no. 10, pp. 6684–6689, 2002.

[74] C. Reardon and D. M. McKay, "TGF-β suppresses IFN-γ-STAT1-dependent gene transcription by enhancing STAT1-PIAS1 interactions in epithelia but not monocytes/macrophages," *Journal of Immunology*, vol. 178, no. 7, pp. 4284–4295, 2007.

[75] M. K. Lee, C. Pardoux, M. C. Hall et al., "TGF-β activates Erk MAP kinase signalling through direct phosphorylation of ShcA," *EMBO Journal*, vol. 26, no. 17, pp. 3957–3967, 2007.

[76] J. Yue and K. M. Mulder, "Requirement of Ras/MAPK pathway activation by transforming growth factor β for transforming growth factor β1 production in a Smad-dependent pathway," *Journal of Biological Chemistry*, vol. 275, no. 40, pp. 30765–30773, 2000.

[77] K. Yamaguchi, K. Shirakabe, H. Shibuya et al., "Identification of a member of the MAPKKK family as a potential Mediator of TGF-β signal transduction," *Science*, vol. 270, no. 5244, pp. 2008–2011, 1995.

[78] M. Takekawa, K. Tatebayashi, F. Itoh, M. Adachi, K. Imai, and H. Saito, "Smad-dependent GADD45β expression mediates delayed activation of p38 MAP kinase by TGF-β," *EMBO Journal*, vol. 21, no. 23, pp. 6473–6482, 2002.

[79] P. G. Santamaria and A. R. Nebreda, "Deconstructing ERK signaling in tumorigenesis," *Molecular Cell*, vol. 38, no. 1, pp. 3–5, 2010.

[80] J. H. Zuo, W. Zhu, M. Y. Li et al., "Activation of EGFR promotes squamous carcinoma SCC10A cell migration and invasion via inducing EMT-like phenotype change and MMP-9-mediated degradation of E-cadherin," *Journal of Cellular Biochemistry*, vol. 112, no. 9, pp. 2508–2517, 2011.

[81] J. P. Thiery, "Cell adhesion in development: a complex signaling network," *Current Opinion in Genetics and Development*, vol. 13, no. 4, pp. 365–371, 2003.

[82] J. Zavadil, M. Bitzer, D. Liang et al., "Genetic programs of epithelial cell plasticity directed by transforming growth factor-β," *Proceedings of the National Academy of Sciences of the United States of America*, vol. 98, no. 12, pp. 6686–6691, 2001.

[83] M. Davies, M. Robinson, E. Smith, S. Huntley, S. Prime, and I. Paterson, "Induction of an epithelial to mesenchymal transition in human immortal and malignant keratinocytes by TGF-β1 involves MAPK, Smad and AP-1 signalling pathways," *Journal of Cellular Biochemistry*, vol. 95, no. 5, pp. 918–931, 2005.

[84] R. U. De Iongh, E. Wederell, F. J. Lovicu, and J. W. McAvoy, "Transforming growth factor-β-induced epithelial-mesenchymal transition in the lens: a model for cataract formation," *Cells Tissues Organs*, vol. 179, no. 1-2, pp. 43–55, 2005.

[85] J. Zavadil and E. P. Böttinger, "TGF-β and epithelial-to-mesenchymal transitions," *Oncogene*, vol. 24, no. 37, pp. 5764–5774, 2005.

[86] L. Xie, B. K. Law, A. M. Chytil, K. A. Brown, M. E. Aakre, and H. L. Moses, "Activation of the Erk pathway is required for TGF-β1-induced EMT in vitro," *Neoplasia*, vol. 6, no. 5, pp. 603–610, 2004.

[87] R. Strippoli, I. Benedicto, M. L. P. Lozano, A. Cerezo, M. López-Cabrera, and M. A. Del Pozo, "Epithelial-to-mesenchymal transition of peritoneal mesothelial cells is regulated by an ERK/NF-κB/Snail1 pathway," *Disease Models and Mechanisms*, vol. 1, no. 4-5, pp. 264–274, 2008.

[88] A. Cano, M. A. Pérez-Moreno, I. Rodrigo et al., "The transcription factor Snail controls epithelial-mesenchymal transitions by repressing E-cadherin expression," *Nature Cell Biology*, vol. 2, no. 2, pp. 76–83, 2000.

[89] P. A. Pérez-Mancera, I. González-Herrero, M. Pérez-Caro et al., "SLUG in cancer development," *Oncogene*, vol. 24, no. 19, pp. 3073–3082, 2005.

[90] J. Choi, S. Y. Park, and C. K. Joo, "Transforming growth factor-β1 represses E-cadherin production via Slug expression in lens epithelial cells," *Investigative Ophthalmology and Visual Science*, vol. 48, no. 6, pp. 2708–2718, 2007.

[91] K. Lehmann, E. Janda, C. E. Pierreux et al., "Raf induces TGFβ production while blocking its apoptotic but not invasive responses: a mechanism leading to increased malignancy in epithelial cells," *Genes and Development*, vol. 14, no. 20, pp. 2610–2622, 2000.

[92] L. Xie, B. K. Law, M. E. Aakre et al., "Transforming growth factor beta-regulated gene expression in a mouse mammary gland epithelial cell line," *Breast Cancer Research*, vol. 5, no. 6, pp. R187–R198, 2003.

[93] R. S. Frey and K. M. Mulder, "Involvement of extracellular signal-regulated kinase 2 and stress- activated protein kinase/Jun N-terminal kinase activation by transforming growth factor β in the negative growth control of breast cancer cells," *Cancer Research*, vol. 57, no. 4, pp. 628–633, 1997.

[94] N. A. Bhowmick, R. Zent, M. Ghiassi, M. McDonnell, and H. L. Moses, "Integrin β1 signaling is necessary for transforming growtn factor-β activation of p38MAPK and epithelial plasticity," *Journal of Biological Chemistry*, vol. 276, no. 50, pp. 46707–46713, 2001.

[95] J. H. Shim, C. Xiao, A. E. Paschal et al., "TAK1, but not TAB1 or TAB2, plays an essential role in multiple signaling pathways in vivo," *Genes and Development*, vol. 19, no. 22, pp. 2668–2681, 2005.

[96] R. Strippoli, I. Benedicto, M. Foronda et al., "p38 maintains E-cadherin expression by modulating TAK1-NF-κB during epithelial-to-mesenchymal transition," *Journal of Cell Science*, vol. 123, no. 24, pp. 4321–4331, 2010.

[97] A. Sorrentino, N. Thakur, S. Grimsby et al., "The type I TGF-β receptor engages TRAF6 to activate TAK1 in a receptor kinase-independent manner," *Nature Cell Biology*, vol. 10, no. 10, pp. 1199–1207, 2008.

[98] M. Yamashita, K. Fatyol, C. Jin, X. Wang, Z. Liu, and Y. E. Zhang, "TRAF6 mediates Smad-independent activation of JNK and p38 by TGF-β," *Molecular Cell*, vol. 31, no. 6, pp. 918–924, 2008.

[99] A. V. Bakin, C. Rinehart, A. K. Tomlinson, and C. L. Arteaga, "p38 mitogen-activated protein kinase is required for TGFβ-mediated fibroblastic transdifferentiation and cell migration," *Journal of Cell Science*, vol. 115, no. 15, pp. 3193–3206, 2002.

[100] I. E. Zohn, Y. Li, E. Y. Skolnik, K. V. Anderson, J. Han, and L. Niswander, "p38 and a p38-interacting protein are critical for downregulation of E-cadherin during mouse gastrulation," *Cell*, vol. 125, no. 5, pp. 957–969, 2006.

[101] Y. Liu, S. El-Naggar, D. S. Darling, Y. Higashi, and D. C. Dean, "Zeb1 links epithelial-mesenchymal transition and cellular senescence," *Development*, vol. 135, no. 3, pp. 579–588, 2008.

[102] J. C. Hedges, M. A. Dechert, I. A. Yamboliev et al., "A role for p38(MAPK)/HSP27 pathway in smooth muscle cell migration," *Journal of Biological Chemistry*, vol. 274, no. 34, pp. 24211–24219, 1999.

[103] S. Edlund, M. Landström, C. H. Heldin, and P. Aspenström, "Transforming growth factor-β-induced mobilization of actin cytoskeleton requires signaling by small GTPases Cdc42 and RhoA," *Molecular Biology of the Cell*, vol. 13, no. 3, pp. 902–914, 2002.

[104] B. R. Hu, C. L. Liu, and D. J. Park, "Alteration of MAP kinase pathways after transient forebrain ischemia," *Journal of Cerebral Blood Flow and Metabolism*, vol. 20, no. 7, pp. 1089–1095, 2000.

[105] Z. -M. Lv, Q. Wang, Q. Wan et al., "The role of the p38 MAPK signaling pathway in high glucose-induced epithelial-mesenchymal transition of cultured human renal tubular epithelial cells," *PLoS One*, vol. 6, no. 7, Article ID e22806, 2011.

[106] M. Mariasegaram, G. H. Tesch, S. Verhardt, L. Hurst, H. Y. Lan, and D. J. Nikolic-Paterson, "Lefty antagonises TGF-β1 induced epithelial-mesenchymal transition in tubular epithelial cells," *Biochemical and Biophysical Research Communications*, vol. 393, no. 4, pp. 855–859, 2010.

[107] B. Herrera, M. Fernández, C. Roncero et al., "Activation of p38MAPK by TGF-β in fetal rat hepatocytes requires radical oxygen production, but is dispensable for cell death," *FEBS Letters*, vol. 499, no. 3, pp. 225–229, 2001.

[108] D. Y. Rhyu, Y. Yang, H. Ha et al., "Role of reactive oxygen species in TGF-β1-induced mitogen-activated protein kinase activation and epithelial-mesenchymal transition in renal tubular epithelial cells," *Journal of the American Society of Nephrology*, vol. 16, no. 3, pp. 667–675, 2005.

[109] H. Wu, X. Wang, S. Liu et al., "Sema4C participates in myogenic differentiation in vivo and in vitro through the p38 MAPK pathway," *European Journal of Cell Biology*, vol. 86, no. 6, pp. 331–344, 2007.

[110] R. P. Kruger, J. Aurandt, and K. L. Guan, "Semaphorins command cells to move," *Nature Reviews Molecular Cell Biology*, vol. 6, no. 10, pp. 789–800, 2005.

[111] J. R. Basile, A. Barac, T. Zhu, K. L. Guan, and J. S. Gutkind, "Class IV semaphorins promote angiogenesis by stimulating Rho-initiated pathways through plexin-B," *Cancer Research*, vol. 64, no. 15, pp. 5212–5224, 2004.

[112] R. J. Pasterkamp, J. J. Peschon, M. K. Spriggs, and A. L. Kolodkin, "Semaphorin 7A promotes axon outgrowth through integrins and MAPKs," *Nature*, vol. 424, no. 6947, pp. 398–405, 2003.

[113] K. Suzuki, A. Kumanogoh, and H. Kikutani, "Semaphorins and their receptors in immune cell interactions," *Nature Immunology*, vol. 9, no. 1, pp. 17–23, 2008.

[114] R. Zeng, M. Han, Y. Luo et al., "Role of Sema4C in TGF-β1-induced mitogen-activated protein kinase activation and epithelialmesenchymal transition in renal tubular epithelial cells," *Nephrology Dialysis Transplantation*, vol. 26, no. 4, pp. 1149–1156, 2011.

[115] P. Momeni, G. Glöckner, O. Schmidt et al., "Mutations in a new gene, encoding a zinc-finger protein, cause trichorhino-phalangeal syndrome type I," *Nature Genetics*, vol. 24, no. 1, pp. 71–74, 2000.

[116] Z. Gai, G. Zhou, S. Itoh et al., "Trps1 functions downstream of Bmp7 in kidney development," *Journal of the American Society of Nephrology*, vol. 20, no. 11, pp. 2403–2411, 2009.

[117] R. Derynck, R. J. Akhurst, and A. Balmain, "TGF-β signaling in tumor suppression and cancer progression," *Nature Genetics*, vol. 29, no. 2, pp. 117–129, 2001.

[118] P. M. Siegel and J. Massagué, "Cytostatic and apoptotic actions of TGF-β in homeostasis and cancer," *Nature Reviews Cancer*, vol. 3, no. 11, pp. 807–821, 2003.

[119] M. P. De Caestecker, E. Piek, and A. B. Roberts, "Role of transforming growth factor-β signaling in cancer," *Journal of the National Cancer Institute*, vol. 92, no. 17, pp. 1388–1402, 2000.

[120] R. C. Bates and A. M. Mercurio, "Tumor necrosis factor-α stimulates the epithelial-tomesenchymal transition of human colonic organoids," *Molecular Biology of the Cell*, vol. 14, no. 5, pp. 1790–1800, 2003.

[121] R. J. Orton, O. E. Sturm, V. Vyshemirsky, M. Calder, D. R. Gilbert, and W. Kolch, "Computational modelling of the receptor-tyrosine-kinase-activated MAPK pathway," *Biochemical Journal*, vol. 392, no. 2, pp. 249–261, 2005.

15

Crosstalk between p53 and TGF-β Signalling

Rebecca Elston and Gareth J. Inman

Division of Cancer Research, Medical Research Institute, Ninewells Hospital and Medical School, University of Dundee, Dundee DD1 9SY, UK

Correspondence should be addressed to Gareth J. Inman, g.j.inman@dundee.ac.uk

Academic Editor: Herman P. Spaink

Wild-type p53 and TGF-β are key tumour suppressors which regulate an array of cellular responses. TGF-β signals in part via the Smad signal transduction pathway. Wild-type p53 and Smads physically interact and coordinately induce transcription of a number of key tumour suppressive genes. Conversely mutant p53 generally subverts tumour suppressive TGF-β responses, diminishing transcriptional activation of key TGF-β target genes. Mutant p53 can also interact with Smads and this enables complex formation with the p53 family member p63 and blocks p63-mediated activation of metastasis suppressing genes to promote tumour progression. p53 and Smad function may also overlap during miRNA biogenesis as they can interact with the same components of the Drosha miRNA processing complex to promote maturation of specific subsets of miRNAs. This paper investigates the crosstalk between p53 and TGF-β signalling and the potential roles this plays in cancer biology.

1. Introduction

Transforming growth factor beta (TGF-β) is a pleiotropic cytokine responsible for the regulation of nearly every human cell type. Under normal conditions, TGF-β functions in a context specific manner to maintain tissue homeostasis largely via transcriptional regulation of genes involved in proliferation, cell survival and cytostasis, differentiation, cell motility and the cellular microenvironment [1–8]. Unsurprisingly, the function of this habitual tumour suppressor is commonly found to be perturbed in cancer cells via receptor and pathway component mutations and oncogene crosstalk [1, 4, 9]. Paradoxically, TGF-β can also act as a tumour promoter as tumourigenesis progresses [1, 3, 4, 10–12].

TGF-β signalling is mediated through binding of a TGF-β isoform (TGF-β1, 2 or 3) to a transmembrane heterotetrameric complex of the serine/threonine kinase receptors TβRII and TβRI [13–15]. Activation of the TGF-β receptors results in the downstream phosphorylation of transcription factors Smad2 and 3, which subsequently dissociate from the receptor before binding their constitutive co-smad, Smad4 (Figure 1) [1, 5, 16–18]. The active Smad complex accumulates in the nucleus where it functions to regulate transcription of a myriad of target genes including p21 and proapoptotic BH3-only members of the BCL2 family (Figure 1) [6, 8, 19, 20].

As well as the activation of the Smad dependent signalling pathway, TGF-β can also regulate non-Smad pathways such as the JNK/p38, Ras-ERK, PI3K/Akt, and RhoA pathways [2, 21, 22]. These pathways can then act to regulate many cellular proteins including Smad interacting coactivators and corepressors and thereby contribute to the context specificity of TGF-β signalling (Figure 1) [2]. Regulation of biological processes by TGF-β signalling is consequently brought to fruition by integration of these signalling cascades with other physiological pathways operating in the target cell.

Renowned as the "Guardian of the Genome" p53 has a critical role in maintaining the genetic integrity of proliferating cells thereby preventing malignant transformation [23–25]. p53 acts primarily as a transcription factor [26]. In response to stress signals for example, genotoxic stress, DNA damage, oncogene activation, and hypoxia, p53 is stabilised resulting in its accumulation and subsequent recruitment to p53 binding sites in chromatin [23, 27–29]. Once chromatin bound, p53 promotes transcriptional activation of numerous target genes responsible for apoptosis for example, BH3-only family members and cytostasis for example, p21, [30–33]. More recently p53 has been found to have a much broader range of functions stimulating DNA repair, cell adhesion, cell motility, membrane functioning, and metabolism [23, 34].

With its central role in tumour suppression, p53 is the most commonly mutated gene in cancer with over 50% of tumours expressing a mutant variant [35, 36]. Mutations are particularly prominent in the central DNA binding domain with 74% occurring here, 30% of which occur at six hotspot codons [35]. Mutation of p53 can result in a gain of function acting to promote tumourigenesis [23, 36, 37]. Additionally once mutated p53 may have a dominant negative effect over its wild-type counterpart acting to induce chromosomal instability, a feature of tumour progression, and suppress genes involved in cell cycle control, apoptosis, and DNA repair pathways [36, 38, 39].

2. TGF-β and Wild-Type p53 Pathway Convergence

Under normal phenotypic conditions, both TGF-β and activated p53 act as gene-specific transcription factors to each regulate a multitude of gene targets producing tumour-suppressive effects. Due to the broad ranging nature of these proteins, overlap of cellular functions occurs in the regulation of cytostasis, apoptosis, and autophagy indicating several potential points of convergence. The initial link between the wild-type p53 and TGF-β pathway was proposed in 1991 by Wyllie et al. Inactivation of wild-type p53 by the SV40 virus resulted in loss of response to TGF-β treatment implying that loss of p53 may prelude resistance to the tumour-suppressive effects of TGF-β [55]. More recently several studies have demonstrated the convergence of p53 and Smad signalling pathways.

2.1. Unearthing the Interaction. p53 has been identified as a gene-specific partner for Smads important for the formation and stabilisation of Smad-DNA complexes. The suggestion of such a partnership was first revealed by functional assays in Xenopus embryos searching for modulators of TGF-β family signalling regulated processes during early development [47, 56]. In both screens, p53 was found to regulate development and that this activity required Smad proteins operating through regulation of specific target genes such as Mix2 [47, 56]. Upon TGF-β/Activin, signalling FAST-1 forms a complex with Smads at the Mix2 promoter thereby facilitating gene transcription [57]. Using the Xenopus embryo model system, Cordenonsi et al. demonstrated that in the presence of a p53 isoform (p53AS) along with FAST-1, TGF-β induces a robust increase in the transcription of Mix2 and importantly this effect was diminished upon p53 knock down [47]. In the same study, Cordenonsi et al. used the mammalian HEK293T cell line to further elucidate the mechanism of this p53-Smad interaction. Both Smad2 and 3, but not Smad4, were found to directly bind immobilised wild-type p53 and p73 [47]. Specifically, binding occurs through the phosphorylated N-terminal domain of activated p53 and the N-terminal MH1 domain of Smad2/3 with the

C-terminal MH2 domain free to interact with Smad4 [47]. Coupling of these proteins is dependent upon the phosphorylation of p53 at Serine 6 and 9 of the N-terminal transactivational domain. Phosphorylation of these residues typically occurs in response to DNA damage. However, the Ras/MAPK cascade acting via casein kinase 1 (CK1) δ and ε can also promote this phosphorylation as demonstrated in mammalian H1299 cells [46]. Crucially, inhibition of the Ras/MAPK effector MEK abrogated p53 phosphorylation and subsequently diminished induction of key TGF-β cytostatic genes p21 and p15 thus indicating that p53 serves to integrate crosstalk between Ras/MAPK and TGF-β signalling [46]. This interaction of p53 with Smads 2 and 3 occurs in a TGF-β dependent fashion [47]. However, to induce a robust increase in TGF-β mediated gene transcription p53 must contact its own cognate site within the gene promoter [46–48]. Deletion or point mutation of the DNA binding domain of p53 blocks its biological activity as demonstrated in Xenopus assays and thereby impedes complex formation of the protein with Smads [47, 48, 56]. Thus Smad2/3 may act as a bridge between p53, bound at the p53 binding-element and the Smad complex, bound at the TGF-β responsive-element, allowing synergistic activation of transcription (Figure 2) [46–48].

Synergism between p53 and TGF-β occurs only with a subset of TGF-β target genes with p53 presence having no effect on the inducibility of others for example, TIEG-1/2 [47]. In spite of this, bioinformatic screening of 800 TGF-β target regulatory sequences versus a genomic database of putative p53 DNA-binding sites revealed in excess of 200 genes could be potentially coregulated [48]. However, clustering analysis of these genes predicted only growth inhibitory and extracellular matrix functions to be under joint regulatory control [48]. In support of this, TGF-β target genes such as p21 and p15 (growth inhibition), PAI-1 and MMP2 (extracellular matrix) require wild-type p53 for full activation [46, 47]. Interestingly, in the context of cytostasis wild-type p63 can compensate for p53 mutation having a functional overlap in regulating at least the p21 gene which is required for cell cycle arrest [47]. A prime example is the TGF-β responsive HaCaT cell line, which is p53 mutant but expresses high levels of p63. Following p63 directed siRNA p21 induction by TGF-β was reduced [47]. However more recently, mutant p53 and TGF-β have been found to complex and induce TGF-β-induced metastasis suggesting coregulation of additional cell responses may also occur [53] (see below).

2.2. Smad and Wild-Type p53 miRNA Crossover. MicroRNAs (miRNAs) are small, noncoding RNAs that regulate protein expression by inhibiting translation and increasing degradation of mRNA [58–60]. Primary (pri-) miRNA is transcribed as a long transcript, which folds back to form a hairpin structure [61]. Inside the nucleus DROSHA processes primiRNAs cleaving the 5′ Cap and 3′ Poly (A) tail to form precursor (pre-) miRNAs which are then transported to the cytoplasm via exportin 5 where cleavage by DICER produces mature miRNAs [58, 59, 62]. Once matured miRNAs are

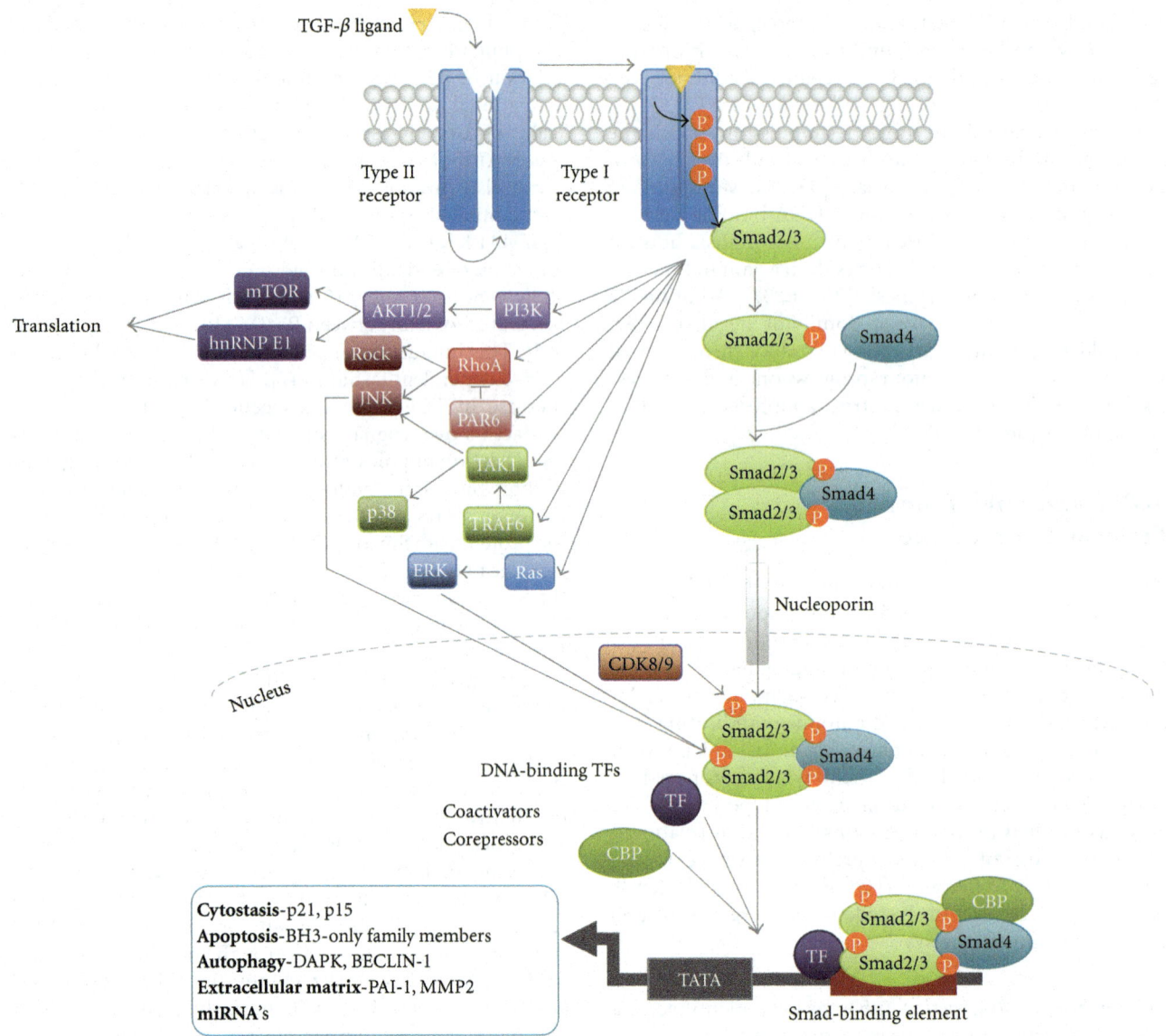

FIGURE 1: Canonical and Noncanonical TGF-β signalling. Initiation of the TGF-β signalling cascade occurs via binding of active TGF-β ligand to the TGF-β type 2 receptor (TGF-βRII) [1, 5]. Once bound TGF-βRII is then able to activate its partner the TGF-β type 1 (TGF-βRI)/ALK5 receptor via phosphorylation [1, 14]. Phosphorylation of TGF-βRI results in a conformational change by which the kinase repressive N-terminal GS domain is flipped to act as a docking site for Receptor Smad (R-smad) proteins for example, Smad2 and 3 and in turn facilitates signal transduction by activation of the catalytic kinase domain [1, 16]. TGF-βRI phosphorylates Smad2 and 3, which associate with their co-smad Smad4 to form the active Smad complex, which accumulates in the nucleus via nucleoporin-mediated transport [5, 40]. Phosphorylation acts to inhibit the constant nucleocytoplasmic recycling of Smads resulting in nuclear accumulation [41]. Smads associate with DNA via binding at target gene DNA-Smad Binding Element's (DNA-SBE), with a optimal conserved sequence of 5'-CAGAC-3' [17, 42]. However, the Smad complex has only relatively weak DNA-binding affinity. Thus, association with numerous DNA-binding transcription factors for example, Zinc-fingers, homeobox and bHLH families, coactivators (e.g., CBP-300), corepressors (e.g., RBL1) and chromatin remodeling factors (e.g., Histone Deacetylase (HDAC)) allows the complex to achieve specific cell responses [17, 42, 43]. In addition activated TGF-βRI can also activate multiple noncanonical pathways. These Smad independent pathways can function autonomously to achieve a wide array of cellular responses in a transcription-independent manner [21]. In addition activation of the JNK, ERK, and CDK8/9 pathways regulate Smad linker phosphorylation to regulate Smad activity [22, 44].

incorporated into the RNA-Induced Silencing Complex (RISC), which positions the miRNA with its target mRNA at the 3′UTR to mediate inhibition [58–60, 63].

The downregulation of mature miRNAs either at the genomic level, by epigenetic modifications or by impaired biogenesis is observed in human malignancies resulting in the promotion of cellular transformation and tumourigenesis [64–66]. Extracellular signals can influence the maturation of specific miRNAs, for example TGF-β and p53 have been found to positively regulate their biogenesis [49, 50].

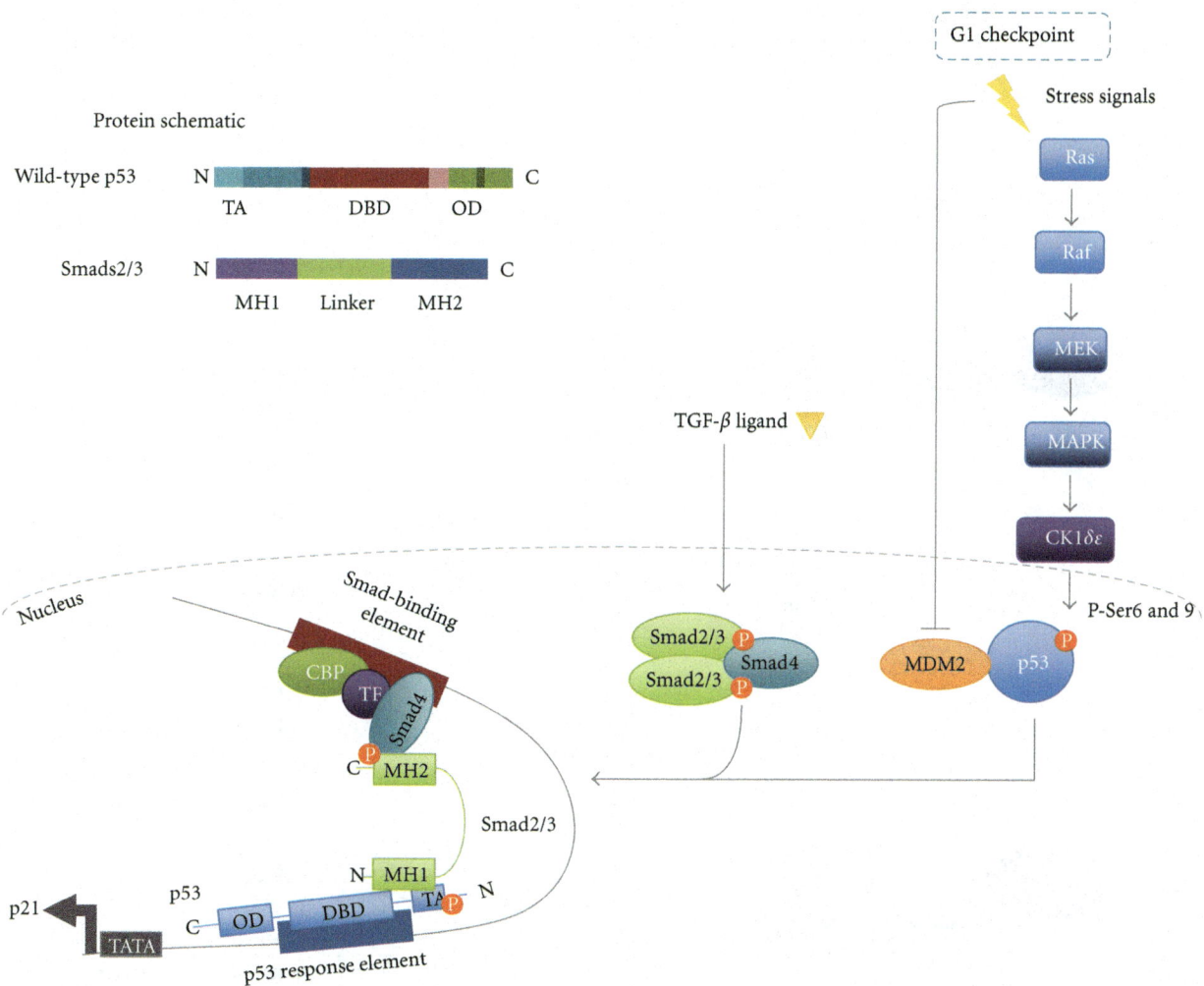

FIGURE 2: Coregulation of gene transcription by p53 and Smad complexes. In the absence of cellular stress p53 is maintained at a low concentration by its negative regulator MDM2 [27, 28, 45]. MDM2 acts to poly-ubiquitinate p53, which targets the tumour suppressor to the proteasome for degradation. In response to DNA damage p53 is phosphorylated at defined Ser/Thr residues resulting in its stabilisation and dissociation from MDM2 [29]. In addition signalling via the Ras/MAPK pathway CK1δ/ε can also result in the activating phosphorylation of p53 [46]. Activated wild-type p53 can act synergistically with Smads to increase the transcription of a subset of genes for example, p21, PAI-1 [46, 47]. The model depicted was originally proposed by Piccolo and colleagues and elegantly demonstrates how p53 and Smads may interact [46–48]. For synergism to occur, the target gene must possess both a DNA-SBE and a p53 response element (RE) to which the activated Smad complex and p53 bind respectively. Once bound at their respective sequences a direct interaction between Smads and p53 may occur in which the N-terminal MH1 domain of Smads2/3 binds the N-terminal transactivational domain (TA) of p53 [46–48]. Association within the gene promoter acts to maximally induce gene transcription.

Such positive regulation on biogenesis may act in a tumour suppressive manner for example, TGF-β and p53 induce miR-215, which acts to induce growth arrest and decrease cell proliferation [51, 67, 68]. Conversely, a positive regulation on biogenesis may also lead to tumour progression for example, TGF-β increases miR-21 maturation [51], which can act to inhibit PTEN and Sprouty 1 key negative regulators of the Akt and Ras/MAPK pathways allowing their aberrant activity [69, 70].

Both p53 and TGF-β can act transcriptionally to regulate the expression of miRNAs by binding at their response elements within target promoters. It is plausible that p53 and TGF-β may converge via the p53-Smad interaction as earlier described to synergistically regulate miRNA transcription.

However, whether such an interaction at miRNA promoters does in fact occur is yet to be described.

In response to TGF-β signalling miRNA microarray profiling of PASMCs revealed mature levels of 20 miRNAs, including miR-21, that were induced in excess of 1.6-fold [51]. Of these miRNAs analysis by Davis et al. revealed 85% contained a conserved stem sequence (CAGAC) homologous to that of the SMAD-binding element present in DNA (Figure 3) [51]. This RNA Smad-binding element (R-SBE) was absent in non-TGF-β-induced miRNA's [51]. In C3H 10T1/2 cells mutation of more than 2 bp in the R-SBE sequence abolished the production of these mature miRNAs revealing that Smads must associate with these miRNAs directly for upregulation to occur [51].

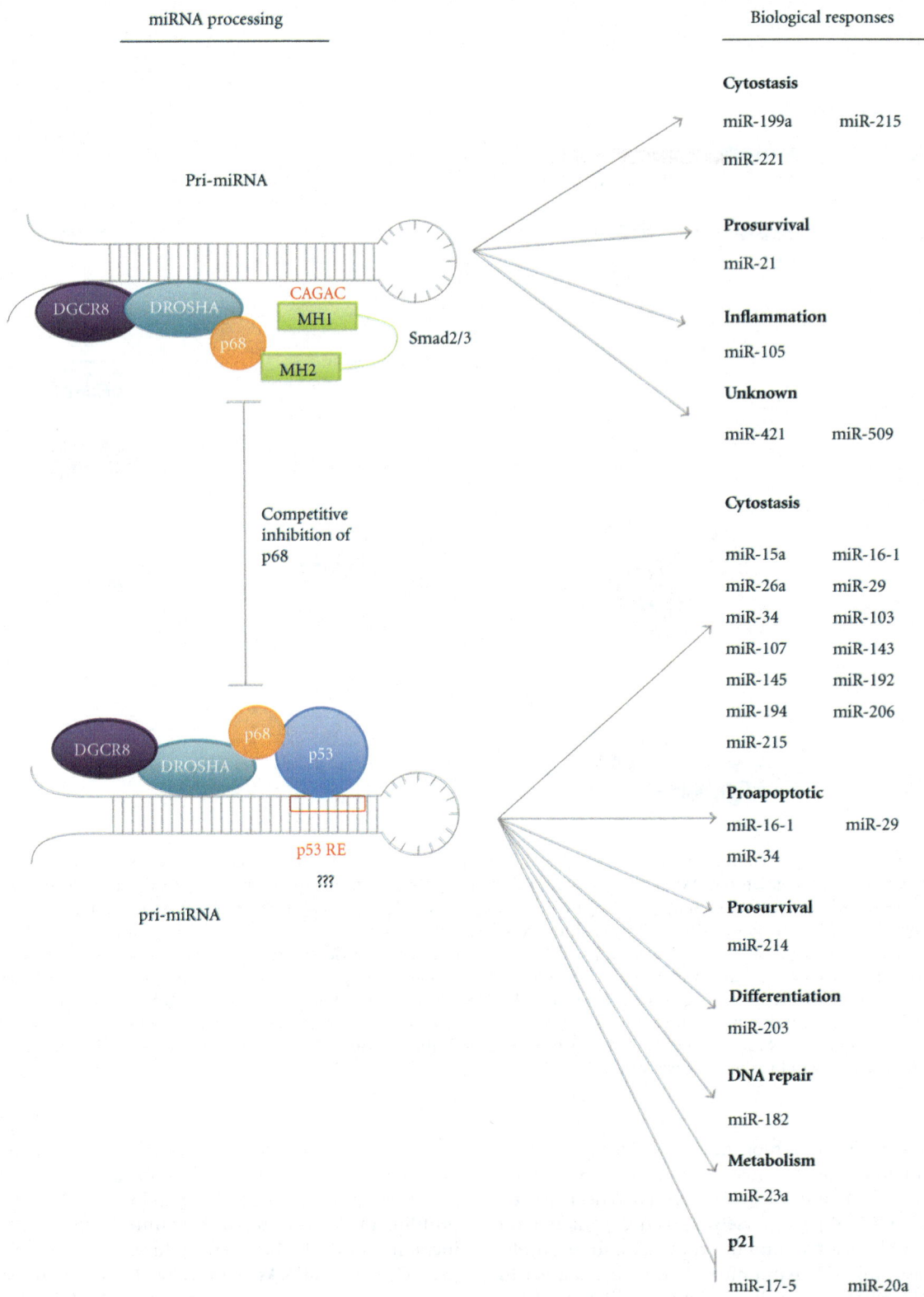

miRNA processing

Biological responses

FIGURE 3: Potential overlapping functions of TGF-β and p53 in microRNA processing. Smads and p53 act to increase the posttranscriptional maturation of a subset of miRNAs via direct binding of the DROSHA-associated helicase p68 [49–52]. These miRNAs have crucial roles in tumour suppression acting in cytostasis and DNA repair. Interestingly pro-survival miRNAs are also upregulated indicating a possible mechanism for protumourigenesis by inhibition of key tumour suppressors. However, upregulation of these prosurvival miRNAs may also facilitate the induction of senescence, protecting cells from cell death induced by tumour suppressor genes. In addition to acting as a molecular tag to direct DROSHA activity binding of Smads and p53 may act to promote p68 helicase activity, which could act to induce conformational changes in pri-miRNA structure making it accessible for DROSHA cleavage. As proposed by Davis et al. competition may occur between Smads and p53 for binding to p68 upon which binding of one protein results in the inhibition of p68 association with other [51]. Binding of Smads to microRNAs is mediated by association with CAGAC Smad DNA-binding-like elements (SBEs) and a similar p53 response-element- (RE) mediated mechanism may also occur for p53. Potential RE and SBE sequence overlap may also occur adding a potential further layer of cross-regulation.

Posttranscriptionally Davis et al. defined how Smad's enhance miRNA maturation. Following TGF-β treatment of PASMC cells the induction of both pre- and mature miR-21 was observed, however, no change in expression of pri-miR-21 was seen indicating TGF-β components must act posttranscriptionally with DROSHA [49, 51]. Use of recombinant GST-Smad fusion proteins demonstrated that the MH1 domain of Smads is responsible for binding of the R-SBE in miRNAs with this domain binding and pulling down 18-fold more pri-miR-21 than GST, whereas the MH2 domain did not bind at all [51]. The association of Smads with miRNAs is unable to facilitate their maturation, instead Smad binding is proposed to act as a molecular tag-promoting interactions with the processing machinery [51]. Both Davis et al. and Warner et al. reported that the MH2 domain of TGF-β Smad2/3 (but not Smad4) interacts with the RNA helicase p68 (Figure 3) [49, 52]. p68 is part of the DROSHA multicomponent processing complex and may function to recognise and bind specific pri-miRNA structures and thus localise DROSHA for cleavage [71]. Further investigation in PASMCs by Davis et al. revealed that siRNA of p68 inhibited the TGF-β-mediated induction of pre- and mature miR-21 thereby demonstrating it's essential role in potentiating DROSHA processing [49]. The enhancement in miRNA maturation may facilitate TGF-β tumour-promoting functions. For example miR-21 is highly expressed in several breast tumour cell lines including, MCF7 and MDA-MB-468 cells where it acts to suppress the apoptotic tumour suppressor programmed cell death 4 (PDCD4) [49].

In response to DNA damage activated wild-type p53 can transcriptionally upregulate miRNAs via direct binding at target promoters for example, miR-34. In addition activated p53 can also act post-transcriptionally to promote the maturation of a subset of miRNAs important in the regulation of cell cycle and proliferative genes for example, K-Ras and CDK6 [50]. Notably these miRNAs are distinct from those induced by TGF-β having no R-SBE. Suzuki et al. determined that like the Smads p53 interacts with the RNA helicases p68 and p72 to facilitate DROSHA processing (Figure 3) [50]. Mutation of p53 also results in decreased miRNA maturation, however, as mutant p53 still associates with p68 suppression must occur in a transcription-dependent manner [50].

As both p53 and Smads can interact with the same components of the Drosha complex it is possible that activation of these transcription factors may result in competition for Drosha complex components and may therefore cross-regulate each other's responses. Indeed Davis et al. noted that maturation of Smad-regulated miRNAs is enhanced in cells with loss of p53 function, for example the mutant p53 cell line MDA-MB-468 versus the wild-type p53 PASMCs [51].

3. Inhibition of TGF-β Tumour Suppressor Function by p53 Mutation

3.1. Transcriptional Activation of TGF-β Target Genes. p53 mutants have been found to affect numerous stages of

the TGF-β pathway; by repressing of the TGF-βRII gene, delaying or reducing phosphorylation of Smad2 by TGF-βRI, and interfering with Smad2/3 and Smad4 association and inhibiting Smad translocation to the nucleus [72]. By affecting the TGF-β pathway Smad-dependent transcription of target genes is ablated and thus TGF-β mediated cellular responses. In addition p53 mutation can result in a loss of DNA-binding capacity thereby inhibiting coupling with Smad's at gene-specific promoters for example, Mix2, PAI-1, and p21 and thus transcriptional induction of these genes is diminished [46, 72]. p21, a cyclin-dependent kinase inhibitor, acts to induce a functional G_1 arrest via the inhibition of downstream cell cycle regulators CDK4/Cyclin D1 and CDK2/Cyclin E. Inhibition results in the hypophosphorylation of the retinoblastoma (Rb) protein preventing its release from E2F, a key transcription factor for DNA replication and thus blocking G_1 to S phase progression. Plasminogen activator inhibitor 1 (PAI-1) acts to inhibit both the degradation of collagen and the catalytic activation of matrix metalloproteinases (MMP) 1 and 10 [73]. When active, these MMPs play a crucial role in the invasion of malignant cells across the basal lamina. The degradation of collagen also mediates this invasion as well as invasion into local blood vessels allowing cells to metastasise. Consequently diminished activation of these genes may aid tumourigenesis inducing limitless replicative potential from a failure to growth arrest by p21 and through MMP activity tissue invasion and metastasis both key hallmarks of cancer [74].

Inactivation of p53 results in aberrant behaviour of cancer cells and may therefore represent a mechanism by which loss of TGF-β tumour suppression occurs [75]. In support Cordenonsi et al. found that reintroduction of the wild-type p53 isoform p53AS in conjunction with Smad2 induced a TGF-β-mediated cytostatic response within the normally unresponsive p53 null SAOS-2 cell line [47].

3.2. Metastasis. Recently Adorno et al. demonstrated that the mutational status of p53 determines the nature of the cellular response to TGF-β. Introduction of wild-type p53 into p53 null H1299 cells resulted in a TGF-β-induced growth arrest via p21 [53]. In contrast reconstitution with mutant p53 caused cells to change from an epithelial to mesenchymal morphology, enabling a promigratory TGF-β response [53]. Under normal conditions metastasis is inhibited by the p53 family member p63 which acts to transcriptionally upregulate key metastatic suppressor genes for example, Sharp-1 and Cyclin G2 [53]. In conjunction with Smads mutant p53 can usurp p63 functioning via ternary complex formation. For example in metastatic D3S2 carcinoma cells, TGF-β treatment resulted in complex formation of nearly all the p63 with mutant p53 thereby facilitating a TGF-β metastatic response. Formation of this complex was found to be dependent on Smads becoming undetectable post-transfection of Smad2/3 siRNA in HaCaT cells. To determine the structural association of Smads in this complex GST-pull down experiments were carried out using immobilised GST-Smad3 and structural isoforms of p63 resulting in the

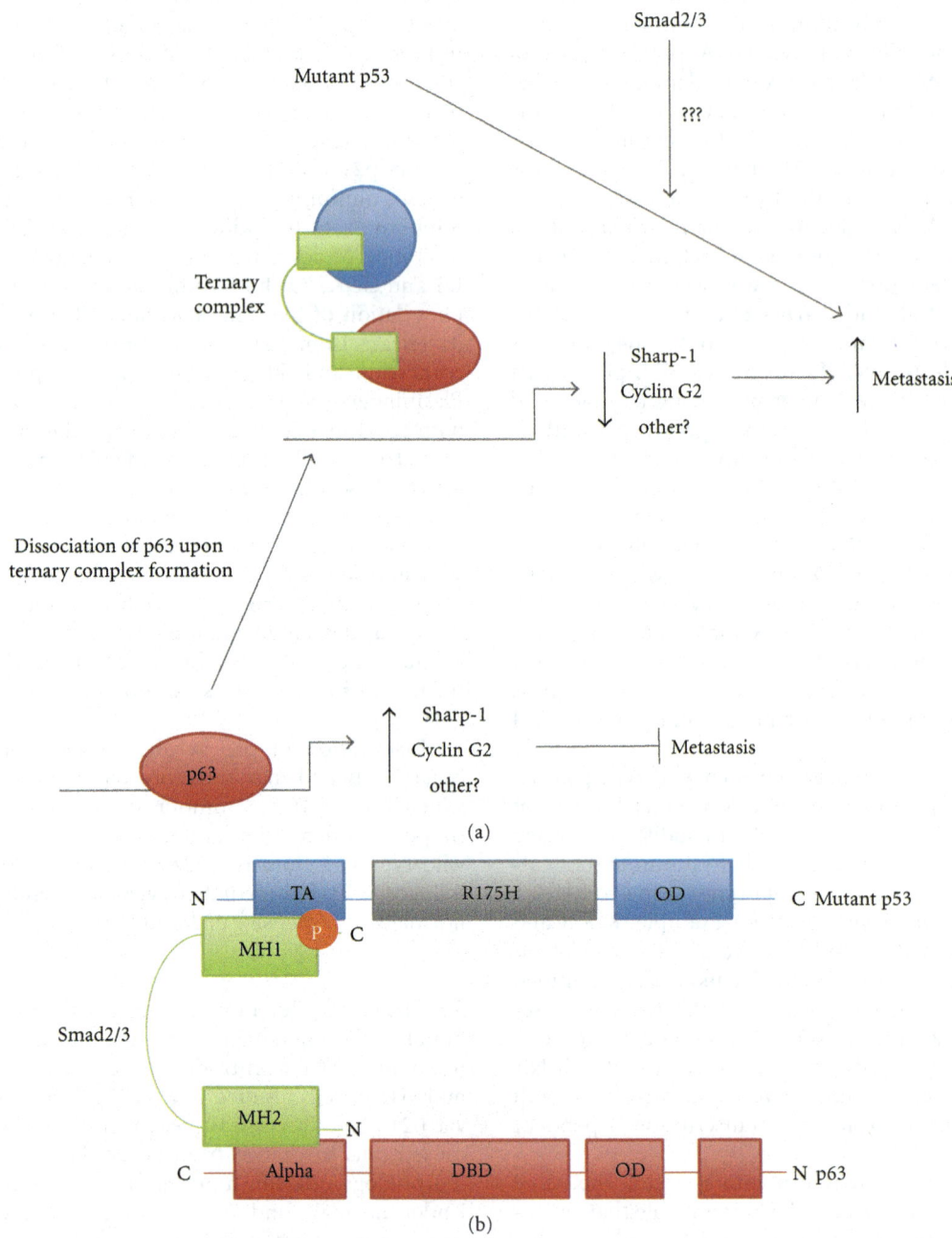

FIGURE 4: Regulation of metastasis by mutant p53 and Smads. (a) p63 has a crucial role in the transcriptional activation of genes which function in the inhibition of metastasis. Mutant p53 can act to inhibit the anti-metastatic functioning of p63 but is dependent upon the formation of a ternary complex with Smads2/3 as described below [53]. Formation of a ternary complex inhibits the binding of p63 to the DNA at target gene promoters thereby inhibiting transcription of these key antimetastatic genes and subsequently increased metastasis of malignant cells is observed [53]. In addition mutant p53 can promote invasion and metastasis independently. For example mutant p53 can suppress p63 in the context of integrin recycling [54]. It is yet unknown whether Smads are involved for these other routes of induction. (b) Mutant p53 is able to inhibit p63 activity by the formation of a ternary complex. Formation of this complex is dependent on receptor Smad2/3 acting as a molecular bridge between the proteins. The C-terminal MH1 domain of Smads2/3 binds the transactivational (TA) domain at the N-terminus of mutant p53 [53]. The N-terminal MH2 domain binds at the C-terminal alpha domain of p63 [53]. Association of p63 in this complex inhibits its capacity to bind DNA thus blocking transcriptional functions of the protein.

identification of two Smad interaction sites within p63 at the transactivational and alpha domains [38]. Importantly the vast majority of p63 is expressed as the ΔNp63 isoform, which lacks an N-terminal transactivation domain [38]. As a result Adorno et al. hypothesised a structure in which R-Smads acting as a bridge between the C-terminal alpha domain of p63 and the N-terminal domain of p53 via respective binding of Smad MH2 and MH1 domains (Figure 4) [53].

Similarly increased invasion is observed in the context of integrin recycling in which mutant p53 expression again inhibits p63 functioning. Here inhibition of p63 promotes the association of Rab-coupling protein with $\alpha5\beta1$ integrin which acts to chaperone the integrin to the plasma membrane where it then acts to promote tumour cell motility [54]. There is no evidence that these processes are influenced by TGF-β signalling and Smad interactions but this warrants further investigation.

3.3. miRNA Biogenesis. In cells harbouring mutant p53 TGF-β stimulation results in greater induction of TGF-β-regulated miRNAs [51]. Davis et al. proposed that Smads and p53 might directly compete for p68 binding and hence loss of p53/p68 interaction may release more p68 for Smad-directed miRNA maturation (Figure 3). In addition to this proposed mechanism of p53/Smad crosstalk in miRNA biogenesis, it is also possible that competition between p53 and Smad complexes for direct RNA binding in the Pri-miRNA seed sequence may occur. Smads regulate a subset of miRNAs via interaction with the SBE consensus AGAC sequence. p53 regulates target genes via binding to the p53 RE which consists of 2 motifs, 5′-PuPuPuC(A/T)(T/A)GPyPyPy-3′, separated by a ≤13 bp spacer [76]. Computational analysis has previously revealed these binding sites to be conserved at the miR34b/c promoters [77]. By assuming a 5′ sequence of 5′-AGAC-3′, this motif has the potential to overlap with the core consensus at Smad-binding-elements [78]. In this case, binding of wild-type p53 at its cognate DNA may result in the displacement of Smads thereby inhibiting Smad-p68 interaction or vice versa. This intriguing possibility and the consequence of p53 mutation on this potential crosstalk warrants future investigation.

4. Concluding Remarks

Establishment of TGF-β-p53 pathway crossover brings new complexity to the regulatory functioning of these proteins. Currently TGF-β and p53 convergence has only been found in cytostasis, extracellular matrix functioning, and metastasis [48, 53]. However, it will be interesting to ascertain whether such crossover occurs in other TGF-β and p53 functions namely apoptosis, proliferation, and autophagy and if such responses are dependent on the presence or phenotypic status of both proteins.

The recent study of Adorno et al. demonstrated how the mutational status of p53 can interfere with TGF-β switching it's functioning from tumour suppressive to protumorigenic [53]. In concurrence Davis et al. shows mutant p53 confers

the ability of TGF-β to promote miRNA maturation for example, miR-21 which can act to inhibit tumour suppressors such as PDCD4 [49]. Such findings suggest that mutant p53 may potentiate tumour-promoting functions of TGF-β thus allowing cancer cells to proliferate and invade leading to advanced tumours.

TGF-β has been implicated in the induction of EMT in breast cancer stem cells and plays an essential role in maintaining the pluripotency of these stem cells [79]. In the Adorno et al. study p63 acts to suppress TGF-β induced EMT [53]. However, in the presence of mutant p53 formation of the ternary complex with p63 in conjunction with Smads acts to inhibit this p63 suppression facilitating TGF-β induced EMT [53]. This raises the interesting question of whether TGF-β/Smads and p53 family members may also cooperate to regulate tumour stem cells.

Further complexities between crosstalk of p53 family members and their multiple splice variants [80] with TGF-β signalling pathways are likely to be unveiled in the near future. For example in MCF10A cells expression of ΔNp63γ results in TGF-β-dependent EMT and subsequently increases the expression of both TGF-β and downstream Smads2/3/4 [81]. A systematic evaluation of the effects of activation of the p53 family and TGF-β signal transduction pathways in different biological situations is likely to shed considerable light and add further intrigue into the crosstalk between these fundamentally important regulators of biology.

Acknowledgment

The authors acknowledge support from Cancer Research UK, The Association for International Cancer Research, and the University of Dundee.

References

[1] J. Massagué, "TGFβ in cancer," *Cell*, vol. 134, no. 2, pp. 215–230, 2008.

[2] R. Derynck and Y. E. Zhang, "Smad-dependent and Smad-independent pathways in TGF-β family signalling," *Nature*, vol. 425, no. 6958, pp. 577–584, 2003.

[3] R. L. Elliott and G. C. Blobe, "Role of transforming factor β in human cancer," *Journal of Clinical Oncology*, vol. 23, no. 9, pp. 2078–2093, 2005.

[4] H. Ikushima and K. Miyazono, "TGFβ singalling: a complex web in cancer progression," *Nature Reviews Cancer*, vol. 10, no. 6, pp. 415–424, 2010.

[5] Y. Shi and J. Massagué, "Mechanisms of TGF—β signaling from cell membrane to the nucleus," *Cell*, vol. 113, no. 6, pp. 685–700, 2003.

[6] P. M. Siegel and J. Massagué, "Cytostatic and apoptotic actions of TGF-β in homeostasis and cancer," *Nature Reviews Cancer*, vol. 3, no. 11, pp. 807–821, 2003.

[7] B. Bierie and H. L. Moses, "Tumour microenvironment: TGFβ: the molecular Jekyll and Hyde of cancer," *Nature Reviews Cancer*, vol. 6, no. 7, pp. 506–520, 2006.

[8] C. H. Heldin, M. Landstrom, and A. Moustakas, "Mechanism of TGF-β signaling to growth arrest, apoptosis, and epithelial-mesenchymal transition," *Current Opinion in Cell Biology*, vol. 21, no. 2, pp. 166–176, 2009.

[9] L. Levy and C. S. Hill, "Alterations in components of the TGF-β superfamily signaling pathways in human cancer," *Cytokine and Growth Factor Reviews*, vol. 17, no. 1-2, pp. 41–58, 2006.

[10] A. B. Roberts and L. M. Wakefield, "The two faces of transforming growth factor β in carcinogenesis," *Proceedings of the National Academy of Sciences of the United States of America*, vol. 100, no. 15, pp. 8621–8623, 2003.

[11] E. Meulmeester and P. T. Dijke, "The dynamic roles of TGF-β in cancer," *Journal of Pathology*, vol. 223, no. 2, pp. 205–218, 2011.

[12] G. J. Inman, "Switching TGFβ from a tumor suppressor to a tumor promoter," *Current Opinion in Genetics & Development*, vol. 21, no. 1, pp. 93–99, 2011.

[13] T. Huang, L. David, V. Mendoza et al., "TGF-β signalling is mediated by two autonomously functioning TβRI: TβRII pairs," *The EMBO Journal*, vol. 30, no. 7, pp. 1263–1276, 2011.

[14] J. Massagué, "A very private TGF-β receptor embrace," *Molecular Cell*, vol. 29, no. 2, pp. 149–150, 2008.

[15] J. Groppe, C. S. Hinck, P. Samavarchi-Tehrani et al., "Cooperative assembly of TGF-β superfamily signaling complexes is mediated by two disparate mechanisms and distinct modes of receptor binding," *Molecular Cell*, vol. 29, no. 2, pp. 157–168, 2008.

[16] J. Massagué, J. Seoane, and D. Wotton, "Smad transcription factors," *Genes and Development*, vol. 19, no. 23, pp. 2783–2810, 2005.

[17] C. H. Heldin and A. Moustakas, "Role of Smads in TGFβ signaling," *Cell and Tissue Research*, vol. 347, no. 1, pp. 21–26, 2012.

[18] X. H. Feng and R. Derynck, "Specificity and versatility in TGF-β signaling through smads," *Annual Review of Cell and Developmental Biology*, vol. 21, pp. 659–693, 2005.

[19] S. Ramesh, X. J. Qi, G. M. Wildey et al., "TGFβ-mediated BIM expression and apoptosis are regulated through SMAD3-dependent expression of the MAPK phosphatase MKP2," *EMBO Reports*, vol. 9, no. 10, pp. 990–997, 2008.

[20] L. C. Spender, D. I. O'Brien, D. Simpson et al., "TGF-β induces apoptosis in human B cells by transcriptional regulation of BIK and BCL-XL," *Cell Death and Differentiation*, vol. 16, no. 4, pp. 593–602, 2009.

[21] Y. Zhang, "Non-Smad pathways in TGF-β signaling," *Cell Research*, vol. 19, no. 1, pp. 128–139, 2009.

[22] Y. Mu, S. K. Gudey, and M. Landstrom, "Non-Smad signaling pathways," *Cell and Tissue Research*, vol. 347, no. 1, pp. 11–20, 2012.

[23] K. H. Vousden and C. Prives, "Blinded by the light: the growing complexity of p53," *Cell*, vol. 137, no. 3, pp. 413–431, 2009.

[24] D. P. Lane, "p53, guardian of the genome," *Nature*, vol. 358, no. 6381, pp. 15–16, 1992.

[25] A. J. Levine and M. Oren, "The first 30 years of p53: growing ever more complex," *Nature Reviews Cancer*, vol. 9, no. 10, pp. 749–758, 2009.

[26] R. Beckerman and C. Prives, "Transcriptional regulation by p53," *Cold Spring Harbor Perspectives in Biology*, vol. 2, no. 8, p. a000935, 2010.

[27] Y. Haupt, R. Maya, A. Kazaz, and M. Oren, "Mdm2 promotes the rapid degradation of p53," *Nature*, vol. 387, no. 6630, pp. 296–299, 1997.

[28] M. H. Kubbutat, S. N. Jones, and K. H. Vousden, "Regulation of p53 stability by Mdm2," *Nature*, vol. 387, no. 6630, pp. 299–303, 1997.

[29] A. Hock and K. H. Vousden, "Regulation of the p53 pathway by ubiquitin and related proteins," *International Journal of Biochemistry and Cell Biology*, vol. 42, no. 10, pp. 1618–1621, 2010.

[30] K. Nakano and K. H. Vousden, "PUMA, a novel proapoptotic gene, is induced by p53," *Molecular Cell*, vol. 7, no. 3, pp. 683–694, 2001.

[31] J. Yu, L. Zhang, P. M. Hwang, K. W. Kinzler, and B. Vogelstein, "PUMA induces the rapid apoptosis of colorectal cancer cells," *Molecular Cell*, vol. 7, no. 3, pp. 673–682, 2001.

[32] W. S. El-Deiry, T. Tokino, V. E. Velculescu et al., "WAF1, a potential mediator of p53 tumor suppression," *Cell*, vol. 75, no. 4, pp. 817–825, 1993.

[33] E. Oda, R. Ohki, H. Murasawa et al., "Noxa, a BH3-only member of the Bcl-2 family and candidate mediator of p53-induced apoptosis," *Science*, vol. 288, no. 5468, pp. 1053–1058, 2000.

[34] O. D. Maddocks and K. H. Vousden, "Metabolic regulation by p53," *Journal of Molecular Medicine*, vol. 89, no. 3, pp. 237–245, 2011.

[35] T. Soussi, "TP53 mutations in human cancer: database reassessment and prospects for the next decade," *Advances in Cancer Research*, vol. 110, pp. 107–139, 2011.

[36] A. M. Goh, C. R. Coffill, and D. P. Lane, "The role of mutant p53 in human cancer," *Journal of Pathology*, vol. 223, no. 2, pp. 116–126, 2011.

[37] M. Oren and V. Rotter, "Mutant p53 gain-of-function in cancer," *Cold Spring Harbor Perspectives in Biology*, vol. 2, no. 2, p. a001107, 2010.

[38] H. Song, M. Hollstein, and Y. Xu, "p53 gain-of-function cancer mutants induce genetic instability by inactivating ATM," *Nature Cell Biology*, vol. 9, no. 5, pp. 573–580, 2007.

[39] A. Willis, E. J. Jung, T. Wakefield, and X. Chen, "Mutant p53 exerts a dominant negative effect by preventing wild-type p53 from binding to the promoter of its target genes," *Oncogene*, vol. 23, no. 13, pp. 2330–2338, 2004.

[40] L. Xu, Y. Kang, S. Col, and J. Massagué, "Smad2 nucleocytoplasmic shuttling by nucleoporins CAN/Nup214 and Nup153 feeds TGFβ signaling complexes in the cytoplasm and nucleus," *Molecular Cell*, vol. 10, no. 2, pp. 271–282, 2002.

[41] G. J. Inman, F. J. Nicolas, and C. S. Hill, "Nucleocytoplasmic shuttling of Smads 2, 3, and 4 permits sensing of TGF-β receptor activity," *Molecular Cell*, vol. 10, no. 2, pp. 283–294, 2002.

[42] S. Ross and C. S. Hill, "How the Smads regulate transcription," *International Journal of Biochemistry and Cell Biology*, vol. 40, no. 3, pp. 383–408, 2008.

[43] H. Ikushima and K. Miyazono, "Cellular context—dependent "colors" of transforming growth factor—β signaling," *Cancer Science*, vol. 101, no. 2, pp. 306–312, 2010.

[44] C. Alarcon, A. I. Zaromytidou, Q. Xi et al., "Nuclear CDKs drive Smad transcriptional activation and turnover in BMP and TGF-β pathways," *Cell*, vol. 139, no. 4, pp. 757–769, 2009.

[45] I. Ringshausen, C. C. O'Shea, A. J. Finch, L. B. Swigart, and G. I. Evan, "Mdm2 is critically and continuously required to suppress lethal p53 activity in vivo," *Cancer Cell*, vol. 10, no. 6, pp. 501–514, 2006.

[46] M. Cordenonsi, M. Montagner, M. Adorno et al., "Integration of TGF-β and Ras/MAPK signaling through p53 phosphorylation," *Science*, vol. 315, no. 5813, pp. 840–843, 2007.

[47] M. Cordenonsi, S. Dupont, S. Maretto, A. Insinga, C. Imbriano, and S. Piccolo, "Links between tumor suppressors: p53 is required for TGF-β gene responses by cooperating with Smads," *Cell*, vol. 113, no. 3, pp. 301–314, 2003.

[48] S. Dupont, L. Zacchigna, M. Adorno et al., "Convergence of p53 and TGF-β signaling networks," *Cancer Letters*, vol. 213, no. 2, pp. 129–138, 2004.

[49] B. N. Davis, A. C. Hilyard, G. Lagna, and A. Hata, "SMAD proteins control DROSHA-mediated microRNA maturation," *Nature*, vol. 454, no. 7200, pp. 56–61, 2008.

[50] H. I. Suzuki, K. Yamagata, K. Sugimoto, T. Iwamoto, S. Kato, and K. Miyazono, "Modulation of microRNA processing by p53," *Nature*, vol. 460, no. 7254, pp. 529–533, 2009.

[51] B. N. Davis, A. C. Hilyard, P. H. Nguyen, G. Lagna, and A. Hata, "Smad proteins bind a conserved RNA sequence to promote MicroRNA maturation by Drosha," *Molecular Cell*, vol. 39, no. 3, pp. 373–384, 2010.

[52] D. R. Warner, V. Bhattacherjee, X. Yin et al., "Functional interaction between Smad, CREB binding protein, and p68 RNA helicase," *Biochemical and Biophysical Research Communications*, vol. 324, no. 1, pp. 70–76, 2004.

[53] M. Adorno, M. Cordenonsi, M. Montagner et al., "A mutant-p53/Smad complex opposes p63 to empower TGFβ-induced metastasis," *Cell*, vol. 137, no. 1, pp. 87–98, 2009.

[54] P. A. Muller, P. T. Caswell, B. Doyle et al., "Mutant p53 drives invasion by promoting integrin recycling," *Cell*, vol. 139, no. 7, pp. 1327–1341, 2009.

[55] F. S. Wyllie, T. Dawson, J. Bond et al., "Correlated abnormalities of transforming growth factor-β1 response and p53 expression in thyroid epithelial cell transformation," *Molecular and Cellular Endocrinology*, vol. 76, no. 1–3, pp. 13–21, 1991.

[56] K. Takebayashi-Suzuki, J. Funami, D. Tokumori et al., "Interplay between the tumor suppressor p53 and TGFβ signaling shapes embryonic body axes in Xenopus," *Development*, vol. 130, no. 17, pp. 3929–3939, 2003.

[57] X. Chen, E. Weisberg, V. Fridmacher, M. Watanabe, G. Naco, and M. Whitman, "Smad4 and FAST-1 in the assembly of activin-responsive factor," *Nature*, vol. 389, no. 6646, pp. 85–89, 1997.

[58] R. W. Carthew and E. J. Sontheimer, "Origins and mechanisms of miRNAs and siRNAs," *Cell*, vol. 136, no. 4, pp. 642–655, 2009.

[59] D. P. Bartel, "MicroRNAs: target recognition and regulatory functions," *Cell*, vol. 136, no. 2, pp. 215–233, 2009.

[60] M. Inui, G. Martello, and S. Piccolo, "MicroRNA control of signal transduction," *Nature Reviews Molecular Cell Biology*, vol. 11, no. 4, pp. 252–263, 2010.

[61] D. P. Bartel, "MicroRNAs: genomics, biogenesis, mechanism, and function," *Cell*, vol. 116, no. 2, pp. 281–297, 2004.

[62] Y. Lee, C. Ahn, J. Han et al., "The nuclear RNase III Drosha initiates microRNA processing," *Nature*, vol. 425, no. 6956, pp. 415–419, 2003.

[63] R. S. Pillai, C. G. Artus, and W. Filipowicz, "Tethering of human Ago proteins to mRNA mimics the miRNA-mediated repression of protein synthesis," *RNA*, vol. 10, no. 10, pp. 1518–1525, 2004.

[64] M. S. Kumar, J. Lu, K. L. Mercer, T. R. Golub, and T. Jacks, "Impaired microRNA processing enhances cellular transformation and tumorigenesis," *Nature Genetics*, vol. 39, no. 5, pp. 673–677, 2007.

[65] A. Esquela-Kerscher and F. J. Slack, "Oncomirs—MicroRNAs with a role in cancer," *Nature Reviews Cancer*, vol. 6, no. 4, pp. 259–269, 2006.

[66] H. I. Suzuki and K. Miyazono, "Dynamics of microRNA biogenesis: crosstalk between p53 network and microRNA processing pathway," *Journal of Molecular Medicine*, vol. 88, no. 11, pp. 1085–1094, 2010.

[67] C. J. Braun, X. Zhang, I. Savelyeva et al., "p53-responsive microRNAs 192 and 215 are capable of inducing cell cycle arrest," *Cancer Research*, vol. 68, no. 24, pp. 10094–10104, 2008.

[68] S. A. Georges, M. C. Biery, S. Y. Kim et al., "Coordinated regulation of cell cycle transcripts by p53-inducible microRNAs, miR-192 and miR-215," *Cancer Research*, vol. 68, no. 24, pp. 10105–10112, 2008.

[69] F. Meng, R. Henson, H. Wehbe-Janek, K. Ghoshal, S. T. Jacob, and T. Patel, "MicroRNA-21 regulates expression of the PTEN tumor suppressor gene in human hepatocellular cancer," *Gastroenterology*, vol. 133, no. 2, pp. 647–658, 2007.

[70] C. Polytarchou, D. Iliopoulos, M. Hatziapostolou et al., "Akt2 regulates all Akt isoforms and promotes resistance to hypoxia through induction of miR-21 upon oxygen deprivation," *Cancer Research*, vol. 71, no. 13, pp. 4720–4731, 2011.

[71] T. Fukuda, K. Yamagata, S. Fujiyama et al., "DEAD-box RNA helicase subunits of the Drosha complex are required for processing of rRNA and a subset of microRNAs," *Nature Cell Biology*, vol. 9, no. 5, pp. 604–611, 2007.

[72] E. Kalo, Y. Buganim, K. E. Shapira et al., "Mutant p53 attenuates the SMAD-dependent transforming growth factor β1 (TGF-β1) signaling pathway by repressing the expression of TGF-β receptor type II," *Molecular and Cellular Biology*, vol. 27, no. 23, pp. 8228–8242, 2007.

[73] C. E. Wilkins-Port, Q. Ye, J. E. Mazurkiewicz, and P. J. Higgins, "TGF-β1 + EGF-initiated invasive potential in transformed human keratinocytes is coupled to a plasmin/mmp-10/mmp-1-dependent collagen remodeling axis: role for PAI-1," *Cancer Research*, vol. 69, no. 9, pp. 4081–4091, 2009.

[74] D. Hanahan and R. A. Weinberg, "The hallmarks of cancer," *Cell*, vol. 100, no. 1, pp. 57–70, 2000.

[75] A. Atfi and R. Baron, "p53 brings a new twist to the Smad signaling network," *Science Signaling*, vol. 1, no. 26, p. pe33, 2008.

[76] W. S. El-Deiry, S. E. Kern, J. A. Pietenpol, K. W. Kinzler, and B. Vogelstein, "Definition of a consensus binding site for p53," *Nature Genetics*, vol. 1, no. 1, pp. 45–49, 1992.

[77] D. C. Corney, A. Flesken-Nikitin, A. K. Godwin, W. Wang, and A. Y. Nikitin, "MicroRNA-34b and MicroRNA-34c are targets of p53 and cooperate in control of cell proliferation and adhesion-independent growth," *Cancer Research*, vol. 67, no. 18, pp. 8433–8438, 2007.

[78] D. S. Wilkinson, S. K. Ogden, S. A. Stratton et al., "A direct intersection between p53 and transforming growth factor β pathways targets chromatin modification and transcription repression of the α-fetoprotein gene," *Molecular and Cellular Biology*, vol. 25, no. 3, pp. 1200–1212, 2005.

[79] K. Polyak and R. A. Weinberg, "Transitions between epithelial and mesenchymal states: acquisition of malignant and stem cell traits," *Nature Reviews Cancer*, vol. 9, no. 4, pp. 265–273, 2009.

[80] M. P. Khoury and J. C. Bourdon, "The isoforms of the p53 protein," *Cold Spring Harbor Perspectives in Biology*, vol. 2, no. 3, p. a000927, 2010.

[81] J. Lindsay, S. S. McDade, A. Pickard, K. D. McCloskey, and D. J. McCance, "Role of δNp63γ in epithelial to mesenchymal transition," *Journal of Biological Chemistry*, vol. 286, no. 5, pp. 3915–3924, 2011.

16

Focal Adhesion Kinases in Adhesion Structures and Disease

Pierre P. Eleniste and Angela Bruzzaniti

Department of Oral Biology, Indiana University School of Dentistry, DS241, 1121 W. Michigan Street, Indianapolis, IN 46202, USA

Correspondence should be addressed to Angela Bruzzaniti, abruzzan@iupui.edu

Academic Editor: Donna Webb

Cell adhesion to the extracellular matrix (ECM) is essential for cell migration, proliferation, and embryonic development. Cells can contact the ECM through a wide range of matrix contact structures such as focal adhesions, podosomes, and invadopodia. Although they are different in structural design and basic function, they share common remodeling proteins such as integrins, talin, paxillin, and the tyrosine kinases FAK, Pyk2, and Src. In this paper, we compare and contrast the basic organization and role of focal adhesions, podosomes, and invadopodia in different cells. In addition, we discuss the role of the tyrosine kinases, FAK, Pyk2, and Src, which are critical for the function of the different adhesion structures. Finally, we discuss the essential role of these tyrosine kinases from the perspective of human diseases.

1. Introduction

The extracellular matrix (ECM) is an insoluble supra-structure comprised of a variety of matrix components including fibronectin, glycosaminoglycans, chrondronectin, osteonectin, collagens, laminin, proteoglycans, and growth factors [1–6]. The ECM provides the scaffold for cell attachment which is necessary for several diverse cellular activities, including cytoskeletal remodeling, polarization, differentiation, migration, and invasion [7–9]. Binding to the ECM is regulated by various signaling pathways that control the assembly and disassembly of three distinct, but functionally related actin and integrin-containing adhesion structures known as focal adhesions, podosomes, and invadopodia. In this review, we will discuss our current understanding of the similarities and differences between focal adhesions, podosomes, and invadopodia. We also will highlight several important tyrosine kinases and other signaling proteins that are known to control the formation and function of these adhesion structures, and we will discuss their role in pathophysiology.

2. Focal Adhesions

Focal adhesion formation and turnover has been used as a model system for understanding the mechanisms of cellular adhesion. Although focal adhesions, podosomes, and invadopodia share common signaling proteins, they are distinct in cellular architecture and function (summarized in Table 1). Focal adhesions, also known as "focal contacts," were identified over 30 years ago by electron microscopy and described as electron-dense plaques associated with actin filament bundles [10]. Focal adhesions can be considered to be large protein assembly complexes that spread mechanical forces from sites of cell adhesion to the cell body. In addition, focal adhesions regulate intracellular signaling pathways necessary for cell migration, growth, proliferation, embryogenesis, wound healing, and tissue repair [11–14]. Focal adhesions are comprised of a wide range of signaling proteins [15], such as the tyrosine kinases Pyk2 [16, 17], FAK [18, 19], Src [20, 21], Abl [22], and integrin-linked kinase [23]; the phosphatases PTP-PEST [24] and PTP1B [25]; the actin-binding proteins paxillin [26, 27], talin [23, 28–30], vinculin [23, 28–30] and tensin [31], the GTPases dynamin [32] and Cdc42/Rho [33, 34], as well as scaffolding proteins p130Cas [35] and Crk [27]. Many of these proteins have been shown to play predominantly a structural role or are involved in signal transduction [36].

Several protein kinases are recruited to focal adhesions upon cell attachment. These protein platforms recruit adaptor proteins and lead to the activation of complex network of signaling cascades that regulate basic cellular functions

Vinculin   Paxillin   Composite

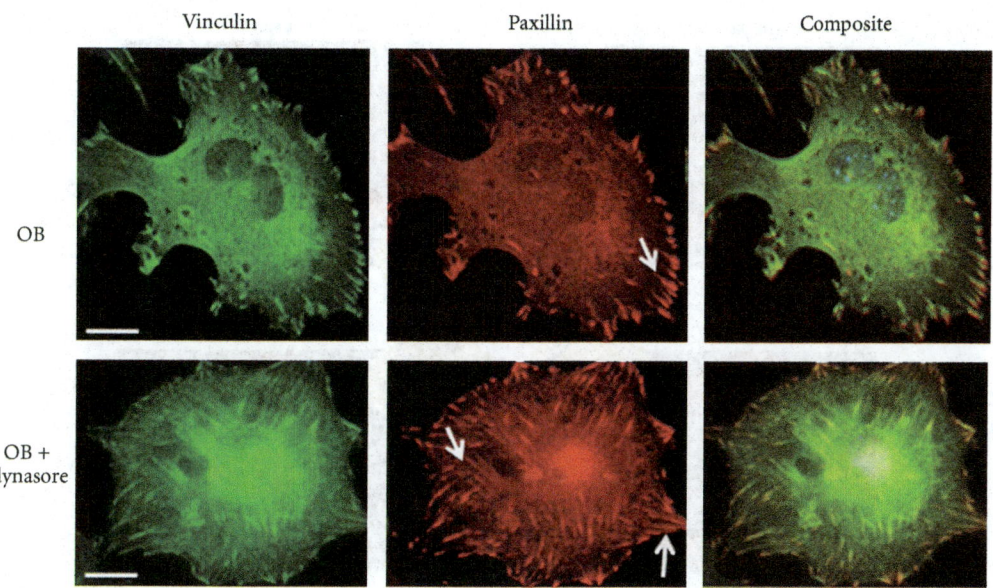

OB

OB +
dynasore

FIGURE 1: Inhibition of dynamin increases focal adhesions. Calvarial-derived osteoblasts (OBs) were treated with dynasore (90 μM) or vehicle for 1 hr and labeled for vinculin (green) or paxillin (red). Green and red channels were merged to form the composite image. Scale bar indicates 10 μm. Arrows show location of focal adhesions.

[16, 36]. An important tyrosine kinase found in focal adhesions is the focal adhesion kinase (FAK). FAK is a 125 kDa cytoplasmic tyrosine kinase that is activated upon integrin engagement and controls signaling pathways crucial for cell proliferation, migration, and survival [37]. The C-terminal domain of FAK is known as the focal adhesion targeting domain (FAT). As its name implies, the FAT domain is involved in directing FAK to focal adhesion complexes in a variety of cells [38]. In contrast, the N-terminal domain of FAK is known as the FERM domain (F for the 4.1 protein, Ezrin, Radixin, and Moesin). The central kinase domain of FAK, which itself is activated by phosphorylation, directs the phosphorylation of several signaling protein such as paxillin, Grb2 and p130Cas [39]. *In vitro* studies have shown that the FERM binds directly to the intracellular domain of the β1-integrin subunit and regulates FAK kinase activity [40]. It was also discovered that blocking β1-integrin function leads to FAK dephosphorylation, which in turn increases the sensitivity of malignant tumors to ionizing radiation and delays the growth of human head and neck squamous cell carcinoma cell lines [41].

FAK and the tyrosine kinase Src play a central regulatory role in focal adhesion turnover, and deletion of either of these kinases increases focal adhesion stability [42]. In addition, it has been shown that FAK and Src work in concert with the GTPase dynamin to regulate microtubule-induced focal adhesion disassembly [43]. In studies by Ezratty and colleagues, FAK−/− fibroblasts exhibited reduced dynamin accumulation around focal adhesions compared to controls [43], suggesting that FAK regulates dynamin localization and recruitment to focal adhesions. In addition, Wang and others demonstrated that Src phosphorylates dynamin at tyrosine residues, which promotes the translocation of dynamin to focal adhesions by FAK [32]. Disruption of the Src-FAK-dynamin complex blocked focal adhesion disassembly and

fibroblast migration [32]. Using bone-forming osteoblasts as our model system, we also found that dynamin is expressed in osteoblasts and inhibition of its GTPase activity with the chemical inhibitor dynasore, increased the number of vinculin and paxillin-positive focal adhesions in osteoblasts, compared to control cells (Figure 1). Interestingly, we found that dynamin is also localized to actin-rich podosomes, in bone-resorbing osteoclasts [44, 45]. Moreover, dynamin knockdown with shRNA or overexpression of a GTPase-inactive dynamin mutant increased podosome stability and the thickness of the podosome belt and decreased osteoclast bone resorbing activity [44]. Together, these studies reveal that dynamin's GTPase activity is necessary for both focal adhesion turnover in osteoblasts as well as podosome turnover in osteoclasts. Furthermore, these findings suggest potential similarities in the mechanism of turnover of focal adhesions and podosomes, which is likely to be dependent on the complement of signaling and scaffolding proteins present in different cell types.

3. Podosomes

Podosomes are highly dynamic adhesion structures found in a wide variety of migratory cells including macrophages, osteoclasts, endothelial cells [46–50], transformed fibroblasts [51], and carcinoma cell lines [52]. They were first identified in the 1980s in v-Src-transformed fibroblasts [53, 54]. Podosomes and focal adhesions are both cell-matrix adhesion sites, but they differ in their structural design and turnover rates [55–59] (Table 1) despite sharing a large number of common signaling proteins, such as FAK, dynamin, talin, paxillin, Wasp, and vinculin [60]. Podosomes turnover occurs very rapidly with an apparent half-life of 2–12 min and involves the polymerization

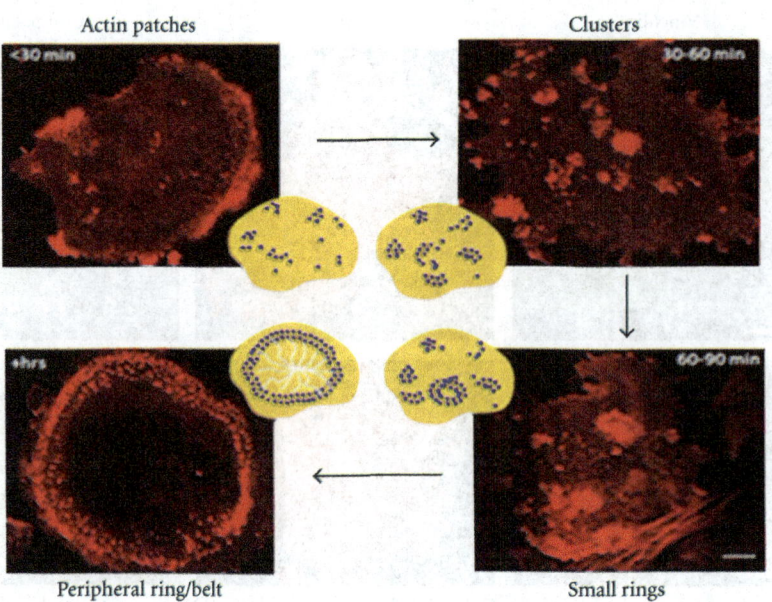

FIGURE 2: Dynamics of podosome organization in osteoclasts. Osteoclasts were generated from mouse bone marrow and plated on FBS-treated coverslips for various times. Cells were fixed and stained with rhodamine phalloidin. Actin patches are found soon after osteoclast attachment. Actin patches then reorganize into small rings and then into a peripheral podosome belt. The podosome belt is stabilized by the microtubule network. Scale bar is 10 μm.

TABLE 1: Common and unique features of focal adhesions, podosomes, and invadopodia. See text for details.

	Focal adhesion	Podosomes	Invadopodia
Appearance	dense plaques of F-actin	F-actin bundle core surrounded by actin cloud	F-actin bundle core surrounded by actin cloud
Size	width: 2–6 μm	width: 0.5–2 μm length: 0.5–2 μm	width: 0.5–2 μm length: >2 μm
Duration (half-life)	hours	minutes	hours
Cell expression	numerous nonmigrating fibroblastic cells	monocytic cells osteoclasts endothelial cells smooth muscle cells Src-transformed fibroblasts	carcinoma cells Src-transformed fibroblasts
Location	often found at leading edge of cell	ventral side of the cellular membrane	ventral side of the cellular membrane
Extracellular matrix degradation	no	yes	yes
Common signaling molecules	focal adhesion proteins GTPases actin regulators motor proteins tyrosine kinases phosphatases scaffolding molecules	focal adhesion proteins GTPases actin regulators motor proteins tyrosine kinases phosphatases scaffolding molecules	focal adhesion proteins GTPases actin regulators motor proteins tyrosine kinases phosphatases scaffolding molecules
Distinct Features	integrin receptors	Integrin receptors matrix-degrading enzymes	matrix-degrading enzymes

and depolymerization of the central F-actin core [50, 61]. Podosomes first appear as small actin dots which are then reorganized into small rings or rosettes with a diameter of 0.5–1 μm and a depth of 0.2–0.4 μm [62, 63] (Figure 2). The assembly of podosomes in macrophages and osteoclasts is dependent on an intact microtubule system [49, 64]. The central core of F-actin is surrounded

by a ring of molecules that are involved in adhesion, matrix degradation, or migration. These proteins include the tyrosine kinases Pyk2 and Src [13], actin-associated proteins [51, 65], integrins [66], and their associated proteins [50], intermediate filaments [47], motor proteins [67] and metalloproteases [50, 68]. In vitro studies demonstrated that RhoA, Rac1, and Cdc42 are also involved in the regulation of podosomes turnover [69, 70] and perhaps in recruiting podosomes to the leading edge of cells following microtubule-dependent cell polarization [64, 69, 71–73].

In contrast to focal adhesions, podosomes are found at sites of ECM degradation [51, 74]. The metalloproteases MT1-MMP and MMP-9 have been localized to podosomes, strongly supporting a role for podosomes in ECM degradation [56, 68, 75] in addition to adhesion [76]. This is well illustrated in osteoclasts, the primary bone-resorbing cells found in the body. In mature osteoclasts, podosomes are organized into a ring or belt-like structure at the cell periphery (referred to as the sealing zone) [50, 77]. This unique actin- and integrin-rich structure functions to dock osteoclasts to ECM proteins in bone and seals off the bone-resorbing compartment. This allows for the localized secretion of acidifying protons, chloride ions, and bone matrix-degrading metalloproteases [70].

In response to integrin engagement, and in the presence of intracellular calcium, Pyk2 is autophosphorylated at tyrosine residue Y402, which is essential for its catalytic activity [37, 78, 79] and for downstream signaling via p130Cas, Src, Cbl, integrins, gelsolin, and paxillin and the tyrosine phosphatase PTP-PEST [24, 80–82]. Pyk2 is expressed at high levels in the nervous system and in various hematopoietic cells [57, 83]. Pyk2 is expressed in osteoblasts [84, 85] and osteoclasts [45, 64]. Deletion of Pyk2 in osteoblasts affects differentiation, migration, and actin remodeling [84, 85]. In osteoclasts, Pyk2 is localized to the podosome belt and deletion of Pyk2 leads to a decrease in osteoclast bone resorption, which contributes to the osteopetrotic phenotype observed in Pyk2-deficient mice [64, 84]. Whereas deletion of Pyk2 in osteoblasts affects focal adhesion turnover (our unpublished findings), osteoclasts lacking Pyk2 exhibit structurally disorganized podosomes [64]. Src has also been shown to be indispensable for osteoclast function and is necessary for podosome assembly/disassembly [86, 87]. Osteoclasts lacking Src exhibit abnormal podosome rings, resulting in a dysfunctional sealing zone [88]. Leupaxin is a member of the focal adhesion-associated adaptor proteins and has been found to be associated with the podosome-belt (sealing zone) in osteoclasts [89, 90]. It was also demonstrated that leupaxin forms a signaling complex with Pyk2, c-Src, and PTP-PEST which regulates the migration of prostate cancer cells [91]. Finally, as discussed above, the GTPase dynamin regulates podosome assembly and dynamics in osteoclasts [44, 63, 92] in a process that involves Src [44]. These studies and others demonstrate that distinct signaling proteins work in concert to regulate podosome organization and turnover in osteoclasts, and perhaps in podosome-containing migratory cells.

The tyrosine kinase Pyk2 is a homolog of FAK and shares 45% overall sequence identity and 60% amino acid identity within the catalytic domain. Structurally, Pyk2 also contains an N-terminal FERM domain, a central catalytic core, several proline rich domains (PRDs), and a C-terminal FAT domain [64, 79, 93]. The FERM domain is involved in localizing Pyk2 to the plasma membrane and facilitates Pyk2 binding to phosphatidylinositol bisphosphate (PIP2)

[94, 95]. Although structural similarities exist between FAK and Pyk2, these proteins appear to exhibit unique effects on adhesion structures in different cells. Recently, it was reported that deletion of FAK in osteoclasts leads to the formation of peripheral podosome belt, whereas deletion of Pyk2 resulted in small podosome rings [96]. In addition, deletion of FAK but not Pyk2, in lung carcinoma CL1-5 cells resulted in decreased formation of podosomes rosettes [96]. These findings suggest that FAK and Pyk2 may regulate different patterning of podosome organization in osteoclasts [96]. Although the mechanism is unknown, the recruitment of downstream effector proteins is likely to be important in the differential roles of these kinases.

4. Invadopodia

Invadopodia appear as dynamic protrusions of the plasma membrane, containing a central actin core surrounded by adhesion proteins, signaling molecules, and scaffolding proteins [59]. In addition, invadopodia are sites of ECM degradation and are often observed in highly migratory metastatic cancer cells [57]. Invadopodia share, overlapping features with podosomes, especially with regards to their intracellular localization, composition of proteins, and cell types in which they are found [55, 59, 62, 97–99] (see Table 1). However, differences between invadopodia and podosomes do exist. In particular, podosomes are short lived (minutes) and found in phagocytic cells such as osteoclasts, whereas invadopdia persist for hours and found primarily in cancer cells [97, 100]. Like podosomes, invadopodia are regulated by a multitude of signaling proteins such as the Src-family kinases, protein kinase C [55, 101–104], cdc42, N-WASP, and Arp2/3 [105, 106]. Dynamin has also been shown to participate in focal extracellular matrix degradation by invasive cells [107]. Although integrin signaling in the initiation of podosome formation is well established, the role of integrins in invadopodia is not yet clear [108].

The life cycle of invadopodia involves initiation, extension, ECM degradation, and disassembly. Each of these steps involves F-actin remodeling and the activation/deactivation of signaling proteins around the central actin core. The initiation of invadopodia is known to be stimulated by EGF, PDGF and reactive oxygen species (ROS) [76]. Following initiation by EGF receptor activation, Src and the tyrosine kinase Abl (Abelson) are recruited and activated [102, 105, 109]. This results in an increase in actin polymerization and cortactin phosphorylation within the elongating invadopodium [102, 105, 109]. Microscopic imaging has shown that cortactin accumulates in invadopodia prior to F-actin nucleation [101], matrix metalloprotease accumulation, and matrix degradation [55], suggesting that cortactin isan early player in this process. In addition to the filamentous actin network, microtubules and intermediate filaments also participate in the elongation and extension of invadopodia [110], with the resulting structure resembling the arrangement of actin filaments in podosomes. The growing protrusive membrane is supplied by vesicular trafficking to sites of invadopodia extension and is controlled by the Golgi apparatus and by F-bar proteins such as CIP4 (cdc42 interacting protein) [107, 111] and the Ena/VASP family protein, Mena [112–114]. Membrane fusion and actin remodeling by dynamin have also been shown to be involved in invadopodia formation [115, 116]. Like podosomes, the formation and stabilization of invadopodia involves microtubule-dependent transport [108, 110]. The third step in the life cycle of invadopodia, and the major function of these structures, is ECM degradation. This function is shared with podosomes but is absent in focal adhesions. ECM degradation is facilitated by secretion of a variety of matrix metalloproteases and serine proteases [56, 112, 117, 118] and is thought to be regulated by cortactin, an actin regulating protein [55]. The secreted proteases act to degrade components of the ECM, thereby facilitating cellular migration and invasion [119, 120]. Finally, the disassembly of invadopodia involves depolymerization of the actin core [121] and has been shown to be regulated by ERK, paxillin, and the calcium-dependent cysteine protease, calpain, which degrades cortactin [121, 122].

The Src family kinases have been demonstrated to be critical for invadopodia formation and maturation. However, several lines of evidence support a role for Src in focal adhesion and podosome stability [123–125]. Similarly, as discussed above, FAK is important for focal adhesion turnover [126] but deletion of FAK has been also shown to increase invadopodia formation [6, 18] and suppress podosomes rosettes formation n fibroblasts [96]. Moreover, FAK has been shown to regulate a switch from phosphotyrosine-containing proteins at focal adhesions to invadopodia through the temporal regulation of active Src [6]. In the same study, it was shown that FAK-Src signaling also plays a significant role in cancer cell invasion [6, 116]. The apparent overlapping role of FAK and Src in different adhesion structures can be explained by the formation of dynamic proteins complexes between these molecules. For example, the major autophosphorylation site in FAK is Y397 (Y402 in Pyk2) which serves as an SH2-binding site, allowing Src to bind FAK (or Pyk2) [127]. The binding of Src leads to release of its own autoinhibitory catalytic domain, leading to the full activation of Src and to the activation of distinct downstream signaling cascades [128].

5. Adhesion Proteins and Human Disease

In the following section, and summarized in Table 2, we provide an overview of the role of key focal adhesion proteins and their potential link to human diseases.

5.1. Skeletal Disease. Bones provide structural rigidity to the skeleton and are constantly remodeled to maintain calcium and mineral homeostasis and repair skeletal damage. Bone architectural integrity relies in part on the rate of apoptosis of bone-forming osteoblasts. The activity of Pyk2 is also linked with a variety of metabolic conditions, including the regulation of bone mass. Deletion of Pyk2 leads to increased bone mass in mice [64, 84] due in part to defects in focal adhesion signaling in osteoblasts (our unpublished findings)

as well as changes in podosome dynamics in osteoclasts [14, 87]. Src is also important for osteoclast function [129]. Deletion of Src impairs osteoclast bone resorbing activity and mice lacking Src exhibit severe osteopetrosis and exhibit defects in tooth eruption [129]. Studies have shown that disruption of the interaction of α-actinin with integrins at focal adhesions increases osteoblast apoptosis, which shifts the balance in favor of osteoclast activity, resulting in bone loss [130].

5.2. Role in Cancer. As discussed above, invadopodia formation is tightly linked with cancer metastasis. For example, recently, it was demonstrated that the transcription factor Twist1, a central regulator of the epithelial mesenchymal transition, promotes invadopodia formation through upregulation of platelet-derived growth factor receptor expression and activity, which play significant role in human breast cancer metastasis [120]. Invadopodia formation and therefore cancer invasion also involves the adaptor proteins TKS4 and TKS5 (tyrosine kinase substrate 4 and 5) [131]. It was also found that TKS5 colocalizes to invadopodia in different human cancer cells and that decreased TKS5 expression leads to decreased podosome formation and to reduced tumor metastasis [132]. Thus, TKS4 and TKS5 could potentially be used as therapeutic targets for the treatment of certain types of cancer. Other studies have demonstrated that loss of function of the *Fgd1* gene, which encodes a GTP-exchange factor, was associated with a rare inherited human developmental disease called faciogenital dysplasia. Fgd1 mutations in humans cause skeletal and neurological effects. However, Fgd1 was also shown to be involved in invadopodia biogenesis and ECM degradation [133], and to be expressed in human prostate and breast cancer cells, suggesting it may also be critical for cancer progression and tumorigenesis.

Several independent studies have demonstrated a critical role for FAK in tumor progression and invasion. Elevated FAK phosphorylation has been observed in several cancers, including breast, colon, thyroid, prostate, oral, neck, and ovarian cancer [134, 135]. Deletion of FAK from tumor cells or breast cancer cells resulted in decreased tumor progression [136, 137], while in endothelial-specific tamoxifen-inducible FAK knockout mice, tumor growth and angiogenesis were reduced [138], indicating that FAK may be important for tumorigenesis. In addition, quantitative real-time PCR has shown an elevation of FAK expression in malignant gastrointestinal stromal tumors [139]. Increased FAK expression was also detected in esophageal squamous cell carcinomas and was associated with cell differentiation, tumor invasiveness, and lymph node metastasis [140]. Also, it was found that FAK was overexpressed in esophageal squamous cell carcinoma which have led to cell differentiation, tumor invasiveness, and lymph node metastasis [140]. *In vitro* evidence also demonstrates that Src-FAK signaling is associated with elevated tumor cell metastases, invadopodia formation, and promotes cell invasion [141, 142]. The Src family of tyrosine kinases are important for embryonic stem cell self-renewal and are key regulators of signal transduction in various cells, including cancer

TABLE 2: Signaling proteins and their link to adhesion structures and disease. [+]Humans mutations are associated with disease. Mutations in dynamin are linked to centronuclear myopathy and Charcot-Marie-Tooth neuropathy in humans. *Bone mass regulation is based on knockout mice studies. Other disease indications are predicted based on animal studies and *in vitro* studies. n/d: not determined. See text for details.

Adhesion protein	Cell type	Adhesion structure	Disease indication
FAK	osteoblasts	focal adhesions	regulation of bone density*
	osteoclasts	podosomes	regulation of bone density*
	endothelial cells	podosomes?	angiogenesis
	lung carcinoma cells	podosomes	cancer metastasis
	various cancer cells	invadopodia	cancer metastasis
Pyk2	osteoblasts	focal adhesions	regulation of bone density*
	osteoclasts	podosomes	regulation of bone density*
	endothelial cells	podosomes?	angiogenesis
	various cancer cells	invadopodia	cancer metastasis
Src	osteoblasts	focal adhesions	regulation of bone density*
	osteoclasts	podosomes	regulation of bone density*
	various cancer cells	invadopodia	cancer metastasis
Dynamin	fibroblasts	focal adhesions	n/d
	osteoblasts	focal adhesions	regulation of bone density*
	osteoclasts	podosomes	regulation of bone density*
	neurons	n/d	neuropathy[+]
Twist1	epithelial cells	invadopodia	cancer metastasis
TKS4/5	human cancer cells	invadopodia	cancer metastasis
Leupaxin	osteoclasts	podosomes	regulation of bone density*
	cancer cells	invadopodia	cancer metastasis
Fgd1	osteoblasts	focal adhesions?	skeletal abnormalities[+]
	cancer cells	invadopodia	prostate and breast cancer metastasis

cells [143, 144]. Collectively, these findings provide strong evidence that overexpression of FAK and other proteins localized to invadopodia are important for invadopodia formation and tumor metastasis. Although there is a strong correlation between the expression of FAK and Src in invadopodia and the potential link of these kinases in cancer progression and invasion, it is not yet clear if Src-FAK signaling specifically in invadopodia is critical role for tumor growth. Nevertheless, FAK may be a useful biomarker for cancer cell metastasis and inhibitors to FAK or Src may be useful to limit disease progression [145]. To this end, the FAK inhibitor PND-1186 was found to dramatically decrease FAK activity in breast carcinoma cells, resulting in tumor cell apoptosis [146].

Lung cancer is considered to be one of the leading causes of mortality among the malignant tumors worldwide. It has been reported that small cell lung cancers (SCLCs) constitute 15–25% of all newly diagnosed primary lung cancers [147]. In the same study, it was shown that inhibition of Pyk2 by lentiviral RNAi or Src using a chemical inhibitor (PP2) reduced SCLC survival and proliferation in liquid culture and in soft agar [147]. In addition, it was demonstrated that Pyk2 also plays an important role in human non-small cell lung cancer (NSCLC) [148]. This was based on the detection of higher levels of Pyk2, as determined by Western blotting and immunohistochemistry, in NSCLC biopsies compared to nontumors [148]. In other studies, FAK signaling was shown

to be important in the early stages of mammary adenocarcinoma lung metastasis [149]. It was further demonstrated that the dominant-negative FAK inhibitor, FRNK, blocked lung metastasis if added one day before tumor cell injection, but had no effect if given several days after tumor cell injection [149]. Furthermore, it was demonstrated that depletion of FAK, but not Pyk2, in lung carcinoma CL1-5 cells, decreased the formation of podosome rosette structures and decreased cell invasion [96]. Nevertheless, despite strong *in vitro* and *ex vivo* evidence linking FAK, Pyk2, and Src to various cancers, a direct link between kinase activity, effects on podosome/invadopodia formation, and cancer cell metastasis/function is currently lacking.

Several studies also suggest a link between the adhesion kinases and prostate cancer. For example, it has been shown that metastatic prostate cancer cells express elevated FAK mRNA levels and protein phosphorylation [150]. More recent studies also suggest that inhibition of Pyk2 and FAK may be an important therapeutic strategy to decrease prostate cancer progression [151]. Sun et al. used a mouse xenograft model injected with a chemical inhibitor of FAK and Pyk2 (PF-562,271) [151]. After two weeks of treatment with PF-562,271 (25 mg/kg), the mouse xenograft model showed a 62% decrease in tumor growth, compared to control mice [151]. Leupaxin was found to associate with Pyk2, c-Src, and PTP-PEST. *In vitro* studies also suggest that the migration of prostate cancer cells (PC-3) may be regulated by protein complexes involving leupaxin, Pyk2, and the tyrosine phosphatase PTP-PEST, which dephosphorylates Pyk2 [91, 152]. Furthermore, it was shown that invasion of PC3 cells in a gelatin matrix is controlled by invadopodia and ECM degradation [153].

Astrocytomas represent the most common intracranial neoplasms accounting for 60% of all primary brain tumors. In separate studies, FAK and Pyk2 expressions have been shown to elevated in human brain astrocytomas [154–156]. In addition, a novel kinase inhibitor of FAK (TAE226) has been shown to increase tumor cell apoptosis in brain tumors [157]. Finally, others have demonstrated that administration of Src family kinase inhibitors, PP1 and Dasatinib, results in a dramatic increase in apoptosis of several pediatric brain tumor cell lines, compared to control cell lines was observed [158]. Collectively, the above findings suggest that inhibition of Pyk2 and FAK and other signaling molecules impair tumor migration by blocking the biogenesis of invadopodia which are important for ECM degradation.

5.3. Pulmonary and Other Diseases. Pyk2 was identified as a central regulator for angiogenesis of pulmonary vascular endothelial cells [159]. Additional studies show that Pyk2 is essential in regulating airway inflammation, Th2 cytokine secretion, and airway hyper-responsiveness in ovalbumin-sensitized mice during antigen challenge *in vivo* [160]. Inhibition of Pyk2 blocked broncho-alveolar lavage, eosinophilia, mucous gland hyperplasia, and airway hyper-responsiveness, conditions that are also characteristic of the asthmatic state in humans. In addition, deletion of Pyk2 leads to developmental defects, abnormal macrophage activity, obesity, and insulin resistance under a high-fat diet [161, 162]. Pyk2 activity in the heart may also protect against arrhythmia [163]. Although the mechanism by which Pyk2 regulates these physiological processes is still unknown, therapeutic strategies that target Pyk2 might be a novel approach for the treatment of a variety of metabolic and pathological diseases. Finally, it has been shown that dynamin mutations are associated with human centronuclear myopathy and Charcot-Marie-Tooth neuropathy [164–166]. These diseases are currently attributed to defects in dynamin-mediated endocytosis. However, it is interest to note that dynamin plays an important role in actin remodeling, which is linked to its function in membrane endocytosis [115, 116]. Therefore, it is possible that dynamin's role in actin remodeling and adhesion structure turnover [43, 44, 63, 92, 107] may also be involved in these pathologies, although this remains to be determined.

6. Summary and Perspectives

In summary, focal adhesions, podosomes, and invadopodia facilitate adhesion to the matrix and cellular migration. In addition to adhesion, podosomes and invadopodia have evolved the unique function of ECM degradation. The focal adhesion kinases, FAK and Pyk2, exhibit overlapping and unique roles in the biogenesis, stability, and disassembly of these different adhesion structures. There is currently a growing body of evidence linking these and other kinases to the biogenesis of different adhesion structures. In addition, a great deal of studies suggests a link between the expression levels of these kinases and several human diseases, especially cancer (see Table 2). Finally, emerging evidence suggests that disrupting the activity of the adhesion kinases not only disrupts the formation of the adhesion structures, but it may also be useful in the treatment of serious medical conditions such as cancer and osteoporosis. A greater understanding of the function of adhesion kinases and the adhesion structures they control will offer future avenues for therapeutic interventions against several human diseases.

Abbreviations

ECM: Extracellular matrix
OC: Osteoclast
OB: Osteoblast
FAK: Focal adhesion kinase
SCLC: Small cell lung cancer
NSCLC: Nonsmall cell lung cancer.

References

[1] E. Hohenester and J. Engel, "Domain structure and organisation in extracellular matrix proteins," *Matrix Biology*, vol. 21, no. 2, pp. 115–128, 2002.

[2] R. O. Hynes, "The extracellular matrix: not just pretty fibrils," *Science*, vol. 326, no. 5957, pp. 1216–1219, 2009.

[3] P. D. Yurchenco and B. L. Patton, "Developmental and pathogenic mechanisms of basement membrane assembly," *Current Pharmaceutical Design*, vol. 15, no. 12, pp. 1277–1294, 2009.

[4] B. Geiger, A. Bershadsky, R. Pankov, and K. M. Yamada, "Transmembrane extracellular matrix-cytoskeleton crosstalk," *Nature Reviews Molecular Cell Biology*, vol. 2, no. 11, pp. 793–805, 2001.

[5] H. C. Slavkin, "Combinatorial process for extracellular matrix influences on gene expression: a hypothesis," *Journal of Craniofacial Genetics and Developmental Biology*, vol. 2, no. 2, pp. 179–189, 1982.

[6] K. T. Chan, C. L. Cortesio, and A. Huttenlocher, "Fak alters invadopodia and focal adhesion composition and dynamics to regulate breast cancer invasion," *The Journal of Cell Biology*, vol. 185, no. 2, pp. 357–370, 2009.

[7] E. D. Hay, "Extracellular matrix," *The Journal of Cell Biology*, vol. 91, no. 3, part 2, pp. 205s–223s, 1981.

[8] C. H. Damsky, "Extracellular matrix-integrin interactions in osteoblast function and tissue remodeling," *Bone*, vol. 25, no. 1, pp. 95–96, 1999.

[9] A. De Arcangelis and E. Georges-Labouesse, "Integrin and ECM functions: roles in vertebrate development," *Trends in Genetics*, vol. 16, no. 9, pp. 389–395, 2000.

[10] M. Abercrombie, J. E. M. Heaysman, and S. M. Pegrum, "The locomotion of fibroblasts in culture. IV. Electron microscopy of the leading lamella," *Experimental Cell Research*, vol. 67, no. 2, pp. 359–367, 1971.

[11] M. A. Wozniak, K. Modzelewska, L. Kwong, and P. J. Keely, "Focal adhesion regulation of cell behavior," *Biochimica et Biophysica Acta*, vol. 1692, no. 2-3, pp. 103–119, 2004.

[12] R. O. Hynes, "Integrins: versatility, modulation, and signaling in cell adhesion," *Cell*, vol. 69, no. 1, pp. 11–25, 1992.

[13] M. A. Schwartz, M. D. Schaller, and M. H. Ginsberg, "Integrins: emerging paradigms of signal transduction," *Annual Review of Cell and Developmental Biology*, vol. 11, pp. 549–599, 1995.

[14] L. H. Romer, K. G. Birukov, and J. G. N. Garcia, "Focal adhesions: paradigm for a signaling nexus," *Circulation Research*, vol. 98, no. 5, pp. 606–616, 2006.

[15] R. Zaidel-Bar, S. Itzkovitz, A. Ma'ayan, R. Iyengar, and B. Geiger, "Functional atlas of the integrin adhesome," *Nature Cell Biology*, vol. 9, no. 8, pp. 858–867, 2007.

[16] E. Zamir and B. Geiger, "Components of cell-matrix adhesions," *Journal of Cell Science*, vol. 114, no. 20, pp. 3577–3579, 2001.

[17] Q. S. Du, X. R. Ren, Y. Xie, Q. Wang, L. Mei, and W. C. Xiong, "Inhibition of PYK2-induced actin cytoskeleton reorganization, PYK2 autophosphorylation and focal adhesion targeting by FAK," *Journal of Cell Science*, vol. 114, no. 16, pp. 2977–2987, 2001.

[18] D. Ilic, Y. Furuta, S. Kanazawa et al., "Reduced cell motility and enhanced focal adhesion contact formation in cells from FAK-deficient mice," *Nature*, vol. 377, no. 6549, pp. 539–544, 1995.

[19] H. B. Wang, M. Dembo, S. K. Hanks, and Y. L. Wang, "Focal adhesion kinase is involved in mechanosensing during fibroblast migration," *Proceedings of the National Academy of Sciences of the United States of America*, vol. 98, no. 20, pp. 11295–11300, 2001.

[20] D. M. Suter and P. Forscher, "Transmission of growth cone traction force through apCAM-cytoskeletal linkages is regulated by Src family tyrosine kinase activity," *The Journal of Cell Biology*, vol. 155, no. 4, pp. 427–438, 2001.

[21] M. C. Frame, V. J. Fincham, N. O. Carragher, and J. A. Wyke, "v-Src's hold over actin and cell adhesions," *Nature Reviews Molecular Cell Biology*, vol. 3, no. 4, pp. 233–245, 2002.

[22] E. Zamir and B. Geiger, "Molecular complexity and dynamics of cell-matrix adhesions," *Journal of Cell Science*, vol. 114, no. 20, pp. 3583–3590, 2001.

[23] C. Grashoff, I. Thievessen, K. Lorenz, S. Ussar, and R. Fässler, "Integrin-linked kinase: integrin's mysterious partner," *Current Opinion in Cell Biology*, vol. 16, no. 5, pp. 565–571, 2004.

[24] A. Angers-Loustau, J. F. Côté, A. Charest et al., "Protein tyrosine phosphatase-PEST regulates focal adhesion disassembly, migration, and cytokinesis in fibroblasts," *The Journal of Cell Biology*, vol. 144, no. 5, pp. 1019–1031, 1999.

[25] A. Bourdeau, N. Dubé, and M. L. Tremblay, "Cytoplasmic protein tyrosine phosphatases, regulation and function: the roles of PTP1B and TC-PTP," *Current Opinion in Cell Biology*, vol. 17, no. 2, pp. 203–209, 2005.

[26] C. E. Turner, "Paxillin and focal adhesion signalling," *Nature Cell Biology*, vol. 2, no. 12, pp. E231–E236, 2000.

[27] H. Yano, H. Uchida, T. Iwasaki et al., "Paxillin α and Crk-associated substrate exert opposing effects on cell migration and contact inhibition of growth through tyrosine phosphorylation," *Proceedings of the National Academy of Sciences of the United States of America*, vol. 97, no. 16, pp. 9076–9081, 2000.

[28] K. A. DeMali, C. A. Barlow, and K. Burridge, "Recruitment of the Arp2/3 complex to vinculin: coupling membrane protrusion to matrix adhesion," *The Journal of Cell Biology*, vol. 159, no. 5, pp. 881–891, 2002.

[29] I. D. Campbell and M. H. Ginsberg, "The talin-tail interaction places integrin activation on FERM ground," *Trends in Biochemical Sciences*, vol. 29, no. 8, pp. 429–435, 2004.

[30] D. R. Critchley, "Genetic, biochemical and structural approaches to talin function," *Biochemical Society Transactions*, vol. 33, no. 6, pp. 1308–1312, 2005.

[31] S. H. Lo, "Tensin," *The International Journal of Biochemistry and Cell Biology*, vol. 36, no. 1, pp. 31–34, 2004.

[32] Y. Wang, H. Cao, J. Chen, and M. A. McNiven, "A direct interaction between the large GTPase dynamin-2 and FAK regulates focal adhesion dynamics in response to active Src," *Molecular Biology of the Cell*, vol. 22, no. 9, pp. 1529–1538, 2011.

[33] C. D. Nobes and A. Hall, "Rho, Rac, and Cdc42 GTPases regulate the assembly of multimolecular focal complexes associated with actin stress fibers, lamellipodia, and filopodia," *Cell*, vol. 81, no. 1, pp. 53–62, 1995.

[34] K. Burridge and K. Wennerberg, "Rho and Rac take center stage," *Cell*, vol. 116, no. 2, pp. 167–179, 2004.

[35] L. A. Cary, D. C. Han, T. R. Polte, S. K. Hanks, and J. L. Guan, "Identification of p130(Cas) as a mediator of focal adhesion kinase-promoted cell migration," *The Journal of Cell Biology*, vol. 140, no. 1, pp. 211–221, 1998.

[36] B. Geiger, J. P. Spatz, and A. D. Bershadsky, "Environmental sensing through focal adhesions," *Nature Reviews Molecular Cell Biology*, vol. 10, no. 1, pp. 21–33, 2009.

[37] S. K. Mitra, D. A. Hanson, and D. D. Schlaepfer, "Focal adhesion kinase: in command and control of cell motility," *Nature Reviews Molecular Cell Biology*, vol. 6, no. 1, pp. 56–68, 2005.

[38] J. D. Hildebrand, M. D. Schaller, and J. T. Parsons, "Identification of sequences required for the efficient localization of the focal adhesion kinase, pp125(FAK), to cellular focal adhesions," *The Journal of Cell Biology*, vol. 123, no. 4, pp. 993–1005, 1993.

[39] J. W. Thomas, M. A. Cooley, J. M. Broome et al., "The role of focal adhesion kinase binding in the regulation of tyrosine phosphorylation of paxillin," *The Journal of Biological Chemistry*, vol. 274, no. 51, pp. 36684–36692, 1999.

[40] M. D. Schaller, C. A. Otey, J. D. Hildebrand, and J. T. Parsons, "Focal adhesion kinase and paxillin bind to peptides mimicking β integrin cytoplasmic domains," *The Journal of Cell Biology*, vol. 130, no. 5, pp. 1181–1187, 1995.

[41] I. Eke, Y. Deuse, S. Hehlgans et al., "β(1) Integrin/FAK/cortactin signaling is essential for human head and neck cancer resistance to radiotherapy," *The Journal of Clinical Investigation*, vol. 122, no. 4, pp. 1529–1540, 2012.

[42] M. G. Yeo, M. A. Partridge, E. J. Ezratty, Q. Shen, G. G. Gundersen, and E. E. Marcantonio, "Src SH2 arginine 175 is required for cell motility: specific focal adhesion kinase targeting and focal adhesion assembly function," *Molecular and Cellular Biology*, vol. 26, no. 12, pp. 4399–4409, 2006.

[43] E. J. Ezratty, M. A. Partridge, and G. G. Gundersen, "Microtubule-induced focal adhesion disassembly is mediated by dynamin and focal adhesion kinase," *Nature Cell Biology*, vol. 7, no. 6, pp. 581–590, 2005.

[44] A. Bruzzaniti, L. Neff, A. Sanjay, W. C. Horne, P. De Camilli, and R. Baron, "Dynamin forms a Src kinase-sensitive complex with Cbl and regulates podosomes and osteoclast activity," *Molecular Biology of the Cell*, vol. 16, no. 7, pp. 3301–3313, 2005.

[45] A. Bruzzaniti, L. Neff, A. Sandoval, L. Du, W. C. Horne, and R. Baron, "Dynamin reduces Pyk2 Y402 phosphorylation and Src binding in osteoclasts," *Molecular and Cellular Biology*, vol. 29, no. 13, pp. 3644–3656, 2009.

[46] P. A. Amato, E. R. Unanue, and D. L. Taylor, "Distribution of actin in spreading macrophages: a comparative study on

living and fixed cells," *The Journal of Cell Biology*, vol. 96, no. 3, pp. 750–761, 1983.

[47] P. C. Marchisio, D. Cirillo, L. Naldini, M. V. Primavera, A. Teti, and A. Zambonin-Zallone, "Cell-substratum interaction of cultured avian osteoclasts is mediated by specific adhesion structures," *The Journal of Cell Biology*, vol. 99, no. 5, pp. 1696–1705, 1984.

[48] J. Wang, Y. Taba, J. Pang, G. Yin, C. Yan, and B. C. Berk, "GIT1 mediates vegf-induced podosome formation in endothelial cells. Critical role for PLCγ," *Arteriosclerosis, Thrombosis, and Vascular Biology*, vol. 29, no. 2, pp. 202–208, 2009.

[49] S. Linder, K. Hufner, U. Wintergerst, and M. Aefelbacher, "Microtubule-dependent formation of podosomal adhesion structures in primary human macrophages," *Journal of Cell Science*, vol. 113, no. 23, pp. 4165–4176, 2000.

[50] O. Destaing, F. Saltel, J. C. Géminard, P. Jurdic, and F. Bard, "Podosomes display actin turnover and dynamic self-organization in osteoclasts expressing actin-green fluorescent protein," *Molecular Biology of the Cell*, vol. 14, no. 2, pp. 407–416, 2003.

[51] K. Mizutani, H. Miki, H. He, H. Maruta, and T. Takenawa, "Essential role of neural Wiskott-Aldrich syndrome protein in podosome formation and degradation of extracellular matrix in Src-transformed fibroblasts," *Cancer Research*, vol. 62, no. 3, pp. 669–674, 2002.

[52] H. M. Kocher, J. Sandle, T. A. Mirza, N. F. Li, and I. R. Hart, "Ezrin interacts with cortactin to form podosomal rosettes in pancreatic cancer cells," *Gut*, vol. 58, no. 2, pp. 271–284, 2009.

[53] W. T. Chen, "Proteolytic activity of specialized surface protrusions formed at rosette contact sites of transformed cells," *Journal of Experimental Zoology*, vol. 251, no. 2, pp. 167–185, 1989.

[54] G. Tarone, D. Cirillo, and F. G. Giancotti, "Rous-sarcoma virus-transformed fibroblasts adhere primarily at discrete protrusions of the ventral membrane called podosomes," *Experimental Cell Research*, vol. 159, no. 1, pp. 141–157, 1985.

[55] V. V. Artym, Y. Zhang, F. Seillier-Moiseiwitsch, K. M. Yamada, and S. C. Mueller, "Dynamic interactions of cortactin and membrane type 1 matrix metalloproteinase at invadopodia: defining the stages of invadopodia formation and function," *Cancer Research*, vol. 66, no. 6, pp. 3034–3043, 2006.

[56] E. S. Clark, A. S. Whigham, W. G. Yarbrough, and A. M. Weaver, "Cortactin is an essential regulator of matrix metalloproteinase secretion and extracellular matrix degradation in invadopodia," *Cancer Research*, vol. 67, no. 9, pp. 4227–4235, 2007.

[57] S. Linder and P. Kopp, "Podosomes at a glance," *Journal of Cell Science*, vol. 118, no. 10, pp. 2079–2082, 2005.

[58] M. Gimona, R. Buccione, S. A. Courtneidge, and S. Linder, "Assembly and biological role of podosomes and invadopodia," *Current Opinion in Cell Biology*, vol. 20, no. 2, pp. 235–241, 2008.

[59] D. A. Murphy and S. A. Courtneidge, "The "ins" and "outs" of podosomes and invadopodia: characteristics, formation and function," *Nature Reviews Molecular Cell Biology*, vol. 12, no. 7, pp. 413–426, 2011.

[60] M. R. Block, C. Badowski, A. Millon-Fremillon et al., "Podosome-type adhesions and focal adhesions, so alike yet so different," *European Journal of Cell Biology*, vol. 87, no. 8-9, pp. 491–506, 2008.

[61] P. Jurdic, F. Saltel, A. Chabadel, and O. Destaing, "Podosome and sealing zone: specificity of the osteoclast model," *European Journal of Cell Biology*, vol. 85, no. 3-4, pp. 195–202, 2006.

[62] R. Buccione, J. D. Orth, and M. A. McNiven, "Foot and mouth: podosomes, invadopodia and circular dorsal ruffles," *Nature Reviews Molecular Cell Biology*, vol. 5, no. 8, pp. 647–657, 2004.

[63] M. A. McNiven, M. Baldassarre, and R. Buccione, "The role of dynamin in the assembly and function of podosomes and invadopodia," *Frontiers in Bioscience*, vol. 9, pp. 1944–1953, 2004.

[64] H. Gil-Henn, O. Destaing, N. A. Sims et al., "Defective microtubule-dependent podosome organization in osteo-clasts leads to increased bone density in Pyk2$^{-/-}$ mice," *The Journal of Cell Biology*, vol. 178, no. 6, pp. 1053–1064, 2007.

[65] Y. Furuta, D. Ilic, S. Kanazawa, N. Takeda, T. Yamamoto, and S. Aizawa, "Mesodermal defect in late phase of gastrulation by a targeted mutation of focal adhesion kinase, FAK," *Oncogene*, vol. 11, no. 10, pp. 1989–1995, 1995.

[66] M. Pfaff and P. Jurdic, "Podosomes in osteoclast-like cells: structural analysis and cooperative roles of paxillin, proline-rich tyrosine kinase 2 (Pyk2) and integrin $\alpha V\beta 3$," *Journal of Cell Science*, vol. 114, no. 15, pp. 2775–2786, 2001.

[67] V. Betapudi, "Myosin II motor proteins with different functions determine the fate of lamellipodia extension during cell spreading," *PLoS ONE*, vol. 5, no. 1, Article ID e8560, 2010.

[68] T. Sato, M. D. C. Ovejero, P. Hou et al., "Identification of the membrane-type matrix metalloproteinase MT1-MMP in osteoclasts," *Journal of Cell Science*, vol. 110, no. 5, pp. 589–596, 1997.

[69] S. Burns, A. J. Thrasher, M. P. Blundell, L. Machesky, and G. E. Jones, "Configuration of human dendritic cell cytoskeleton by Rho GTPases, the WAS protein, and differentiation," *Blood*, vol. 98, no. 4, pp. 1142–1149, 2001.

[70] C. Itzstein, F. P. Coxon, and M. J. Rogers, "The regulation of osteoclast function and bone resorption by small GTPases," *Small GTPases*, vol. 2, no. 3, pp. 117–130, 2011.

[71] S. F. G. van Helden and P. L. Hordijk, "Podosome regulation by Rho GTPases in myeloid cells," *European Journal of Cell Biology*, vol. 90, no. 2-3, pp. 189–197, 2011.

[72] S. Ory, H. Brazier, G. Pawlak, and A. Blangy, "Rho GTPases in osteoclasts: orchestrators of podosome arrangement," *European Journal of Cell Biology*, vol. 87, no. 8-9, pp. 469–477, 2008.

[73] G. Giannone, G. Jiang, D. H. Sutton, D. R. Critchley, and M. P. Sheetz, "Talin1 is critical for force-dependent reinforcement of initial integrin-cytoskeleton bonds but not tyrosine kinase activation," *The Journal of Cell Biology*, vol. 163, no. 2, pp. 409–419, 2003.

[74] V. V. Artym, K. M. Yamada, and S. C. Mueller, "ECM degradation assays for analyzing local cell invasion," *Methods in Molecular Biology*, vol. 522, pp. 211–219, 2009.

[75] J. M. Delaissé, M. T. Engsig, V. Everts et al., "Proteinases in bone resorption: obvious and less obvious roles," *Clinica Chimica Acta*, vol. 291, no. 2, pp. 223–234, 2000.

[76] S. Linder and M. Aepfelbacher, "Podosomes: adhesion hot-spots of invasive cells," *Trends in Cell Biology*, vol. 13, no. 7, pp. 376–385, 2003.

[77] S. Hu, E. Planus, D. Georgess et al., "Podosome rings generate forces that drive saltatory osteoclast migration," *Molecular Biology of the Cell*, vol. 22, no. 17, pp. 3120–3126, 2011.

[78] I. Dikic, G. Tokiwa, S. Lev, S. A. Courtneidge, and J. Schlessinger, "A role for Pyk2 and Src in linking G-protein-coupled receptors with MAP kinase activation," *Nature*, vol. 383, no. 6600, pp. 547–550, 1996.

[79] H. Avraham, S. Y. Park, K. Schinkmann, and S. Avraham, "RAFTK/Pyk2-mediated cellular signalling," *Cellular Signalling*, vol. 12, no. 3, pp. 123–133, 2000.

[80] D. Davidson and A. Veillette, "PTP-PEST, a scaffold protein tyrosine phosphatase, negatively regulates lymphocyte activation by targeting a unique set of substrates," *The EMBO Journal*, vol. 20, no. 13, pp. 3414–3426, 2001.

[81] Y. Shen, G. Schneider, J. F. Cloutier, A. Veillette, and M. D. Schaller, "Direct association of protein-tyrosine phosphatase PTP-PEST with paxillin," *The Journal of Biological Chemistry*, vol. 273, no. 11, pp. 6474–6481, 1998.

[82] C. E. Turner, "Paxillin interactions," *Journal of Cell Science*, vol. 113, no. 23, pp. 4139–4140, 2000.

[83] S. Avraham, R. London, Y. Fu et al., "Identification and characterization of a novel related adhesion focal tyrosine kinase (RAFTK) from megakaryocytes and brain," *The Journal of Biological Chemistry*, vol. 270, no. 46, pp. 27742–27751, 1995.

[84] L. Buckbinder, D. T. Crawford, H. Qi et al., "Proline-rich tyrosine kinase 2 regulates osteoprogenitor cells and bone formation, and offers an anabolic treatment approach for osteoporosis," *Proceedings of the National Academy of Sciences of the United States of America*, vol. 104, no. 25, pp. 10619–10624, 2007.

[85] M. A. Kacena, P. P. Eleniste, Y. H. Cheng et al., "Megakaryocytes regulate expression of Pyk2 isoforms and caspase-mediated cleavage of actin in osteoblasts," *The Journal of Biological Chemistry*, vol. 287, no. 21, pp. 17257–17268, 2012.

[86] L. T. Duong, P. T. Lakkakorpi, I. Nakamura, M. Machwate, R. M. Nagy, and G. A. Rodan, "PYK2 in osteoclasts is an adhesion kinase, localized in the sealing zone, activated by ligation of $\alpha(v)\beta3$ integrin, and phosphorylated by Src kinase," *Journal of Clinical Investigation*, vol. 102, no. 5, pp. 881–892, 1998.

[87] A. Sanjay, A. Houghton, L. Neff et al., "Cbl associates with Pyk2 and Src to regulate Src kinase activity, $\alpha v \beta3$ integrin-mediated signaling, cell adhesion, and osteoclast motility," *The Journal of Cell Biology*, vol. 152, no. 1, pp. 181–195, 2001.

[88] O. Destaing, A. Sanjay, C. Itzstein et al., "The tyrosine kinase activity of c-Src regulates actin dynamics and organization of podosomes in osteoclasts," *Molecular Biology of the Cell*, vol. 19, no. 1, pp. 394–404, 2008.

[89] A. Gupta, B. S. Lee, M. A. Khadeer et al., "Leupaxin is a critical adaptor protein in the adhesion zone of the osteoclast," *Journal of Bone and Mineral Research*, vol. 18, no. 4, pp. 669–685, 2003.

[90] S. N. Sahu, M. A. Khadeer, B. W. Robertson, S. M. Núñez, G. Bai, and A. Gupta, "Association of leupaxin with Src in osteoclasts," *American Journal of Physiology*, vol. 292, no. 1, pp. C581–C590, 2007.

[91] S. N. Sahu, S. Nunez, G. Bai, and A. Gupta, "Interaction of Pyk2 and PTP-PEST with leupaxin in prostate cancer cells," *American Journal of Physiology*, vol. 292, no. 6, pp. C2288–C2296, 2007.

[92] G. C. Ochoa, V. I. Slepnev, L. Neff et al., "A functional link between dynamin and the actin cytoskeleton at podosomes," *The Journal of Cell Biology*, vol. 150, no. 2, pp. 377–389, 2000.

[93] S. Han, A. Mistry, J. S. Chang et al., "Structural characterization of proline-rich tyrosine kinase 2 (PYK2) reveals a unique (DFG-out) conformation and enables inhibitor design," *The Journal of Biological Chemistry*, vol. 284, no. 19, pp. 13193–13201, 2009.

[94] A. H. Chishti, A. C. Kim, S. M. Marfatia et al., "The FERM domain: a unique module involved in the linkage of cytoplasmic proteins to the membrane," *Trends in Biochemical Sciences*, vol. 23, no. 8, pp. 281–282, 1998.

[95] K. Hamada, T. Shimizu, T. Matsui, S. Tsukita, S. Tsukita, and T. Hakoshima, "Structural basis of the membrane-targeting and unmasking mechanisms of the radixin FERM domain," *The EMBO Journal*, vol. 19, no. 17, pp. 4449–4462, 2000.

[96] Y. R. Pan, C. L. Chen, and H. C. Chen, "FAK is required for the assembly of podosome rosettes," *The Journal of Cell Biology*, vol. 195, no. 1, pp. 113–129, 2011.

[97] I. Ayala, M. Baldassarre, G. Caldieri, and R. Buccione, "Invadopodia: a guided tour," *European Journal of Cell Biology*, vol. 85, no. 3-4, pp. 159–164, 2006.

[98] S. Linder, "The matrix corroded: podosomes and invadopodia in extracellular matrix degradation," *Trends in Cell Biology*, vol. 17, no. 3, pp. 107–117, 2007.

[99] S. Linder, "Invadosomes at a glance," *Journal of Cell Science*, vol. 122, no. 17, pp. 3009–3013, 2009.

[100] M. Vicente-Manzanares and A. R. Horwitz, "Cell migration: an overview," *Methods in Molecular Biology*, vol. 769, pp. 1–24, 2011.

[101] I. Ayala, M. Baldassarre, G. Giacchetti et al., "Multiple regulatory inputs converge on cortactin to control invadopodia biogenesis and extracellular matrix degradation," *Journal of Cell Science*, vol. 121, no. 3, pp. 369–378, 2008.

[102] S. Tehrani, N. Tomasevic, S. Weed, R. Sakowicz, and J. A. Cooper, "Src phosphorylation of cortactin enhances actin assembly," *Proceedings of the National Academy of Sciences of the United States of America*, vol. 104, no. 29, pp. 11933–11938, 2007.

[103] M. Marzia, R. Chiusaroli, L. Neff et al., "Calpain is required for normal osteoclast function and is down-regulated by calcitonin," *The Journal of Biological Chemistry*, vol. 281, no. 14, pp. 9745–9754, 2006.

[104] S. S. Stylli, T. T. I. Stacey, A. M. Verhagen et al., "Nck adaptor proteins link Tks5 to invadopodia actin regulation and ECM degradation," *Journal of Cell Science*, vol. 122, no. 15, pp. 2727–2740, 2009.

[105] C. C. Mader, M. Oser, M. A. O. Magalhaes et al., "An EGFR-Src-Arg-cortactin pathway mediates functional maturation of invadopodia and breast cancer cell invasion," *Cancer Research*, vol. 71, no. 5, pp. 1730–1741, 2011.

[106] T. Uruno, J. Liu, P. Zhang et al., "Activation of Arp2/3 complex-mediated actin polymerization by cortactin," *Nature Cell Biology*, vol. 3, no. 3, pp. 259–266, 2001.

[107] M. Baldassarre, A. Pompeo, G. Beznoussenko et al., "Dynamin participates in focal extracellular matrix degradation by invasive cells," *Molecular Biology of the Cell*, vol. 14, no. 3, pp. 1074–1084, 2003.

[108] S. Linder, C. Wiesner, and M. Himmel, "Degrading devices: invadosomes in proteolytic cell invasion," *Annual Review of Cell and Developmental Biology*, vol. 27, pp. 185–211, 2011.

[109] F. Kimura, K. Iwaya, T. Kawaguchi et al., "Epidermal growth factor-dependent enhancement of invasiveness of squamous cell carcinoma of the breast," *Cancer Science*, vol. 101, no. 5, pp. 1133–1140, 2010.

[110] M. Schoumacher, R. D. Goldman, D. Louvard, and D. M. Vignjevic, "Actin, microtubules, and vimentin intermediate filaments cooperate for elongation of invadopodia," *The Journal of Cell Biology*, vol. 189, no. 3, pp. 541–556, 2010.

[111] C. S. Pichot, C. Arvanitis, S. M. Hartig et al., "Cdc42-interacting protein 4 promotes breast cancer cell invasion and formation of invadopodia through activation of N-WASp," *Cancer Research*, vol. 70, no. 21, pp. 8347–8356, 2010.

[112] R. Buccione, G. Caldieri, and I. Ayala, "Invadopodia: specialized tumor cell structures for the focal degradation of

the extracellular matrix," *Cancer and Metastasis Reviews*, vol. 28, no. 1-2, pp. 137–149, 2009.

[113] C. Albiges-Rizo, O. Destaing, B. Fourcade, E. Planus, and M. R. Block, "Actin machinery and mechanosensitivity in invadopodia, podosomes and focal adhesions," *Journal of Cell Science*, vol. 122, no. 17, pp. 3037–3049, 2009.

[114] U. Philippar, E. T. Roussos, M. Oser et al., "A Mena invasion isoform potentiates EGF-induced carcinoma cell invasion and metastasis," *Developmental Cell*, vol. 15, no. 6, pp. 813–828, 2008.

[115] D. A. Schafer, "Regulating actin dynamics at membranes: a focus on dynamin," *Traffic*, vol. 5, no. 7, pp. 463–469, 2004.

[116] G. Eitzen, "Actin remodeling to facilitate membrane fusion," *Biochimica et Biophysica Acta*, vol. 1641, no. 2-3, pp. 175–181, 2003.

[117] M. Egeblad and Z. Werb, "New functions for the matrix metalloproteinases in cancer progression," *Nature Reviews Cancer*, vol. 2, no. 3, pp. 161–174, 2002.

[118] M. Seiki, "Membrane-type 1 matrix metalloproteinase: a key enzyme for tumor invasion," *Cancer Letters*, vol. 194, no. 1, pp. 1–11, 2003.

[119] F. Saltel, T. Daubon, A. Juin, I. E. Ganuza, V. Veillat, and E. Génot, "Invadosomes: intriguing structures with promise," *European Journal of Cell Biology*, vol. 90, no. 2-3, pp. 100–107, 2011.

[120] M. A. Eckert and J. Yang, "Targeting invadopodia to block breast cancer metastasis," *Oncotarget*, vol. 2, no. 7, pp. 562–568, 2011.

[121] C. Badowski, G. Pawlak, A. Grichine et al., "Paxillin phosphorylation controls invadopodia/podosomes spatiotemporal organization," *Molecular Biology of the Cell*, vol. 19, no. 2, pp. 633–645, 2008.

[122] C. L. Cortesio, K. T. Chan, B. J. Perrin et al., "Calpain 2 and PTP1B function in a novel pathway with Src to regulate invadopodia dynamics and breast cancer cell invasion," *The Journal of Cell Biology*, vol. 180, no. 5, pp. 957–971, 2008.

[123] L. C. Kelley, A. G. Ammer, K. E. Hayes et al., "Oncogenic Src requires a wild-type counterpart to regulate invadopodia maturation," *Journal of Cell Science*, vol. 123, no. 22, pp. 3923–3932, 2010.

[124] L. Li, M. Okura, and A. Imamoto, "Focal adhesions require catalytic activity of Src family kinases to mediate integrin-matrix adhesion," *Molecular and Cellular Biology*, vol. 22, no. 4, pp. 1203–1217, 2002.

[125] S. Granot-Attas, C. Luxenburg, E. Finkelshtein, and A. Elson, "Protein tyrosine phosphatase epsilon regulates integrin-mediated podosome stability in osteoclasts by activating Src," *Molecular Biology of the Cell*, vol. 20, no. 20, pp. 4324–4334, 2009.

[126] D. J. Webb, K. Donais, L. A. Whitmore et al., "FAK-Src signalling through paxillin, ERK and MLCK regulates adhesion disassembly," *Nature Cell Biology*, vol. 6, no. 2, pp. 154–161, 2004.

[127] H. Sasaki, K. Nagura, M. Ishino, H. Tobioka, K. Kotani, and T. Sasaki, "Cloning and characterization of cell adhesion kinase β, a novel protein- tyrosine kinase of the focal adhesion kinase subfamily," *The Journal of Biological Chemistry*, vol. 270, no. 36, pp. 21206–21219, 1995.

[128] R. Baron, "Molecular mechanisms of bone resorption: therapeutic implications," *Revue du Rhumatisme (English Edition)*, vol. 63, no. 10, pp. 633–638, 1996.

[129] T. Miyazaki, A. Sanjay, L. Neff, S. Tanaka, W. C. Horne, and R. Baron, "Src kinase activity is essential for osteoclast

[130] J. W. Triplett and F. M. Pavalko, "Disruption of α-actinin-integrin interactions at focal adhesions renders osteoblasts susceptible to apoptosis," *American Journal of Physiology*, vol. 291, no. 5, pp. C909–C921, 2006.

[131] S. A. Courtneidge, "Cell migration and invasion in human disease: the Tks adaptor proteins," *Biochemical Society Transactions*, vol. 40, no. 1, pp. 129–132, 2012.

[132] B. Blouw, D. F. Seals, I. Pass, B. Diaz, and S. A. Courtneidge, "A role for the podosome/invadopodia scaffold protein Tks5 in tumor growth in vivo," *European Journal of Cell Biology*, vol. 87, no. 8-9, pp. 555–567, 2008.

[133] I. Ayala, G. Giacchetti, G. Caldieri et al., "Faciogenital dysplasia protein Fgd1 regulates invadopodia biogenesis and extracellular matrix degradation and is up-regulated in prostate and breast cancer," *Cancer Research*, vol. 69, no. 3, pp. 747–752, 2009.

[134] G. W. McLean, N. O. Carragher, E. Avizienyte, J. Evans, V. G. Brunton, and M. C. Frame, "The role of focal-adhesion kinase in cancer—a new therapeutic opportunity," *Nature Reviews Cancer*, vol. 5, no. 7, pp. 505–515, 2005.

[135] V. G. Brunton and M. C. Frame, "Src and focal adhesion kinase as therapeutic targets in cancer," *Current Opinion in Pharmacology*, vol. 8, no. 4, pp. 427–432, 2008.

[136] H. Lahlou, V. Sanguin-Gendreau, D. Zuo et al., "Mammary epithelial-specific disruption of the focal adhesion kinase blocks mammary tumor progression," *Proceedings of the National Academy of Sciences of the United States of America*, vol. 104, no. 51, pp. 20302–20307, 2007.

[137] M. Luo, H. Fan, T. Nagy et al., "Mammary epithelial-specific ablation of the focal adhesion kinase suppresses mammary tumorigenesis by affecting mammary cancer stem/progenitor cells," *Cancer Research*, vol. 69, no. 2, pp. 466–474, 2009.

[138] B. Tavora, S. Batista, L. E. Reynolds et al., "Endothelial FAK is required for tumour angiogenesis," *EMBO Molecular Medicine*, vol. 2, no. 12, pp. 516–528, 2010.

[139] N. Koon, R. Schneider-Stock, M. Sarlomo-Rikala et al., "Molecular targets for tumour progression in gastrointestinal stromal tumours," *Gut*, vol. 53, no. 2, pp. 235–240, 2004.

[140] T. Miyazaki, H. Kato, M. Nakajima et al., "FAK overexpression is correlated with tumour invasiveness and lymph node metastasis in oesophageal squamous cell carcinoma," *British Journal of Cancer*, vol. 89, no. 1, pp. 140–145, 2003.

[141] C. R. Hauck, D. A. Hsia, X. S. Puente, D. A. Cheresh, and D. D. Schlaepfer, "FRNK blocks v-Src-stimulated invasion and experimental metastases without effects on cell motility or growth," *The EMBO Journal*, vol. 21, no. 23, pp. 6289–6302, 2002.

[142] C. R. Hauck, D. A. Hsia, D. Ilic, and D. D. Schlaepfer, "v-Src SH3-enhanced interaction with focal adhesion kinase at β1 integrin-containing invadopodia promotes cell invasion," *The Journal of Biological Chemistry*, vol. 277, no. 15, pp. 12487–12490, 2002.

[143] C. Annerén, C. A. Cowan, and D. A. Melton, "The Src family of tyrosine kinases is important for embryonic stem cell self-renewal," *The Journal of Biological Chemistry*, vol. 279, no. 30, pp. 31590–31598, 2004.

[144] S. J. Parsons and J. T. Parsons, "Src family kinases, key regulators of signal transduction," *Oncogene*, vol. 23, no. 48, pp. 7906–7909, 2004.

[145] J. M. Su, L. Gui, Y. P. Zhou, and X. L. Zha, "Expression of focal adhesion kinase and α5 and β1 integrins in

carcinomas and its clinical significance," *World Journal of Gastroenterology*, vol. 8, no. 4, pp. 613–618, 2002.

[146] I. Tanjoni, C. Walsh, S. Uryu et al., "PND-1186 FAK inhibitor selectively promotes tumor cell apoptosis in three-dimensional environments," *Cancer Biology and Therapy*, vol. 9, no. 10, pp. 764–777, 2010.

[147] S. Roelle, R. Grosse, T. Buech, V. Chubanov, and T. Gudermann, "Essential role of Pyk2 and Src kinase activation in neuropeptide-induced proliferation of small cell lung cancer cells," *Oncogene*, vol. 27, no. 12, pp. 1737–1748, 2008.

[148] S. Zhang, X. Qiu, Y. Gu, and E. Wang, "Up-regulation of proline-rich tyrosine kinase 2 in non-small cell lung cancer," *Lung Cancer*, vol. 62, no. 3, pp. 295–301, 2008.

[149] M. J. van Nimwegen, S. Verkoeijen, L. van Buren, D. Burg, and B. van de Water, "Requirement for focal adhesion kinase in the early phase of mammary adenocarcinoma lung metastasis formation," *Cancer Research*, vol. 65, no. 11, pp. 4698–4706, 2005.

[150] L. Tremblay, W. Hauck, A. G. Aprikian, L. R. Begin, A. Chapdelaine, and S. Chevalier, "Focal adhesion kinase (pp125FAK) expression, activation and association with paxillin and p50CSK in human metastatic prostate carcinoma," *International Journal of Cancer*, vol. 68, no. 2, pp. 164–171, 1996.

[151] H. Sun, S. Pisle, E. R. Gardner, and W. D. Figg, "Bioluminescent imaging study: FAK inhibitor, PF-562,271, preclinical study in PC3M-luc-C6 local implant and metastasis xenograft models," *Cancer Biology and Therapy*, vol. 10, no. 1, pp. 38–43, 2010.

[152] P. P. Eleniste, L. Du, M. Shivanna, and A. Bruzzaniti, "Dynamin and PTP-PEST cooperatively regulate Pyk2 dephosphorylation in osteoclasts," *The International Journal of Biochemistry & Cell Biology*, vol. 44, no. 5, pp. 790–800, 2012.

[153] B. Desai, T. Ma, and M. A. Chellaiah, "Invadopodia and matrix degradation, a new property of prostate cancer cells during migration and invasion," *The Journal of Biological Chemistry*, vol. 283, no. 20, pp. 13856–13866, 2008.

[154] A. Gutenberg, W. Brück, M. Buchfelder, and H. C. Ludwig, "Expression of tyrosine kinases FAK and Pyk2 in 331 human astrocytomas," *Acta Neuropathologica*, vol. 108, no. 3, pp. 224–230, 2004.

[155] Z. Li, X. Yuan, Z. Wu, Z. Guo, P. Jiang, and Z. Wen, "Expressions of FAK and Pyk2 in human astrocytic tumors and their relationship with angiogenesis," *Chinese-German Journal of Clinical Oncology*, vol. 7, no. 11, pp. 658–660, 2008.

[156] T. P. Hecker, J. R. Grammer, G. Y. Gillespie, J. Stewart Jr., and C. L. Gladson, "Focal adhesion kinase enhances signaling through the Shc/extracellular signal-regulated kinase pathway in anaplastic astrocytoma tumor biopsy samples," *Cancer Research*, vol. 62, no. 9, pp. 2699–2707, 2002.

[157] Q. Shi, A. B. Hjelmeland, S. T. Keir et al., "A novel low-molecular weight inhibitor of focal adhesion kinase, TAE226, inhibits glioma growth," *Molecular Carcinogenesis*, vol. 46, no. 6, pp. 488–496, 2007.

[158] A. H. Sikkema, S. H. Diks, W. F. A. den Dunnen et al., "Kinome profiling in pediatric brain tumors as a new approach for target discovery," *Cancer Research*, vol. 69, no. 14, pp. 5987–5995, 2009.

[159] S. M. Weis, S. T. Lim, K. M. Lutu-Fuga et al., "Compensatory role for Pyk2 during angiogenesis in adult mice lacking endothelial cell FAK," *The Journal of Cell Biology*, vol. 181, no. 1, pp. 43–50, 2008.

[160] Y. Duan, J. Learoyd, A. Y. Meliton, B. S. Clay, A. R. Leff, and X. Zhu, "Inhibition of Pyk2 blocks airway inflammation and hyperresponsiveness in a mouse model of asthma," *American Journal of Respiratory Cell and Molecular Biology*, vol. 42, no. 4, pp. 491–497, 2010.

[161] Y. Yu, S. A. Ross, A. E. Halseth et al., "Role of PYK2 in the development of obesity and insulin resistance," *Biochemical and Biophysical Research Communications*, vol. 334, no. 4, pp. 1085–1091, 2005.

[162] M. Okigaki, C. Davis, M. Falascat et al., "Pyk2 regulates multiple signaling events crucial for macrophage morphology and migration," *Proceedings of the National Academy of Sciences of the United States of America*, vol. 100, no. 19, pp. 10740–10745, 2003.

[163] D. Lang, A. V. Glukhov, T. Efimova, and I. R. Efimov, "Role of Pyk2 in cardiac arrhythmogenesis," *American Journal of Physiology Heart and Circulatory Physiology*, vol. 301, no. 3, pp. H975–H983, 2011.

[164] G. M. Fabrizi, M. Ferrarini, T. Cavallaro et al., "Two novel mutations in dynamin-2 cause axonal Charcot-Marie-Tooth disease," *Neurology*, vol. 69, no. 3, pp. 291–295, 2007.

[165] J. Böhm, V. Biancalana, E. T. Dechene et al., "Mutation spectrum in the large GTPase dynamin 2, and genotype-phenotype correlation in autosomal dominant centronuclear myopathy," *Human Mutation*, vol. 33, no. 6, pp. 949–959, 2012.

[166] P. N. M. Sidiropoulos, M. Miehe, T. Bock et al., "Dynamin 2 mutations in Charcot-Marie-Tooth neuropathy highlight the importance of clathrin-mediated endocytosis in myelination," *Brain*, vol. 135, no. 5, pp. 1395–1411, 2012.

17

DNA Methylation, Histone Modifications, and Signal Transduction Pathways: A Close Relationship in Malignant Gliomas Pathophysiology

Raúl Alelú-Paz, Nadia Ashour, Ana González-Corpas, and Santiago Ropero

Department of Biochemistry and Molecular Biology, School of Medicine, University of Alcalá,
Carretera Madrid-Barcelona Km. 33.6, 28871 Madrid, Spain

Correspondence should be addressed to Santiago Ropero, santiago.ropero@uah.es

Academic Editor: Laura Cerchia

Gliomas are the most common type of primary brain tumor. Although tremendous progress has been achieved in the recent years in the diagnosis and treatment, its molecular etiology remains unknown. In this regard, epigenetics represents a new approach to study the mechanisms that control gene expression and function without changing the sequence of the genome. In the present paper we describe the main findings about the alterations of cell signaling pathways in the most aggressive glioma in the adult population, namely, glioblastoma, in which epigenetic mechanisms and the emerging role of cancer stem cell play a crucial function in the development of new biomarkers for its detection and prognosis and the corresponding development of new pharmacological strategies.

1. Introduction

The majority of Central Nervous System (CNS) tumors have a glial origin. From a clinical point of view, gliomas can be classified into four grades on the basis of its histology and prognosis, encompassing three different tissue types: astrocytomas (about 70%), oligodendrogliomas (10–30%), and ependymomas (less than 10%). In this clinical scale, glioblastoma (GBM) corresponds to grade IV astrocytoma and represents the most aggressive glioma in the adult population, with a median overall survival between 9 and 12 months after the diagnosis, characterized by rapid growth and diffuse invasiveness into the adjacent brain parenchyma.

2. Epigenetic Mechanisms in Normal Cells

Epigenetics can be defined as the study of mechanisms that control gene expression in a potentially heritable way [1]. In humans, the most widely studied epigenetic modification is the methylation of cytosine residues at the carbon 5 position (5 mC) within the CpG dinucleotides [2] mediated by DNA methyltransferases (DNMTs), a family of enzymes that catalyze the transfer of a methyl group from S-adenosyl methionine to the DNA. In mammals, there are three main DNMTs: DNMT1, DNMT3a, and DNMT3b. DNMT1 is the most abundant DNMT in the cell and is transcribed mostly during the S phase of the cell cycle [1]. Its activity is focused on the faithfully preservation of DNA methylation patterns, acting preferably on the hemimethylated DNA generated during semiconservative DNA replication. DNMT3a and-3b are thought to be responsible for establishing the pattern of methylation during embryonic development showing a high expression in embryonic stem cells and a downregulation in differentiated cells, although its function is not only restricted to the novo methylation; both contribute to the methylation of the sites missed by DNMT1 at the replication fork [3].

As we have already mentioned, DNA methylation occurs mainly at CpG dinucleotides, which are not randomly distributed throughout the human genome but are concentrated in regions called CpG islands, preferentially located at the promoter region of about 60% of human genes. These CpG island are usually unmethylated in normal tissues allowing gene expression when the appropriate transcription

DNA Methylation, Histone Modifications, and Signal Transduction Pathways: A Close Relationship in
Malignant Gliomas Pathophysiology

199

factors are present. Methylation of promoter CpG islands is associated with a closed chromatin structure and transcriptional silence of the associated genes. Although CpG islands are usually unmethylated in normal tissues, some physiological processes require DNA methylation, such as genomic imprinting, the inactivation of X chromosome in females, the regulation of germline-specific genes, and, finally, in the silencing of tissue-specific genes in cell types in which they should not be expressed [4–6]. Among other mechanisms, gene silencing is carried out by the recruitment of methyl-CpG-binding domain proteins (MBD) that leads the recruitment of histone-modifying and chromatin-remodeling complexes.

Despite of the DNA methylation has been described preferably at CpG islands, this epigenetic mechanism is not exclusive of these regions. CpG island shores and regions of lower CpG density close to CpG islands (~2 kb) are associated with transcriptional inactivation, focusing its activity in the regulation of tissue-specific gene expression. On the contrary, in gene bodies this epigenetic mechanism is common in ubiquitously expressed genes and is positively correlated with gene expression involved in elongation efficiency and prevention of spurious initiations of transcription [1]. Finally DNA methylation is present in repetitive elements in order to protect chromosomal integrity preventing the reactivation of endoparasitic sequences.

Histone modifications are the other major epigenetic modification, which consist in dynamic and reversible post-translational modifications of the residues at N-terminal tails of histones that are mediated by sets of enzymatic complexes that site-specifically attach or remove the corresponding chemical groups [7]. The core histones H2A, H2B, H3, and H4 group into two H2.A-H2.B dimers and one H3-H4 tetramer to form the nucleosome that is the basic unit of the chromatin. Around the histone octamer, a 147-bp segment of DNA wrapped in 1.65 turns and neighboring nucleosomes are separated by, on average, ~50 bp of free DNA [1].

The histone modifications described so far include acetylation, methylation, phosphorylation, ubiquitination, SUMOylation, and ADP-ribosylation, having a main role in important cellular processes such as DNA repair, DNA replication, alternative splicing, and chromosome condensation. In regard to gene expression regulation, histone modifications have been associated with both transcriptional repression and activation. Histone acetylation results from the balance of the activities of HATs (histone acetyltransferases) and HDACs (histone deacetylases) and in general is associated with a less-condensed chromatin state and transcriptionally active gene status [8], while histone deacetylation increases ionic interactions between the positively charged histones and negatively charged DNA, which yields a more compact chromatin structure and represses gene transcription by limiting the accessibility of the transcription machinery. Histone acetylation also plays an important role in regulation of DNA replication and DNA repair [9]. Histone methylation is regulated by histone methyltransferases (HMTs) and is both associated with transcriptional activation and repression, so gene expression is associated with high levels of trimethylated H3K4, H3K36, and H3K79 and, on the

contrary, transcriptional repression is characterized by high levels of H3K9, H3K27, and H4K20 methylation.

These epigenetic modifications do not work alone; histones can be modified at different sites simultaneously, giving rise the cross-talk among the different histone marks. Thus, combination of all these marks in a nucleosome or region together with the DNA methylation pattern specifies chromatin structure and so transcriptional activity.

3. Epigenetics in the Human Central Nervous System

Dynamic relationships between epigenetic marks described in the previous section reach the higher levels of complexity in the CNS. The brain develops in a well-programmed order, which begins as a sheet of neural stem cells that lead to the formation of neurons at the embryonic stage and the appearance of glial cells at a later embryonic stage and postnatal period [10]. In both populations, epigenetic marks determine the potential of gene transcriptional activity.

Although the epigenetic mechanisms that regulate the gene expression in the CNS are the same as other organs, the human brain is a complex structure that made it necessary the introduction of new variables in its study, that is, an epigenetic connection to brain anatomy. In this regard, it has been described different epigenetic signatures depending on the brain area analyzed [11], so the DNA methylation patterns vary from one region to another, between cell types and, even, among its different subpopulations (i.e., astrocytes and oligodendrocytes). Moreover, the analysis of the DNA methylation in the human brain could not be restricted to the promoter region of the gene; a recent study suggest the necessity to look beyond promoters, specifically to the intragenic regions and its effects on the gene regulation processes in each cell types and brain regions [12].

Finally, it is important to highlight the role of 5-hydroxymethylcytosine (5 hmC) in the DNA methylation-related plasticity in the human brain. This epigenetic mark derives from an enzymatical modification of 5 mC by Tet family proteins through Fe(II) α-KG-dependent hydroxylation [13]. The levels of 5 hmC in the CNS are higher in comparison with other tissues and approximately tenfold greater than those seen in embryonic stem cells [14]; although little is know about the function of this new epigenetic mark, it has been suggested that it plays a critical role in postnatal neurodevelopment and aging, as well as in different human neurological disorders [12].

4. The Epigenetics of Malignant Gliomas

The signaling network in cancer follows a pattern of stochastic and complex interactions responsible for different processes that form its pathophysiology. These processes involve genetic and epigenetic changes that disturb the normal function of signal transduction pathways regulating cellular processes such as cell proliferation, adhesion, migration, and differentiation. In recent years, a great number of DNA methylation markers have been identified in cancer through the use of the target candidate gene and whole genome approaches, providing a valuable information about the etiology of cancer, and enabling us to the development of new strategies for assessing cancer risk status, detecting tumors as early as possible, monitoring prognosis, and instituting more accurate tumor staging, along with the monitoring of prevention strategies. Four major cancer clinical areas could benefit from DNA methylation markers: cancer detection, tumor behavior, prediction of response to treatment, and therapies that target methylated tumor suppressor genes.

As other types of tumorigenesis, malignant gliomas involve both activation of oncogenes and inactivation of tumor suppressor genes [15]. In this regard, it has been described different genetic alterations related with GBM involved in several processes as control of cell cycle, growth, apoptosis, invasion, and neovascularization. Although tremendous progress has been achieved in the understanding of the molecular mechanisms involved in the genesis and progression of GBM, its epigenetics regulation remains unclear. Keeping in mind that distinct epigenetic signatures has been associated with different GBM subsets, in this paper we will focus on the epigenetic modifications of those genes that have been traditionally related with the pathophysiology of the disease.

5. DNA Hypomethylation in GBM

There are two major DNA methylation phenomena associated with cancer development: hypomethylation and hypermethylation. DNA hypomethylation has been reported mainly in repetitive sequences such as satellite sequences and pericentromeric regions, producing genomic instability and reactivation of transposable elements, events that have been related to the development of several cancers including GBM. Moreover, in a study using a multistage skin cancer progression model, the authors found that DNA hypomethylation is an early event in tumor development, and a biomarker of tumor aggressiveness [16]. In particular, DNA global hypomethylation has been described to occur at high frequency (85%) in primary GBM (Figure 1).

This phenomenon also affects single-copy loci promoting the expression of cancer-related genes such as the melanoma antigen gene (MAGE1), that belongs to a group of germline specific genes that become transcriptionally activated in multiple tumors including GBM and low-grade astrocytoma. In these tumors types, MAGE1 expression has been related with DNA hypomethylation.

The signal transduction pathway regulated by insulin-like growth factor 2 (IGF2) is also dysregulated by DNA hypomethylation. IGF2 gain of function by loss of imprinting is a common event in several tumor types including GBM. IGF2 promotes cellular growth through the insulin-like growth factor receptor 1 and phosphoinositide-3-kinase regulating subunit 3 (PIK3R3). In particular, IGF2-PIK3R3 signaling pathway promote the growth of a subclass of highly aggressive GBM that lack epidermal growth factor receptor (EGFR) amplification [17].

6. Promoter Hypermethylation and Signal-Transduction Pathways in GBM

Until now, the driving force of DNA methylation research in cancer has been focused on CpG island hypermethylation. In cancer, numerous genes have been identified that have undergone CpG island hypermethylation. These genes include most of the well-established tumor suppressor genes that regulate almost all cellular functions, such as cell cycle ($p16^{INK4}$, $p15^{INK4b}$, RB, and $p14^{ARF}$), DNA repair (BRCA1, hMLH1, MGMT, and WRN), cell-adherence and invasion (CDH1, CDH13, EXT1, SLIT2, and EMP3), apoptosis (DAPK, TMS1, and SFRP1), carcinogen-metabolism (GSTP1), hormonal response (RARB2, ER, PRL, and TSH receptors), and Ras signaling (RASSF1A and NOREIA), microRNAs [18].

In glioma cells, however, gene silencing by DNA hypermethylation can occur at genes that are not expressed in the brain, indicating that not all instances of CpG island hypermethylation are functionally relevant for tumor development and progression. With this consideration, a number of signal-transduction pathways have been found dysregulated by DNA methylation changes in gliomas (Figure 1). For example, promoter hypermethylation of $p16^{INK4}$, $p14^{ARF}$, RB, PTEN and p53 affects the function of RB, PI3K and p53 signaling pathways.

The signaling $p16^{INK4}$/RB pathway is considered one of the most frequently altered in GBM [19]. RB is considered as a tumor suppressor gene since functions as inhibitor of cell cycle progression. The RB gene product, pRB, has a key role during G1 phase of the cell cycle by binding to the E2F family of transcription factors and generally repressing the target genes by epigenetic mechanism, through the recruitment of corepressor complexes that regulate chromatin structure and function. pRb phosphorylation by mitogen-activated cyclin-dependent kinases (CDKs) impairs the binding to E2F transcription factors and culminate in cell cycle deregulation. pRb also acts in the cell cycle through the inhibition the S phase progression by attenuating cyclin A/Cdk2 activity, resulting in disruption of PCNA function and DNA replication. RB gene promoter hypermethylation is the major mechanism underlying loss of RB expression in GBM, and this is an early event in tumor progression since RB hypermethylation is more frequent in secondary GBM [20]. $p16^{ink4}$ is located on chromosome 9p21, a region that shows frequent loss of heterozygosity in II–IV gliomas but not in low-grade gliomas. This gene acts as a tumor suppressor gene through its product, $p16^{ink4}$, that binds to $CDK4^2$ and CDK6 to prevent their interaction with cyclin D, keeping RB unphosphorylated and avoiding the cell cycle progression. $p16^{ink4}$ gene silencing by promoter hypermethylation is also found in gliomas [21].

The cellular signaling regulated by $p14^{ARF}$/p53 is also deregulated by epigenetic mechanism in cancer. p53 is a tumor suppressor gene involved in the control of the cell cycle and apoptosis, whose mutation has been described in several neoplasms including GBM. Although the main gene inactivation mechanism for p53 is through the mutation plus deletion of this gene, its reduced expression has also

DNA Methylation, Histone Modifications, and Signal Transduction Pathways: A Close Relationship in
Malignant Gliomas Pathophysiology

201

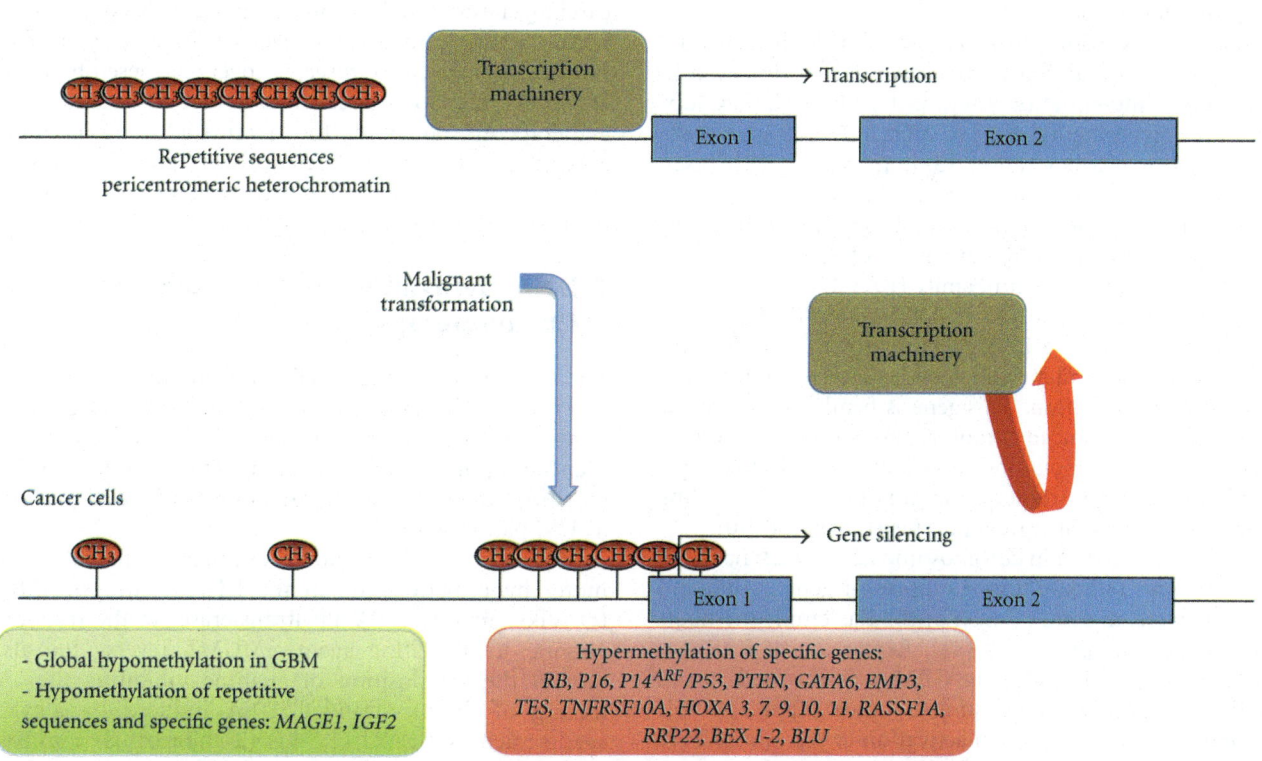

FIGURE 1: Summary of the changes in the DNA methylation at the repetitive sequences and CpG island associated with GBM.

been associated with hypermethylation of its promoter region, whereas the inactivation of $p14^{ARF}$, a stabilizer of $p53$, is mostly associated with DNA methylation rather than mutational activity [22]. The loss of $p53$ function by DNA hypermethylation of itself or $p14^{ARF}$ produces the loss of cellular response to DNA damage or oncogenic transformation that is mediated by $p14^{ARF}/p53$ signaling pathway.

Other important signal-transduction pathway dysregulated by epigenetic mechanisms is the PI3K/Akt pathway, in which *PTEN* has a main role. The *PTEN* suppressor gene is located at 10q23.3 and encodes a protein with homology to the catalytic domain of tyrosine phosphatases. Its mutations are frequent in primary GBM, and the methylation of its promoter region has been described in different human neoplasms, including GBM [23]. PTEN dephosphorylates phosphatidylinositol (3,4,5)-triphosphate (PtdIns-3,4,5-P3 or PIP-3), an intracellular second messenger related to the activation of Akt pathway. Since AKT pathway is involved in cell growth, cell differentiation and survival, the loss of *PTEN* function by promoter hypermethylation results in increased cell proliferation, cell survival, and tumor invasion [23].

Other genes silenced by promoter hypermethylation and regulating important pathways in cellular homeostasis maintenance have been involved in the processes that underlie the pathophysiology of the GBM (Figure 1). Those genes include *GATA6, EMP3, TES, TNFRSF10A, HOXA, RASSF1A, RRP22, BEX1, BEX2,* and *BLU. GATA6* is one of the six

members of the *GATA* family of transcription factors, which interact with a canonical DNA motif through two highly conserved zinc finger DNA-binding domains [24] with a tissue-specific expression regulating cell-restricted programs of gene expression [25]. Methylation of the *GATA6* has been involved in different cancer types, as lung and ovarian cancer and, in GBM, is considered as a tumor suppressor gene associated with the formation of the tumor [24].

Epithelial membrane protein 3 (*EMP3*) is a myelin-related gene associated with cell-cell interactions and cell proliferation. *EMP3* promoter has been found hypermethylated and, so, silenced in primary gliomas and neuroblastoma, showing similar features than a tumor suppressor gene [26–29].

TES encodes a Sertoli cell secretory protein that contains three LIM domains (double zinc-finger motifs) and mediate protein-protein interactions between transcription factors, cytoskeletal and signaling proteins. It is involved in different processes as cell growth, cell adhesion, and cell spreading acting as a tumor suppressor. Hypermethylation of *TES* in GBM has been described both by pharmacological inhibition of DNA coupled with gene expression microarray profiles and in a microarray-based DNA methylation study [25, 30].

TNFRSF10A encodes a protein member of the TNF-receptor superfamily activated by tumor necrosis factor-related apoptosis inducing ligand (TNFSF10/TRAIL), transducing cell death signal, and inducing cell apoptosis. *TNFRSF10A* gene silencing by promoter hypermethylation has been related with osteosarcomas [31], gastric carcinoma [32], and GBM, where it presents a hypermethylation pattern in its promoter region [25, 33].

HOXA genes belong to *HOX* gene family that encodes homeodomain-containing transcription factors involved in cell growth, differentiation [34], and embryonic development [35]. Hypermethylation of *HOXA 11* has previously been found in ovarian cancer [36]. In regard with brain cancer, hypermethylation of this gene plus *HOXA 3, 7, 9,* and *10* has been related with GBM, establishing two of them (9 and 10) as biomarkers for the prognosis of the disease [37].

Ras-Association Domain Family (RASSF) comprises ten members termed RASSF1 to RASSF10. *RASSF1A* encodes a protein similar to the RAS effector proteins required for death receptor-dependent apoptosis, cell-cycle control, and microtubule stabilization. This gene is firmly established as an epigenetically silenced tumor suppressor gene in a wide variety of cancers, including GBM, due to selective CpG methylation of the promoter upstream of the exon encoding the unique N-terminal segment of the isoform [38–40].

Ras-related protein in chromosome 22 (*RRP22*) has been suggested as a candidate tumor suppressor gene in different human cancers, in spite of most of the Ras family members possess oncogenic properties [41]. Expression of *RRP22* is restricted to the CNS [42]; in GBM it is involved in cell growth and apoptosis, suggesting a tumor suppressor role although its relevance and inactivation mechanisms have not been fully assessed so far [41]. A recent study suggests that mRNA *RRP22* levels are decreased in GBM due to the methylation of its promoter region [41].

BEX 1 and BEX 2 aremembers of the brain expressed X-linked gene family which have 91% sequence similarity which each other. *BEX 1* encodes a signaling adapter molecule involved in p75NTR/NGFR signaling, playing an important role in cell cycle progression and in the inhibition of neuronal differentiation in response to nerve growth factor. *BEX 2* regulates mitochondrial apoptosis and G1 cell cycle in breast cancer. Both are considered as tumor suppressor genes silenced by methylation of its promoter region in GBM [43].

Finally, hypermethylation of *BLU* gene promoter has been described both for glioma cell lines and astrocytomas [44]. This gene is located immediately centromeric to *RASSF1* locus and contains a predicted MYND domain at its C-terminus essential to the function of many transcription regulatory proteins involved in important transcriptional regulation pathways [44]. In GBM, it has been proposed that *BLU* acts as a tumor suppressor gene in which its hypermethylation together with an unmethylated *CASP8* is associated with prolonged time to tumor progression [45].

Epigenetic changes and in particular DNA methylation are, therefore, as etiologically relevant as the sequences changes that occur via genetic alterations such as point mutations and translocations. Since there is a delicate profile of CpG islands hypermethylation in human tumors, the detection of hypermethylated CpG islands may offer one of the most promising approaches for assessing cancer risk status, to achieve the earliest tumor detection and monitoring prognosis, and to institute more accurate tumor stating,

along with the monitoring of prevention strategies. DNA methylation changes have been reported to occur early in the carcinogenesis and, therefore, are potentially good indicators both of existing disease, and even of risk assessment for the future development of disease. Together, these observations encourage us to consider the use of DNA methylation as a therapeutic target for the treatment of cancer. In fact, azacitidine is the first DNA methyltransferase inhibitor to be approved by the US Food and Drug Administration for the treatment of myelodysplastic syndromes.

7. DNA Methylation and Resistance to Chemotherapy

The sensitivity of cancer cells to chemotherapy and radiotherapy can be also affected by the epigenetic silencing of different genes. In particular, the reactivation of the silenced suppressor of cytokine signaling I (*SOCS1*) in GBM sensitized these tumors to radiation via inactivation of the *MAPK* pathway [46].

However, the best-known example is the role of promoter hypermethylation of the DNA-repair gene *MGMT* (O^6-alkylguanine-DNA alkyltransferase) in the response of gliomas to alkylating agents. *MGMT* reverse the alkylation at the O^6 position of guanine inhibiting the cross-linking of double-stranded DNA induced by alkylating agents such as BCNU (1,3-bis (2-chloroethyl)-1-nitrosourea), ACNU (1-(4-amino-2-methyl-5-pyrimidinyl) methyl-3-(2-chloroethyl)-3-nitrosourea), procarbazine (N-methylhydrazine), and temozolomide (TMZ, SCHS2.365) [47, 48]. MGMT mRNA expression varies among different types of gliomas, lacking in approximately 30% of them. This loss of expression is due to *MGMT* promoter hypermethylation [49]. The loss of MGMT expression and function by DNA methylation increases the DNA damage induced by alkylating agents. Thus, *MGMT* methylation increases the sensitivity of GBM patients to alkylating drugs treatment, increasing the overall survival and the time to progression of disease [50]. Interestingly, *MGMT* was found hypermethylated in all long-term survivors (LTS) GBM patients, defined as those patients with a median survival time of more than 3 years [51], proving the study of this gene as a clinically relevant predictor of response to treatment in glioma patients [52]. These results are limited to the adult population in view of the fact that it has been reported the incidence of methylation of *MGMT* promoter in pediatric GBM is rare, losing the prognosis value in this population [53].

8. Histone Modifications in GBM

As we have described in a previous section, in addition to DNA promoter hypermethylation, histone modifications are key players in gene expression regulation network. For example, silenced CpG island promoters are characterized by the lost of H3K9 acetylation together with H3K9 methylation. Thus, changes in the histone modifications patterns play a key role in gene expression dysregulation and so in cancer development. The loss of acetylated Lys16 and trimethylated Lys20 of histone H4 is a common event in

DNA Methylation, Histone Modifications, and Signal Transduction Pathways: A Close Relationship in
Malignant Gliomas Pathophysiology

203

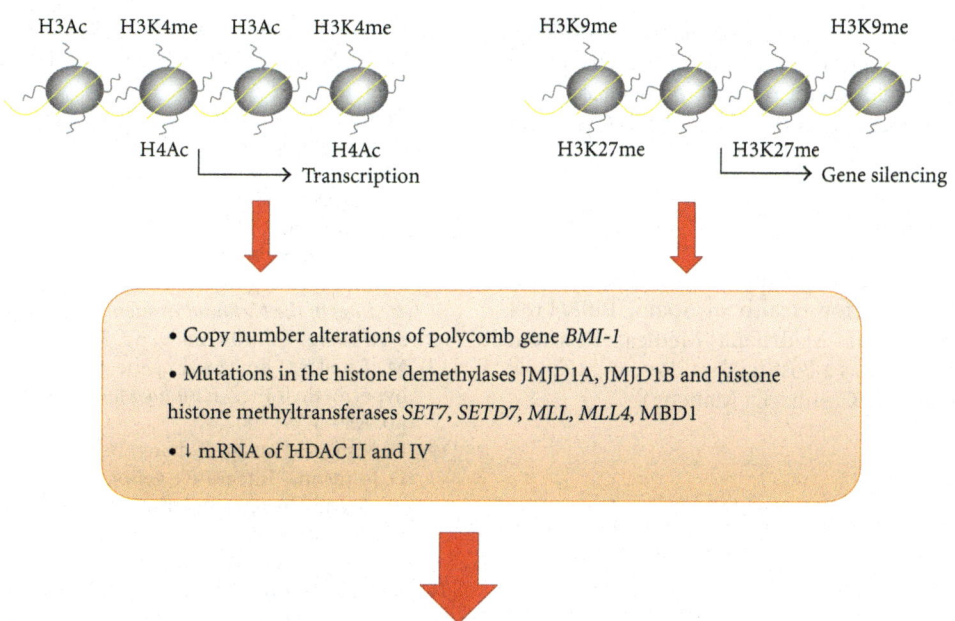

FIGURE 2: Summary of the alterations in the histone modifiers genes associated with gene expression deregulation in GBM. Ac (acetylation);
me (methylation).

human cancer [54] that is associated with the hypomethylation of repetitive sequences. These changes can be explained by genetic alterations and/or deregulated expression of genes encoding histone-modifying enzymes. In acute promyelocytic leukemias, for example, a genetic characteristic is the chromosomal translocation that produces the fusion proteins containing RAR-PML and RAR-PLZF. These fusion proteins bind to retinoic acid-responsive elements (RAREs) and recruit the HDAC repressor complex with a high affinity, preventing the binding of retinoic acid, and repressing the expression of genes that regulate normal differentiation and proliferation of myeloid cells. Mutations resulting in altered Class I HDACs expression and activity also occur in cancer. Mutation of the gene encoding HDAC2, for example, occurs in sporadic tumors with microsatellite instability. This mutation produces the loss of HDAC2 expression and activity and leads to a global gene expression deregulation, characterized by the upregulation of transforming genes suggesting a role of HDAC2 mutations in human tumorigenesis [55, 56].

Until now there is few evidence for the deregulation of the histone modifying enzymes in GBM (Figure 2). In particular, alteration of the copy number of BMI-1 gene, that codifies for a protein regulating H3K27 methylation, is a frequent event in low- and high-grade gliomas [57]. Mutations in other histone-modifying enzymes have been found in GBM such as the histone demethylases JMJD1A and JMJD1B, the histone methyltransferases SET7, SETD7, MLL, MLL4, and MBD1 [58]. Other proteins, as histone deacetylases, are also altered in GBM; class II and IV deacetylases show a decrease in mRNA expression in GBM in comparison with low-grade astrocytomas and normal brain [28]. The coexistence of histone repressive marks and DNA hypermethylation patterns is well represented in one of the genes previously described; methylation of MGMT promoter, a frequent event in GBM, is accompanied by H3K9 dimethylation and deacetylation, two other markers of gene silencing [9].

9. Future Directions: Cancer Stem Cells and Malignant Gliomas

In the last years, several reports have suggested that an important percentage of the cancer cells within certain tumors have the properties of cancer stem cells (CSCs) [59]. These types of cells have the ability to generate tumors after implantation in animal hosts, to self renew and to give rise to nonstem cells [60]. The cancer stem cell model suggests that the epigenetic changes characteristics of normal stem or progenitor cells are the earliest events in cancer initiation [61]. We can found a link between this event, cancer initiation, and stem cell biology in the function of polycomb (PcG) and trithorax (TrxG) group proteins that provide epigenetic signatures to stem cell identity [62]. These groups affect covalent modifications of histone tails and the position or composition of nucleosomes, as well as DNA methylation, so they have the ability to affect chromatin transcriptional status. In general, PcG repress gene expression, whereas, TrxG proteins activate it. In this regard, the gain of PcG and loss of TrXG in cancer demonstrate the oncogenic and tumor suppressor roles, respectively, of these complexes [63], having many tumors a reactivation in the expression of stem cell-associated genes, such as Hox genes, one of the targets of PcG and TrxG proteins. Unraveling the role of

CSCs in the pathophysiology of cancer opens up possibilities for discovering new biomarkers for cancer detection and prognosis and the development of new pharmacological strategies that incorporate agents that target both CSCs and non-CSCs.

Acknowledgments

S. Ropero's Group is financially supported by the Spanish Ministry of Health (Fund for Health of Spain, PI08/1184 Grant) and by the Mutua Madrileña Medical Research Foundation. R. Alelú-Paz has a Postdoctoral Research Fellow (Junta de Comunidades de Castilla-La Mancha).

References

[1] A. Portela and M. Esteller, "Epigenetic modifications and human disease," *Nature Biotechnology*, vol. 28, no. 10, pp. 1057–1068, 2010.

[2] P. W. Laird, "Principles and challenges of genome-wide DNA methylation analysis," *Nature Reviews Genetics*, vol. 11, no. 3, pp. 191–203, 2010.

[3] Z. X. Chen, J. R. Mann, C. L. Hsieh, A. D. Riggs, and F. Chédin, "Physical and functional interactions between the human DNMT3L protein and members of the de novo methyltransferase family," *Journal of Cellular Biochemistry*, vol. 95, no. 5, pp. 902–917, 2005.

[4] W. Reik, W. Dean, and J. Walter, "Epigenetic reprogramming in mammalian development," *Science*, vol. 293, no. 5532, pp. 1089–1093, 2001.

[5] M. Esteller, "The necessity of a human epigenome project," *Carcinogenesis*, vol. 27, no. 6, pp. 1121–1125, 2006.

[6] T. Straub and P. B. Becker, "Dosage compensation: the beginning and end of generalization," *Nature Reviews Genetics*, vol. 8, no. 1, pp. 47–57, 2007.

[7] R. G. Urdinguio, J. V. Sanchez-Mut, and M. Esteller, "Epigenetic mechanisms in neurological diseases: genes, syndromes, and therapies," *The Lancet Neurology*, vol. 8, no. 11, pp. 1056–1072, 2009.

[8] P. A. Grant, "A tale of histone modifications," *Genome Biology*, vol. 2, no. 4, article 3, 2001.

[9] R. Burgess, R. Jenkins, and Z. Zhang, "Epigenetic changes in gliomas," *Cancer Biology and Therapy*, vol. 7, no. 9, pp. 1326–1334, 2008.

[10] X. Qian, Q. Shen, S. K. Goderie et al., "Timing of CNS cell generation: a programmed sequence of neuron and glial cell production from isolated murine cortical stem cells," *Neuron*, vol. 28, no. 1, pp. 69–80, 2000.

[11] C. Ladd-Acosta, J. Pevsner, S. Sabunciyan et al., "DNA methylation signatures within the human brain," *American Journal of Human Genetics*, vol. 81, no. 6, pp. 1304–1315, 2007.

[12] A. K. Maunakea, R. P. Nagarajan, M. Bilenky et al., "Conserved role of intragenic DNA methylation in regulating alternative promoters," *Nature*, vol. 466, no. 7303, pp. 253–257, 2010.

[13] K. E. Szulwach, X. Li, Y. Li et al., "5-hmC-mediated epigenetic dynamics during postnatal neurodevelopment and aging," *Nature Neuroscience*, vol. 14, no. 12, pp. 1607–1616, 2011.

[14] D. Globisch, M. Münzel, M. Müller et al., "Tissue distribution of 5-hydroxymethylcytosine and search for active demethylation intermediates," *PLoS ONE*, vol. 5, no. 12, Article ID e15367, 2010.

[15] M. M. Lino and A. Merlo, "PI3Kinase signaling in glioblastoma," *Journal of Neuro-Oncology*, vol. 103, no. 3, pp. 417–427, 2011.

[16] M. F. Fraga, M. Herranz, J. Espada et al., "A mouse skin multistage carcinogenesis model reflects the aberrant DNA methylation patterns of human tumors," *Cancer Research*, vol. 64, no. 16, pp. 5527–5534, 2004.

[17] L. Soroceanu, S. Kharbanda, R. Chen et al., "Identification of IGF2 signaling through phosphoinositide-3-kinase regulatory subunit 3 as a growth-promoting axis in glioblastoma," *Proceedings of the National Academy of Sciences of the United States of America*, vol. 104, no. 9, pp. 3466–3471, 2007.

[18] M. Esteller, "Epigenetic gene silencing in cancer: the DNA hypermethylome," *Human Molecular Genetics*, vol. 16, no. 1, pp. R50–R59, 2007.

[19] H. Kim, W. Huang, X. Jiang, B. Pennicooke, P. J. Park, and M. D. Johnson, "Integrative genome analysis reveals an oncomir/oncogene cluster regulating glioblastoma survivorship," *Proceedings of the National Academy of Sciences of the United States of America*, vol. 107, no. 5, pp. 2183–2188, 2010.

[20] M. Nakamura, Y. Yonekawa, P. Kleihues, and H. Ohgaki, "Promoter hypermethylation of the RB1 gene in glioblastomas," *Laboratory Investigation*, vol. 81, no. 1, pp. 77–82, 2001.

[21] J. F. Costello, M. S. Berger, H. J. S. Huang, and W. K. Cavenee, "Silencing of p16/CDKN2 expression in human gliomas by methylation and chromatin condensation," *Cancer Research*, vol. 56, no. 10, pp. 2405–2410, 1996.

[22] M. J. Bello and J. A. Rey, "The p53/Mdm2/p14ARF cell cycle control pathway genes may be inactivated by genetic and epigenetic mechanisms in gliomas," *Cancer Genetics and Cytogenetics*, vol. 164, no. 2, pp. 172–173, 2006.

[23] N. Baeza, M. Weller, Y. Yonekawa, P. Kleihues, and H. Ohgaki, "PTEN methylation and expression in glioblastomas," *Acta Neuropathologica*, vol. 106, no. 5, pp. 479–485, 2003.

[24] G. Cecener, B. Tunca, U. Egeli et al., "The promoter hypermethylation status of GATA6, MGMT, and FHIT in glioblastoma," *Cellular and Molecular Neurobiology*, vol. 32, no. 2, pp. 237–244, 2011.

[25] R. Martinez, J. I. Martin-Subero, V. Rohde et al., "A microarray-based DNA methylation study of glioblastoma multiforme," *Epigenetics*, vol. 4, no. 4, pp. 255–264, 2009.

[26] M. Alaminos, V. Dávalos, S. Ropero et al., "EMP3, a myelin-related gene located in the critical 19q13.3 region, is epigenetically silenced and exhibits features of a candidate tumor suppressor in glioma and neuroblastoma," *Cancer Research*, vol. 65, no. 7, pp. 2565–2571, 2005.

[27] C. A. Scrideli, C. G. Carlotti, O. K. Okamoto et al., "Gene expression profile analysis of primary glioblastomas and non-neoplastic brain tissue: identification of potential target genes by oligonucleotide microarray and real-time quantitative PCR," *Journal of Neuro-Oncology*, vol. 88, no. 3, pp. 281–291, 2008.

[28] R. P. Nagarajan and J. F. Costello, "Epigenetic mechanisms in glioblastoma multiforme," *Seminars in Cancer Biology*, vol. 19, no. 3, pp. 188–197, 2009.

[29] S. Zheng, E. A. Houseman, Z. Morrison et al., "DNA hypermethylation profiles associated with glioma subtypes and EZH2 and IGFBP2 mRNA expression," *Neuro-Oncology*, vol. 13, no. 3, pp. 280–289, 2011.

[30] W. Mueller, C. L. Nutt, M. Ehrich et al., "Downregulation of RUNX3 and TES by hypermethylation in glioblastoma," *Oncogene*, vol. 26, no. 4, pp. 583–593, 2007.

[31] B. Sadikovic, M. Yoshimoto, S. Chilton-MacNeill, P. Thorner, J. A. Squire, and M. Zielenska, "Identification of interactive

DNA Methylation, Histone Modifications, and Signal Transduction Pathways: A Close Relationship in Malignant Gliomas Pathophysiology

205

networks of gene expression associated with osteosarcoma oncogenesis by integrated molecular profiling," *Human Molecular Genetics*, vol. 18, no. 11, pp. 1962–1975, 2009.

[32] K. H. Lee, S. W. Lim, H. G. Kim et al., "Lack of death receptor 4 (DR4) expression through gene promoter methylation in gastric carcinoma," *Langenbeck's Archives of Surgery*, vol. 394, no. 4, pp. 661–670, 2009.

[33] R. Martinez, G. Schackert, and M. Esteller, "Hypermethylation of the proapoptotic gene TMS1/ASC: prognostic importance in glioblastoma multiforme," *Journal of Neuro-Oncology*, vol. 82, no. 2, pp. 133–139, 2007.

[34] C. Cillo, M. Cantile, A. Faiella, and E. Boncinelli, "Homeobox genes in normal and malignant cells," *Journal of Cellular Physiology*, vol. 188, no. 2, pp. 161–169, 2001.

[35] W. J. Gehring and Y. Hiromi, "Homeotic genes and the homeobox," *Annual Review of Genetics*, vol. 20, pp. 147–173, 1986.

[36] H. Fiegl, G. Windbichler, E. Mueller-Holzner et al., "HOXA11 DNA methylation—a novel prognostic biomarker in ovarian cancer," *International Journal of Cancer*, vol. 123, no. 3, pp. 725–729, 2008.

[37] A. Di Vinci, I. Casciano, E. Marasco et al., "Quantitative methylation analysis of *HOXA3, 7, 9*, and *10* genes in glioma: association with tumor WHO grade and clinical outcome," *Journal of Cancer Research and Clinical Oncology*, vol. 138, no. 1, pp. 35–47, 2011.

[38] H. Donninger, M. D. Vos, and G. J. Clark, "The RASSF1A tumor suppressor," *Journal of Cell Science*, vol. 120, no. 18, pp. 3163–3172, 2007.

[39] J. Avruch, R. Xavier, N. Bardeesy et al., "Rassf family of tumor suppressor polypeptides," *Journal of Biological Chemistry*, vol. 284, no. 17, pp. 11001–11005, 2009.

[40] A. Lorente, W. Mueller, E. Urdangarín et al., "RASSF1A, BLU, NORE1A, PTEN and MGMT expression and promoter methylation in gliomas and glioma cell lines and evidence of deregulated expression of de novo DNMTs," *Brain Pathology*, vol. 19, no. 2, pp. 279–292, 2009.

[41] N. Schmidt, S. Windmann, G. Reifenberger, and M. J. Riemenschneider, "DNA hypermethylation and histone modifications downregulate the candidate tumor suppressor gene RRP22 on 22q12 in human gliomas," *Brain Pathology*, vol. 22, no. 1, pp. 17–25, 2011.

[42] J. Zucman-Rossi, P. Legoix, and G. Thomas, "Identification of new members of the Gas2 and Ras families in the 22q12 chromosome region," *Genomics*, vol. 38, no. 3, pp. 247–254, 1996.

[43] G. Foltz, G. Y. Ryu, J. G. Yoon et al., "Genome-wide analysis of epigenetic silencing identifies BEX1 and BEX2 as candidate tumor suppressor genes in malignant glioma," *Cancer Research*, vol. 66, no. 13, pp. 6665–6674, 2006.

[44] L. Hesson, I. Bièche, D. Krex et al., "Frequent epigenetic inactivation of RASSF1A and BLU genes located within the critical 3p21.3 region in gliomas," *Oncogene*, vol. 23, no. 13, pp. 2408–2419, 2004.

[45] R. Martinez, F. Setien, C. Voelter et al., "CpG island promoter hypermethylation of the pro-apoptotic gene caspase-8 is a common hallmark of relapsed glioblastoma multiforme," *Carcinogenesis*, vol. 28, no. 6, pp. 1264–1268, 2007.

[46] H. Zhou, R. Miki, M. Eeva et al., "Reciprocal regulation of SOCS1 and SOCS3 enhances resistance to ionizing radiation in glioblastoma multiforme," *Clinical Cancer Research*, vol. 13, no. 8, pp. 2344–2353, 2007.

[47] W. J. Bodell, T. Aida, M. S. Berger, and M. L. Rosenblum, "Increased repair of O6-alkylguanine DNA adducts in glioma-derived human cells resistant to the cytotoxic and cytogenetic effects of 1,3-bis(2-chloroethyl)-1-nitrosourea," *Carcinogenesis*, vol. 7, no. 6, pp. 879–883, 1986.

[48] M. Colvin and J. Hilton, "Pharmacology of cyclophosphamide and metabolites," *Cancer Treatment Reports*, vol. 65, no. 3, pp. 89–95, 1981.

[49] C. Balana, C. Carrato, J. L. Ramirez et al., "Tumour and serum MGMT promoter methylation and protein expression in glioblastoma patients," *Clinical and Translational Oncology*, vol. 13, no. 9, pp. 677–685, 2011.

[50] M. Esteller, J. Garcia-Foncillas, E. Andion et al., "Inactivation of the DNA-repair gene MGMT and the clinical response of gliomas to alkylating agents," *The New England Journal of Medicine*, vol. 343, no. 19, pp. 1350–1354, 2000.

[51] R. Martinez, G. Schackert, R. Yaya-Tur, I. Rojas-Marcos, J. G. Herman, and M. Esteller, "Frequent hypermethylation of the DNA repair gene MGMT in long-term survivors of glioblastoma multiforme," *Journal of Neuro-Oncology*, vol. 83, no. 1, pp. 91–93, 2007.

[52] M. Uno, S. M. Oba-Shinjo, A. A. Camargo et al., "Correlation of MGMT promoter methylation status with gene and protein expression levels in glioblastoma," *Clinics*, vol. 66, no. 10, pp. 1747–1755, 2011.

[53] J. Y. Lee, C. K. Park, S. H. Park, K. C. Wang, B. K. Cho, and S. K. Kim, "MGMT promoter gene methylation in pediatric glioblastoma: analysis using MS-MLPA," *Child's Nervous System*, vol. 27, no. 11, pp. 1877–1883, 2011.

[54] M. F. Fraga, E. Ballestar, A. Villar-Garea et al., "Loss of acetylation at Lys16 and trimethylation at Lys20 of histone H4 is a common hallmark of human cancer," *Nature Genetics*, vol. 37, no. 4, pp. 391–400, 2005.

[55] S. Ropero, M. F. Fraga, E. Ballestar et al., "A truncating mutation of HDAC2 in human cancers confers resistance to histone deacetylase inhibition," *Nature Genetics*, vol. 38, no. 5, pp. 566–569, 2006.

[56] S. Ropero, E. Ballestar, M. Alaminos, D. Arango, S. Schwartz, and M. Esteller, "Transforming pathways unleashed by a HDAC2 mutation in human cancer," *Oncogene*, vol. 27, no. 28, pp. 4008–4012, 2008.

[57] V. Häyry, M. Tanner, T. Blom et al., "Copy number alterations of the polycomb gene BMI1 in gliomas," *Acta Neuropathologica*, vol. 116, no. 1, pp. 97–102, 2008.

[58] D. W. Parsons, S. Jones, X. Zhang et al., "An integrated genomic analysis of human glioblastoma multiforme," *Science*, vol. 321, no. 5897, pp. 1807–1812, 2008.

[59] P. B. Gupta, C. L. Chaffer, and R. A. Weinberg, "Cancer stem cells: mirage or reality?" *Nature Medicine*, vol. 15, no. 9, pp. 1010–1012, 2009.

[60] M. F. Clarke, J. E. Dick, P. B. Dirks et al., "Cancer stem cells—perspectives on current status and future directions: AACR workshop on cancer stem cells," *Cancer Research*, vol. 66, no. 19, pp. 9339–9344, 2006.

[61] A. P. Feinberg, R. Ohlsson, and S. Henikoff, "The epigenetic progenitor origin of human cancer," *Nature Reviews Genetics*, vol. 7, no. 1, pp. 21–33, 2006.

[62] M. Spivakov and A. G. Fisher, "Epigenetic signatures of stem-cell identity," *Nature Reviews Genetics*, vol. 8, no. 4, pp. 263–271, 2007.

[63] A. A. Mills, "Throwing the cancer switch: reciprocal roles of polycomb and trithorax proteins," *Nature Reviews Cancer*, vol. 10, no. 10, pp. 669–682, 2010.

Permissions

The contributors of this book come from diverse backgrounds, making this book a truly international effort. This book will bring forth new frontiers with its revolutionizing research information and detailed analysis of the nascent developments around the world.

We would like to thank all the contributing authors for lending their expertise to make the book truly unique. They have played a crucial role in the development of this book. Without their invaluable contributions this book wouldn't have been possible. They have made vital efforts to compile up to date information on the varied aspects of this subject to make this book a valuable addition to the collection of many professionals and students.

This book was conceptualized with the vision of imparting up-to-date information and advanced data in this field. To ensure the same, a matchless editorial board was set up. Every individual on the board went through rigorous rounds of assessment to prove their worth. After which they invested a large part of their time researching and compiling the most relevant data for our readers. Conferences and sessions were held from time to time between the editorial board and the contributing authors to present the data in the most comprehensible form. The editorial team has worked tirelessly to provide valuable and valid information to help people across the globe.

Every chapter published in this book has been scrutinized by our experts. Their significance has been extensively debated. The topics covered herein carry significant findings which will fuel the growth of the discipline. They may even be implemented as practical applications or may be referred to as a beginning point for another development. Chapters in this book were first published by Hindawi Publishing Corporation; hereby published with permission under the Creative Commons Attribution License or equivalent.

The editorial board has been involved in producing this book since its inception. They have spent rigorous hours researching and exploring the diverse topics which have resulted in the successful publishing of this book. They have passed on their knowledge of decades through this book. To expedite this challenging task, the publisher supported the team at every step. A small team of assistant editors was also appointed to further simplify the editing procedure and attain best results for the readers.

Our editorial team has been hand-picked from every corner of the world. Their multi-ethnicity adds dynamic inputs to the discussions which result in innovative outcomes. These outcomes are then further discussed with the researchers and contributors who give their valuable feedback and opinion regarding the same. The feedback is then collaborated with the researches and they are edited in a comprehensive manner to aid the understanding of the subject.

Apart from the editorial board, the designing team has also invested a significant amount of their time in understanding the subject and creating the most relevant covers. They scrutinized every image to scout for the most suitable representation of the subject and create an appropriate cover for the book.

The publishing team has been involved in this book since its early stages. They were actively engaged in every process, be it collecting the data, connecting with the contributors or procuring relevant information. The team has been an ardent support to the editorial, designing and production team. Their endless efforts to recruit the best for this project, has resulted in the accomplishment of this book. They are a veteran in the field of academics and their pool of knowledge is as vast as their experience in printing. Their expertise and guidance has proved useful at every step. Their uncompromising quality standards have made this book an exceptional effort. Their encouragement from time to time has been an inspiration for everyone.

The publisher and the editorial board hope that this book will prove to be a valuable piece of knowledge for researchers, students, practitioners and scholars across the globe.

List of Contributors

Delira Robbins and Yunfeng Zhao
Department of Pharmacology, Toxicology & Neuroscience, Louisiana State University Health Sciences Center, Shreveport, LA 71130, USA

Joel D. Pearson, Jason K.H. Lee, Julinor T. C. Bacani and Robert J. Ingham
Department of Medical Microbiology and Immunology, University of Alberta, Edmonton, AB, Canada T6G 2E1

Raymond Lai
Department of Laboratory Medicine and Pathology, University of Alberta, Edmonton, AB, Canada T6G 2B7

Cristina Bertocchi and Megha Vaman Rao
Mechanobiology Institute Singapore, National University of Singapore, Singapore 117411

Ronen Zaidel-Bar
Mechanobiology Institute Singapore, National University of Singapore, Singapore 117411
Department of Bioengineering, Faculty of Engineering, National University of Singapore, Singapore 119077

Gonzalo Rodríguez-Berriguete, Benito Fraile, Ricardo Paniagua and Mar Royuela
Department of Cell Biology and Genetics, University of Alcal´a, Alcal´a de Henares, 28871 Madrid, Spain

Pilar Martínez-Onsurbe and Gabriel Olmedilla
Department of Pathology, Pr´ıncipe de Asturias Hospital, Alcal´a de Henares, 28806 Madrid, Spain

Takashi W. Ijiri and Ken-ichi Sato
Laboratory of Cell Signaling and Development, Department of Molecular Biosciences, Faculty of Life Sciences, Kyoto Sangyo University, Kyoto 603-8555, Japan

A. K. M. Mahbub Hasan
Laboratory of Cell Signaling and Development, Department of Molecular Biosciences, Faculty of Life Sciences, Kyoto Sangyo University, Kyoto 603-8555, Japan
Laboratory of Gene Biology, Department of Biochemistry and Molecular Biology, University of Dhaka, Dhaka 1000, Bangladesh

Utchariya Anantamongkol
Department of Physiology and Biophysics, University of Illinois at Chicago, Chicago, IL 60612, USA2Department of Physiology, Faculty of Science, Mahidol University, Bangkok 10400, Thailand

Mei Ao and Mrinalini C. Rao
Department of Physiology and Biophysics, University of Illinois at Chicago, Chicago, IL 60612, USA

Jayashree Sarathy nee Venkatasubramanian
Department of Physiology and Biophysics, University of Illinois at Chicago, Chicago, IL 60612, USA
Department of Biological Sciences, Benedictine University, Lisle, IL 60532, USA

Y. Sangeeta Devi
Department of Physiology and Biophysics, University of Illinois at Chicago, Chicago, IL 60612, USA
Obstetrics, Gynecology and Reproductive Biology, Michigan State University, Grand Rapids, MI 49503, USA

Nateetip Krishnamra
Department of Physiology, Faculty of Science, Mahidol University, Bangkok 10400, Thailand

Haruhiko Kanasaki, Indri Purwana, Aki Oride, Tselmeg Mijiddorj and Kohji Miyazaki
Department of Obstetrics and Gynecology, Faculty of Medicine, Shimane University, Izumo 693-8501, Japan

Linda Yu, Alicia B.Moore, Lysandra Castro, Xiaohua Gao, Hoang-Long C. Huynh, Michelle Klippel and Darlene Dixon
Molecular Pathogenesis Group, National Toxicology Program (NTP) Laboratory, NTP, Department of Health and Human Services (DHHS), National Institute of Environmental Health Sciences (NIEHS), National Institutes of Health (NIH), Research Triangle Park, NC 27709, USA

Norris D. Flagler
Cellular and Molecular Pathology Branch, NTP, Department of Health and Human Services (DHHS), National Institute of Environmental Health Sciences (NIEHS), National Institutes of Health (NIH), Research Triangle Park, NC 27709, USA

Yi Lu and Grace E. Kissling
Biostatistics Branch, Department of Health and Human Services (DHHS), National Institute of Environmental Health Sciences (NIEHS), National Institutes of Health (NIH), Research Triangle Park, NC 27709, USA

Mohamed Kodiha and Ursula Stochaj
Department of Physiology, McGill University, Montreal, QC, Canada H3G 1Y6

Karin F. K. Ejendal and Val J. Watts
Department of Medicinal Chemistry and Molecular Pharmacology, College of Pharmacy, Purdue University, 575 Stadium Mall Drive, West Lafayette, IN 47907-2051, USA

Carmen W. Dessauer
Department of Integrative Biology and Pharmacology, University of Texas Health Science Center at Houston, Houston, TX 77030, USA

Terence E. Hébert
Department of Pharmacology Therapeutics, McGill University, McIntyre Medical Sciences Building, Montr'eal, QC, Canada H3G 1Y6

Akihiro Fujii, Yuko Kase, Chiaki Suzuki, Akihito Kamizono and Teruaki Imada
Japan Blood Products Organization, Central Research Laboratory, Protein Pharmacology Research Section, 1-5-2 Minatojima Minami-machi, Chuo-ku, Kobe, Hyogo 650-0047, Japan

Yannick D. Benoit
Departement d'Anatomie et Biologie Cellulaire, Facult'e de M'edecine et des Sciences de la Sant'e, Universit'e de Sherbrooke, Sherbrooke, QC, Canada J1H 5N4
Pharmacology Department, Weill Cornell Medical College, New York, NY 10065, USA

Jean-François Groulx, David Gagné and Jean-François Beaulieu
Departement d'Anatomie et Biologie Cellulaire, Facult'e de M'edecine et des Sciences de la Sant'e, Universit'e de Sherbrooke, Sherbrooke, QC, Canada J1H 5N4

Heather L. Watt, Zakaria Rachid and Bertrand J. Jean-Claude
Cancer Drug Research Laboratory, Division of Oncology, Department of Medicine, McGill University Health Centre, Royal Victoria Hospital, Montreal, QC, Canada H3A 1A1

Ting Gui, Yujing Sun, Aiko Shimokado and Yasuteru Muragaki
First Department of Pathology, Wakayama Medical University School of Medicine, 811-1 Kimiidera, Wakayama 641-0012, Japan

Rebecca Elston and Gareth J. Inman
Division of Cancer Research, Medical Research Institute, Ninewells Hospital and Medical School, University of Dundee, Dundee DD1 9SY, UK

Pierre P. Eleniste and Angela Bruzzaniti
Department of Oral Biology, Indiana University School of Dentistry, DS241, 1121 W. Michigan Street, Indianapolis, IN 46202, USA

Raúl Alelú-Paz, Nadia Ashour, Ana González-Corpas and Santiago Ropero
Department of Biochemistry and Molecular Biology, School of Medicine, University of Alcal´a, Carretera Madrid-Barcelona Km. 33.6, 28871 Madrid, Spain

CPSIA information can be obtained
at www.ICGtesting.com
Printed in the USA
LVOW05*1500260917

550132LV00004B/20/P

9 781632 420909